Neuropsychiatric Disorders: Clinical Perspectives

Neuropsychiatric Disorders: Clinical Perspectives

Editor: Saul Jones

AMERICAN
MEDICAL PUBLISHERS
www.americanmedicalpublishers.com

AMERICAN
MEDICAL PUBLISHERS
www.americanmedicalpublishers.com

Cataloging-in-Publication Data

Neuropsychiatric disorders : clinical perspectives / edited by Saul Jones.
p. cm.
Includes bibliographical references and index.
ISBN 978-1-63927-319-5
1. Neurobehavioral disorders. 2. Neurobehavioral disorders--Treatment.
3. Brain--Diseases. 4. Mental illness. I. Jones, Saul.
RC386 .N48 2022
616.8--dc23

American Medical Publishers,
41 Flatbush Avenue,
1st Floor, New York,
NY 11217, USA

ISBN 978-1-63927-319-5 (Hardback)

Contents

Preface

The disorders which are classified as organic brain diseases and which show psychiatric symptoms are known as neuropsychiatric disorders. They can cause cognitive impairment such as personality-behavioral changes, dementia and amnesic syndrome. These are studied within the field of neuropsychiatry, which in turn falls under the umbrella of psychiatry. The study of the complex interrelationship between brain function and behavior through the viewpoints of psychiatry, neurology and psychology is undertaken under this field. Advances in the study of neuropsychiatric disorders helps in the improvement of diagnosis, facilitates the development of new and more efficient interventions, and assists in treatment selection. This book contains some path-breaking studies in the field of neuropsychiatric disorders. It consists of contributions made by international experts. As the research in this field is emerging at a rapid pace, the contents of this book will help the readers understand the modern concepts and aspects of the subject.

Various studies have approached the subject by analyzing it with a single perspective, but the present book provides diverse methodologies and techniques to address this field. This book contains theories and applications needed for understanding the subject from different perspectives. The aim is to keep the readers informed about the progresses in the field; therefore, the contributions were carefully examined to compile novel researches by specialists from across the globe.

Indeed, the job of the editor is the most crucial and challenging in compiling all chapters into a single book. In the end, I would extend my sincere thanks to the chapter authors for their profound work. I am also thankful for the support provided by my family and colleagues during the compilation of this book.

Editor

1

Resignation Syndrome: Catatonia? Culture-Bound?

Edited by:
Raymond C. K. Chan, Chinese Academy of Sciences, China

***Correspondence:**
Karl Sallin
karl.sallin@ki.se

Karl Sallin [1,2]*, Hugo Lagercrantz [2], Kathinka Evers [1], Ingemar Engström [3], Anders Hjern [4] and Predrag Petrovic [5]

[1] Centre for Research Ethics and Bioethics (CRB), Uppsala University, Uppsala, Sweden, [2] Department of Women's and Children's Health, Division of Neonatology, Karolinska Institute, Solna, Sweden, [3] School of Health and Medical Sciences, Örebro University, Örebro, Sweden, [4] Centre for Health and Equity Studies (CHESS), Karolinska Institute and Stockholm University, Stockholm, Sweden, [5] Department of Clinical Neuroscience, Karolinska Institute, Solna, Sweden

Resignation syndrome (RS) designates a long-standing disorder predominately affecting psychologically traumatized children and adolescents in the midst of a strenuous and lengthy migration process. Typically a depressive onset is followed by gradual withdrawal progressing via stupor into a state that prompts tube feeding and is characterized by failure to respond even to painful stimuli. The patient is seemingly unconscious. Recovery ensues within months to years and is claimed to be dependent on the restoration of hope to the family. Descriptions of disorders resembling RS can be found in the literature and the condition is unlikely novel. Nevertheless, the magnitude and geographical distribution stand out. Several hundred cases have been reported exclusively in Sweden in the past decade prompting the Swedish National Board of Health and Welfare to recognize RS as a separate diagnostic entity. The currently prevailing stress hypothesis fails to account for the regional distribution and contributes little to treatment. Consequently, a re-evaluation of diagnostics and treatment is required. Psychogenic catatonia is proposed to supply the best fit with the clinical presentation. Treatment response, altered brain metabolism or preserved awareness would support this hypothesis. Epidemiological data suggests culture-bound beliefs and expectations to generate and direct symptom expression and we argue that culture-bound psychogenesis can accommodate the endemic distribution. Last, we review recent models of predictive coding indicating how expectation processes are crucially involved in the placebo and nocebo effect, delusions and conversion disorders. Building on this theoretical framework we propose a neurobiological model of RS in which the impact of overwhelming negative expectations are directly causative of the down-regulation of higher order and lower order behavioral systems in particularly vulnerable individuals.

Keywords: catatonia, migration, culture-bound syndrom, pervasive refusal, psychogenic, apathy, hopelessness, predictive coding

INTRODUCTION

In Sweden, apathy has been the colloquial term for a condition characterized by global and severe loss of function affecting children and adolescents seeking asylum or undergoing migration process. Typically prodromal anxiousness and depressive symptoms, in particular lethargy, progresses into stupor and finally complete lack of any response behavior even to painful stimulus.

At this stage patients are seemingly unconscious and tube feeding life sustaining. After months to years remission ensues with gradual return to what appears to be normal function.

From January 1st 2003 to April 31st 2005, 424 cases were reported (Hessle and Ahmadi, 2006) and out of the 6547 asylum applications submitted for children (0–17 years) in Sweden in 2004 (Von Folsach and Montgomery, 2006), 2.8% were thus diagnosed. No cases reported from other countries, the phenomenon appears unique to Sweden.

The nature and prevalence of the condition has been subject to intense public debate. Malingering or Munchausen syndrome by proxy has been proposed. Opposing views have labelled these hypotheses xenophobic and instead suggested the migratory process, purportedly unpredictable and long, to precipitate the putatively stress-induced condition affecting traumatized individuals. An asserted "questioning attitude", in particular within the health care system, it has been claimed, may constitute a "perpetuating retraumatization possibly explaining the endemic" distribution (Bodegård, 2014).

An official inquiry (Hessle and Ahmadi, 2006) and an expert committee (Rydelius, 2006) have both proposed multifactorial explanatory models involving individual vulnerability, traumatization, migration, culturally conditioned reaction patterns and parental dysfunction or pathological adaption to a caregiver's expectations to interplay in pathogenesis. Severe depression or conversion/dissociation disorder has been suggested (Rydelius, 2006) and malingering or factitious disorder remain unsupported (Aronsson et al., 2009).

January 1st 2014, the Swedish National Board of Health and Welfare recognized the novel diagnostic entity *resignation syndrome* (RS; Socialstyrelsen, 2013). Implying a psychological etiology, its appropriateness remains to be demonstrated. In this presentation, the term will be used; however, should be interpreted free from theory.

As of today, diagnostic criteria are undetermined, pathogenesis uncertain and the regional distribution unexplained. New cases are presenting, 22 in the Stockholm area in 2014 (Schiller, 2015, Personal Communication), and effective treatment is lacking.

In this article we address three questions in relation to RS: What is it? Why is it locally distributed? And how can it arise? First we summarize and analyze the literature on RS. Then we argue: (1) that RS should be perceived as catatonia, a hypothesis readily testable by either neuroimaging or evaluation of treatment response; (2) that culturally transmitted and sanctioned beliefs may, through psychogenesis, account for the regional distribution; and (3) on a mechanistic level, that cultural and contextual influence may fundamentally change expectations and priors on the bodily functions inducing failure to activate both higher order and lower order behaviors in vulnerable individuals. To support this claim we frame it in a predictive coding context that has been suggested to be causally involved in placebo and nocebo effects, delusions and conversion disorders.

BACKGROUND

Clinical Observations and Treatment

In a material of 23 patients, Bodegård (2005b) described the typical patient as "totally passive, immobile, lacks tonus, withdrawn, mute, unable to eat and drink, incontinent and not reacting to physical stimuli or pain". He further noted that "[p]eriods of panicky refusal and/or anxiety can proceed or intervene with the stuporous state" and that "[s]econdary symptoms may appear, such as tachycardia, rise in temperature, weight gain, oedema, profuse sweating, reactivation (?) of latent viral infection, skin ulcers and muscular atrophy" (Bodegård, 2005b). Later reports and current observations find less evidence of "panicky refusal" and "secondary symptoms". The persisting impression is that of symptoms progressing on a continuum from introversion and lethargy to stupor, lack of response and seeming unconsciousness.

Typically, non-negotiable symptoms, such as inability to ingest, elicit contact with the health care system. Sometimes a possible trigger incident, such as a negative asylum decision, can be identified. Patients may be admitted after a few days marked by rapid deterioration and stupor. On other occasions a more gradual presentation of anxiety, dysphoria, sleeping disturbances, social withdrawal and other symptoms are subsequently supplemented by mutism, failure to participate in activities such as school and play, failure to communicate altogether, and finally, to initiate motor activity and respond to stimulus leaving the patient in a supine position seemingly unconscious and generally with eyes closed (for clinical characteristics, see **Box 1**). At this stage, RS prompts tube feeding and full ADL-support (Bodegård, 2005b; Aronsson et al., 2009; Ascher and Hjern, 2013; Forslund and Johansson, 2013).

Routine work-up includes toxic screening and anamnestic interviewing via interpreter. Neuroradiology, neurophysiological examinations and lumbar puncture are considered optional (Socialstyrelsen, 2013). Electroencephalogram (EEG) and computed tomography of the skull have generally been unimpressive as well as laboratory screenings (Bodegård, 2004; Aronsson et al., 2009; Forslund and Johansson, 2013). Magnetic resonance tomography (MRT) is recommended (Rydelius, 2006) however, rarely performed.

Once stabilized, somatic illness excluded and the parent(s) comfortable administering tube feeding, the patient is discharged and subsequent treatment given in a home setting with regular ambulatory visits to the clinic. In previous years long-term hospitalization was common and there is still a lacking consensus regarding level of care (Lindberg and Sundelin, 2005). Although Bodegård (2006) finds support for hospitalization in one report out-patient care aiming for family involvement is presently the preferred model.

Apart from life-sustaining tube feeding, treatment amounts to promoting and maintaining a secure and hopeful environment, encouraging a sense of coherence. Several authors stress the importance of a permanent residency permit (PRP; Lindberg and Sundelin, 2005; Ascher and Gustavsson, 2008) although a permit

BOX 1 | Clinical characteristics of RS.

Prodromal
Anxiety
Dysphoria
Sleeping disturbances
Social withdrawal

Deterioration
Mutism
Failure to participate in activities
Failure in non verbal communication

Fully developed
Stupor
Unresponsiveness/negativism
Immobility
Incontinence
No reaction to pain stimulus including reflex
Dependent on tube-feeding and full ADL assistance
Tachycardia
Elevated temperature
Occasional profuse sweating
Occasional hyperventilation
Muscular atrophy
Periods of excitability, anxiety, "refusal"
Generally normal routine neurologic examination
Hypotonicity (sometimes coded as flaccid paralysis)
Reflexes generally responding but weak
Eyes open or closed not permitting passive opening
Pupils reactive to light and occasionally responsive to threat
Eyes divert from examiner and appear unseeing
Jerks
Indications of preserved awareness
Electroencephalogram (EEG), CT of skull and brain, laboratory sampling including toxicology all unimpressive

Remission
Generally in an ordered pattern (hand squeeze or eye opening without eye contact; eye contact; nodding and active partaking in feeding; gross motor skills; fine motor skills; verbal communication)
Indications of varying degrees of amnesia
Full recovery without remaining symptoms or deficits

Based on own experience and reports (Bodegård, 2005b; Aronsson et al., 2009; Ascher and Hjern, 2013; Forslund and Johansson, 2013).

in itself neither is sufficient for remission nor precludes debut (Bodegård, 2006). Alongside care given by the family, nurses, psychologists, physiotherapists and occupational therapists are responsible for day-to-day care. A pediatrician and a child and adolescent psychiatrist are involved at regular intervals. One center employed individualized sense stimulation (Forslund and Johansson, 2013). No reports of successful pharmacological treatment, including antidepressants, or attempted electroconvulsive therapy (ECT) exist.

The duration of tube-feeding ranges from months to years. In one study ($n = 29$) the mean duration was 10, 6 months (1.1–24.5; Aronsson et al., 2009) and in another, inpatient study ($n = 5$), 27 weeks (10–60; Forslund and Johansson, 2013). Bodegård (2006) ($n = 25$) reports duration of tube feeding to covariate, in particular, with level of care (in favor of hospitalization); however, also with time elapsed between hospitalization and PRP being granted.

One study ($n = 29$) described remission following a similarly ordered pattern in 22 patients; hand squeeze or eye opening without eye contact was followed by eye contact, nodding and active partaking in feeding, return of gross motor skills, return of fine motor skills and verbal communication (Aronsson et al., 2009).

One survey ($n = 5$) report full recovery 1–8 years after discharge (Forslund and Johansson, 2013). At present, in relation to available data, the generally held assumption of "full recovery" remains poorly supported.

Epidemiology

The patient group as hitherto described comprises of children and adolescents 7–19 years of age (mean 14.3) with 2:3 female predominance (Bodegård, 2004; Aronsson et al., 2009; Söndergaard et al., 2012; Forslund and Johansson, 2013). All described cases are refugees often belonging to a political or ethnic minority (Bodegård, 2005a, 2014; Forslund and Johansson, 2013). A disproportionally large share of patients originate from former Soviet republics or former Yugoslavia (Von Folsach and Montgomery, 2006) but cases from Bangladesh and Africa have been reported (Lindberg and Sundelin, 2005). The Uighur ethnic group is reported to be overrepresented among those affected (Rydelius, 2006). Traumatization in terms of physical abuse, harassment or by witnessing violence and abuse in the close family, is prevalent in half to all affected individuals (Bodegård, 2005b; Godani et al., 2008; Aronsson et al., 2009; Forslund and Johansson, 2013). Purported pre-morbid personality traits such as conscientiousness and high achieving have been reported (Forslund and Johansson, 2013).

To our knowledge, no cases have been established outside of Sweden. An accurate estimate of the total number of cases is challenging due to varying quality in reported materials. In 2002, 65 cases were reported and in 2004, 130. A national effort in 2003–2005 recognized 424 cases. In 2006 a temporary refugee amnesty easing asylum approval was enforced and later considered to contribute to a subsequent decrease (Socialstyrelsen, 2013). In 2005–2007, 70 patients were included in the rehabilitation programme in the Stockholm area alone (Aronsson et al., 2009), in 2013, 15 and in 2014, 22 (Schiller, 2015, Personal Communication). The prevalence as stated by the national effort 2003–2005 probably represents an exaggeration (Billing, 2014, Personal Communication). In an official inquiry from 2006 extensive interviewing, register inventories and field studies conducted in relevant countries and regions yielded no information of reaction patterns, nor of circumstances, such as cultural peculiarities, that could account for the phenomenon (Hessle and Ahmadi, 2006).

Apathy

In relation to the epidemiological data it is not entirely unreasonable to at least speculate in a novel pathogenic entity. However, historic accounts of similar symptom panoramas exist arguably precluding this interpretation.

In 1913, Jaspers characterized apathy: "[t]his is the term given to absence of feeling" where "there is no incentive to act"

BOX 2 | "Apathy" according to Jaspers (1913/1993).

"This is the term given to absence of feeling. If this absence is complete, as can happen in acute psychoses, the patient is fully conscious and oriented, sees, hears, observes and remembers, but he lets everything pass him by with the same total indifference; happiness, pleasure, something positive in which he is involved, danger, sorrow, annihilation are all the same. He remains "dead with wakeful eyes". In this condition there is no incentive to act; apathy brings about aboulia. It seems as if that one aspect of psychic life we call object-awareness has become isolated; there is only the mere grasp of reason on the world as an object. We can compare it to a photographic plate. Reason can portray its environment but cannot appreciate it. This absence of feeling shows itself objectively in the patient not taking food, in a passive indifference to being hurt, burnt, etc. The patient would die if we did not keep him alive with feeding and nursing care. The apathy of these acute states must be distinguished from the dullness of certain abnormal personalities who are constantly at the mercy of innumerable feelings, only crude in quality."

(Jaspers, 1913/1993)

manifested "objectively in the patient not taking food, in a passive indifference to being hurt, burnt, etc. The patient would die if we did not keep him alive with feeding and nursing care" (Jaspers, 1913/1993; see **Box 2**).

Children exhibiting lethargy and apathy with resemblance to depressive stupor or catatonia in connexion to traumatic events (Annell, 1958) and reaction patterns in catastrophes and war involving reduced contact and "apathic introversion" along with other symptoms interpreted to be psychosomatic (Otto, 1982), have been described.

Numerous phenomena resembling RS have been reported by physicians and anthropologists across contexts, cultures and time periods suggesting a common psychosomatic mechanism (Kihlbom, 2013). Acute as well as prolonged death ensuing real or magical threat of death is known from cultures on most continents (see e.g., Lester, 2009). "Epidemics" of dying in war and captivity where no hope remains has been described (Kihlbom, 2013). Nostalgia has been examined in relation to deterioration, apathy and dying (Johannisson, 2001). The concentration camp term "muselmann" denoted those void of all hope exhibiting resignation behavior (Kertész, 1998) claimed to sustain for weeks without nutrition in a state of "archaic autohypnosis" (Kihlbom, 2013). Unexpected and unexplainable sudden death following cancer diagnosis has been termed "self-willed death" (Milton, 1973). Sudden nocturnal death in Hmong immigrants in the USA (Adler, 1994) is hypothesized to result from sleep paralysis-type panic attacks involving punishment by spiritual encounter inspired by folk tales.

Resignation, apathy and eventually death in response to severe unavoidable threat is a consistent finding throughout history and across cultures.

Diagnostic Conceptualizations

A wide range of diagnostic alternatives have been considered; various neurological disorders, anorexia nervosa, selective mutism, school refusal, social phobia, other anxiety states, states of conversion and dissociation, chronic fatigue syndrome, depression, catatonic states, and malingering. Among these none, according to Bodegård (2005a), fully exhaust the clinical picture including presentation, course and recovery. He therefore coined the term *Depressive Devitalization* (DD) only to later argue the condition, in its most severe form, to be identical to *Pervasive Refusal Syndrome* (PRS; Bodegård, 2005b) as introduced by Lask et al. (1991) and designating a child's "dramatic social withdrawal and determined refusal to walk, talk, eat, drink, or care for themselves in any way".

The similarities and differences between DD and PRS have been discussed (Von Folsach and Montgomery, 2006); PRS involves active refusal, DD in all its forms does not, and further, PRS does not manifest "flaccid paralysis and generalized sensory loss", DD does. Accordingly, DD and PRS have been suggested to be subgroups of "the same refusal syndrome" (Von Folsach and Montgomery, 2006).

In a re-conceptualization of PRS, yet another term—*Pervasive Arousal-Withdrawal Syndrome* (PAWS)—was introduced together with an hypothesis of hyper-arousal in the sympathetic and parasympathetic autonomic nervous systems resulting in a "deadlock" manifesting itself in refusal, on this account re-conceptualized as a combination of "extreme anxiety avoidance" and "behavioral paralysis" mirroring the autonomic responses respectively. The authors predict high energy consumption as well as activity shifts in amygdala and insula to be present (Nunn et al., 2014). Interestingly, indirect calorimetry demonstrated energy expenditure below the requirement of basal metabolism in two patients suggesting an equivalent of hibernation (Jeppsson, 2013).

In contrast to the novel diagnostic entities such as DD, PRS and PAWS stand accounts relying on established diagnoses.

Several authors discuss stress-induced conditions such as *posttraumatic stress disorder* (PTSD) yet refrain, due to lack of diagnostic fit, from adopting these (Lindberg and Sundelin, 2005; Söndergaard et al., 2012; Bodegård, 2014).

An expert committee (Rydelius, 2006) identified severe depression or conversion/dissociation disorder to be the best diagnostic alternatives. Engström (2013), a member of the committee, argued traditional diagnostic entities sufficient in the majority of cases. He recognized RS as *severe major depressive disorder with psychotic features specified as catatonic* (DSM-IV 296.24), or in the ICD-10 taxonomy; as a *severe depressive episode with psychotic symptoms, in particular stupor* (F32.3).

January 1st 2014 the Swedish National Board of Health and Welfare, for epidemiological purposes, recognized *RS* (*uppgivenhetssyndrom*, ICD-10 F32.3A) and the specifier *problem adhering to status as refugee and asylum seeking* (Z65.8A). From a diagnostic viewpoint the introduction has been argued unnecessary (Engström, 2013). RS classified among the depressive entities (F32–33) should be interpreted as pragmatic solution to controversies regarding the nature of the phenomenon (Socialstyrelsen, 2013). Diagnostic criteria remain undetermined.

Etiological Conceptualizations

An expert committee suggested six etiological conceptualizations (Rydelius, 2006). These included: (1) the *medical model of disorder* according to which a disorder affects vulnerable individuals under certain circumstances; (2) the *family model* stressing family psychology system theory; (3) the *psychological model* emphasizing effects of uncontrollability; (4) the *political model* identifying political decisions governing the asylum process; (5) the *cultural model* proposing the symptoms to instantiate a phenomenon belonging to either the patients' cultural, religious or existential descent or to that of the country to which they migrate. Implicit in the cultural model lays the notion of secondary illness gain; and (6) according to the *intended model* an intentional decision made by the family or by the child explains the symptoms.

A Stress Hypothesis

Several authors endorse a stress hypothesis arguing a sustained stress response to be, if not the explanation, at least a contributing factor in pathogenesis (Lindberg and Sundelin, 2005; Söndergaard et al., 2012; Bodegård, 2014). Hypothetically, a sufficient and sustained "discrepancy between what is expected and what really exists" (Ursin and Eriksen, 2010) eliciting a stress response could precipitate debut in individuals predisposed by genetic, comorbid (depression, anxiety, neuropsychiatric disorders), premorbid (personality traits or adverse life events) or other unknown factors. Early symptoms accord with a stress induced condition (Lindberg and Sundelin, 2005) and altered autonomic function (tachycardia and rise in temperature) may be interpreted in analogy. The impact of a PRP on remission is taken to support the stress hypothesis and obtaining it is therefore considered an essential element in treatment (Lindberg and Sundelin, 2005).

Trauma and stressful events interplay with coping. This conjunction in turn impact on risk and resilience with regards to psychopathology (Ursin and Eriksen, 2010). Relatedly, one RS report (n = 29) surveyed predisposing, precipitating and perpetuating factors (Godani et al., 2008). In the neonatal period, 15 children exhibited predisposing factors associated with attachment (preterm birth, obstetric or neonatal complications, malformations, severe infection, congenital hip dysplasia etcetera). In the toddler period 25 had exhibited behavioral anomalies or had been subject to stressors (migration, loss of primary carer, severe illness, starvation, war, threat, death in family etcetera). Only a few individuals failed to demonstrate predisposing factors altogether. Putatively precipitating factors of either having witnessed or been subject to traumatization by threat, violence, rape or witnessing death, were demonstrated in all but one child. Indications of perpetuating factors, such as insufficient maternal care and ability to supply security, including previous maternal psychiatric illness and traumatization by assault, rape, murder of relative etcetera were, taken together, present in the majority of cases. The fathers' contribution could not be studied due to insufficient data. Findings support predisposing and perpetuating factors being of considerable importance. Traumatization of mothers and children correlate inversely with time spent in Sweden prior to debut and directly with length of tube-feeding dependency (Godani et al., 2008). The material was biased towards advanced cases, and controls were lacking altogether.

In concordance with the stress hypothesis diminished diurnal variation of cortisol measured in saliva has been demonstrated, however in a small sample (n = 4; Godani et al., 2008). In another study (n = 11), patterns of endogenous steroids imply negative association of concentrations of cortisol and cortisone, and positive association with pregnenolone, 17-hydroxypregnenolone and dehydroepiandrosterone (DHEA) with severity of symptoms and the time of recovery (Söndergaard et al., 2012). No statistically significant difference in cortisol levels at entry and after recovery was shown. Elevated levels of DHEA and pregnenolone was demonstrated and suggested to support a *neurosteroid hypothesis of stress* (Söndergaard et al., 2012).

The reported overrepresentation within the Uighur ethnic group (Rydelius, 2006), it may be hypothesized, could result from a predisposing genetic or epigenetic factor. However, no cases of RS or similar phenomena were confirmed in the regions from which the Uighurs migrate (Hessle and Ahmadi, 2006).

The stress hypothesis suggests the condition to be present in comparable populations and in particular other refugee populations. To our knowledge no such reports exist. Personal communication with the child and adolescent psychiatrist Dr Abdulbaghi Ahmad, founding director of Metin Health House, a child mental health center in Duhok, Kurdistan, reveals no cases in the Duhok refugee camps accommodating approximately 100,000 people of Syrian decent and more than 600,000 internally displaced people from Iraq, among which about 28% are 5–14 years of age. Dr Ahmad, with expertise in childhood trauma, from Sweden and Kurdistan (Ahmad, 2008; Ahmad et al., 2008), reports various stress-induced conditions in the camps but none resembling RS. To account for the regional distribution, the stress hypothesis would need an auxiliary hypothesis.

A Psychodynamic Interpretation

A model implicating the mother's predicament as the driving force behind RS has been proposed (Bodegård, 2005a). Inspired by the hypothesized mechanisms underpinning PRS (Nunn and Thompson, 1996), Bodegård suggests a psychodynamic interpretation.

The majority of mothers in Bodegård's material had been subject to physical and or sexual abuse (Bodegård, 2005a; Godani et al., 2008) and were described as severely traumatized. Their attitude was signified by a lack of trust, rejection of medical information excluding physical illness as causing the condition and resistance to rehabilitation and treatment on the child's behalf. On Bodegård's interpretation, this attitude and the corresponding behavior may be perceived as parts of a coping strategy by which the mother's traumatized depressed situation and need for consolation is projected from herself and onto her child. She creates a "delusive fantasy of the child as dying" and the child acting to maintain the right to be its mother's child, a folie à deux implicating the idea of a serious illness is staged. By "lethal mothering" the mother unconsciously creates and maintains an alternative reality in which she finds meaning in caring for a child imagined as dying in turn affecting the child and promoting debut and progression of the disorder.

The situation can be related to a Munchausen by proxy scenario in which the mother's delusion, aimed at concealing her own desperate situation by projecting it to the imagined disorder of the child, distorts not only her reality but also that of the child which in the process is abandoned and forced into adapting the role of dying or, "devitalized". From the child's perspective the prospect of rejection by the mother is more frightening (on a subconscious level) than adopting the delusion which protects not only from rejection itself but also from the emotional trauma of failing mothering. In relation to this interplay the child's deterioration, withdrawal, stupor and finally, full blown DD, may be conceptualized on a psychodynamic interpretation according to Bodegård (2005a).

Other authors fail to report evidence of inadequate mothering or disadvantageous maternal coping strategies. The hypothesis would suggest the phenomenon to be present in comparable populations. Such reports have failed to reach the research community.

Interestingly, a notion of expectancy as a contributor in pathogenesis is invoked. The staging of the child as dying and it acting accordingly, would serve to illustrate how a propagated set of beliefs may govern reaction patterns. Also, Bodegård's proposal involves a family system perspective attractive in relation to the observation that, to our knowledge, RS in unaccompanied minors have not been observed.

HYPOTHESES

In relation to the nature and regional distribution of RS neither of the two examined hypotheses—the stress hypothesis and the psychodynamic hypothesis—are sufficient. Both, although possibly of importance, fail to account for the regional distribution and predict the disorder to be present in populations where it is not. We now proceed to argue that catatonia satisfyingly fits the clinical characteristics of RS and that the regional distribution can be explained by invoking a notion of culture-bound psychogenesis.

RS is Catatonia

Rather than a lack of awareness, RS is characterized by an inability to initiate motor response, a finding also present in catatonia and conversion disorder. On the basis of substantial clinical overlap, we argue that RS should be perceived as catatonia. As catatonia promptly responds to a test dose of lorazepam (or equivalent) and is validated by positive treatment effect with benzodiazepines and/or ECT (Fink and Taylor, 2003); and as neuroimaging may indicate altered brain activity in catatonia (De Tiége et al., 2003), as well as preserved awareness (Vanhaudenhuyse et al., 2010) the hypothesis is testable.

Arousal and Awareness in RS

At its most advanced stage RS patients appear unconscious. The eyes of the patients are generally closed and remain so despite stimulation. If passively opened eyes sometimes diverge away from the examiner. Further, patients exhibit (what has been interpreted as) flaccid paralysis or hypotonicity and complete lack of pain response (sternal rub, supraorbital pressure, nail-bed pressure) as well as reaction to extraction or insertion of nasogastric tube. We are unaware of caloric testing having been performed in order to determine physiological nystagmus indicative of wakefulness. An "Amytal interview"[1] (Iserson, 1980; Posner et al., 2007) or a benzodiazepine challenge[2] (Fink and Taylor, 2003) has to our knowledge not been exploited in order to reveal a psychogenic state. Interestingly, however, Bodegård (2005a) reports of two patients temporarily normalizing following midazolam administration prior to insertion of a nasogastric tube. Nevertheless, a condition lacking both arousal and awareness is the general impression when examining RS patients.

The general impression needs however be questioned. Sleep-wake cycles are indicated by hypnagogic jerks and confirmed by EEG-recordings (Bodegård, 2005a). Language acquisition in the seemingly unaware state, tear excretion in otherwise detached faces, self-report of inclination to console parents in despair as well as of blurred visions including "fairies" all testify to preserved awareness (Engström, 2013). Bodegård claims full awareness (n = 5) during the course of the disorder and negates amnesia (Bodegård, 2005a). Another study reports varying degrees of amnesia (Forslund and Johansson, 2013).

According to these reports RS exhibits a combination of inability to respond to any stimulation and maintained, perhaps fluctuating, awareness, as well as preserved arousal. Neither arousal nor awareness thus appear impaired to an extent explaining the lack of response to painful stimulus. Accepting this line of argument, the inability to initiate motor activity would have to account for unresponsiveness, which indeed has been proposed (Engström, 2013). On this interpretation, RS is consistent with psychogenic unresponsiveness possibly on the basis of catatonia or conversion disorder both known to generate motor symptoms of either inhibitory or excitatory nature (Posner et al., 2007).

Catatonia

Recently a considerable shift has occurred in the conception of catatonia (Tandon et al., 2013). For a long period considered a sub group within schizophrenia, in DSM-IV catatonia was partly separated from this hierarchy by the addition of a new class; *Catatonia secondary to medical condition*. Successful treatment in catatonia exhibiting little or no effect in schizophrenia, and catatonia occurring in relation to other psychiatric as well as somatic disorders motivated the separation, which in DSM-5 was finalized by the deletion of *schizophrenia, catatonic type* altogether. Currently catatonia is conceived of as a neuropsychiatric syndrome associated with systemic illness (Fink, 2013; Fink et al., 2015).

In DSM-5, catatonia is defined as the presence of three or more symptoms out of a list of twelve (**Table 1**). Among

[1] Under the slow intravenous injection of amobarbital, continuous interviewing and evaluation of symptoms, patients with psychogenic impairment of consciousness exhibit symptom relief.

[2] A modern version of the Amytal interview in which lorazepam or diazepam is used.

TABLE 1 | Catatonia in DSM-5.

Catatonia is defined as the presence of three or more of the following:

1.	Catalepsy	Passive induction of a posture held against gravity
2.	Waxy flexibility	Slight and even resistance to positioning by examiner
3.	Stupor	No psychomotor activity; not actively relating to environment
4.	Agitation	(Not influenced by external stimuli)
5.	Mutism	No, or very little, verbal response (not applicable if there is an established aphasia)
6.	Negativism	Opposing or not responding to instructions or external stimuli
7.	Posturing	Spontaneous and active maintenance of a posture against gravity
8.	Mannerisms	Odd caricature of normal actions
9.	Stereotypies	Repetitive, abnormally frequent, non-goal directed movements
10.	Grimacing	
11.	Echolalia	Mimicking another's speech
12.	Echopraxia	Mimicking another's movements

American Psychiatric Association (2013)

these, stupor, mutism and negativism are all general finding in RS (**Box 1**). Diagnostic criteria apply regardless of age. Nevertheless, pediatric catatonia has been suggested to consist of three cardinal symptoms; immobility, mutism and withdrawal or refusal to ingest (Takaoka and Takata, 2003). Depending on clinical presentation, either the specifier *with catatonia* together with major depressive disorder, or, the separate entity *catatonic disorder NOS* (*not otherwise specified*; Tandon et al., 2013) would be applicable to RS. From a phenomenological perspective, applying these diagnostic labels should meet no resistance.

Posner et al. (2007) characterize catatonic stupor (as opposed to the excited form): the patient's eyes are usually open apparently unseeing, or sometimes, tightly closed resisting passive opening. Skin is pale and acne or oily skin common. Pulse is rapid (90–120) and temperature often elevated (1.0–1.5°C). Spontaneous movement is rare and unawareness the impression. Pupils are dilated and reactive to light, alternating anisochoria is common and opticokinetic response present, however, patients' may fail to blink to visual threat. Doll's eye test is negative and caloric testing produces normal ocular nystagmus. Increased salivation is sometimes noted. Incontinence may be present. Urinary retention may require catheterization. Extremities are relaxed or rigid resisting passive movements. Catalepsy (waxy muscular/postural rigidity and reduced responsiveness) is present in 30%. Choreiform jerks of the extremities and grimaces are common. Reflexes are normal. Consciousness is preserved although the appearance is the opposite. On recovering, the patient is often, but not always, able to recall events that occurred during illness. Normal neurological examination and self-reports after recovery attest preserved consciousness.

Further, inability to speak despite urge to do so, as reported in an RS patient (Engström, 2013), has been reported in Catatonia (Fink, 2013) and after remission, catatonic patients recover fully which appears to be the case also in RS patients (Forslund and Johansson, 2013) although this finding need to be confirmed. "Panicky refusal" (Bodegård, 2005b) may be interpreted as agitation, a common finding in the exited form of Catatonia (Fink and Taylor, 2003).

Reviewing the symptoms of RS and catatonia, (**Box 1, Table 1**) resemblance is undeniable. Clinical characteristics of RS match the diagnostic criteria of catatonia. Dhossche et al. (2012) argue pediatric catatonia to be the genuine diagnosis in both RS and PRS and find evidence of deprivation, abuse and trauma to precipitate catatonia in children and adolescents. Shorter (2012) contests the prevailing belief that pediatric catatonia is a rare disorder; other diagnostic labels have obscured the condition (**Table 2**), which, prior to Kahlbaum coining the term in 1874, was only natural. An extensive review of catatonia in all age groups supports Shorter's analysis (Fink, 2013). Cohen et al. (1999), based on a literature review, report 42 cases of adolescent catatonia among which 19 were associated with mood disorder. Posner et al. (2007) suggest catatonic stupor to be rare due to effective treatment. This is of course only applicable if the condition is recognized and treated.

Demonstrating Catatonia

In acute catatonia, treatment effect verifies the diagnosis: prompt response to a benzodiazepine challenge implies catatonia and treatment effect with benzodiazepines and/or ECT validates the diagnosis (Fink and Taylor, 2003). As already noted, Bodegård (2005a) observed two patients temporarily normalizing in response to midazolam. In acute catatonia, 60–90% responds to lorazepam (Northoff, 2002; Fink and Taylor, 2003). Chronic cases may fail to respond (Northoff, 2002). Amantadine may have effect in these cases and ECT, considered the most potent alternative, exhibits effect in 80–100% of all cases (Luchini et al., 2015).

Pediatric catatonia is typically treated with benzodiazepines and ECT (Dhossche et al., 2009; Weiss et al., 2012; Wachtel et al., 2013). In a pediatric population ECT is considered effective and safe. There are no studies indicating deleterious side-effect and the fear of inflicting damage to the developing brain finds no support (Wachtel et al., 2011). Interestingly, the first five patients receiving treatment with convulsive therapy in 1934 were stuporous and had required tube-feeding for

TABLE 2 | Diagnostic labels that have historically obscured Catatonia as an independent disease according to Shorter (2012).

Pre 1850s	Stupor
	Catalepsy
	Stupidité
	Death spells
1869	Neurasthenia
	Hysteria (dissociated from Catatonia in 1920s)
1871	Hebephrenia
1874	Catatonia
1899	Dementia praecox
1903	Psychasthenia
1908	Schizophrenia
1920s	Encephalitis lethargica
1934	"Brain stem" changes (precursor to ADHD)
1943	Autism
1991	Pervasive refusal syndrome
2007	Anti-NMDA receptor encephalitis

several months; repeated intramuscular injection of camphor precipitating seziures were effective in all patients (Luchini et al., 2015).

Posner et al. (2007) conceive of catatonia as psychogenic unresponsiveness (which is not to say it is imagined). In the clinical context, psychologically induced neurological symptoms usually exhibit normal EEG and MRI findings (Posner et al., 2007); however, using positron emission tomography (PET) technology, regional metabolic abnormalities have been demonstrated including reduced metabolism in the prefrontal cortex (the anterior cingulate, the medial prefrontal and dorsolateral cortices) in a 14 year old girl diagnosed with akinetic catatonia in the context of Bipolar type 1 disorder (De Tiége et al., 2003). Interestingly, anterior cingulate cortex (ACC) lesions are known to contribute to a range of behavioral disorders including akinetic mutism, diminished self-awareness, impaired motor initiation and reduced pain response (Devinsky et al., 1995). Posner et al. (2007) predict abnormal brain metabolism in *psychogenic coma*. Evaluation of prefrontal metabolism in RS patients is an attractive, so far unexplored, diagnostic alternative.

Demonstrating Awareness in RS

If RS is catatonia, consciousness should be preserved. In RS the general impression is that of a condition void of arousal as well as awareness, which by definition implies unconsciousness, yet indications of the opposite exist (Bodegård, 2005a; Engström, 2013). The unresponsive RS patient exhibiting only *that* behavior, bedside tests are inadequate. A similar situation faces the clinician examining patients suffering from *disorders of consciousness* (DOC) where residual awareness may be impossible to determine with traditional methods (Giacino et al., 2009). However, through analysis of brain resting state activity a further means of discriminating between the unaware and aware patient has been made possible (Owen et al., 2006; Vanhaudenhuyse et al., 2010; Evers and Sigman, 2013).

Aberrant activity in the *default mode network* (DMN) has been demonstrated to correlate with a number of psychiatric and neurological disorders (Zhang and Raichle, 2010) as well as with physiological and induced variations in level of consciousness (Heine et al., 2012). Importantly, the level of consciousness in patients suffering from DOC have been described vis-à-vis activity in the DMN: functional as well as structural connectivity, established by exploiting fMRI BOLD-signal and diffusion tensor imaging (DTI) respectively, have been demonstrated to correlate with levels of consciousness thus discriminating between unaware and aware patients (Vanhaudenhuyse et al., 2010; Fernández-Espejo et al., 2012).

RS, like the DOC, may benefit from characterization by means of fMRI-BOLD resting state analysis. Undoubtedly different mechanisms generate DOC and RS. Nevertheless, the covariance between level of consciousness and DMN connectivity also in anesthesia (Ramani, 2015), hypnosis (Vanhaudenhuyse et al., 2014) and sleep (Horovitz et al., 2009) implies the DMN connectivity of interest in relation to level of consciousness regardless of cause. Resting state analysis could indicate to what extent RS patients are conscious and demonstration of preserved awareness would indirectly support RS being catatonia. It would also imply feasibility of neuro-technological communication (Owen et al., 2006; Evers and Sigman, 2013).

Interim Summary

Catatonia is from a phenomenological and clinical perspective an adequate label of what has been labelled RS. The reluctance to this attribution may be explained by unwillingness to ECT in children in Sweden (Shorter, 2012) and the up until recently prevailing view of catatonia as a sub group within schizophrenia. Catatonia prompts ECT or benzodiazepines. To our knowledge no RS patients have received such treatment. Residual hesitance may be overcome by at test dose of a benzodiazepine or by performing a PET examination to objectify suggested reduced prefrontal metabolism. Clinical observations implying preserved awareness may be evaluated further by resting state network analysis. The reconceptualization of catatonia invites to a re-evaluation of RS, more so now than ever, and its correspondence to catatonia.

Culture-Bound Psychogenesis Explains the Regional Distribution of RS

Regardless of the relationship between catatonia and RS, the question remains how to explain the regional distribution of RS. Expressions of distress are constrained by brain function upon which beliefs and expectations impact. Evolving and transpiring within cultural contexts, beliefs and expectations readily serve as vehicles of *idioms of distress*. Culture-bound psychogenesis, it will be argued, may explain the regional distribution of RS. Genetic or environmental factors are conceivable in accounting for the regional distribution, nevertheless; such commendable analyses are beyond the scope of this article.

Clinical Traditions

Differences in diagnostics and treatment across countries conceivably supply explanations for the endemic distribution of RS. Provided the condition is promptly reversed, patients would not reach the prolonged stuporous state RS exhibits. This hypothesis predicts the incidences of catatonia—and/or other similar disorders—and RS to correspond.

In 2003–2005, the estimated annual incidence of RS was 2.8% in 0–17 year old asylum seekers. Catatonia incidence has been examined in two pediatric and adolescent psychiatric materials and found to be 0.6 and 5.5% respectively (Cohen et al., 1999; Thakur et al., 2003). The general incidence in the young population was estimated at 0.16% in Paris (Cohen et al., 1999). Estimated RS incidence is thus comparable to that of catatonia in psychiatric materials but does not correspond to that in a general material.

This discrepancy could reflect the vulnerability refugees as a group exhibit and the high incidence interpreted accordingly. Similar incidences would then be expected in comparable populations—in particular refugees populations—which, to our knowledge, remains to be surveyed in this respect. However, were the incidence of catatonia in young refugees in the vicinity of 2.8%, it would most likely have been reported, and; thus, differences in clinical practice are not likely to account for the regional distribution of RS. Possibly, however unlikely, other diagnostic entities could obscure RS in other refugee populations.

Billing (2014, Personal Communication) proposed too liberal diagnostic inclusion could explain the peak in incidence 2003–2005. However, this proposal does not explain the regional distribution *per se*. Instead, it illustrates the importance of perceiving a diagnosis as more than the label of a clinical entity. It invites the discussion of the diagnosis as a culturally influenced construct and an analysis of its application within a cultural context.

Culture-Bound

Yap (1962), in order to unify and retain traditional nosology, proposed the class "atypical culture-bound psychogenic psychoses" (later culture-bound syndromes) on recognizing the "pathoplastic influence" effected by culture to generate in "exotic psychoses". Consequently, *Latah*, *Susto*, *Koro*, *Dhat* etcetera, were conceptualized as, and grouped among, the "reactive psychoses (psychogenic reactions)" (Yap, 1967). By *culture-bound* it was implied that "[w]ith respect to the psychogenic reactions, significant etiological factors are commonly to be found at the social and psychosocial level rather than the anatomical and biochemical" (Yap, 1967).

Although transcultural differences in psychiatry are controversial (Kleinman, 1987; Prince and Tcheng-Laroche, 1987; Keshavan, 2014; Ventriglio et al., 2015) they are evident; the incidence, symptoms, course and outcomes in schizophrenia (Myers, 2011); clinical presentation of depression and anxiety (Kirmayer, 2001), and; symptoms, self-perception, help-seeking behavior and treatment in relation to war trauma (Miller et al., 2009; Hinton and Lewis-Fernández, 2010; Shannon et al., 2015) vary across cultures. In recognition, all mental distress is, in DSM-5, considered culturally framed and populations expected to display culturally determined differences in communicating distress as well as in relation to explanations of causality, coping-methods and help-seeking behaviors (American Psychiatric Association, 2013). Consequently, culture-bound syndromes are recognized and grouped within the *cultural concepts of distress* defined as "ways cultural groups experience, understand, and communicate suffering, behavioral problems, or troubling thoughts and emotions" (American Psychiatric Association, 2013).

By *culture-bound* we recognize the impact exerted by socio-culturally transferable beliefs and expectations on an individual or population.

Many consider dualism an out-dated metaphysical basis for psychiatry (Shorter, 2006). In cognitive neuroscience the connexion between psychology, brain physiology and behavior is nevertheless indisputable and everyday life as well as clinical experience informs of the relevance of psychological processes to behavior. To demonstrate the impact of culture and context on symptom generation and presentation we draw on an account of psychogeninc illness (Shorter, 1992) exemplified by "La Grand Hystérie", epidemic hysteria and suggestion. These phenomena are presented to illustrate the likelihood of RS being culture-bound.

"La Grande Hystérie"

Shorter, in an extensive analysis of the history of psychogenic illness, explores the relationship between physicians, patients and conceptions of disease throughout centuries (Shorter, 1992). In essence, he argues that cultural context–in particular diagnostic techniques, medical paradigms, familial expectation and social roles–influences what symptoms are legitimate and illegitimate by associating to them underlying organic disease for which the patient cannot be blamed, and; that unconsciously, in response to stress, trauma or suggestion, symptoms are assimilated from the "symptom pool" of legitimate symptoms and perceived as genuine indicators of an organic disorder or dysfunction by patients and physicians alike.

In treating patients with "hystero-epilepsy" at La Salpêtrière hospital in Paris, Jean-Martin Charcot developed a theory asserting that hysteria was an inherited, life-long, disease of the nervous system with sensory (headache, loss of sensation etcetera) and motor (tremor, paralysis etcetera) stigmata accompanied by reoccurring fits characterized by four phases presenting in a law-like manner: (1) the epileptiod period; (2) the "period of contortions and grande mouvements" during which the patients flung themselves about, crying and adopting improbable postures like "arc-de-cercles"; (3) the period of "impassioned poses" like prayer, crucifixion etcetera; and (4) a "terminal period" where anything could happen. Ovary tenderness at debut of fits was considered pathognomonic as well as hypnotisability.

Treatment—consisting of "metallotherapy" and hypnosis—and patient demonstrations, attended by students, visiting physicians, journalists and the general public, produced "a climate of suggestion" prompting patients to exhibit symptoms in accordance with the "laws of hysteria". Scientific and journalistic reports paralleled the spread and increase of cases with predicted symptomatology. Eventually patients were referred from other continents.

On observing startle shock and suggestion by hypnosis precipitating the symptoms, Charcot later came to recognize psychological factors as possible inducers of hysteria. This shift Shorter interprets as the beginning of the end for "Charcot's Hysteria". No longer an organic disorder—and patients less prone to unconsciously select and present symptoms indicating a problem "merely in the head"—the incidence dropped. Also, Charcot's successor, attributing the "epidemic" to iatrogenic suggestion, prohibited mention of hysteric symptoms in front of patients and ferociously challenged those exhibiting fits. Babinski, a student of Charcot's—and the discoverer of a clinical procedure useful in distinguishing hysteric from organic paralysis—later characterized hysteria in La Salpêtrière as "any symptom that could be induced by suggestion [understood as medical or cultural] and abolished by persuasion [including hypnosis and psychotherapy]".

"La Grand Hystérie" illustrates how psychogenic symptoms evolve over time, transpire epidemically and affect by suggestion. According to Shorter, the content of the symptom pool evolve constantly, through the continuous negotiation between physicians and patients immersed in cultural context, and is reflected in "pathoplasticity", the changing psychogenic symptomatology. Current negotiations are affected in particular by media, and the contemporary expressions—controversially—include *chronic fatigue syndrome* and *environmental hypersensitivity* (Stewart, 1990; Shorter, 1992).

Epidemic Hysteria

Epidemic hysteria (Boss, 1997) of *mass sociogenic illness*—the rapid spread of unconsciously exhibited symptoms indicative of excitation, loss or alteration of neurological function without corresponding etiology in a cohesive group—exhibit contagious characteristics, and has been asserted, due to surface heterogeneity, to represent an under-appreciated, social problem (Bartholomew and Wessley, 2002).

Examples include regionally dispersed "dancing mania"—known as the St Vitus dance—reoccurring throughout the Middle Ages; motor hysteria outbreaks in nunneries or, more recently, boarding schools (reported from Malaysia during the 1980s), and; *mass hysteria*—often in poor working environment and related to mysterious odors (Boss, 1997). Continuous anxiety or stress in segregated highly controlled groups has been suggested to engender dissociation and hyper-suggestibility eliciting delusions reflecting the Zeitgeist, epidemic hysteria thus mirroring its time (Bartholomew and Wessley, 2002).

Recent reports include mass psychogenic illness (n = 170) attributed to toxic exposure at a high school (Jones et al., 2000); an outbreak of conversion disorder (n = 5) among Amish adolescent girls (Cassady et al., 2005), and; acute stridor (n = 12) in a female cohort of students in preparation for national exams (Powell et al., 2007).

Suggestion

Socio-cultural impact on individual psychogenic expressions has also been studied. Patients present symptoms in relation to social surroundings, iatrogenic suggestion (Fallik and Sigal, 1971) and following hypnosis (Halligan et al., 2000). Also, symptom attribution varies with "trendy diagnoses": In 1985, most patients with environmental hypersensitivity disorder (n = 50), also attributed their problems to food and synthetics, in 1986 to Candida albicans, and in 1987 to chronic Epstein-Barr virus (Stewart, 1990). Contemporary fixed illness attributions have been suggested to align with media reports, and controversially, *chronic fatigue syndrome*, *myalgic encephalomyelitis* and *environmental hypersensitivity* are examples from our time (Shorter, 1992).

RS is Culture-Bound

Psychogenic symptom expression paralleling progression in medicine and culture (Shorter, 1992; North, 2015), discrete episodes of epidemic hysteria (Levy and Nail, 1993; Boss, 1997; Bartholomew and Wessley, 2002) and intra-individual presentation as well as progression of psychogenic illness attributions relating to trends (Stewart, 1990; Shorter, 1992) suggest culture-bound psychogenesis to be a robust and important phenomenon. The acknowledgment of transcultural differences (American Psychiatric Association, 2013), idioms of distress (Ventriglio et al., 2015) and varying psychogenic illness presentation supply indirect evidence culture-bound transfer of psychopathology and symptom induction by hypnosis (Halligan et al., 2000) provide direct evidence.

Mass psychogenic illness, traditionally *epidemic hysteria*, exhibit certain characteristics (Levy and Nail, 1993; Boss, 1997; Bartholomew and Wessley, 2002). Highly segregated groups where stress, control or obligations are evident and inescapable are predisposed and historically in particular religious settings are overrepresented. Female patients predominate. Patients below 20 years of age are overrepresented. Epidemics involve typical symptoms, including fatigue and unconsciousness, without demonstrable organic lesions. Relapse is common. "Compensational" issues have been reported of importance. Media reports are known to enable transmission of illness behavior.

RS mostly afflicts individuals of the same ethnic group, language community and previous, as well as present, cultural context (Rydelius, 2006) in which psychological and or physical trauma as well as stress are prevalent (Godani et al., 2008). Helplessness and hopelessness—equivalents of inescapability—are generally asserted (Bodegård, 2005a; Lindberg and Sundelin, 2005). Uighurs early trust children with high responsibility (Rydelius, 2006) something the predicaments of migration and asylum seeking may reinforce creating more of control and obligations. The male to female ratio is 2:3, mean age 14.3 years old and relapses have occurred. Symptoms imply a central nervous affliction, however, none have been demonstrated. A secondary illness gain may be assumed, as severe illness hypothetically generate in increased chances of asylum approval. On a different level the seemingly unconscious state may *per se* be perceived as a secondary illness gain offering relief. The estimated peak in RS cases was paralleled by extensive media reports, popularization and an infected debate—regarding in particular etiology, malingering and level of care—and involving, in a transparent way, also the medical profession (Hacking, 2010) supplying ample opportunities for the negotiation and transpiration of legitimate symptoms.

The RS endemic fails to demonstrate a clear index case (which there nevertheless may have been), an identifiable trigger event (although individual presentation sometimes is preceded by e.g., a negative asylum decision) and it is uncertain to which degree individual cases have been in contact prior to presentation. These factors are generally seen in epidemic hysteria (Boss, 1997).

Not described in other parts of the world and overrepresented in ethnic minorities from certain parts of the world, RS respects national borders and to some extent, ethnicity and/or language community. These peculiar circumstances are difficult to explain without reference to culture and context and we therefore assert RS to be culture-bound.

Psychogenesis

In the previous section the notion of psychogenesis was inherent and served to transform culturally transpiring idioms of distress into generation of corresponding symptoms. Such neurological dysfunction in the absence of demonstrable organic lesion has been know to physicians since ancient times as *hysteria*. Grouped either among *conversion disorders* (DSM-5) or *dissociative disorders* (ICD-10), symptoms encompass loss, excitation or alteration of motor and sensory functions, including altered states of consciousness, sometimes in conjunction. Symptoms are genuine, sometimes disabling, and common–in one study functional and psychological symptoms were found to account for 16% of diagnosis in neurology units (Stone et al., 2010). Importantly, the symptoms are also involuntary, a fact not consistently recognized.

From Latin "hysterus", hysteria originally implied an etiology involving dysfunction or displacement of the uterus. Charcot recognized suggestion or psychogenic shock to precipitate symptoms—treatable with hypnosis—and proposed abnormal or absent "mental imagery" to result in corresponding neurological dysfunctions (Shorter, 1992; Gelder, 2001). Janet, invoked traumatic narrowing of attention with subsequent *dissociation* and disintegration of mental processes creating unconscious yet processed mental realms (Gelder, 2001). Breuer and Freud (1956/1893) adopted this notion in their psychodynamic theory of *conversion* in which negative emotions ensuing "psychical trauma" were hypothesized to convert into symbolic physical symptoms resulting in *primary* and *secondary illness gain*. Invoking "a morbid condition of emotion, of idea and emotion, or of idea alone" in pathogenesis, Reynolds (1869) appreciated emotive as well as cognitive dysfunction.

The most commonly reported symptoms—*psychogenic non-epileptic seizures* (PNES), loss of consciousness and motor symptoms (Brown and Lewis-Fernández, 2011)—imitate organic disorders. Prevalence is increased following brain injury (Eames, 1992), prior to debut of, and parallel to, epilepsy (Devinsky et al., 2011), with depression, PTSD (Ballmaier and Schmidt, 2005), anxiety and borderline personality disorder (Brown and Lewis-Fernández, 2011). Although transculturally understudied (Brown and Lewis-Fernández, 2011), functional disorders have been claimed to vary little in incidence and semiology across cultures (Carota and Calabrese, 2014). Importantly, complex behavior, such as pseudo-labor, Genser syndrome, anorexia nervosa and catatonia, has been attributed to conversion (Jensen, 1984; Lyman, 2004; Jiménez Gómez and Quintero, 2012; Shah et al., 2012; Goldstein et al., 2013) implicating also higher order processes. Moreover, *de facto* organic findings in conversion disorder (Ballmaier and Schmidt, 2005; Vuilleumier, 2005, 2014; García-Campayo et al., 2009) indicate, contrary to the traditional conception, the possibility of a neurocognitive mechanism answering to symptom generation, and conversion disorder thus being a phenomenon, also, of the brain.

Reflecting the multitude of mechanisms and etiologies suggested, current DSM and ICD nosology is "widely regarded as unsatisfactory" (Gelder, 2001) in particular with regards to clinical overlap between conversion, dissociation and somatization (Brown and Lewis-Fernández, 2011; North, 2015), and mechanistic as well as etiological bias involving unconscious mental states and psychological stress or trauma, with undecided, little, or no empirical relation to symptoms (Roelofs and Spinhoven, 2007; Brown and Lewis-Fernández, 2011). Although the DSM-5 criterion involving identification of a specific psychological cause has been abandoned and *functional neurologic symptom disorder* (FNSD) introduced as an alternate term to conversion disorder (American Psychiatric Association, 2013), more extensive reclassification has been proposed (Brown et al., 2007; North, 2015).

In the previous section culturally determined expectations and beliefs were demonstrated of importance to symptom generation of culture-bound phenomena (Stewart, 1990; Shorter, 1992; Levy and Nail, 1993; Boss, 1997; Hinton and Lewis-Fernández, 2010; Medeiros De Bustos et al., 2014). Even so, a dogmatic psychological approach has been asserted "misguided and unhelpful" (Edwards and Bhatia, 2012) as psychological factors, particularly understood as trauma or internal conflict, not consistently are supported clinically or in epidemiological studies (Roelofs and Spinhoven, 2007; Brown and Lewis-Fernández, 2011). Moreover, inorganic genesis has been denied altogether (Slater, 1965) perhaps signaling dualism to some an out-dated metaphysical basis for psychiatry (Shorter, 2006). In cognitive neuroscience the connexion between psychology, brain physiology and behavior is nevertheless indisputable and everyday life as well as clinical experience informs of the relevance of psychological processes to behavior.

In general, the presupposition of physical symptoms occurring unattended by demonstrable organic findings, where there are strong evidence or presumptions that the symptoms are linked to psychological factors, seems to force an unwarranted and unfortunate mutually excluding, dichotomy creating a divide between neurological and psychological mechanisms. Either it is in the mind or, it is in the body. This starting point is infertile and so, denying *psychogenesis*—understood as implying psychological impact on symptom generation and precipitation—altogether, is equally absurd as is the opposite.

However, as the controversies regarding mechanisms and etiologies indicate fundamental difficulties in conceiving of the pathophysiology (Gelder, 2001; Roelofs and Spinhoven, 2007; Brown and Lewis-Fernández, 2011; North, 2015), an analysis of psychogenesis, relying on current nosology, is from the outset likely to perpetuate previous unhelpful conceptions. Ultimately, a model appreciating the impact of beliefs and expectations in directing and generating symptoms is the ambition. Consequently, although aspiring to neutrality, also *culture-bound psychogenesis* should be considered preliminary and any mechanistic analysis of symptom generation preferably be unbiased even in relation to, although not inconsistent with, psychological causation.

Relying on a framework of predictive coding, a mechanism answering to the protean nature of phenomena attributed to psychogenesis, we argue, may be attained. Importantly, such a mechanism permits also organic genesis of symptoms. Nevertheless, in relation to the present context—the notion of culture-bound serving to explain the regional distribution of RS—it should be emphasized that a description solely on the level of the brain is unlikely to be successful.

A PREDICTIVE CODING MODEL

The effect of expectations on biological systems has been shown to be a decisive factor in both health and disease. The common denominator may be found in the models of predictive coding as a fundamental way the brain processes information. The general idea that the models of the world harnessed within the brain impact how we experience the world itself have been proposed more than a hundred years ago by Helmholtz (Helmholtz, 1866; Frith, 2007). Modern predictive coding theories suggest that Bayesian inference describe these processes (Friston, 2005; Frith, 2007).

Conceptually, such predictive coding hypotheses suggest that the brain constructs models of the world on different hierarchical levels. The models also act as expectations or predictors (priors) of the external and internal worlds. When a signal reaches the brain in a primary sensory region it will be compared with the priors, and if it does not match (in that the expectations are different as compared to the signal) it will produce an error signal. This error is proportional to the difference between prior and input, and will be propagated to the next hierarchical level where it is compared to priors on the intermediate levels. If these priors fail to explain the error signal it will continue its propagation to higher order hierarchies. The error signal may be used to change the priors or models of the world. However, the priors and the models may also change the way input is processed or perceived. Thus, a percept is determined both by the input and by the model. In Bayesian terms the models are conceptualized as *priors* and input as *observation* while the percept (thus dependent on both the prior and the observation) is often referred to as the *posterior*.

Research on placebo and nocebo treatment effects has suggested that expectation processes are crucially involved in the underlying mechanism (Petrovic et al., 2010; Büchel et al., 2014). For any given treatment, expectations about its effect will be built up in the subject or the patient. Verbal information about the effectiveness of the treatment is one source of information affecting the expectations. Other contextual factors in treatment may also change the expectations—including how invasive the treatment is (e.g., injections seems to be more effective than giving a pill). Importantly, also low-level conditioning effects are important for determining the expectation effect (Amanzio and Benedetti, 1999; Jensen et al., 2012, 2015), albeit in lower levels of the hierarchical network. Thus, placebo effects are not dependent on conscious mechanism. In more formal terms all these sources of information processing change the priors of the brain in different hierarchical levels, all of which are thought to contribute to the placebo effect.

The underlying neural mechanism of the placebo effect has mostly been studies with regards to pain, where also the underlying opioid system has been proposed of importance (Petrovic et al., 2002; Zubieta et al., 2005; Wager et al., 2007). Further, placebo treatment has been suggested to change the neural processing underlying emotions (Petrovic et al., 2005) depression (Mayberg et al., 2002) and Parkinson's disease (de la Fuente-Fernández et al., 2001). Moreover, similar manipulations of expectations have been shown to change how visual stimuli are processed (Sterzer et al., 2008; Schmack et al., 2013) in line with the idea that any type of perception is perceived in relation to the expectations of the systems.

How profoundly can expectation change the experience of the world? It has been suggested that extremely powerful priors are essentially the cause of hallucinations and delusions in psychosis (Frith, 2007; Fletcher and Frith, 2009; Adams et al., 2013). In line with this idea, manipulations of higher order expectations have shown that delusion prone individuals will experience the world more in line with those expectations (Schmack et al., 2013; Teufel et al., 2015).

A common theme, apart from the involvement of expectations, is dopamine system involvement in different aspects of placebo responses (de la Fuente-Fernández et al., 2001; Scott et al., 2008). As a main contributor also in psychosis, it may have a specific role in the balance between priors and observation.

Thus, in a predictive coding framework, priors change the way information is processed, even to the extent that delusions may arise in realms beyond control and awareness. Moreover, certain personality traits, such as delusion proneness, may explain why some individuals are more likely to develop pathogenic priors.

Interestingly, it has furthermore been suggested that functional sensory or motor symptoms in somatization and conversion disorder may be initiated and maintained by strong, although not necessarily conscious, priors (Edwards et al., 2012). In the sensory domain, the results of strong priors are well formed precepts, which may or may not be accurate representations of the world. In the motor domain, strong priors will elicit motor behavior, or its absence, through top-down influence on motor reflex arcs which, involuntarily generated, is perceived as abnormal behavior and symptoms of a neurological disorder.

The interoceptive system has been proposed to be likewise affected by expectation (Barrett and Simmons, 2015). Thus, the experienced bodily state will be determined not only by input from different interoceptive channels but also by expectations regarding the state itself. In particular, homeostatic cues from the hormonal, immune, metabolic and autonomic nervous systems have been suggested to generate error signals resulting in either bottom-up adjustment of predictions, or, top-down influence over physiological homeostasis (Seth, 2013; Barrett and Simmons, 2015). Thus, by predictive coding, the brain not only acquires and adjusts to homeostatically relevant information; it also orchestrates the adaption of the organism in relation to physiological needs instructed by priors. In particular, according to the model, the latter occurs in parts of the system where priors are strong and observations weak or imprecise, a balance likely to be of importance in homeostatic systems relying on fixed parameters to maintain the organism within a physiological state.

It is hypothesized (Seth, 2013; Barrett and Simmons, 2015) that not only basic homeostasis—converging particularly on the anterior insular cortex (AIC)—but also higher order self-related representations of emotion, agency, self-narration and body-ownership—subserved in ACC, posterior ventromedial PFC, posterior OFC—and supporting conscious self-perception and attentional control, are implicated in a wider interoceptive predictive coding system instantiated by the brain. Through the multisensory representation of in particular homeostatically relevant predictions distributed in the AIC and ACC, modulation of attentional, sensory and behavioral responses, is attained and transmitted in the wider system. Through these channels higher order functions may be recruited in minimizing prediction error by adjusting priors or instructing behavior on the conscious level.

Thus, by engaging physiological control mechanisms at the core of the organism, as well as attentional, sensory and behavioral responses also under the influence of higher cognitive processing, a powerful and integrated system answering to ecological needs of the organism is running, orchestrated within a predictive coding framework, in the brain.

Here we propose that a multitude of factors—psychological and or physical trauma, helplessness and hopelessness, familial expectations and obligations, the predicaments of migration and asylum seeking, including negative expectations regarding chances of obtaining a PRP—are crucial for setting inner priors of the interoceptive system to extreme levels in predisposed individuals. These priors may include (conscious or non-conscious) models untenable for bodily function under massive external stress thus eliciting a vulnerable state evolving into RS.

A situation of extreme stress and negative prospects (nocebo) is under normal circumstances not detrimental as interoceptive and exteroceptive input generates prediction errors driving physiological and behavioral change aimed at overcoming the situation. On the contrary, when strong priors are set "low", due to previous experience projecting to the present, the same nocebo situation will only accord with the predictions and adjustment will be absent thus perpetuating negative predictions with corresponding physiological, attentional, sensory and behavioral consequences.

Moreover, even if the interoceptive and exteroceptive input improve, prediction error may—provided priors are sufficiently strong, or sensory input imprecise—drive adjustment not of the model, but instead towards the prediction, in which case homeostatic mechanisms are directed top-down to attain a physiological state in correspondence with the prediction so as to minimize prediction error. The corresponding percept of the internal state represented in the AIC and the ACC is through the wider system responsible for modulation of cognitive, emotive and behavioral processes thus unlocking the full potential of the organism's predictive capacity resulting also in a mind-set corresponding to the prediction.

At this stage, negative predictions having generalized in higher and lower levels of the hierarchy, and physiological systems threatening homeostasis, the organism, at some point, adopts a behavior which elicits support from its surroundings; an idiom of distress.

Within a predictive coding framework this may be interpreted either as an attempt at minimizing prediction error by projecting the interocepted state onto the world as to affect it to accord with the prediction, in which case the intended result is the prevention of help from the surrounding; or, as a change in strategy and if so presumably driven by another set of priors corresponding to a rescue attempt from an inexorably escalating development. Interestingly, Seth (2013) finds support for an extended Bayesian framework encompassing also social interaction. Drawing on evidence from psychosis, behavior such as loss or alteration of general function may be as powerful as a delusion. Importantly, the response from the surrounding may on this hypothesis not only contribute to perpetuation of an illness-state but also possibly hold the key to its resolve.

We thus propose that RS may be conceived within a predictive coding framework, as a condition where predisposing and contextual factors generate in negative expectations and beliefs instantiated in fixed priors, which drives homeostatic and behavioral effects as well as self-perception, towards the prediction, minimizing prediction error, however at the cost of pushing the physiological, cognitive and emotional state further away from that which sustains life. The resulting behavior—described in terms of apathy, RS or catatonia—may be interpreted as, an outwardly broadcasted self-representation functioning as to minimize prediction error by extending also into the world the interocepted state in order to affect it accordingly, or, as a behavior serving to elicit support from the surrounding. In either case, the particular behavior, intended for a specific purpose, is conceivably one corresponding to culturally sanctioned expectations of what that behavior entails. Consequently, culture-bound reaction patterns are predicted by the model.

DISCUSSION

With regards to the phenomenon referred to as RS, our analysis has suggested catatonia to supply the best fit with clinical data, culture-bound psychogenesis to account for the regional distribution and predictive coding to supply a promising context in which to express a mechanistic model. We have purposely omitted to develop an account of the neural components instantiating the Bayesian machinery in the brain and instead direct the reader to recent conceptualizations (Edwards et al., 2012; Seth, 2013; Barrett and Simmons, 2015).

Our analysis has lead us to a proposal that catatonia in certain instances may be culture-bound, which, considering the organic presentation of the disorder and its historical relation to schizophrenia, is highly controversial. Nevertheless, the current conception of catatonia as a neuropsychiatric syndrome associated with systemic illness (Fink et al., 2015) implies the possibility of a heterogeneous etiology.

Relatedly, an analysis of catatonia and Parkinson's disease—conceived as movement disorders—at the level of the brain, has been suggested should invoke a "principle of double way", asserting that "function of the same anatomical apparatus may be disturbed by both organic lesions and psychological alterations". Hypothetically, the same motor loop may be abnormally affected either by psychological (cortical) top-down regulation, or, by aberrant (subcortical) bottom-up regulation illustrated by akinetic catatonia and Parkinson's disease functionally affecting the same "motor loop", however, by different mechanisms originating in the orbitofrontal cortex (OFC) and the substantia nigra respectively (Northoff, 2002). Even though this proposal is not set in a predictive coding framework, it may be reinterpreted in relation to motor predictions and proprioceptive input generating error signals eliciting top-down directed (absence of) movement or bottom-up adjustments of predictions, both converging on intermediate levels of the hierarchy and eliciting motor symptoms in accordance with a recent proposal by Edwards et al. (2012).

Catatonia has further been conceived of as a disorder resulting from abnormal emotional processing. Catatonic patients ($n = 10$) exhibited altered activity in mOFC and mPFC as well as abnormal orbitofrontal and premotor/motor cortical functional connectivity on exposure to negative emotional images and compared to psychiatric and healthy controls. Also, catatonic behavioral and affective symptoms correlated with deactivation in OFC whereas motor symptoms correlated with mPFC activation (Northoff et al., 2004). It was suggested that abnormal emotional processing and deactivation of OFC—through connections to the basal nucleus of amygdala implicated in affective inhibition by cognitive control—result in subsequent altered activity in medial prefrontal and premotor/motor function generating affective, behavioral and motor symptoms of catatonia. Response to anxiolytic drugs and self-report of overwhelming uncontrollable emotions—both notably reported also in RS (Bodegård, 2005b; Engström, 2013)—is taken to support the hypothesis (Northoff et al., 2004). Supplying an adequate fit with the data, this hypothesis nevertheless lacks in sufficient precision to allow anything but a very general reconceptualization within a predictive coding framework amounting to an analysis involving inadequate priors generating prediction errors the system adapts to by actions on intermediate levels involving lower as well as higher processing nevertheless below the conscious level.

An alternate exploration of catatonia recognizes connexion with anxiety or fear states on the basis of immediate treatment response to anxiolytics drugs, taken to support a limbic system pathophysiology (Daniels, 2009). Deficits in akinetic catatonia, such as stupor, mutism and negativism, are however consistent also with an underlying motivational deficit suggesting that suppression of incentive salience ("wanting"; Berridge and Robinson, 2003), mediated in dopaminergic mesolimbic structures projecting into prefrontal areas could account for core symptoms. Dopamine, of importance in placebo (Scott et al., 2008) and delusions (Adams et al., 2013) may interplay in shifting the balance between prior and observation also generating catatonic symptoms in relation to predictions.

Other than reconceptualizations of previous findings complying with a Bayesian analysis, there are clinical evidence of a multifactorial genesis involving also psychogenic generation of catatonia. Case-reports attributing catatonia to conversion (Jensen, 1984; Shah et al., 2012) and catatonia ($n = 10$) as well as conversion ($n = 5$) successfully confirmed through a common method of Amytal interviewing (Iserson, 1980) are found in support. Moreover, catatonic presentation varying throughout history (Shorter, 2006, 2012) attributes to it a characteristic generally considered a hallmark of conversion disorder and Shorter (2012) asserts "It is important to understand that cultural suggestion can cause patients to present catatonic symptoms in some epochs, but not in others, whereas changes in diagnostic fashion determine whether physicians make the diagnosis or not". Thus, it does not seem unlikely that the brain, influenced by "cultural suggestion", could generate catatonic symptoms and the model here proposed supply a mechanistic account of how this could be instantiated.

Pertaining to RS, there are, as we have here demonstrated, indications that mandate the assertion equating RS with catatonia. Apart from clinical characteristics, in particular reports of normalization in response to midazolam, implies this hypothesis should be evaluated and we have suggested means thereto. As for the regional distribution, considered as a hypothesis, it is difficult to test. In different parts of science, however, different truth-criteria are manifest and from the general point of view, broader involvement in this issue, and in particular an epidemiological effort, is much needed.

Other than treatment already routinely offered in catatonia—which is reported safe and efficient, also in children adolescents—our model predicts no magic bullet. On the contrary, if fixed predictions—laid down by previous experience projecting into the present, in order to tell the future—generate in prediction error denial, with subsequent drive in homeostatic and higher level systems, towards the perpetuation of those malicious predictions, by arranging the inner and outer world so as to accord therewith, the situation indeed seems desperate.

Nevertheless, on the hypothesis that the behavior characterizing RS is a social extension of interoceptive predictions, which serves to either sound the alarm or perpetuate inappropriate priors, the behavioral pattern represents on some level a strategy selected in a social context. (Which is not to say it is in any way voluntary). If this line of reasoning is correct, which indeed is implied by the phenomenon respecting barriers pertaining to language, culture, ethnicity and national borders, measures aimed at pre-empting the unfortunate strategy should be enforced. Certainly, a deepened understanding of the history, culture and situation of risk groups individuals would be necessary in order to reach out to these individuals.

The appeal to culture-bound psychopathology raises an ethical dilemma. The argument we have presented, according to which cultural sanctioning contributes to the generation of specific kinds of behavioral patterns, implies that by offering treatment, to which there is no alternative, we are also, on another level, causing new cases.

CONCLUSION

The regional distribution and the prevalence of RS are challenging to explain. Firstly, we have tried to establish that RS represents a disorder previously described. Historical accounts demonstrate that so is the case. We find no reason to ascribe to this phenomenon a novel diagnostic entity.

Secondly, bearing this in mind, the diagnostic fit to known disorders and hypotheses previously put forward have been evaluated. We have argued catatonia to supply the best fit and suggested means of examining this hypothesis in accordance with clinical practise and by neuroimaging. Catatonia, recently reconceptualized, amounts to a phenomenological description of a clinical entity for which there presumably can be different causes.

Thirdly, the regional distribution, we have argued, is best explained by perceiving RS as culture-bound. Importantly, this does not preclude other factors to interplay in pathogenesis. On the contrary, individual predisposition, traumatization, contextual factors as well as culturally sanctioned beliefs and expectations, may all be involved.

Lastly, we have provided a predictive coding model of RS. On the basis of extreme priors, fixed by previous experiences, the percept of the inner and outer world is stable and skewed. Consequently, error signal minimization is directed towards effecting the inner and outer worlds to accord with the predictions which unharnesses homeostatic and behavioral responses with that objective. This includes, on a social extension, the projection of a culturally sanctioned idiom of distress also interpretable in a predictive coding framework. Accommodating an extensive multilevel involvement of homeostatic, cognitive and emotional systems with deep impact on behavior influenced by cultural expectations, this analysis is compatible with RS being catatonia, culture-bound.

AUTHOR CONTRIBUTIONS

KS: wrote manuscript, responsible of general ideas. PP: contributed in revising. PP and other authors: commented on previous versions of manuscript, helped developing lines of argument.

REFERENCES

Adams, R. A., Stephan, K. E., Brown, H. R., Frith, C. D., and Friston, K. J. (2013). The computational anatomy of psychosis. *Front. Psychiatry* 4:47. doi: 10.3389/fpsyt.2013.00047

Adler, S. R. (1994). Ethnomedical pathogenesis and Hmong immigrants' sudden nocturnal deaths. *Cult. Med. Psychiatry* 18, 23–59. doi: 10.1007/bf01384876

Ahmad, A. (2008). Posttraumatic stress among children in Kurdistan. *Acta Paediatr.* 97, 884–888. doi: 10.1111/j.1651-2227.2008.00873.x

Ahmad, A., von Knorring, A. L., and Sundelin-Wahlsten, V. (2008). Traumatic experiences and post-traumatic stress symptoms in Kurdish children in their native country and in Exile. *Child Adolesc. Ment. Health* 13, 193–197. doi: 10.1111/j.1475-3588.2008.00501.x

Amanzio, M., and Benedetti, F. (1999). Neuropharmacological dissection of placebo analgesia: expectation-activated opioid systems versus conditioning-activated specific subsystems. *J. Neurosci.* 19, 484–494.

American Psychiatric Association. (2013). *Diagnostic and Statistical Manual of Mental Disorders: DSM-5.* Arlington, VA: American Psychiatric Association.

Annell, A.-L. (1958). *Elementär barnpsykiatri.* Stockholm: Sv. bokförl. (Norstedt).

Aronsson, B., Wiberg, C., Sandstedt, P., and Hjern, A. (2009). Asylum-seeking children with severe loss of activities of daily living: clinical signs and course during rehabilitation. *Acta Paediatr.* 98, 1977–1981. doi: 10.1111/j.1651-2227.2009.01499.x

Ascher, H., and Gustavsson, T. (2008). Klargorande konferens om barn med uppgivenhetssymtom. *Läkartidningen* 105, 31–33.

Ascher, H., and Hjern, A. (2013). *Från apati till aktivitet: teori och behandling av flyktingbarn med svår psykisk ohälsa.* Lund: Studentlitteratur.

Ballmaier, M., and Schmidt, R. (2005). Conversion disorder revisited. *Funct. Neurol.* 20, 105–113.

Barrett, L. F., and Simmons, W. K. (2015). Interoceptive predictions in the brain. *Nat. Rev. Neurosci.* 16, 419–429. doi: 10.1038/nrn3950

Bartholomew, R. E., and Wessley, S. (2002). Protean nature of mass sociogenic illness: from possessed nuns to chemical and biological terrorism fears. *Br. J. Psychiatry* 180, 300–306. doi: 10.1192/bjp.180.4.300

Berridge, K. C., and Robinson, T. E. (2003). Parsing reward. *Trends Neurosci.* 26, 507–513. doi: 10.1016/s0166-2236(03)00233-9

Bodegård, G. (2004). [Case reports of devitalization because of depression. Refugee children seeking asylum develop life-threatening losses of function]. *Lakartidningen* 101, 1696–1699.

Bodegård, G. (2005a). Life-threatening loss of function in refugee children: another expression of pervasive refusal syndrome? *Clin. Child Psychol. Psychiatry* 10, 337–350. doi: 10.1177/1359104505053753

Bodegård, G. (2005b). Pervasive loss of function in asylum-seeking children in Sweden. *Acta Paediatr.* 94, 1706–1707. doi: 10.1111/j.1651-2227.2005.tb01841.x

Bodegård, G. (2006). *Vård av Barn med Uppgivenhetssymtom. En Belysning av Behandlingens Utformning Utifrån Erfarenheten av Vården av 25 Asylsökande Barn vid Barnavdelningen Eugenia.* Research Report, No. 23 ISSN 1403-607X. Stockholm, Karolinska Institutet.

Bodegård, G. (2014). Comment on the paper "Pervasive Refusal Syndrome (PRS) 21 years on-a reconceptualization and renaming" by Ken Nunn, Bryan Lask and Isabel Owen. *Eur. Child Adolesc. Psychiatry* 23, 179–181. doi: 10.1007/s00787-013-0435-5

Boss, L. P. (1997). Epidemic hysteria: a review of the published literature. *Epidemiol. Rev.* 19, 233–243. doi: 10.1093/oxfordjournals.epirev.a017955

Breuer, J., and Freud, S. (1956/1893). On the psychical mechanism of hysterical phenomena. *Int. J. Psychoanal.* 37, 8–14.

Brown, R. J., and Lewis-Fernández, R. (2011). Culture and conversion disorder: implications for DSM-5. *Psychiatry* 74, 187–206. doi: 10.1521/psyc.2011.74.3.187

Brown, R. J., Cardeña, E., Nijenhuis, E., Sar, V., and van der Hart, O. (2007). Should conversion disorder be reclassified as a dissociative disorder in DSM V? *Psychosomatics* 48, 369–378. doi: 10.1176/appi.psy.48.5.369

Büchel, C., Geuter, S., Sprenger, C., and Eippert, F. (2014). Placebo analgesia: a predictive coding perspective. *Neuron* 81, 1223–1239. doi: 10.1016/j.neuron.2014.02.042

Carota, A., and Calabrese, P. (2014). Hysteria around the World. *Front. Neurol. Neurosci.* 169–180. doi: 10.1159/000360062

Cassady, J. D., Kirschke, D. L., Jones, T. F., Craig, A. S., Bermudez, O. B., and Schaffner, W. (2005). Case series: outbreak of conversion disorder among amish adolescent girls. *J. Am. Acad. Child Adolesc. Psychiatry* 44, 291–297. doi: 10.1097/00004583-200503000-00014

Cohen, D., Flament, M., Dubos, P. F., and Basquin, M. (1999). Case series: catatonic syndrome in young people. *J. Am. Acad. Child Adolesc. Psychiatry* 38, 1040–1046. doi: 10.1097/00004583-199908000-00021

Daniels, J. (2009). Catatonia: clinical aspects and neurobiological correlates. *J. Neuropsychiatry Clin. Neurosci.* 21, 371–380. doi: 10.1176/appi.neuropsych.21.4.371

de la Fuente-Fernández, R., Ruth, T. J., Sossi, V., Schulzer, M., Calne, D. B., and Stoessl, A. J. (2001). Expectation and dopamine release: mechanism of the placebo effect in Parkinson's disease. *Science* 293, 1164–1166. doi: 10.1126/science.1060937

De Tiége, X., Bier, J. C., Massat, I., Laureys, S., Lotstra, F., Berré, J., et al. (2003). Regional cerebral glucose metabolism in akinetic catatonia and after remission. *J. Neurol. Neurosurg. Psychiatry* 74, 1003–1004. doi: 10.1136/jnnp.74.7.1003

Devinsky, O., Gazzola, D., and LaFrance, W. C., Jr. (2011). Differentiating between nonepileptic and epileptic seizures. *Nat. Rev. Neurol.* 7, 210–220. doi: 10.1038/nrneurol.2011.24

Devinsky, O., Morrell, M. J., and Vogt, B. A. (1995). Contributions of anterior cingulate cortex to behaviour. *Brain* 118, 279–306. doi: 10.1093/brain/118.1.279

Dhossche, D. M., Ross, C. A., and Stoppelbein, L. (2012). The role of deprivation, abuse and trauma in pediatric catatonia without a clear medical cause. *Acta Psychiatr. Scand.* 125, 25–32. doi: 10.1111/j.1600-0447.2011.01779.x

Dhossche, D. M., Shettar, S. M., Kumar, T., and Burt, L. (2009). Electroconvulsive therapy for malignant catatonia in adolescence. *South. Med. J.* 102, 1170–1172. doi: 10.1097/SMJ.0b013e3181b9e39c

Eames, P. (1992). Hysteria following brain injury. *J. Neurol. Neurosurg. Psychiatry* 55, 1046–1053. doi: 10.1136/jnnp.55.11.1046

Edwards, M. J., Adams, R. A., Brown, H., Pareés, I., and Friston, K. J. (2012). A Bayesian account of "hysteria". *Brain* 135, 3495–3512. doi: 10.1093/brain/aws129

Edwards, M. J., and Bhatia, K. P. (2012). Functional (psychogenic) movement disorders: merging mind and brain. *Lancet Neurol.* 11, 250–260. doi: 10.1016/S1474-4422(11)70310-6

Engström, I. (2013). "Diagnostik och differentialdiagnostik," in *Från apati till aktivitet: teori och behandling av flyktingbarn med svår psykisk ohälsa*, eds H. Ascher and A. Hjern (Lund: Studentlitteratur), 117–135.

Evers, K., and Sigman, M. (2013). Possibilities and limits of mind-reading: a neurophilosophical perspective. *Conscious. Cogn.* 22, 887–897. doi: 10.1016/j.concog.2013.05.011

Fallik, A., and Sigal, M. (1971). Hysteria - the choice of symptom site. *Psychother. Psychosom.* 19, 310–318. doi: 10.1159/000286328

Fernández-Espejo, D., Soddu, A., Cruse, D., Palacios, E. M., Junque, C., Vanhaudenhuyse, A., et al. (2012). A role for the default mode network in the bases of disorders of consciousness. *Ann. Neurol.* 72, 335–343. doi: 10.1002/ana.23635

Fink, M. (2013). Rediscovering catatonia: the biography of a treatable syndrome. *Acta Psychiatr. Scand.* 127, 1–47. doi: 10.1111/acps.12038

Fink, M., Fricchione, G., Rummans, T., and Shorter, E. (2015). Catatonia is a systemic medical syndrome. *Acta Psychiatr. Scand.* doi: 10.1111/acps.12510 [Epub ahead of print].

Fink, M., and Taylor, M. A. (2003). *Catatonia A Clinician's Guide to Diagnosis and Treatment.* Cambridge: Cambridge University Press.

Fletcher, P. C., and Frith, C. D. (2009). Perceiving is believing: a Bayesian approach to explaining the positive symptoms of schizophrenia. *Nat. Rev. Neurosci.* 10, 48–58. doi: 10.1038/nrn2536

Forslund, C. M., and Johansson, B. A. (2013). Pervasive refusal syndrome among inpatient asylum-seeking children and adolescents: a follow-up study. *Eur. Child Adolesc. Psychiatry* 22, 251–258. doi: 10.1007/s00787-012-0341-2

Friston, K. (2005). A theory of cortical responses. *Philos. Trans. R Soc. Lond. B Biol. Sci.* 360, 815–836. doi: 10.1098/rstb.2005.1622

Frith, C. (2007). *Making Up the Mind: How the Brain Creates Our Mental World.* Oxford: Blackwell.

García-Campayo, J., Fayed, N., Serrano-Blanco, A., and Roca, M. (2009). Brain dysfunction behind functional symptoms: neuroimaging and somatoform, conversive and dissociative disorders. *Curr. Opin. Psychiatry* 22, 224–231. doi: 10.1097/YCO.0b013e3283252d43

Gelder, M. G. (2001). *Shorter Oxford Textbook of Psychiatry.* Oxford: Oxford University Press.

Giacino, J. T., Schnakers, C., Rodriguez-Moreno, D., Kalmar, K., Schiff, N., and Hirsch, J. (2009). Behavioral assessment in patients with disorders of consciousness: gold standard or fool's gold? *Prog. Brain Res.* 177, 33–48. doi: 10.1016/s0079-6123(09)17704-X

Godani, G., Bodegård, G., and Rydelius, P.-A. (2008). *Bördan de Kom med.* Rapport från forskningsprojektet: Barn i asylprocessen som utvecklade uppgivenhetssymtom i Sverige. Stockholm, Save the Children Sweden. ISBN 978-91-7321-309-7.

Goldstein, M., Madden, S., and Peters, L. (2013). The use of effective treatments: the case of an adolescent girl with anorexia nervosa in the context of a conversion disorder. *Clin. Child Psychol. Psychiatry* 18, 214–223. doi: 10.1177/1359104512447313

Hacking, I. (2010). Pathological withdrawl of refugee children seeking asylum in Sweden. *Stud. Hist. Philos. Biol. Biomed. Sci.* 41, 309–317. doi: 10.1016/j.shpsc.2010.10.001

Halligan, P. W., Athwal, B. S., Oakley, D. A., and Frackowiak, R. S. (2000). Imaging hypnotic paralysis: implications for conversion hysteria. *Lancet* 355, 986–987. doi: 10.1016/s0140-6736(00)99019-6

Heine, L., Soddu, A., Gómez, F., Vanhaudenhuyse, A., Tshibanda, L., Thonnard, M., et al. (2012). Resting state networks and consciousness Alterations of multiple resting state network connectivity in physiological, pharmacological and pathological consciousness states. *Front. Psychology* 3:295. doi: 10.3389/fpsyg.2012.00295

Helmholtz, H. V. (1866). *Handbuch der Physiologischen Optik.* Leipzig: Leopold Voss.

Hessle, M., and Ahmadi, N. (2006). *Asylsökande Barn med Uppgivenhetssymtom – Trauma, Kultur, Asylprocess.* SOU 2006:49. (Statens Offentliga Utredningar).

Hinton, D. E., and Lewis-Fernández, R. (2010). Idioms of distress among trauma survivors: subtypes and clinical utility. *Cult. Med. Psychiatry* 34, 209–218. doi: 10.1007/s11013-010-9175-x

Horovitz, S. G., Braun, A. R., Carr, W. S., Picchioni, D., Balkin, T. J., Fukunaga, M., et al. (2009). Decoupling of the brain's default mode network during deep sleep. *Proc. Natl. Acad. Sci. U S A* 106, 11376–11381. doi: 10.1073/pnas.0901435106

Iserson, K. V. (1980). The emergency amobarbital interview. *Ann. Emerg. Med.* 9, 513–517. doi: 10.1016/s0196-0644(80)80189-2

Jaspers, K. (1913/1993). *General Psychopathology.* Baltimore and London: The Johns Hopkins University Press.

Jensen, P. S. (1984). Case report of conversion catatonia: indication for hypnosis. *Am. J. Psychother.* 38, 566–570.

Jensen, K. B., Kaptchuk, T. J., Kirsch, I., Raicek, J., Lindstrom, K. M., Berna, C., et al. (2012). Nonconscious activation of placebo and nocebo pain responses. *Proc. Natl. Acad. Sci. U S A* 109, 15959–15964. doi: 10.1073/pnas.1202056109

Jensen, K., Kirsch, I., Odmalm, S., Kaptchuk, T. J., and Ingvar, M. (2015). Classical conditioning of analgesic and hyperalgesic pain responses without conscious awareness. *Proc. Natl. Acad. Sci. U S A* 112, 7863–7867. doi: 10.1073/pnas.1504567112

Jeppsson, O. (2013). "Nutritionsbehandling av barn med uppgivenhetssyndrom," in *Från apati till aktivitet: teori och behandling av flyktingbarn med svår psykisk ohälsa*, eds H. Ascher and A. Hjern (Lund: Studentlitteratur), 169–176.

Jiménez Gómez, B., and Quintero, J. (2012). Ganser syndrome: review and case report. *Actas Esp. Psiquiatr.* 40, 161–164.

Johannisson, K. (2001). *Nostalgia: en känslas historia.* Stockholm: Bonnier.

Jones, T. F., Craig, A. S., Hoy, D., Gunter, E. W., Ashley, D. L., Barr, D. B., et al. (2000). Mass psychogenic illness attributed to toxic exposure at a high school. *N Engl. J. Med.* 342, 96–100. doi: 10.1056/nejm200001133420206

Kertész, I. (1998). *Mannen utan öde.* Stockholm: Norstedt.

Keshavan, M. S. (2014). Culture bound syndromes: disease entities or simply concepts of distress? *Asian J. Psychiatr.* 12, 1–2. doi: 10.1016/j.ajp.2014.11.003

Kihlbom, M. (2013). "Apati och uppgivenhetssyndrom är inget nytt fenomen," in *Från apati till aktivitet: teori och behandling av flyktingbarn med svår psykisk ohälsa*, eds H. Ascher and A. Hjern (Lund: Studentlitteratur), 31–43.

Kirmayer, L. J. (2001). Cultural variations in the clinical presentation of depression and anxiety: implications for diagnosis and treatment. *J. Clin. Psychiatry* 62, 22–28.

Kleinman, A. (1987). Anthropology and psychiatry. The role of culture in cross-cultural research on illness. *Br. J. Psychiatry* 151, 447–454. doi: 10.1192/bjp.151.4.447

Lask, B., Britten, C., Kroll, L., Magagna, J., and Tranter, M. (1991). Children with pervasive refusal. *Arch. Dis. Child.* 66, 866–869. doi: 10.1136/adc.66.7.866

Lester, D. (2009). Voodoo death. *Omega (Westport)* 59, 1–18. doi: 10.2190/OM.59.1.a

Levy, D. A., and Nail, P. R. (1993). Contagion: a theoretical and empirical review and reconceptualization. *Genet. Soc. Gen. Psychol. Monogr.* 119, 233–284.

Lindberg, T., and Sundelin, C. (2005). Apatiska barn–var står vetenskapen idag? *Läkartidningen* 102, 1338–1345.

Luchini, F., Medda, P., Mariani, M. G., Mauri, M., Toni, C., and Perugi, G. (2015). Electroconvulsive therapy in catatonic patients: efficacy and predictors of response. *World J. Psychiatry* 5, 182–192. doi: 10.5498/wjp.v5.i2.182

Lyman, D. (2004). Pseudolabor: a new conversion disorder subtype? A case presentation and literature review. *Prim. Care Companion J. Clin. Psychiatry* 6, 61–64. doi: 10.4088/pcc.v06n0203

Mayberg, H. S., Silva, J. A., Brannan, S. K., Tekell, J. L., Mahurin, R. K., McGinnis, S., et al. (2002). The functional neuroanatomy of the placebo effect. *Am. J. Psychiatry* 159, 728–737. doi: 10.1176/appi.ajp.159.5.728

Medeiros De Bustos, E., Galli, S., Haffen, E., and Moulin, T. (2014). Clinical manifestations of hysteria: an epistemological perspective or how historical dynamics illuminate current practice. *Front. Neurol. Neurosci.* 35, 28–43. doi: 10.1159/000360436

Miller, K. E., Omidian, P., Kulkarni, M., Yaqubi, A., Daudzai, H., and Rasmussen, A. (2009). The validity and clinical utility of post-traumatic stress disorder in Afghanistan. *Transcult. Psychiatry* 46, 219–237. doi: 10.1177/1363461509105813

Milton, G. W. (1973). Self-willed death or the bone-pointing syndrome. *Lancet* 1, 1435–1436. doi: 10.1016/s0140-6736(73)91754-6

Myers, N. L. (2011). Update: schizophrenia across cultures. *Curr. Psychiatry Rep.* 13, 305–311. doi: 10.1007/s11920-011-0208-0

North, C. S. (2015). The classification of hysteria and related disorders: historical and phenomenological considerations. *Behav. Sci. (Basel)* 5, 496–517. doi: 10.3390/bs5040496

Northoff, G. (2002). What catatonia can tell us about "top-down modulation": a neuropsychiatric hypothesis. *Behav. Brain Sci.* 25, 555–577; discussion 578–604. doi: 10.1017/s0140525x02000109

Northoff, G., Kötter, R., Baumgart, F., Danos, P., Boeker, H., Kaulisch, T., et al. (2004). Orbitofrontal cortical dysfunction in akinetic catatonia: a functional magnetic resonance imaging study during negative emotional stimulation. *Schizophr. Bull.* 30, 405–427. doi: 10.1093/oxfordjournals.schbul.a007088

Nunn, K. P., Lask, B., and Owen, I. (2014). Pervasive refusal syndrome (PRS) 21 years on: a re-conceptualisation and a renaming. *Eur. Child Adolesc. Psychiatry* 23, 163–172. doi: 10.1007/s00787-013-0433-7

Nunn, K. P., and Thompson, S. L. (1996). The pervasive refusal syndrome: learned helplessness and hopelessness. *Clin. Child Psychol. Psychiatry* 1, 121–132. doi: 10.1177/1359104596011011

Otto, U. (1982). *Katastrof- och Försvarspsykiatri.* Lund: Studentlitteratur.

Owen, A. M., Coleman, M. R., Boly, M., Davis, M. H., Laureys, S., and Pickard, J. D. (2006). Detecting awareness in the vegetative state. *Science* 313:1402. doi: 10.1126/science.1130197

Petrovic, P., Dietrich, T., Fransson, P., Andersson, J., Carlsson, K., and Ingvar, M. (2005). Placebo in emotional processing–induced expectations of anxiety relief activate a generalized modulatory network. *Neuron* 46, 957–969. doi: 10.1016/j.neuron.2005.05.023

Petrovic, P., Kalso, E., Petersson, K. M., Andersson, J., Fransson, P., and Ingvar, M. (2010). A prefrontal non-opioid mechanism in placebo analgesia. *Pain* 150, 59–65. doi: 10.1016/j.pain.2010.03.011

Petrovic, P., Kalso, E., Petersson, K. M., and Ingvar, M. (2002). Placebo and opioid analgesia–imaging a shared neuronal network. *Science* 295, 1737–1740. doi: 10.1126/science.1067176

Posner, J. B., Saper, C. B., and Schiff, N. (2007). *Plum and Posner's Diagnosis of Stupor and Coma.* 4th Edn. New York: Oxford University Press.

Powell, S. A., Nguyen, C. T., Gaziano, J., Lewis, V., Lockey, R. F., and Padhya, T. A. (2007). Mass psychogenic illness presenting as acute stridor in an adolescent female cohort. *Ann. Otol. Rhinol. Laryngol.* 116, 525–531. doi: 10.1177/000348940711600708

Prince, R., and Tcheng-Laroche, F. (1987). Culture-bound syndromes and international disease classifications. *Cult. Med. Psychiatry* 11, 3–19. doi: 10.1007/bf00055003

Ramani, R. (2015). Connectivity. *Curr. Opin. Anaesthesiol.* 28, 498–504. doi: 10.1097/ACO.0000000000000237

Reynolds, J. R. (1869). Remarks on paralysis and other disorders of motion and sensation, dependent on idea. *Br. Med. J.* 2, 483–485. doi: 10.1136/bmj.2.462.483

Roelofs, K., and Spinhoven, P. (2007). Trauma and medically unexplained symptoms towards an integration of cognitive and neuro-biological accounts. *Clin. Psychol. Rev.* 27, 798–820. doi: 10.1016/j.cpr.2007.07.004

Rydelius, P.-A. (2006). *Rapport om de s.k. Apatiska Barnen.* Research Report, No. 25. ISSN 1403-607X. Stockholm, Karolinska Institutet.

Schmack, K., Gòmez-Carrillo de Castro, A., Rothkirch, M., Sekutowicz, M., Rössler, H., and Haynes, J. D. (2013). Delusions and the role of beliefs in perceptual inference. *J. Neurosci.* 33, 13701–13712. doi: 10.1523/JNEUROSCI.1778-13.2013

Scott, D. J., Stohler, C. S., Egnatuk, C. M., Wang, H., Koeppe, R. A., and Zubieta, J. K. (2008). Placebo and nocebo effects are defined by opposite opioid and dopaminergic responses. *Arch. Gen. Psychiatry* 65, 220–231. doi: 10.1001/archgenpsychiatry.2007.34

Seth, A. K. (2013). Interoceptive inference, emotion and the embodied self. *Trends Cogn. Sci.* 17, 565–573. doi: 10.1016/j.tics.2013.09.007

Shah, J. L., Meyer, F. L., Mufson, M. J., Escobar, J. I., and Goisman, R. M. (2012). Catatonia, conversion, culture: an acute presentation. *Harv. Rev. Psychiatry* 20, 160–169. doi: 10.3109/10673229.2012.694325

Shannon, P. J., Wieling, E., McCleary, J. S., and Becher, E. (2015). Exploring the mental health effects of political trauma with newly arrived refugees. *Qual. Health Res.* 25, 443–457. doi: 10.1177/1049732314549475

Shorter, E. (1992). *From Paralysis to Fatigue: A History of Psychosomatic Illness in the Modern Era.* New York: Free Press.

Shorter, E. (2006). Hysteria and catatonia as motor disorders in historical context. *Hist. Psychiatry* 17, 461–468. doi: 10.1177/0957154x06073012

Shorter, E. (2012). Making childhood catatonia visible, separate from competing diagnoses. *Acta Psychiatr. Scand.* 125, 3–10. döi: 10.1111/j.1600-0447.2011.01788.x

Slater, E. (1965). Diagnosis of "Hysteria". *Br. Med. J.* 1, 1395–1399. doi: 10.1136/bmj.1.5447.1395

Socialstyrelsen, B. (2013). *Barn Med Uppgivenhetssyndrom. En vägledning för Personal inom Socialtjänst och Hälso- och Sjukvård.* Stockholm: Socialstyrelsen.

Söndergaard, H. P., Kushnir, M. M., Aronsson, B., Sandstedt, P., and Bergquist, J. (2012). Patterns of endogenous steroids in apathetic refugee children are compatible with long-term stress. *BMC Res. Notes* 5:186. doi: 10.1186/1756-0500-5-186

Sterzer, P., Frith, C., and Petrovic, P. (2008). Believing is seeing: expectations alter visual awareness. *Curr. Biol.* 18, R697–R698. doi: 10.1016/j.cub.2008.06.021

Stewart, D. E. (1990). The changing faces of somatization. *Psychosomatics* 31, 153–158. doi: 10.1016/s0033-3182(90)72188-3

Stone, J., Carson, A., Duncan, R., Roberts, R., Warlow, C., Hibberd, C., et al. (2010). Who is referred to neurology clinics?–the diagnoses made in 3781 new patients. *Clin. Neurol. Neurosurg.* 112, 747–751. doi: 10.1016/j.clineuro.2010.05.011

Takaoka, K., and Takata, T. (2003). Catatonia in childhood and adolescence. *Psychiatry Clin. Neurosci.* 57, 129–137. doi: 10.1046/j.1440-1819.2003.01092.x

Tandon, R., Heckers, S., Bustillo, J., Barch, D. M., Gaebel, W., Gur, R. E., et al. (2013). Catatonia in DSM-5. *Schizophr. Res.* 150, 26–30. doi: 10.1016/j.schres.2013.04.034

Teufel, C., Subramaniam, N., Dobler, V., Perez, J., Finnemann, J., Mehta, P. R., et al. (2015). Shift toward prior knowledge confers a perceptual advantage in early psychosis and psychosis-prone healthy individuals. *Proc. Natl. Acad. Sci. U S A* 112, 13401–13406. doi: 10.1073/pnas.1503916112

Thakur, A., Jagadheesan, K., Dutta, S., and Sinha, V. K. (2003). Incidence of catatonia in children and adolescents in a paediatric psychiatric clinic. *Aust. N. Z. J. Psychiatry* 37, 200–203. doi: 10.1046/j.1440-1614.2003.01125.x

Ursin, H., and Eriksen, H. R. (2010). Cognitive activation theory of stress (CATS). *Neurosci. Biobehav. Rev.* 34, 877–881. doi: 10.1016/j.neubiorev.2009.03.001

Vanhaudenhuyse, A., Laureys, S., and Faymonville, M.-E. (2014). Neurophysiology of hypnosis. *Neurophysiol. Clin.* 44, 343–353. doi: 10.1016/j.neucli.2013.09.006

Vanhaudenhuyse, A., Noirhomme, Q., Tshibanda, L. J., Bruno, M. A., Boveroux, P., Schnakers, C., et al. (2010). Default network connectivity reflects the level of consciousness in non-communicative brain-damaged patients. *Brain* 133, 161–171. doi: 10.1093/brain/awp313

Ventriglio, A., Ayonrinde, O., and Bhugra, D. (2015). Relevance of culture-bound syndromes in the 21st century. *Psychiatry Clin. Neurosci.* doi: 10.1111/pcn.12359 [Epub ahead of print].

Von Folsach, L. L., and Montgomery, E. (2006). Pervasive refusal syndrome among asylum-seeking children. *Clin. Child Psychol. Psychiatry* 11, 457–473. doi: 10.1177/1359104506064988

Vuilleumier, P. (2005). Hysterical conversion and brain function. *Prog. Brain Res.* 150, 309–329. doi: 10.1016/s0079-6123(05)50023-2

Vuilleumier, P. (2014). Brain circuits implicated in psychogenic paralysis in conversion disorders and hypnosis. *Neurophysiol. Clin.* 44, 323–337. doi: 10.1016/j.neucli.2014.01.003

Wachtel, L. E., Dhossche, D. M., and Kellner, C. H. (2011). When is electroconvulsive therapy appropriate for children and adolescents? *Med. Hypotheses* 76, 395–399. doi: 10.1016/j.mehy.2010.11.001

Wachtel, L. E., Schuldt, S., Ghaziuddin, N., and Shorter, E. (2013). The potential role of electroconvulsive therapy in the "Iron Triangle" of pediatric catatonia, autism and psychosis. *Acta Psychiatr. Scand.* 128, 408–409. doi: 10.1111/acps.12158

Wager, T. D., Scott, D. J., and Zubieta, J.-K. (2007). Placebo effects on human mu-opioid activity during pain. *Proc. Natl. Acad. Sci. U S A* 104, 11056–11061. doi: 10.1073/pnas.0702413104

Weiss, M., Allan, B., and Greenaway, M. (2012). Treatment of catatonia with electroconvulsive therapy in adolescents. *J. Child Adolesc. Psychopharmacol.* 22, 96–100. doi: 10.1089/cap.2010.0052

Yap, P. M. (1962). Transcultural studies panel discussion at the third world congress of psychiatry June 10, 1961. *Acta Psychiatr. Scand.* 38, 157–169. doi: 10.1111/j.1600-0447.1962.tb01790.x

Yap, P. M. (1967). Classification of the culture-bound reactive syndromes. *Aust. N. Z. J. Psychiatry* 1, 172–179. doi: 10.3109/00048676709159191

Zhang, D., and Raichle, M. E. (2010). Disease and the brain's dark energy. *Nat. Rev. Neurol.* 6, 15–28. doi: 10.1038/nrneurol.2009.198

Zubieta, J.-K., Bueller, J. A., Jackson, L. R., Scott, D. J., Xu, Y., Koeppe, R. A., et al. (2005). Placebo effects mediated by endogenous opioid activity on mu-opioid receptors. *J. Neurosci.* 25, 7754–7762. doi: 10.1523/jneurosci.0439-05.2005

Conflict of Interest Statement: The authors declare that the research was conducted in the absence of any commercial or financial relationships that could be construed as a potential conflict of interest.

2

Top-Down Dysregulation: From ADHD to Emotional Instability

Edited by:
Raymond C. K. Chan,
Chinese Academy of Sciences, China

***Correspondence:**
Predrag Petrovic
predrag.petrovic@ki.se

Predrag Petrovic[1] and F. Xavier Castellanos[2,3]*

[1] Department of Clinical Neuroscience, Karolinska Institutet, Stockholm, Sweden , [2] Department of Child and Adolescent Psychiatry, The Child Study Center at NYU Langone Medical Center, New York, NY, USA, [3] Nathan Kline Institute for Psychiatric Research, Orangeburg, NY, USA

Deficient cognitive top-down executive control has long been hypothesized to underlie inattention and impulsivity in attention-deficit/hyperactivity disorder (ADHD). However, top-down cognitive dysfunction explains a modest proportion of the ADHD phenotype whereas the salience of emotional dysregulation is being noted increasingly. Together, these two types of dysfunction have the potential to account for more of the phenotypic variance in patients diagnosed with ADHD. We develop this idea and suggest that top-down dysregulation constitutes a gradient extending from mostly non-emotional top-down control processes (i.e., "cool" executive functions) to mainly emotional regulatory processes (including "hot" executive functions). While ADHD has been classically linked primarily to the former, conditions involving emotional instability such as borderline and antisocial personality disorder are closer to the other. In this model, emotional subtypes of ADHD are located at intermediate levels of this gradient. Neuroanatomically, gradations in "cool" processing appear to be related to prefrontal dysfunction involving dorsolateral prefrontal cortex (dlPFC) and caudal anterior cingulate cortex (cACC), while "hot" processing entails orbitofrontal cortex and rostral anterior cingulate cortex (rACC). A similar distinction between systems related to non-emotional and emotional processing appears to hold for the basal ganglia (BG) and the neuromodulatory effects of the dopamine system. Overall we suggest that these two systems could be divided according to whether they process non-emotional information related to the exteroceptive environment (associated with "cool" regulatory circuits) or emotional information related to the interoceptive environment (associated with "hot" regulatory circuits). We propose that this framework can integrate ADHD, emotional traits in ADHD, borderline and antisocial personality disorder into a related cluster of mental conditions.

Keywords: ADHD, emotional instability, top-down regulation, prefrontal, cingulate

INTRODUCTION

Arguably, altered regulation of information processing represents the core underlying mechanism for many psychiatric disorders. Such aberrations can affect multiple dimensions, including both non-emotional and emotional processes. Currently, some disorders are conceptualized as dysfunction of one or the other of these dimensions. For example, attention-deficit/hyperactivity disorder (ADHD) is defined on the basis of dysfunctional regulation of non-emotional information processing (including inattention, impulsivity and hyperactivity), whereas disorders such as borderline personality disorder (BPD), antisocial personality disorder (ASPD) and conduct disorder (CD) entail symptoms reflecting emotional instability associated with dysfunctional regulation of emotional processes. Other disorders involving emotional instability include intermittent explosive disorder and oppositional defiant disorder (ODD). Traditionally, these psychiatric disorders have been studied separately, reflecting their historical categorical divisions, and the tendency of investigators and disciplines to reify such distinctions. However, these historical distinctions are increasingly appreciated as having impeded understanding of specific disorders in relation to each other. In this Hypothesis and Theory article, we propose that dysregulation in these different dimensions can be incorporated into a unified model.

Although disorders that include persistent emotional dysregulation differ in many symptoms, recent neurocognitive research results suggests common features are involved in emotional dysfunction. These "emotional instability disorders" are characterized by emotional hyper-responsiveness in amygdala and insula, regions involved in shaping emotional responses and experience (Blair, 2010; Rubia, 2011; Blair et al., 2014; Glenn and Raine, 2014; Krause-Utz et al., 2014). Structurally, the gray matter volumes of amygdala and insula are often reduced in such disorders (Blair, 2010; Rubia, 2011; Blair et al., 2014; Glenn and Raine, 2014; Krause-Utz et al., 2014). These observations suggest that a more general approach to study emotional instability may reveal insights into common underlying mechanisms. In this article, we will illustrate our thesis by focusing on ADHD and BPD. Less emphasis will be placed on CD and ASPD since these disorders also include sub-populations with callous-unemotional traits that are associated with decreased behavioral and neural responding to emotional stimuli, potentially confounding the contribution from emotional instability traits (Blair, 2010, 2013; Rubia, 2011; Blair et al., 2014). We believe the literature on the neurobiology of ODD and intermittent explosive disorder is currently insufficient to warrant their inclusion in this illustrative essay, although the approaches we highlight should also be applicable in future studies.

Several reviews and theoretical articles have recently discussed how top-down regulation in ADHD differs in comparison to specific emotional instability disorders including BPD (Sebastian et al., 2014) and CD (Rubia, 2011; Blair et al., 2014). The difference between putative regulatory systems involved in classical ADHD and emotional variants of ADHD has also been noted (Castellanos et al., 2006). Here we focus on the relationship between ADHD and emotional instability disorders in general. Instead of emphasizing their many differences, we seek to place these disorders in a common theoretical framework.

In more detail, we will put forward a model in which ADHD and emotional instability disorders are mechanistically related. We will argue that the fundamental problem in both types of disorders is a similar dysfunctional top-down regulation of information processing, in which the difference between the two types of categorical disorders (ADHD vs. emotional instability disorders) is whether the dysfunctional top-down regulation is associated with emotional (and interoceptive) processing or non-emotional (and exteroceptive) processing (*Hypothesis 1*). Given that the disorders are mechanistically related we also hypothesize that the symptoms associated to one type of dysregulation will be overly represented in patients that have the disorder associated with the other type of dysregulation—even when there is no explicit comorbidity (*Hypothesis 2*). Thus, a dimensional approach would better describe the existing phenotypes than categorical distinctions. Finally, if the underlying mechanisms are similar, treatments proven to be efficacious for one category of disorders should also be efficacious for the other category of disorders (*Hypothesis 3*). This could open new important possibilities for treatment.

We first discuss a dimensional approach to psychiatric disorders, as this is central for understanding the relation between emotional and non-emotional dysregulation in clinical populations. We then take up the relation between non-emotional executive functions ("cool" executive functions) and ADHD. Given that executive functions are fundamentally associated with ADHD, we then review the underlying prefrontal networks in the brain mediating such top-down control and show that these systems are altered in ADHD. A similar review will be done for emotion associated ("hot") executive functions and emotional regulation, and their relation to emotional instability disorders as well as for "emotional" traits in ADHD. We then discuss how systems mediating emotional and non-emotional top-down regulation (and dysregulation) relate to each other in prefrontal, striatal and dopamine networks. We will also discuss how this stratification between emotional and non-emotional regulation could be discussed in terms of systems related to interoceptive and exteroceptive processing. Finally, we present a model that can incorporate both ADHD and emotional instability disorders based on the relationship between these top-down regulatory systems.

CATEGORICAL AND DIMENSIONAL APPROACHES TO PSYCHOPATHOLOGY

In psychiatry, the adoption of the third edition of the Diagnostic and statistical manual of mental disorders (DSM; American Psychiatric Association, 1980) initiated the practice of defining psychiatric disorders as present or absent depending on whether a minimum number of clinical criteria were satisfied. This categorical approach enhanced the reliability of psychiatric diagnoses, but it has not advanced our understanding of underlying mechanisms (Insel et al., 2010; Cuthbert and Insel, 2013). One problem is that many psychiatric symptoms are continuously distributed in the general population. Truncating the range of variation by applying arbitrary cut-points impedes an understanding of underlying mechanisms since it does not mirror the true relationship between symptom levels and neurocognitive levels. Moreover, only focusing on psychiatric disorders excludes data from healthy individuals that are not treated with medication nor show any comorbidities—factors that confound categorically based research. Another problem is that defining disorders categorically based on whether criteria cut-points are met increases heterogeneity. Two patients can differ on nearly every symptom and still receive the same diagnosis. Moreover, in existing categorical diagnostic systems such as the 5th edition of the DSM (DSM-5; American Psychiatric Association, 2013) or the 10th edition of the International classification of diseases (ICD-10; World Health Organization, 2011), a particular diagnosis can be partially defined by opposite symptoms. For example, patients with depression can sleep too much or too little, have increased or decreased appetite, or increased or decreased activity levels. Logically, different underlying mechanisms could mediate these behaviors—although an alternative hypothesis is that both extremes become more likely when a regulatory process is dysfunctional (Klein, 1999). Accordingly, investigators are being urged to focus on specific *fundamental behavioral components* that may be altered in multiple psychiatric disorders, such as attention or emotional regulation as a part of the Research Domain Criteria (RDoC) initiated by the USA National Institute of Mental Health (NIHM; Insel et al., 2010; Cuthbert and Insel, 2013). Variation of such functions in the general population has specifically been identified as a promising way to understand dysfunction in these systems.

By focusing on how information is processed on a systems level, cognitive neuroscience has been successful in describing mechanisms underlying normative human perception and behavior (Gazzaniga, 2014). A major challenge for cognitive neuroscience is to translate such basic knowledge of brain function to psychiatric disorders. From a cognitive neuroscience perspective, specific cognitive processes underlie particular behaviors—here we term those *cognitive core processes*. Building on previously given examples of fundamental behavioral components from the RDoC such as attention and emotional regulation, we define cognitive core processes as the underlying neuronal mechanisms, on a system level, needed to produce a given behavior. There are many different attentional and emotional regulation processes and each process may include multiple aspects. For example, ample data suggest that amygdala modulates visual processing of threat cues (Vuilleumier and Driver, 2007; Vuilleumier, 2015). The specific modulation of amygdala on information processing in visual cortex may then be defined as a cognitive core process. Dysfunctions in these processes underpin the fundamental behavioral components that are coupled to different psychiatric states (Insel et al., 2010; Cuthbert and Insel, 2013). Variability between individuals in different cognitive core processes may underlie behavioral differences among healthy individuals but also clinical symptoms beyond the normative range. As cognitive neuroscience often includes analyses of inter-subject variability in cognitive core processes (Bishop, 2009; Indovina et al., 2011), it is well suited to study variation in fundamental behavioral processes (Insel et al., 2010; Cuthbert and Insel, 2013) related to specific psychiatric symptoms.

Studies adopting a neurocognitive endophenotype approach have often compared patients and healthy next-of-a-kin in specific behaviors and underlying structure/processes that are more present in these groups than in controls (Ersche et al., 2010, 2012, 2013; Morein-Zamir et al., 2013). An alternative approach is to directly study variability in the general population. A fundamental question is then how variation in the capacity to process information relates to clinical symptoms. One hypothesis is that the capacity to carry out cognitive core processes is inversely and directly related to certain psychiatric symptoms. From an information-processing viewpoint, cognitive core process capacities vary in the population from extremely efficient to extremely inefficient, depending on underlying genetic composition, learning history and state variables. This variation is often normally distributed (**Figure 1A**), e.g., in executive functions (Zelazo et al., 2013). Since cognitive processes form and shape individual behaviors, suboptimal cognitive core capacity can translate into behavioral symptoms. The frequency and intensity of these symptoms will be continuously distributed in the general population—with most below the threshold for clinical significance (**Figure 1B**). However, increasingly severe symptoms impair functioning, making it difficult for the affected individual to uphold expected social relations, or be occupationally productive. Such loss of functioning is the *sine qua non* of psychiatric disorders. To the extent that psychiatric disorders constitute extremes in variation across the population caused by suboptimal cognitive core process function, dimensional approaches will be a better fit than categorical ones. This has been suggested for several disorders such as ADHD (**Figure 1C**; Das et al., 2012).

"COOL" EXECUTIVE FUNCTIONS AND ADHD

Applying the model described above on dimensional approaches of psychopathology suggests that the worse cognitive capacity an individual possesses, the more symptoms he or she should manifest. Empirically, the general dimensional model seems to hold particularly well for ADHD. For example, in a non-clinical sample of more than 2000 adults, ADHD symptoms were normally distributed (Das et al., 2012). The dimensionality of ADHD symptoms has also been repeatedly observed in patient samples (Levy et al., 1997; Salum et al., 2014). Early models of ADHD posited that ADHD is a disorder of dysfunctional executive functions (e.g., Barkley, 1997). In line with these ideas, ADHD patients as a group tend to perform below average in laboratory tests of executive function capacity (Willcutt et al., 2005). While there is evidence suggesting a dimensionality for both ADHD symptoms and executive function capacity, associating trait-like capacities for executive functions to ADHD symptoms in the general population is not trivial. Namely, test performance can vary across and within individuals as a function of numerous factors including alertness/arousal, motivation, and past experience/exposure. Other clinical conditions such as traumatic brain injury or periodic psychiatric problems (e.g., mood disorders) also may affect executive function performance. Correspondingly, numerous traits may be related to ADHD, only some of which

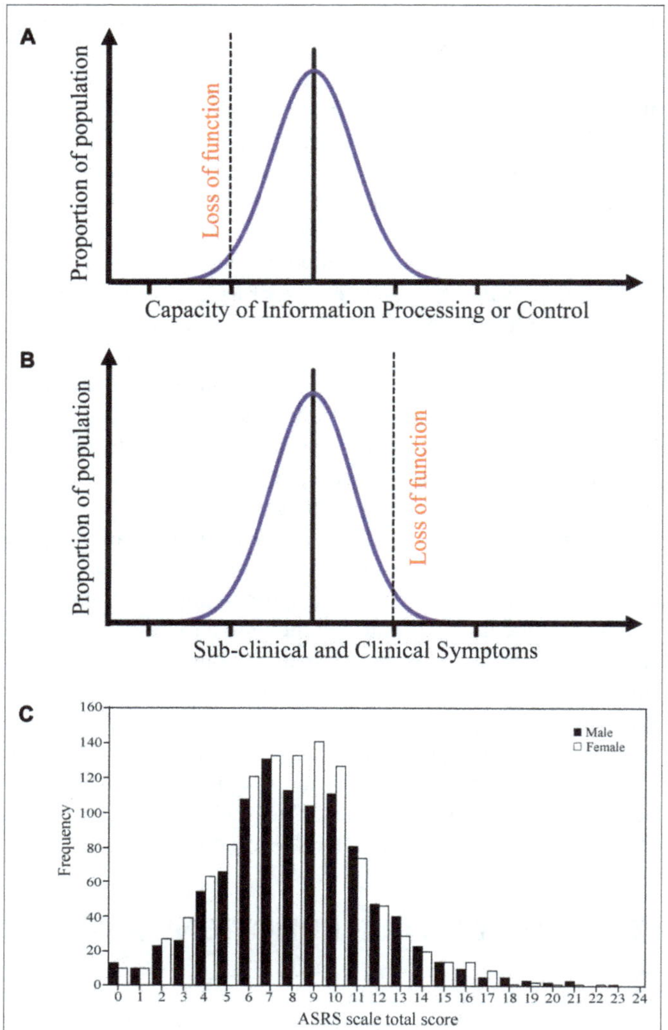

FIGURE 1 | Distribution of processing capacities and symptoms in the general population. (A) A model that suggests that different cognitive core capacities in the population often follows a normal distribution. Extremely low cognitive core capacities will induce a functional loss. Such a distribution is for example observed for executive function capacity. **(B)** The model posits that this capacity is mirrored in different behavioral symptoms, and that the transition from sub-clinical to clinical symptoms is defined by functional loss. **(C)** ADHD symptoms in the general population follows such a distribution. Panel **C** is originally from Das et al. (2012) and reprinted with permission from *PLos One*.

are related to dysfunctional executive functions (Castellanos and Proal, 2012). Finally, different individuals may rate the same behavior differently depending on cultural factors and meta-cognitive capacity. Still, a community study of more than 16,000 children and adolescents provides some support for the dimensionality of ADHD symptoms and their relationship to putative executive function capacity (Crosbie et al., 2013). Specifically, the study reproduced, in a general pediatric population, the normal distribution of ADHD-symptoms (Das et al., 2012). Moreover, rated attentional problems in daily life correlated with putative executive function capacity on the stop signal test. The stop signal test measures capacity to suppress an initiated movement and is frequently used for measuring executive functions in ADHD (Nichols and Waschbusch, 2004; Alderson et al., 2007). The relationship between real life problems and stop signal performance was linear across the entire distribution rather than limited to the children who had been diagnosed with ADHD. Thus, there is evidence that both ADHD symptoms and executive function capacity are normally distributed in the population, and that they are associated with each other. On a more general level this suggests that there is a relation between the capacity of specific *cognitive core processes* and symptom severity in the population extending from healthy individuals to those with frank psychiatric states.

Neuroatonomy of "Cool" Executive Functions

Since executive functions and ADHD symptoms appear to be linked, understanding the underlying neural mechanisms mediating the cognitive processes should help elucidate how related clinical symptoms emerge. Executive functions may be defined as a set of control mechanisms that regulate non-routine information processing including behavioral suppression, task switching, adaption, or change of strategy (Barkley, 2012; Goldstein and Naglieri, 2014). To distinguish classical executive functions from those related to emotional processes, the former have been termed "cool" executive functions. These functions are dependent on the prefrontal cortex (PFC) although they represent distributed network processes encompassing many different brain regions including the basal ganglia (BG) and brainstem neuromodulatory systems. The circuits subserving executive functions also involve thalamus, parietal cortex and cerebellum. However, for simplicity, we abbreviate these complex circuits by referring primarily to the prefrontal and anterior cingulate cortex (ACC). In part resulting from Barkley's (1997) suggestion of the primacy of inhibitory capacity in ADHD, many investigators have examined performance on the stop-signal test (Crosbie et al., 2013) and the Stroop test (Lansbergen et al., 2007), both of which involve inhibitory aspects.

The Stroop test targets the involvement of executive functions in resolution of a cognitive conflict mediated by an incongruent stimulus (see **Figure 2**). This test of executive functions is especially interesting for the model presented here because it can also be used in the emotional domain (Egner et al., 2008; Eippert et al., 2009). A seminal article (Kerns et al., 2004) used the Stroop task to decompose different neuronal aspects of executive functions. This study leveraged the conflict resolution that occurs when the same cognitive conflict condition is repeated (see **Figure 2A**). By presenting two incongruent stimuli in a row, Kerns et al. (2004) differentiated two separate conditions for the same type of incongruent stimulus: (1) when conflict was high and conflict resolution was low (first incongruent stimulus); and (2) when conflict resolution was high and conflict was low (second incongruent stimulus). The first type of stimulus presentation evoked an error signal that could activate prefrontal

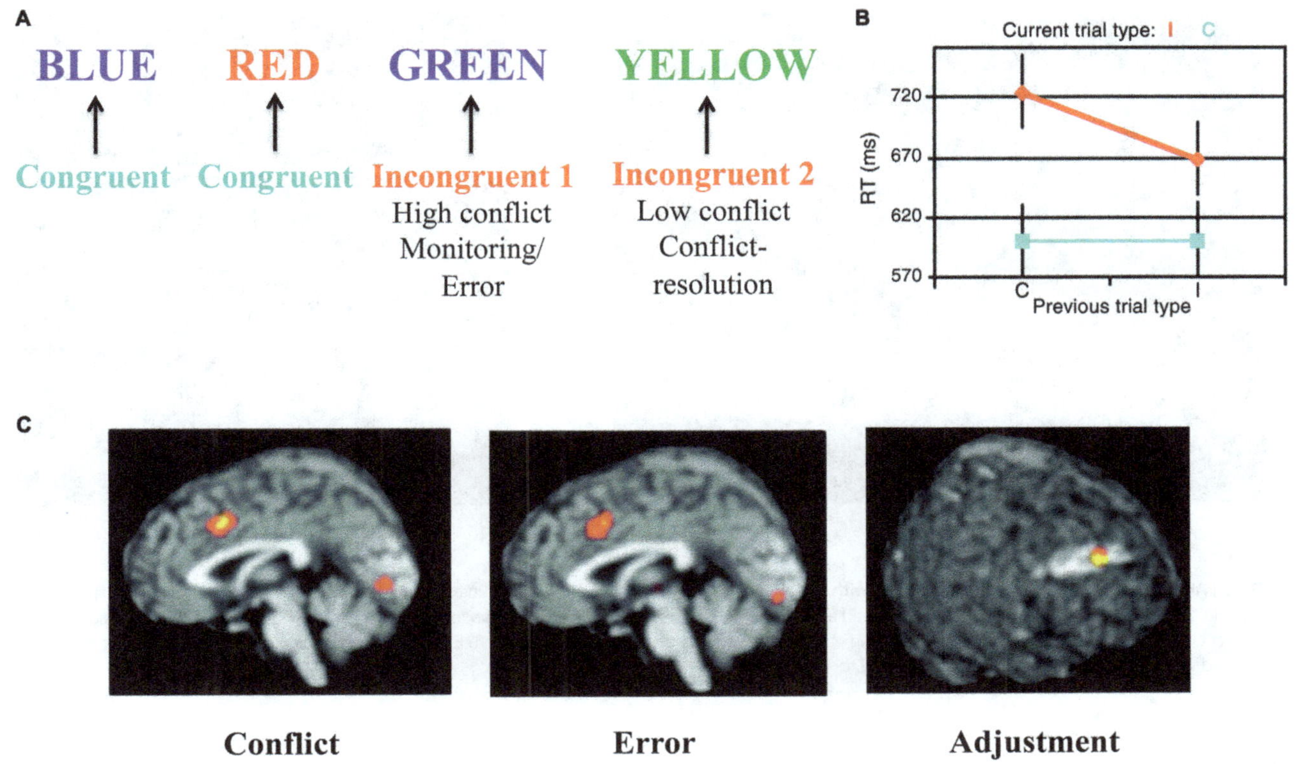

FIGURE 2 | The Stroop task—as an example of "cool" executive function tasks. (A) In the Stroop task colored words are presented where the word itself represents a color. The task is to indicate the color of the word but ignore the word meaning. In some conditions both the color and the word are associated with the same color (congruent condition), while in other conditions the color and the word are associated with different colors (incongruent condition). In the incongruent condition there is a conflict between processes associated with color identification/naming and reading. In order to solve the task, this cognitive conflict has to be regulated using top-down control by suppressing the conflicting process and strengthening the processes associated with the correct response. If two incongruent stimuli are presented in a row, the conflict and error signal is somewhat smaller in the second incongruent condition as conflict-resolution (i.e., adjustment) has been engaged (Kerns et al., 2004). **(B)** Behaviorally, response times mirror the cognitive conflict (red vs. blue) and its resolution (smaller response time in the second incongruent condition vs. the first incongruent condition—both in red). **(C)** These different conditions are mirrored in the underlying brain activations of caudal anterior cingulate cortex (cACC) and dorsolateral prefrontal cortex (dlPFC) representing conflict, error and adjustment. Panels **B,C** are originally from Kerns et al. (2004) and reprinted with permission from AAAS.

conflict resolution systems and decrease conflict in the next stimulus presentation. These manipulations were reflected behaviorally in terms of magnitude of response-time cost of incongruency and in neural signals. Specifically, activation in caudal anterior cingulate cortex (cACC), observed in the first incongruent stimuli condition, was associated with conflict and error-signals (see **Figure 2C**; Kerns et al., 2004) or with initially resolving the conflict (Roelofs et al., 2006; Aarts et al., 2008). Subsequent activation of dorsolateral prefrontal cortex (dlPFC), observed in the second incongruent stimulus condition, was interpreted as reflecting updating the rules used to more effectively solve the conflict (see **Figure 2C**).

Meta-analyses suggest that similar regions including cACC and dlPFC are also involved in other executive function tasks including spatial interference, stop-signal task, go/no-go task, flanker task and Simon task (Nee et al., 2007; Cieslik et al., 2015). Apart from those regions, parietal cortex is also critically involved in executive function tasks as a part of frontoparietal executive control networks. Interestingly, both ventrolateral PFC (vlPFC) and anterior insula are involved in such executive function tasks (Nee et al., 2007; Whelan et al., 2012; Cieslik et al., 2015)—although they often are assigned to emotional processing systems.

Neuroanatomy of "Cool" Executive Functions in ADHD

Dysfunctional executive functions observed in ADHD patients should be mirrored in the underlying structure and function of systems mediating this regulation (Castellanos et al., 2006; Bush, 2010). In line with this idea, maturation of the thickness of the cortex, which follows a normative inverted-U trajectory, was found to be significantly delayed in children with ADHD across nearly the entire cortex, with greatest delays in PFC and ACC (Shaw et al., 2007). In a naturalistic comparison, adolescents taking psychostimulants differed in the rate of change of cortical thickness from those not taking psychostimulants (Shaw et al., 2009), suggesting that medication might ameliorate the delayed development. Thinning in the medial and dlPFC was persistent only in those patients that maintained the full ADHD diagnosis

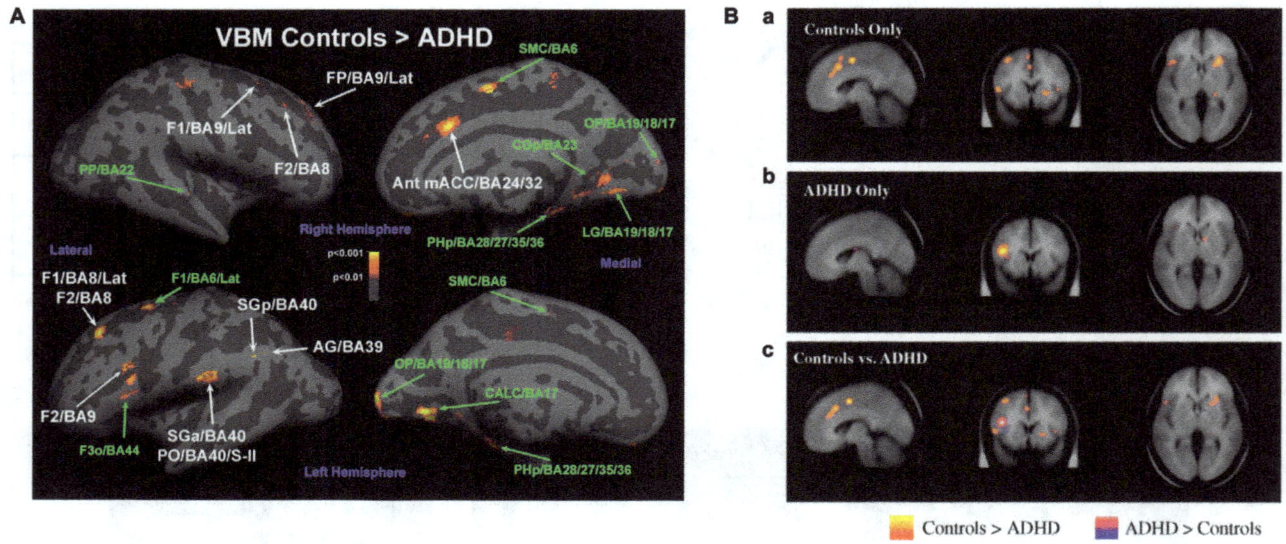

FIGURE 3 | Altered networks in ADHD associated with "cool" executive functions. (A) Some studies have suggested a smaller gray matter volume in cACC and dlPFC (e.g., Seidman et al., 2011), and **(B)** diminished activations in these networks during executive function tasks in patients with ADHD compared to controls (Dickstein et al., 2006). Panel **A** is originally from Seidman et al. (2011) and reprinted with permission from Elsevier. Panel **B** is originally from Dickstein et al. (2006) and reprinted with permission from John Wiley & Sons, Ltd.

in adulthood (Shaw et al., 2013). An earlier and smaller study found that adult patients with ADHD displayed decreased smaller gray matter volumes in both cACC and dlPFC, although the findings were modest and did not survive full brain correction (Seidman et al., 2011; **Figure 3A**).

Similarly, activation of these networks is altered during top-down regulatory tasks in ADHD-patients. Meta-analysis of functional imaging studies reveals decreased activation in patients with ADHD in systems involved in executive functions (e.g., the frontoparietal networks) and attention (e.g., ventral attentional network) in task-based studies (Cortese et al., 2012). When studies were restricted to inhibition or attention tasks, ADHD patients showed reduced activation in similar networks (Dickstein et al., 2006; Hart et al., 2013; **Figure 3B**). While the deficit in inhibition activation was more prominent in right inferior frontal cortex, supplementary motor area (SMA) and ACC, the deficit in attention-activation was more prominent in dlPFC, parietal and cerebellar areas (Hart et al., 2013). Specifically in the Stroop task, dlPFC was less activated for sustained attentional control and the cACC less activated for transient aspects of attentional control (i.e., incongruent trials vs. neutral trials in the incongruent block) in young adults with ADHD vs. controls (Banich et al., 2009).

"HOT" EXECUTIVE FUNCTIONS, EMOTIONAL PROCESSING, AND EMOTIONAL INSTABILITY

Can Emotional Processes be Isolated?

Information processing in the brain is dependent on complex reciprocal interactions between multiple regions in large-scale networks (Mesulam, 1998, 2012; Engel et al., 2001; Dehaene and Changeux, 2011; Siegel et al., 2012). It has therefore been debated whether brain processes associated with "emotion" can be separated from those associated with "cognition" (Pessoa, 2008; Okon-Singer et al., 2015). This question may be rephrased in terms of whether it is possible to separate "emotional" from "non-emotional" processes (and associated regulatory mechanisms), since cognition comprises both emotional and non-emotional information. For example, attention, working-memory and executive-control are not either emotional or non-emotional processes as they operate on both types of information. This point has previously been made for theoretical constructs of attention in distinguishing "cool" executive functions regulating non-emotional processes and "hot" executive functions regulating emotional processes (Zelazo and Mueller, 2002; Kerr and Zelazo, 2004; Castellanos et al., 2006; Rubia, 2011). Therefore, the focus is instead on the possible distinction between emotional processes and non-emotional processes. Clearly, both processes influence each other (Pessoa, 2008; Okon-Singer et al., 2015). In the same vein, any emotional regulatory task will contain non-emotional processes such as holding instructions on line in a working-memory buffer and associated attentional processes.

Nevertheless, the distinction between emotional regulatory systems and non-emotional regulatory systems is useful since there are clinical states in which dysfunction of one pole or the other predominates. Dysregulation is more related to non-emotional processes in classical ADHD while it is more associated with emotional processes in various clinical disorders of emotional instability such as BPD, ASPD or CD. These clinical entities suggest that although emotional and non-emotional processes are both overlapping and interwoven (Pessoa, 2008; Okon-Singer et al., 2015), certain aspects of the involved networks may be more related to emotional or non-emotional dysregulation, respectively. Therefore, to understand the specificity of these disorders, components that are more associated with emotional regulation and non-emotional regulation need to be identified.

Large numbers of emotional regulatory processes have been described (Hartley and Phelps, 2010; Gyurak et al., 2011; Ochsner et al., 2012). While some directly modulate an emotional experience (Ochsner et al., 2012), others are subtler and regulate emotional processes to accomplish a cognitive task (Gyurak et al., 2011), i.e., "hot" executive functions, or are involved in extinction (Schiller and Delgado, 2010; Milad and Quirk, 2012). While processes that regulate emotions are often voluntary and therefore explicit, attentional processes are often automatic and implicit. Here we focus on two fundamental types of emotional regulatory processes that represent different types of top-down control: implicit attentional and explicit cognitive reappraisal processes (Gyurak et al., 2011; Ochsner et al., 2012).

Implicit Attentional Control of Emotional Processes

The attentional dimension in voluntary regulation of emotional experiences has been extensively discussed (Ochsner et al., 2012). However, for the present purpose automatic implicit attentional mechanisms in strictly defined executive function tasks (Gyurak et al., 2011) may be even more interesting since they have the potential to separate emotional from non-emotional components.

Building on the model of decomposing sub-components of executive functions in the Stroop task (Kerns et al., 2004), Etkin et al. (2006) constructed an emotional Stroop task in which affective facial expressions were displayed with overlaid congruent or incongruent words expressing affects (**Figure 4**). The task was to report the facial affect and ignore the overlaid words. This yielded both congruent stimuli (in which the facial expression and the word corresponded to the same emotion) and incongruent stimuli incorporating a conflicting process (in which the affective facial expression and emotion word differed). As in the non-emotional version (Kerns et al., 2004), this task could separate an incongruent stimulus in which conflict remained high (first incongruent stimulus) from an incongruent stimulus in which the conflict level was smaller due to conflict resolution (second incongruent stimulus). There was a reaction time increase for the incongruent condition as compared with the congruent condition, indicating that a conflict was successfully induced. Importantly, this increase was smaller for the second incongruent condition compared with the first incongruent condition, indicating conflict resolution. On a neuronal level, amygdala activation was observed in the high conflict condition reflecting increased influence of the non-relevant emotional incongruent stimuli. However, amygdala activity decreased and activity in rostral ACC (rACC) increased in the low conflict (repeated) incongruent condition. Path-analysis indicated that rACC directly suppressed amygdala activity in this condition.

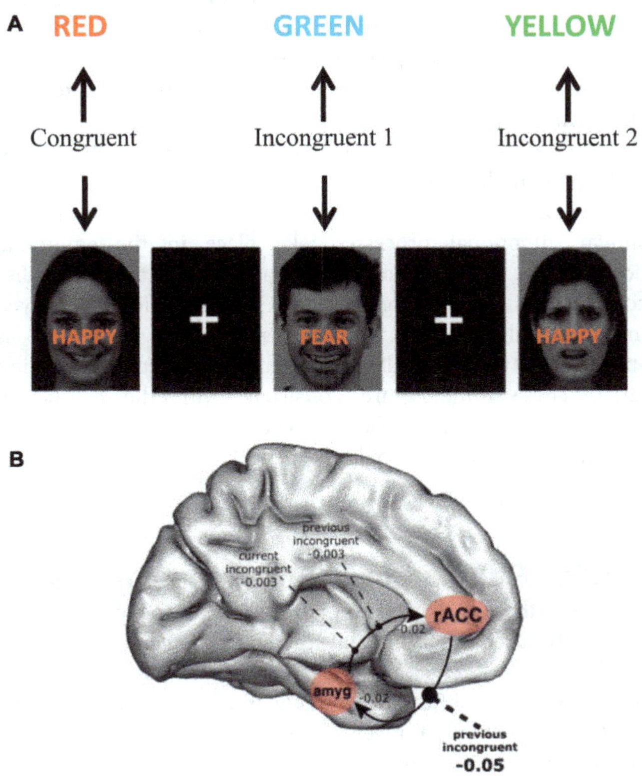

FIGURE 4 | Brain systems underlying the emotional Stroop task. **(A)** The emotional Stroop task has similar features as the original Stroop task including congruent stimuli (without conflict between different processes) and incongruent stimuli (with a conflict between different processes)—but also includes an emotional dimension that needs to be controlled. In the presented example above faces were used from the karolinska directed emotional faces (KDEF; Lundqvist et al., 1998). **(B)** Using a similar version of emotional Stroop task Etkin et al. (2006) showed that higher conflicts increased amygdala involvement and conflict resolution was associated with rostral anterior cingulate cortex (rACC) activation and negative influence on amygdala activity. Panel **B** is orginally from Etkin et al. (2006) and reprinted with permission from Elsevier.

Thus, this study suggests that rACC influences amygdala processing to solve an executive function task with emotional content.

A potential confound in the above study was that non-emotional regulation was not controlled for. Therefore, regulatory mechanisms that were specific to emotional regulation could not be differentiated from mechanisms that are shared with non-emotional regulatory processes. A later study by the same group (Egner et al., 2008) sought to distinguish these two dimensions by presenting the same stimuli in two different tasks, differing in emotional intensity. One task was as described above, and the other involved labeling sex with congruent or incongruent words (i.e., "male" or "female") using the same set of pictures. The original findings were reproduced and survived controlling for the non-emotional regulatory processes. It may be argued that the control for non-emotional regulation was not perfect since both tasks contained affective facial expressions. However, this tradeoff is inevitable since using different types of stimuli in the non-emotional condition would have confounded the task. In sum, this study represents an innovative example of how to control for non-emotional aspects of top-down regulation in automatic attentional tasks.

Other studies on affective interferences in the Stroop test and comparable tasks (Whalen et al., 1998; Ochsner et al., 2009; Rahm et al., 2013) also support the conclusion that similar attentional processes take place in the emotional domain as in the non-emotional domain. The studies converge in highlighting the rACC as specifically involved in emotional executive function tasks, while the cACC is specifically involved in related non-emotional executive function tasks. These findings are consistent with the distinction between "cool" and "hot" executive function processes and their relative regional specificity (Zelazo and Mueller, 2002; Kerr and Zelazo, 2004; Castellanos et al., 2006; Rubia, 2011).

Explicit Regulation of Emotional Processes

Arguably, the cognitive reappraisal task is one of the most frequently used experimental methods to study emotional regulation (Ochsner et al., 2012; Buhle et al., 2014). Cognitive reappraisal tasks differ substantially from Stroop tasks. While Stroop tasks entail a mechanism that implicitly deals with demanding and fast interference that needs to be resolved on-line for the task to be performed, cognitive reappraisal of emotional stimuli involves an explicit in-depth regulation of information processing. In cognitive reappraisal of emotional stimuli, the task is to change the emotional interpretation of a stimulus. In this way it is more explicit and proactive than Stroop tasks. A task can involve reinterpreting the meaning of emotional pictures from negative to neutral or positive valence. For example, the face of a crying woman, which is automatically interpreted as an emotionally negative picture, can be reinterpreted as a woman who is crying from happiness over seeing her son again after a year. Thus, instead of controlling distracting emotional processes (as in an emotional Stroop task) the reappraisal task actually changes the rules for the emotional interpretation of the world. It requires active assignment of different emotional meaning to stimuli.

The inherent problem of cognitive reappraisal tasks is the difficulty of obtaining behavioral measures since these tasks rely on subjective reports. Moreover, subjects have little insight into what they do during the task. Nevertheless, this has been a popular approach to study emotional regulation since it can dramatically change how we experience the world and it is theoretically close to various cognitive therapies. Cognitive reappraisal tasks have been found to modulate the processing of emotional stimuli in regions such as amygdala and the ventral striatum (Buhle et al., 2014).

The emotional Stroop task regularly shows prefrontal activations both in dlPFC and lateral orbitofrontal cortex (lOFC)/vlPFC (Eippert et al., 2007; Wager et al., 2008; Kanske et al., 2011; Golkar et al., 2012; Buhle et al., 2014), although other regions (including the dorsal ACC and the dorsomedial PFC) seem to support other components of the task (Ochsner et al., 2012). It has been suggested that dlPFC is involved in general selective attention and working memory, while the lOFC/vlPFC seems to be important for selecting a goal-appropriate reappraisal (Ochsner et al., 2012). Thus, theoretically the lOFC/vlPFC should be more specifically involved in emotional regulatory components of the task. In a few studies, attempts have been made to tease apart these components (Wager et al., 2008; Golkar et al., 2012). In one of the studies (Wager et al., 2008), when the rated success of emotional regulation was regressed on the cognitive reappraisal of emotion contrast, the dlPFC contribution was smaller and that of the lOFC/vlPFC larger than in the standard subtraction analysis (**Figure 5**). Thus a measurement better reflecting actual emotional regulation was more tightly coupled to lOFC/vlPFC than dlPFC. In another study (Golkar et al., 2012), a neutral control state was introduced which contained non-emotional aspects of the task, and the interaction revealed more specific activation also in the lOFC/vlPFC. Both these studies are examples that suggest that it is possible to partially separate emotional from non-emotional components in the cognitive re-appraisal task and

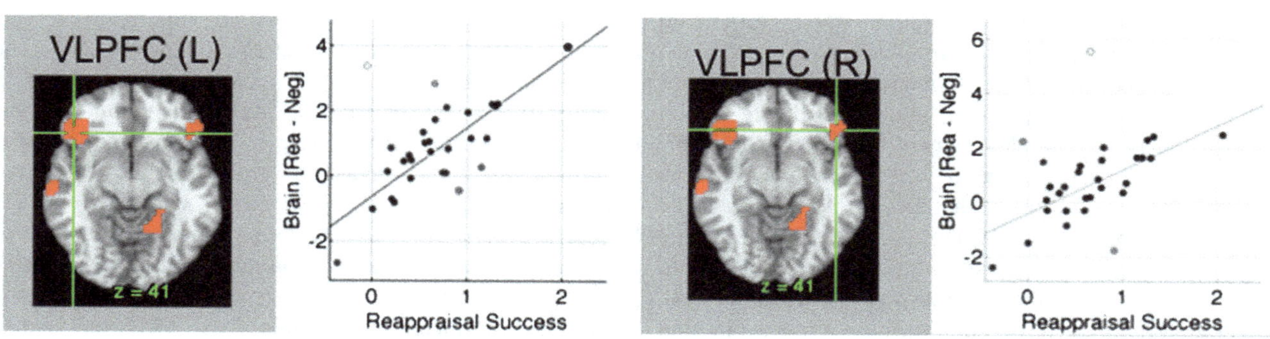

FIGURE 5 | Brain systems underlying cognitive re-appraisal. In cognitive reappraisal studies, typically an emotional picture is presented and the subjects are given a task to explicitly down- or up-regulate the emotional content. In conditions where unpleasant pictures are re-interpreted as more positive, amygdala activity is down-regulated and a network of regions is activated including lateral orbitofrontal cortex (lOFC). lOFC activity correlates closely with re-appraisal success during cognitive re-appraisal (Wager et al., 2008). Figure is originally from Wager et al. (2008) and reprinted with permission from Elsevier.

that indicate greater involvement of the lOFC/vlPFC in the emotional component. Thus, as for rACC there seems to be specificity for lOFC in emotional regulation. This also suggests a possible role for this region in disorders involving emotional dysregulation.

A Role for rACC in Regulation of Emotion and Pain

Previously we have suggested the importance of rACC in implicit attentional regulation in the emotional domain (such as "hot" executive functions). However, a range of other studies suggests a general role for the ACC in emotional regulation. Importantly, although the rACC and cACC differ in their involvement in attentional tasks—as has long been suggested (Bush et al., 2000)—there is little support for a general division between an emotional and a non-emotional cingulate (Etkin et al., 2011; Okon-Singer et al., 2015). In fact, some parts of cACC are highly involved in emotional processes that include negative valence such as pain unpleasantness (Vogt et al., 1993), social exclusion (Eisenberger, 2012) and fear potentiation and appraisal (Etkin et al., 2011; Milad and Quirk, 2012). The cACC is also implicated in behaviors associated with emotional or painful situations and has been viewed as an emotional motor output region (Craig, 2009; Perini et al., 2013). Other influential theories suggest that this part of the cACC has a common role of linking reinforcers to motor centers responsible for expressing negative affect and executing goal-directed behaviors (Shackman et al., 2011) and thereby performing similar fundamental processes for both pain and attention. However, the anatomical and functional relation between ACC involvement in processing of pain/emotion and non-emotional attentional processes is yet to be established.

Studies on placebo analgesia (Petrovic et al., 2002; Wager et al., 2004, 2007; Zubieta et al., 2005; Bingel et al., 2006; Eippert et al., 2009; Wager and Atlas, 2015) and emotional placebo (Petrovic et al., 2005; Ellingsen et al., 2013) have also suggested the rACC is involved in top-down regulation of pain and emotion (see **Figure 6A**). Importantly, this activation remained when controlling for non-emotional attentional aspects of treatment either through interaction or correlation analyses (Petrovic et al., 2002, 2005). The high concentration of opioid receptors expressed in rACC (Vogt et al., 1993; Fields, 2004) has been hypothesized to relate to attentional mechanisms that can suppress pain processing (Petrovic et al., 2002), a suggestion that has received experimental support (Zubieta et al., 2005; Wager et al., 2007; Eippert et al., 2009). In more general terms, specific neuromodulatory systems in the rACC have been suggested to be involved in conflict resolution in the pain or emotion domains when expectations do not match processing of sensory input (Petrovic et al., 2002). The known anatomical connectivity between opioid systems in rACC and the periaqueductal gray (PAG; Vogt et al., 1993) in turn suggests that such modulation acts through regulating opioid systems in the PAG (Petrovic et al., 2002). This was suggested by functional connectivity between rACC and PAG that was opioid and placebo specific (Petrovic et al., 2002) as well as opioid dependent (Eippert et al., 2009; see **Figures 6B,C**). More specific opioid connectivity between these structures was also shown (Wager et al., 2007). Apart from the PAG, other regions such as amygdala and ventral striatum are likely involved in the placebo effect and may be directly controlled by the rACC (Petrovic et al., 2005; Zubieta et al., 2005; Bingel et al., 2006; Wager et al., 2007; Scott et al., 2008; Eippert et al., 2009; Ellingsen et al., 2013). Thus, studies of the placebo effect suggest that rACC is in a position to regulate emotion and pain processes using specific underlying neuromodulatory systems such as the opioid system. Other neuromodulatory systems may also be involved although this is still unknown. Note that more caudal parts of the ACC process pain *per se* (Petrovic et al., 2002), in line with the idea that cACC is involved in processing the unpleasant aspects of pain (Vogt et al., 1993).

A closely related domain of research on conditioning and extinction in both rodents and humans also suggests that ventromedial PFC (vmPFC), an area neighboring rACC, supports extinction while cACC supports increased aversive processing (Milad and Quirk, 2012; see **Figure 7**). The vmPFC is thought to modulate amygdala processing of conditioned fear by suppressing fear responses through a set of amygdala neurons in the intercalated region between the basolateral and central amygdala nucleus (Milad and Quirk, 2012). Different strategies to modify conditioned fear, i.e., extinction, reversal and voluntary regulation of fear, have been shown to activate similar regions in vmPFC/rACC (Schiller and Delgado, 2010). In other words, this line of research mimics placebo research in assigning similar regions in the brain an emotional regulatory function on emotional processes in subcortical regions such as amygdala.

Another line of research has suggested that rACC and the neighboring vmPFC are important in processing the subjective value of rewards (Kable and Glimcher, 2007), which may also be associated with opioid activation (Petrovic et al., 2008). In the neuroeconomics literature, overlapping activity often centered on neighboring vmPFC is thought to integrate anticipated values and costs (from regions such as ventral striatum and amygdala) associated with the different options being converted into a single quantity to guide behavior (Ruff and Fehr, 2014).

In summary, converging lines of evidence (including research on emotional executive functions, placebo research and research on extinction of conditioned fear) suggest that rACC and neighboring vmPFC are specifically involved in emotional regulation of lower-level structures including amygdala, PAG and ventral striatum. This effect seems to be specific for emotion/pain processes and supports the idea of a system sub-specialized for "hot" executive functions and emotional regulation.

A Role for OFC in Regulation of Emotion and Pain

Above we have suggested that OFC has an important role in explicit emotional regulation such as cognitive re-appraisal, in which subjects are asked to modulate the emotions associated with a picture (see above). How does this relate to the

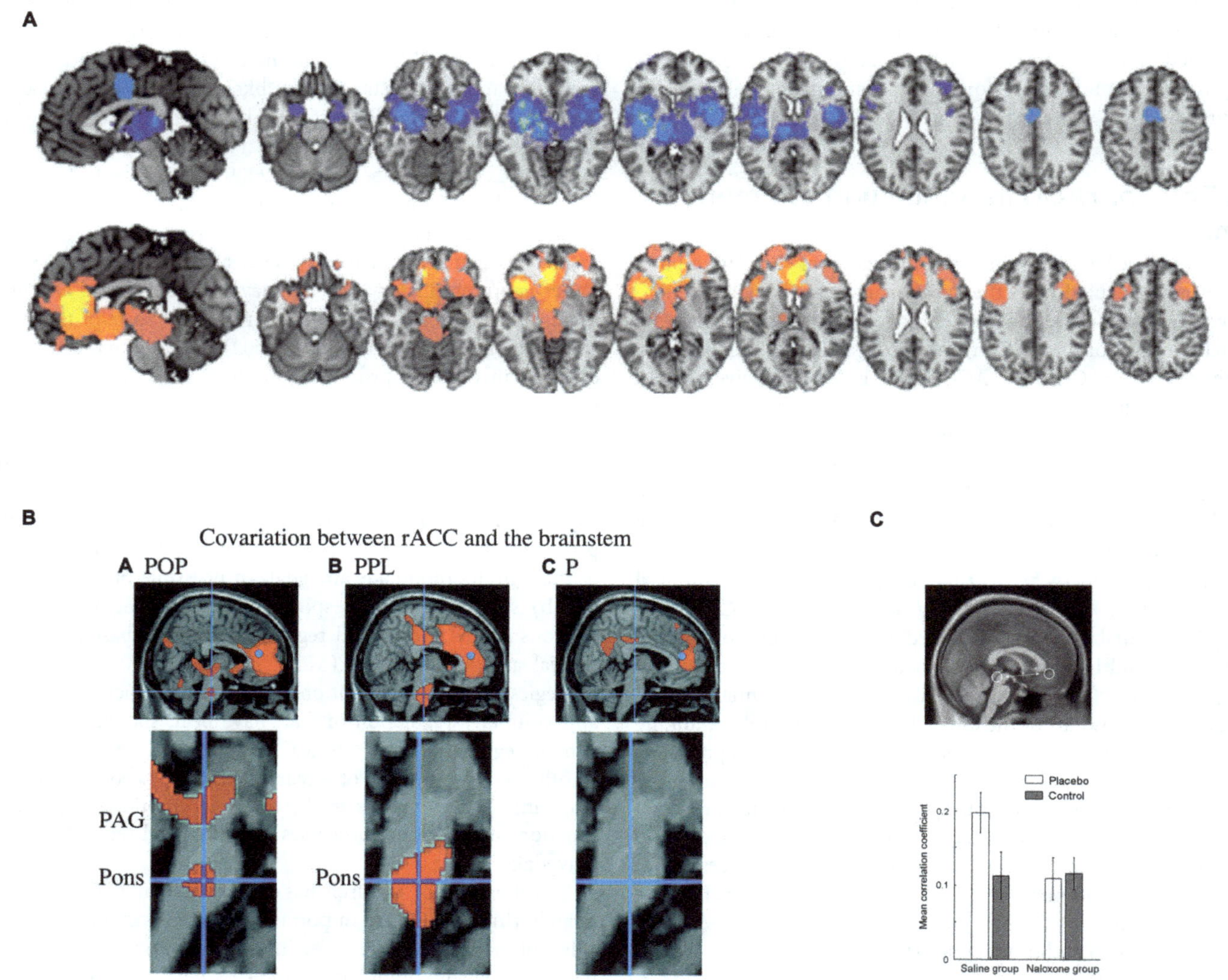

FIGURE 6 | Brain systems underlying the placebo effect. (A) Meta-analysis indicating brain networks showing suppressed activity (blue) and increased activity (yellow/orange) related to placebo analgesia (PPL; Atlas and Wager, 2014). Regions showing increased activity include ventromedial prefrontal cortex (vmPFC)/rACC and lOFC. Note that caudal ACC (cACC) decreases in activity after placebo treatment in association with decreased pain unpleasantness. **(B)** Studies also show that PPL involves opioid dependent interactions between rACC and the brainstem. For example, functional connectivity between rACC (blue dot) and the brainstem was observed in opioid analgesia (POP) and in PPL but not in untreated pain (P; Petrovic et al., 2002). **(C)** This connectivity has been shown to be opioid dependent (Eippert et al., 2009). Panel **A** is originally from Atlas and Wager (2014) and reprinted with permission from Springer. Panel **B** is originally from Petrovic et al. (2002) and reprinted with permission from AAAS. Panel **C** is originally from Eippert et al. (2009) and reprinted with permission from Elsevier.

general function of OFC? The OFC comprises a complex set of regions that may be differentiated along medial-lateral and anterior-posterior gradients (Ongur and Price, 2000; Ongur et al., 2003; Kringelbach and Rolls, 2004; Kringelbach, 2005). Although the OFC receives input from many sensory modalities and may be the most polymodal region in the cortex (Kringelbach and Rolls, 2004), it is notable that many OFC inputs are interoceptive. Thus, the interoceptive needs of the subject are mapped in OFC where they may interact with reward signals and reinforcers from the exteroceptive world. While more primitive unimodal signals seem to be processed posteriorly, more abstract multimodal signals and reinforcers seem to be processed anteriorly (Kringelbach and Rolls, 2004). A lateral orbital network receives inputs from different sensory modalities and a medial network includes regions in ACC and ventro/dorsomedial prefrontal systems and has been suggested to be an important cortical output for visceromotor structures (Ongur and Price, 2000). The medial-lateral distinction has also been observed in human functional imaging of reward processing in which positive feedback and value are mapped to medial OFC while negative feedback is mapped to lOFC (O'Doherty et al., 2001). These results are in line with findings that lOFC represents aversive error-signals (Seymour et al., 2005).

Recent models of a general OFC function emphasize involvement in constructing expected values based on

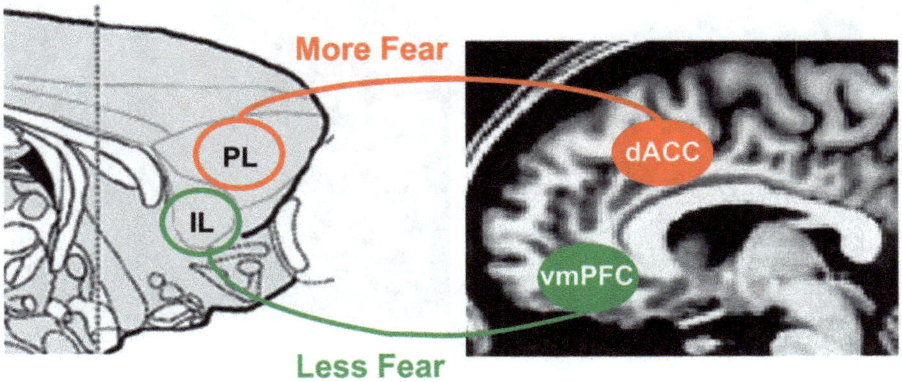

FIGURE 7 | Brain systems underlying fear conditioning. In fear conditioning, vmPFC in humans and infralimbic regions (IL) in rodents is associated with suppressed conditioned fear while cACC (dACC here) in humans and prelimbic regions (PL) in rodents is associated with increased conditioned fear through modulation of amygdala (Milad and Quirk, 2012). Figure is originally published by Milad and Quirk (2012) and reprinted with permission from Annual Reviews.

multimodal inputs (including current internal states) that drive behavior (Schoenbaum and Roesch, 2005; Murray et al., 2007; Schoenbaum et al., 2009; Rudebeck and Murray, 2014). In functional imaging, the association between OFC and complex expected values is illustrated in selective reward devaluation (Small et al., 2001; Gottfried et al., 2003; Kringelbach et al., 2003) and context dependent processing of subjective values (de Araujo et al., 2005; Plassmann et al., 2008).

While the studies above suggest that subjective experience of stimuli may be driven by expectation systems, this has been a principal focus in research on the placebo effect. The lOFC has been activated in several placebo treatment studies (often in co-activation with rACC) as indicated by meta-analysis (Atlas and Wager, 2014; Wager and Atlas, 2015; **Figure 6A**) including placebo analgesia (Petrovic et al., 2002; Lieberman et al., 2004; Wager et al., 2004) and emotional placebo (Petrovic et al., 2005). Interestingly, the lOFC was specifically activated during placebo analgesia but not during opioid-induced analgesia (Petrovic et al., 2002, 2010) suggesting that some cognitive mechanisms are important for the placebo effect but not for opioid-mediated analgesia. Activation in lOFC is believed to represent treatment expectation and the related error-signal between treatment expectation and incoming nociceptive signal (Petrovic et al., 2010) in line with the idea that predictions about different outcomes drive the placebo response (Buchel et al., 2014). Such expectation related processes in the lOFC have been suggested to drive pain and emotion regulatory signals in rACC and are in line with placebo-specific functional connectivity between these regions (Petrovic et al., 2010).

The involvement of lOFC in cognitive reappraisal and placebo can be understood in light of theoretical models of OFC function (Schoenbaum and Roesch, 2005; Murray et al., 2007; Schoenbaum et al., 2009; Rudebeck and Murray, 2014). In cognitive reappraisal, subjects are instructed to shift their expectation about emotional stimuli, which resembles the expectation manipulation performed in response to placebo. The change of expectations in both paradigms involves assigning new values to emotional stimuli by OFC.

"Hot" Executive Functions and Emotional Regulation in Emotional Instability

The need for understanding the specific processes underlying emotional regulation is driven by the clinical symptoms often observed in emotional instability disorders such as BPD, ASPD and CD. Although all these disorders have a high rate of comorbidity with ADHD and with ADHD symptoms, they are unquestionably different from classical DSM-5 ADHD. Symptoms involving frequent variability in experiencing intense emotional states and emotion related behaviors are fundamental to emotional instability disorders but not a necessary component of classic ADHD. A central question is therefore whether networks that are more specifically involved in emotional regulation also are more specifically dysfunctional in these disorders. Given the specific involvement of rACC and lOFC in emotional regulation (as outlined above) it may be questioned whether these regions also differ in structure and function in conditions characterized by emotional instability.

Several studies of brain morphometry have been conducted in emotional instability disorders including BPD, ASPD and CD. Although, they represent initial steps in understanding the underlying pathophysiology, there are two major problems with many of these studies. The first is that most studies have been underpowered, with few patients and controls. The second is that ADHD has not been considered. Nevertheless, two relatively well-powered volumetric studies of BPD (Soloff et al., 2008, 2012) found smaller gray matter volume in rACC and lOFC (**Figures 8A,B**). Smaller lOFC volume was specifically observed in suicide attempters and even more so in high lethality suicide attempters (Soloff et al., 2012). Similar structural abnormalities have also been observed in other emotional instability disorders such as ASPD (Yang and Raine, 2009). However, such findings have not regularly been observed in morphometric studies of ADHD—in fact

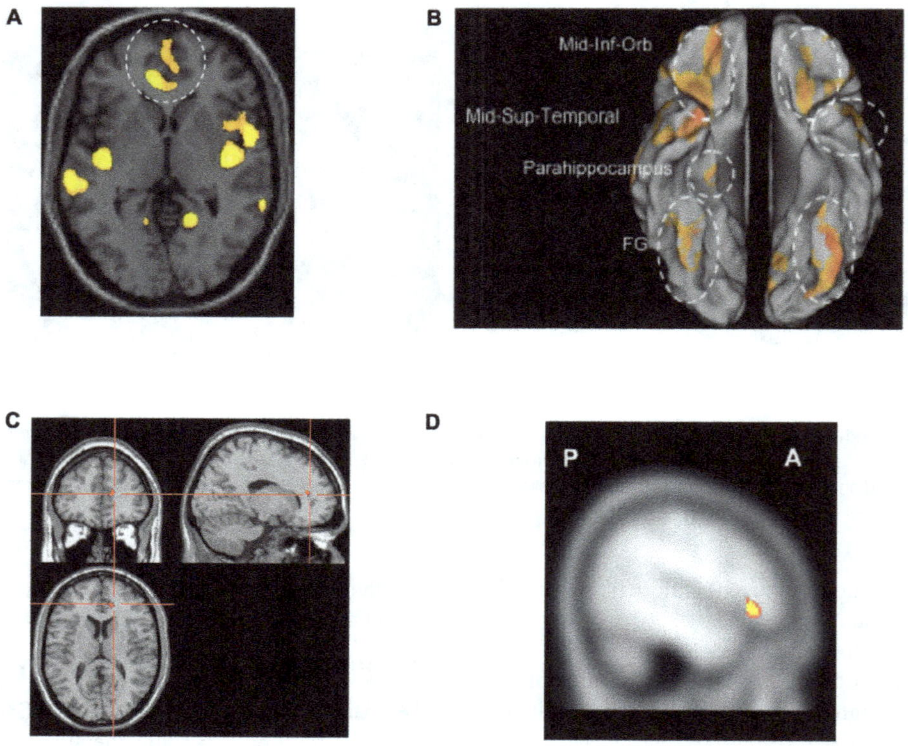

FIGURE 8 | Altered networks in borderline personality disorder (BPD) associated with "hot" executive functions and emotional regulation. **(A,B)** Previous research has suggested smaller gray matter volume in rACC and lOFC in patients with BPD (Soloff et al., 2008, 2012). **(C)** Attenuated activity has been observed in rACC during emotional Stroop (Wingenfeld et al., 2009) in BPD as compared to controls. **(D)** Moreover, lower lOFC activity has been observed during cognitive re-appraisal in BPD as compared to controls (Schulze et al., 2011). Panel **A** is originally from Soloff et al. (2008) and reprinted with permission from Elsevier. Panel **B** is originally from Soloff et al. (2012) and reprinted with permission from Elsevier. Panel **C** is originally from Wingenfeld et al. (2009) and reprinted with permission from Elsevier. Panel **D** is originally from Schulze et al. (2011) and reprinted with permission from Elsevier.

the opposite has been observed (Seidman et al., 2011)—as discussed below. The volume of other regions suggested to be involved in emotional processing in BPD, such as amygdala and insula, was also smaller (Soloff et al., 2008, 2012).

Although structural findings can be suggestive, ultimately, the functionality of regions such as rACC and lOFC in tasks involving emotional regulation must be addressed to better understand emotional instability. Few studies have been published so far that directly test "hot" executive functions and emotional regulation in emotional instability disorders. However, some studies suggest a lower activation of regulatory networks in such disorders. Using a verbal emotional Stroop task, Wingenfeld et al. (2009) observed that BPD patients had overall slower reaction times compared to healthy controls but no increased slowing with emotional interference. However, the BPD patients were not able to recruit rACC when they needed to control for negative words (see **Figure 8C**). Another recent study showed that BPD patients that dissociated were more prone to show greater emotional interference (Winter et al., 2015), although no differences were observed in rACC using a verbal emotional Stroop task. One reason may be that the interference in the verbal emotional Stroop task that was used was too weak, as the controls showed neither a behavioral interference effect nor any rACC activity. By contrast, this was readily observed in Stroop tasks using affective faces (Etkin et al., 2006; Egner et al., 2008). Several other studies using tasks involving emotional conflict control have also shown deficient activations of the subgenual ACC and rACC in patients with BPD (Silbersweig et al., 2007; Enzi et al., 2013; Holtmann et al., 2013; Jacob et al., 2013). Interestingly, in most studies involving patients with BPD in which an emotional conflict must be suppressed, increased activity in amygdala or insula (compared with controls) has been observed, indicating unresolved or heightened emotional conflict (Silbersweig et al., 2007; Krause-Utz et al., 2012; Holtmann et al., 2013; Jacob et al., 2013; Prehn et al., 2013)—but see Smoski et al. (2011). In line with these findings a behavioral study has shown that patients with CD have an impaired Stroop performance under distressing emotional stimulation but no difference under neutral emotional stimulation as compared to controls (Euler et al., 2014). Thus this generalizes the above findings for other emotional instability disorders.

Testing more complex emotional regulation targeting the OFC with cognitive reappraisal of emotional pictures, BPD patients have been found to activate lOFC to a lesser extent than controls while they activated amygdala and insula more (Schulze et al., 2011; **Figure 8D**). A study of cognitive reappraisal of a script-driven emotional induction did not show differences in lOFC but found lower activations in rACC during up- and down-regulation in BPD subjects compared to controls (Lang et al., 2012).

Although the studies above have not corrected for non-emotional ADHD symptoms nor isolated emotion-specific components in the emotional Stroop-task or during cognitive reappraisal, they indicate that rACC and lOFC appear to be activated to a lesser degree during "hot" executive functions and complex emotional regulation, and are structurally smaller in BPD, the paradigmatic emotional instability disorder.

Emotional ADHD and "Hot" Executive Functions

ADHD as defined since DSM-III has considered emotional dysregulation an associated feature, rather than a core component. Instead, ADHD has been considered by many to be synonymous with a disorder of executive function. However, as mentioned previously, laboratory measures of executive function are only moderately correlated with ADHD symptoms and they correspond poorly to measures of real world impairment. Interestingly, the effects of stimulant medications impact laboratory measures of executive function less than rated symptoms (Coghill et al., 2014b; Baroni and Castellanos, 2015). Rather, the main effects seem to be on subjective factors such as motivation. Along these lines, phenomenological studies increasingly point to the profoundly impairing effects of emotional dysregulation among many adolescents and adults with ADHD (Castellanos et al., 2006; Thorell, 2007; Yu et al., 2015). In line with this reasoning, including tests on delay aversion and temporal discounting along with standard executive function tests reveals abnormalities in a large majority of ADHD patients (Castellanos et al., 2006; Thorell, 2007; Yu et al., 2015). These tests show that many subjects with ADHD more often chose a smaller reward immediately than a larger reward later in time as compared to controls. Thus, they indicate that altered reward processing and behavior is another important aspect of ADHD rather than only dysfunctional executive functions. These observations have formed the basis for the notion that the neurobiology of ADHD entails at least two pathways, one related to motivation, emotion and reward, and the other focused on dysregulation of action and thought resulting from poor inhibitory control (Sonuga-Barke, 2002; Thorell, 2007; Coghill et al., 2014a).

Few functional imaging studies have addressed the difference between "non-emotional" and "emotional" ADHD traits. However, we note that one study observed that the strength of functional connectivity (magnitude of correlation in spontaneous activity) between amygdala and rACC and between amygdala and posterior insula were significantly correlated with parent ratings of emotional dysregulation in children with ADHD (Hulvershorn et al., 2014)—suggesting that emotional traits in ADHD may influence information processing. Studies of this type are beginning to link emotional dysregulation and brain circuits in the context of ADHD.

THE RELATION BETWEEN EMOTIONAL AND NON-EMOTIONAL REGULATORY SYSTEMS

In summary, clinical dysfunctions of top-down regulatory networks can be associated to non-emotional control such as in classic DSM-5 ADHD or to emotional control such as in BPD. We propose that this distinction is tenable because certain regulatory components are more linked to one of the two dimensions although emotional and non-emotional processes highly overlap in the brain. As the cognitive core process capacity of these regulatory systems varies in the population, symptoms associated with both non-emotional dysregulation and emotional dysregulation can be found along a continuum—often normally distributed. This suggests that some clinical states could therefore better be described as extremes on this continuum than as categorically defined disorders.

One important question that arises in this comparison is how dysregulation of emotional processes relates to dysregulation of non-emotional processes. It could be argued that the underlying systems are completely independent, and therefore separate in function and dysfunction. In this case there should not be any increased comorbidity between related clinical disorders (as compared to other disorders) nor an increased risk to have dysregulation in another dimension as compared to healthy subjects. However, this is not the case. The comorbidity between ADHD and the different emotional instability disorders is remarkably large. For example, 42% comorbidity between ADHD and BPD was reported in adolescence and 16% in adulthood in a BPD sample (Philipsen et al., 2008) while the prevalence of BPD in a cohort of 81 patients with ADHD was 37% (Anckarsater et al., 2006). Up to 65% of men with ASPD were reported to present comorbid ADHD (Semiz et al., 2008). Comorbidity among ADHD and CD is substantial (Rubia, 2011). The clinical state of emotional ADHD (Castellanos et al., 2006) also suggests a link between non-emotional and emotional dysregulation. Moreover, ADHD is genetically related to emotional instability disorders such as BPD (Distel et al., 2011). Therefore, the emerging picture suggests both common overlapping mechanisms and specific non-overlapping mechanisms.

However, although research suggests a strong association between non-emotional and emotional regulation, recent brain imaging results suggest that the relation is complex. In a reasonably large study on ADHD that specifically excluded patients with affective problems (Seidman et al., 2011) somewhat smaller gray matter volumes were found in dlPFC and cACC as predicted. An exploratory analysis also found tentative evidence of larger gray matter volumes bilaterally in lOFC and rACC in the ADHD group than in the healthy controls (**Figure 9A**). By contrast, well-powered studies of BPD (Soloff et al., 2008, 2012) showed smaller gray matter volumes in rACC and lOFC. Thus,

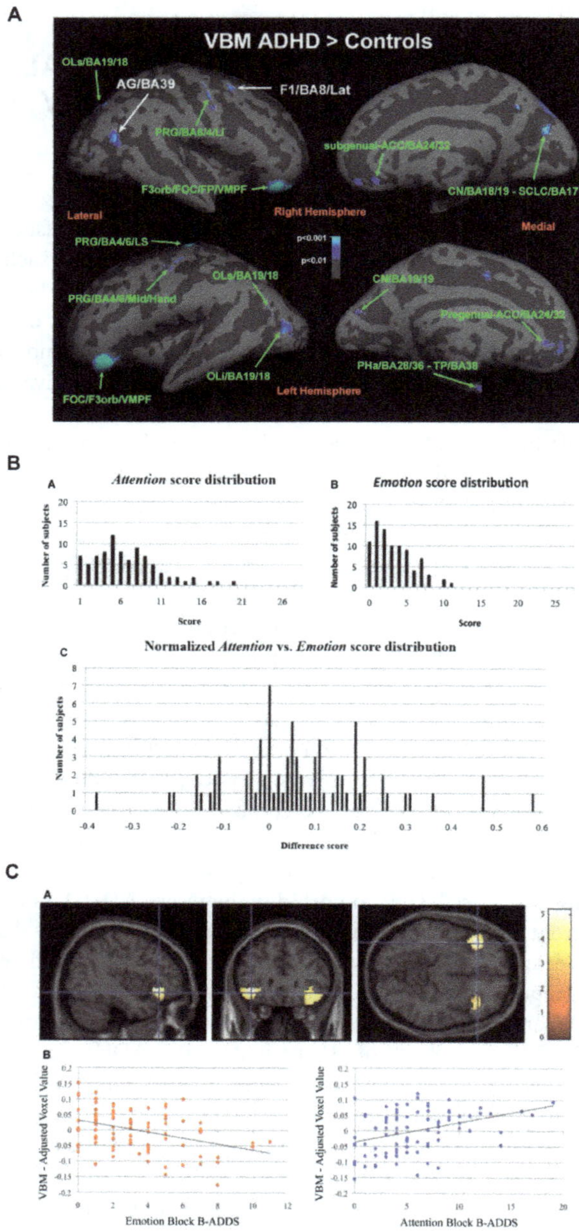

FIGURE 9 | Relation between networks mediating emotional and non-emotional top-down regulation. (A) Patients with ADHD without emotional dysregulation disorders showed larger gray matter volume in lOFC and rACC compared with controls (Seidman et al., 2011). **(B)** Variability observed when healthy subjects rate sub-clinical symptoms associated with non-emotional attentional dysregulation and emotional dysregulation (Petrovic et al., 2015) using the Brown Attention-Deficit Disorder Scales (Brown, 1996). **(C)** Gray matter volume in lOFC was negatively correlated with symptoms related to emotional dysregulation but positively correlated with symptoms related to non-emotional attentional dysregulation (Petrovic et al., 2015). Panel **A** is originally from Seidman et al. (2011) and reprinted with permission from Elsevier. Panels **B,C** are originally from Petrovic et al. (2015) and reprinted with permission from Oxford University Press.

the opposite picture emerges for gray matter volume in these regions in classical ADHD (where the affective component is small) compared to BPD.

These results were partially replicated in a recent study on emotional dysregulation in 87 healthy subjects (Petrovic et al., 2015; see **Figures 9B,C**). In this study, symptoms related to emotional dysregulation correlated negatively with gray matter volume in lOFC bilaterally, while symptoms related to non-emotional attentional dysregulation (i.e., classical ADHD-like symptoms) were positively correlated with gray matter volume in the same region. Thus, it seems that although emotional and non-emotional dysregulation are positively correlated, these dimensions can be inversely related to brain volume in regions that are more involved in non-emotional regulation (such as dlPFC and cACC) and regions that are more involved in emotional regulation (such as lOFC and rACC).

What underlies this puzzling relation between the two regulatory systems is not known. However, these top-down modulatory regions have shown opposite activations during specific attentional tasks (Simpson et al., 2000; Dolcos and McCarthy, 2006; Dolcos et al., 2011)—suggesting mutual active suppression. Moreover, some of these regions such as rACC and cACC tend to correspond to distinct resting state networks that can exhibit anticorrelations during resting state scans (Fox et al., 2005; Fransson, 2005). Although such negative correlations cannot be interpreted as implying mutual inhibition, these robust anti-phase patterns do suggest interactions between emotional and non-emotional regulatory systems in general. We speculate that dysfunction in one regulatory system (e.g., "non-emotional") could promote the other regulatory system (e.g., "emotional") to develop and compensate for the dysfunctional system. This imbalance in development would further inhibit the other system leading to even more protracted development. It would be interesting to study whether larger lOFC/rACC gray matter volumes also suggest better emotional regulation after controlling for the non-emotional components in an experimental task.

The findings that emotional dysregulation and non-emotional dysregulation may be inversely related to brain volume and activation patterns in prefrontal regulatory networks suggest that both dimensions should be assessed simultaneously. Thus, endophenotype dimensions relating to emotional dysregulation and non-emotional dysregulation as well as the emotional vs. non-emotional aspects of different tasks must be taken into consideration. This has rarely been done in studies of BPD and ASPD. However, some research on CD in children has tried to control for ADHD and even directly test for differences between patients with "pure" CD vs. patients with "pure" ADHD (Rubia, 2011). In a set of executive function tasks (Rubia, 2011), children with ADHD activated PFC less than children with CD, while on a reward task, children with CD showed less activation in OFC than children with ADHD, as expected from the neuropsychological profiles of the two disorders.

The balance between emotional and non-emotional processes may also be discussed in relation to specific behaviors that are altered in a set of psychiatric states. For example, impulsivity (measured with self-rating questionnaires or behavioral tests such as stop signal or go-no-go tests) has been studied as a neurocognitive endophenotype marker across disorders (Robbins et al., 2012). This suggests that a common underlying process related to impulse control capacity could underlie different disorders. However, impulse control is not a simply unitary construct (Robbins et al., 2012; Sebastian et al., 2014). For example, in BPD, impulsivity is associated with emotional distress and self-injurious behavior while it is associated with both emotional and non-emotional behaviors in ADHD (Sebastian et al., 2014). Thus, impulse control and impulsivity may exist in both non-emotional and emotional domains and represent different cognitive core processes.

Even in the same cognitive task, different components may fail in individuals with non-emotional dysregulation as compared to individuals with emotional dysregulation. Evidence for this was observed in the Imagen project (Schumann et al., 2010) in which almost 2000 children underwent structural and functional imaging scanning and a battery of cognitive tests and clinical questionnaires. In a functional imaging analysis of the stop-signal task, two main regressors (indicating different phenotypes) were tested separately while controlling for the other. One regressor involved misuse of substances as an indicator of [emotional] impulsivity (associated with emotional dysregulation; $n = 1593$) and the other regressor quantified non-emotional ADHD traits (attentional problems and impulsivity; $n = 342$; Whelan et al., 2012). While there was no behavioral difference in performance on the stop-signal test, the substance abuse regressor was associated with hypoactivation in the lOFC during the stop-success aspect of the trial while the ADHD-associated regressor was linked to hypoactivation of bilateral inferior frontal network and BG network during the stop-fail aspects of the trials. Thus, this study suggests that different strategies are used by subjects with emotional dysregulation tendencies vs. non-emotional attentional dysregulation, possibly mirroring an imbalance in the emotional vs. non-emotional regulatory systems.

A DIVISION BETWEEN EMOTIONAL AND NON-EMOTIONAL REGULATION BEYOND PREFRONTAL AND CINGULATE CORTEX

Neuronal Circuitry—Prefrontal-Basal Ganglia Loops

The PFC and ACC work in close connection with the BG and specific neuromodulatory systems, including the dopamine system, to accomplish cognitive computations such as choosing specific behavioral responses, learning reward associations and behaviors, and transforming new behaviors into habits (Graybiel, 2008; Haber and Knutson, 2010; Haber and Behrens, 2014). If emotional and non-emotional processing can be partially differentiated, then so should prefrontal interactions with BG and neuromodulatory systems. In line with this idea, the distinction between OFC/rACC (including vmPFC) and dlPFC/cACC is mirrored in the circuits linking PFC/ACC with BG (Graybiel, 2008; Haber and Knutson, 2010; Haber and Behrens, 2014). The PFC-BG-thalamus-PFC circuit is organized as parallel loops that are both segregated and integrated (Graybiel, 2008; Haber and Knutson, 2010; Haber and Behrens, 2014). While rACC/vmPFC and OFC are particularly strongly connected with ventral striatum, the cACC and dlPFC are strongly connected with dorsal striatum in a graded manner (Graybiel, 2008; Haber and Knutson, 2010; Haber and Behrens, 2014). This allows a degree of separation between reward processes, non-reward cognitive processes and motor processes. As the loops interconnect, the different dimensions can also interact with each other, as is essential. In this way, this system allows a transformation from reward guided responses and reward learning to behavioral habits and compulsions (Graybiel, 2008; Robbins et al., 2012).

Neuromodulatory Effects of Dopamine and Reward Processing

The dopamine system is especially interesting in relation to ADHD as it is altered in ADHD and the main pharmacological treatments modulate catecholamines, including dopamine (Swanson et al., 2007, 2011; Volkow et al., 2009). A similar division between an "emotional" and a "non-emotional" dimension can also be discerned in the dopamine system as for the prefrontal and BG circuits (Williams and Goldman-Rakic, 1998; Björklund and Dunnett, 2007; Haber and Behrens, 2014; **Figures 10A,B**). Dopamine neurons are organized as tiers of nuclei from the ventral tegmental area (VTA) to the substantia nigra. While VTA neurons tend to reach ventral striatum and the subgenual/rostral ACC (including vmPFC), substantia nigra neurons tend to project to the dorsal striatum and the dlPFC—also in a graded manner. The described system allows for both segregated and integrated processing at multiple levels (midbrain/dopamine, BG and PFC/ACC) and is likely relevant to specific behaviors related to ADHD and emotional instability disorders, respectively.

Both associative and instrumental reward learning are dependent on the ventral striatum, which signals reward prediction errors via the dopamine system (Schultz et al., 1997; Schultz, 2007). Functional imaging studies on humans support this model (O'Doherty et al., 2003, 2006; Pessiglione et al., 2006). The reward anticipation period is an important component of this reward learning system (Haber and Knutson, 2010).

Numerous functional imaging studies have found that ADHD patients show a decreased BOLD response in the ventral striatum during the anticipation of rewards (Scheres et al., 2007; Strohle et al., 2008; Stark et al., 2011; Carmona et al., 2012; Edel et al., 2013; Furukawa et al., 2014; Kappel et al., 2015)—making this one of the most robust paradigms in functional imaging research on ADHD—but see von Rhein et al. (2015) and the following discussion (Plichta and Scheres, 2015). Interestingly, even the degree of subclinical ADHD symptoms has been shown to correlate with striatal hypoactivity during reward anticipation in a non-clinical sample (Stark et al., 2011). At the same time, some studies have found a stronger response to reward outcome either in striatum (Furukawa et al., 2014; von Rhein et al., 2015) or in the OFC (Strohle et al., 2008) in ADHD patients vs. controls. Together with hypofunction during

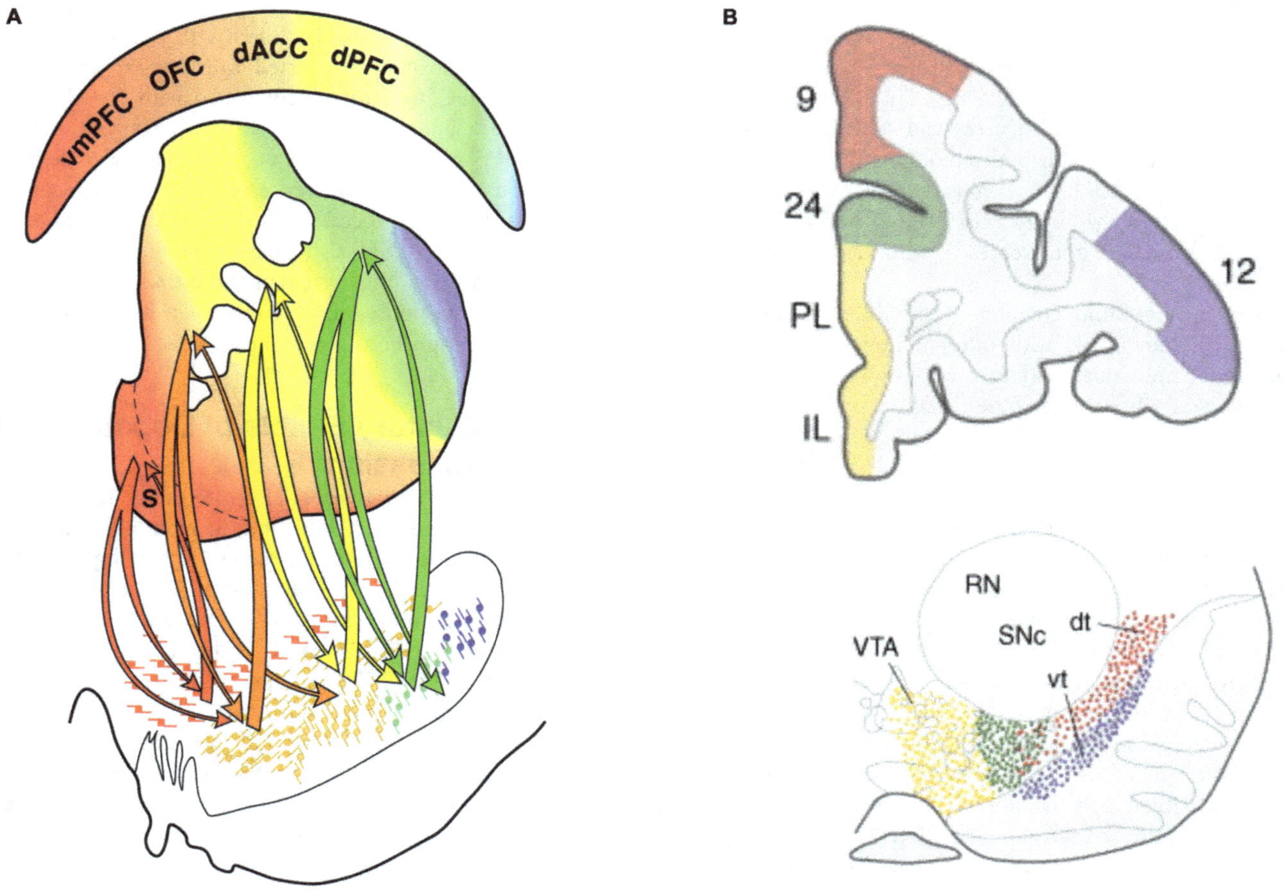

FIGURE 10 | Connectivity between the dopamine system and basal ganglia (BG), and between the dopamine system and PFC. (A) The division between different prefrontal and anterior cingulate cortex systems is mirrored in BG organization and dopamine system projections to BG. Color-coded connectivity is shown between dopamine neurons in the midbrain (lower part of the figure) and different parts of the BG (middle part of the figure; the ventral striatum in is shown in red and dorsal striatum is mainly shown in yellow and green) (Haber and Behrens, 2014). The color-coded upper part of the figure indicates that while vmPFC/rACC and orbitofrontal cortex are more connected to the ventral striatum, caudal ACC (cACC, here designated dACC) and dorsal PFC (dPFC) are more connected to the dorsal striatum. **(B)** In primates a distinction between different prefrontal and anterior cingulate cortex areas is also preserved in the dopamine system projecting directly to the cortex (Williams and Goldman-Rakic, 1998; Björklund and Dunnett, 2007). Panel **A** is originally from Haber and Behrens (2014) and reprinted with permission from Elsevier. Panel **B** is originally from Björklund and Dunnett (2007) and reprinted with permission from Elsevier.

reward anticipation, this suggests that ADHD patients are more affected by immediate rewards than by future rewards. Although a robust finding, the striatal reward anticipation dysfunction observed in ADHD patients must remain tentative as emotional instability traits have not been controlled for in most existing ADHD studies. We speculate that the emotional dimension of ADHD will be more related to the differential processing of reward anticipation than the non-emotional dimensions. Few studies have investigated this issue in emotional instability disorders but initial studies show similar results in BPD and ASPD (Vollm et al., 2007).

The decreased striatal BOLD signal in reward anticipation observed in ADHD may be associated with the abnormalities in delay aversion and temporal discounting that are often observed in ADHD (Castellanos et al., 2006; Thorell, 2007; Yu et al., 2015)—as all are related to processing of future rewards (vs. processing an immediate reward). These processes involve error signals from dopamine neurons in the VTA (Haber and Knutson, 2010), also pointing towards dysfunction in the emotional domain. In line with this reasoning, initial studies have shown that emotional instability in CD is related to increased temporal discounting unrelated to ADHD (White et al., 2014). It would therefore be important to test how reward anticipation relates specifically to the emotional vs. non-emotional dimensions in ADHD. Interestingly, timing deficits are highly problematic in non-emotional tasks in patients with ADHD (Rubia et al., 2009) and may be more related to the "non-emotional" dysregulation traits.

Initial studies suggest that the hypoactivation of ventral striatum observed in reward anticipation is more expressed in inattentive ADHD compared to combined type ADHD in adults (Edel et al., 2013) suggesting that sub-categorization of ADHD may be important in understanding how future rewards are processed. In line with this, non-emotional trait impulsivity in the general population is related to increased striatal activation in the reward anticipation phase in contrast to hypoactivation in ADHD (Plichta and Scheres, 2014). Different models have been evoked to explain this discrepancy (Plichta and Scheres, 2014). However, an unmentioned possibility is that emotional dysregulation may be linked to striatal hypoactivation in ADHD but not to the trait-impulsivity of healthy subjects. This would be in line with the finding that subclinical ADHD symptoms are also associated with lower striatal activation during reward anticipation (Stark et al., 2011). Thus, non-emotional trait impulsivity and ADHD symptoms appear to be dissociated in the general population in relation to reward processing.

INTEROCEPTION VS. EXTEROCEPTION AS AN ALTERNATIVE FRAMEWORK

The differentiation of information processing into an "emotional" domain and a "non-emotional" domain may be criticized in several ways. First, the definition of emotion is at best weak. Emotion pertains to a subjective experience. However, many associated processes that deal with threats, rewards, or social signals are subconscious—but are also referred to as emotional processes. Moreover, some fast behavioral responses that are associated with threat or reward cues that may start even before the emotional experience are also termed emotional responses.

The common theme with all "emotional" processes is that they are directly or indirectly associated with interoceptive systems. While exteroceptive stimuli involve the external world, interoceptive stimuli relate to the state of the body, its needs and threats (Craig, 2002, 2009). Craig (2002, 2009) has suggested that interoceptive information from the body directly reaches posterior insula and cACC. Craig (2002, 2009) views the posterior insula as the primary cortex for interoceptive stimuli ("primary interoceptive representation"), and the cACC as a limbic motor region. The interoceptive signal progresses forward in the insula and is integrated with information from various sensory modalities (via, for example, higher-order sensory regions, the temporal pole and the amygdala) and prefrontal input (including information from OFC) to form a "meta-representation" in the anterior insula. According to this theory, such meta-representations form the moment-to-moment emotional states that we experience subjectively (termed "global emotional moments"). These representations are considered fundamental for emotional experiences.

Apart from interoceptive signals from the body being re-represented to construct a subjective feeling state, emotional states may be produced by top-down mechanisms that directly activate emotional processes in anterior insula and ACC. Similarly, exteroceptive signals may trigger conditioned responses in these systems. It could be argued that such top-down induced processes are closely associated to the interoceptive system by analogy with visual imagination induced by top-down systems. For example, increased activity in anterior insula and ACC in empathy for pain overlaps with the activations induced by nociceptive signals associated with the experience of pain (Singer et al., 2004). The extent to which the top-down induced activity in empathy for pain is related to the processing of bottom-up nociceptive input is under debate (Singer et al., 2004; Wager et al., 2013; Rutgen et al., 2015).

Top-down activated emotional processes may be also indirectly associated to interoceptive systems through the activation of bodily responses and induction of peripheral perceptions (e.g., through emotional expressions and autonomic responses), which in turn can provide interoceptive feedback to "hot" circuits (James, 1890; Damasio, 1993; Craig, 2002, 2009). Thus, there is a tight relation between bottom-up and top-down influences on emotional processes.

While it is not clear to what extent early interoceptive signals are prone to modulation, it has been shown that all parts of insula (posterior, mid and anterior) as well as cACC may be regulated by top-down systems during processing of bottom-up interoceptive input (Atlas and Wager, 2014) and processing of top-down induced activation in the interoceptive stream (Singer et al., 2006; Rutgen et al., 2015).

Apart from insula and ACC, several subcortical regions are important for processing stimuli that are closely associated to the bodily state. External signals related to threat and rewards are not directly generated in the interoceptive environment although they are of fundamental importance for survival. Such signals are dependent on amygdala and ventral striatum, sub-cortical regions that often are co-activated with insula and ACC (Paulus et al., 2005; Paulus and Stein, 2006; Kable and Glimcher, 2007; Milad and Quirk, 2012). Thus, amygdala and ventral striatum form a tight network with cortical interoceptive structures. Apart from a direct interaction with insula and ACC, signals from amygdala and ventral striatum may also re-enter the interoceptive loop through proprioceptive feedback from behavior and autonomic responses related to fear and reward. Therefore, the processing of certain external inputs in these structures, including threats and rewards, may be viewed as highly associated to the interoceptive dimension.

Given the difficulties of differentiating "emotional" and "non-emotional" processing, an alternative is a division into one set of processes related only to the "exteroceptive" dimension and another set of processes associated to the "interoceptive" dimension focused on bodily survival and homeostasis. Importantly, even in this type of division of information processing, we note that exteroceptive information interacts with interoceptive information at many stages of the brain hierarchies.

The division between a network that is mostly focused on exteroceptive processes and a network that is associated with interoceptive processes (such as body states and the needs of the bodily functions related to survival) suggests a demand for two different regulatory functions as well. One proposal would be that cACC and dlPFC regulate processes related to the exteroceptive world, while rACC and lOFC regulate processes related to the interoceptive world and its needs by controlling information processing in insula, cACC, amygdala, ventral striatum and the brainstem. As every individual acts in an external environment, these networks need to interact at multiple levels. The division between interoceptive and exteroceptive networks, including their specific top-down regulatory systems, fits with the observation that some individuals have problems that relate more to a specific dimension of top-down control such as "non-emotional" regulation or "emotional" regulation. A testable hypothesis derived from this reasoning is whether processing of more classical interoceptive input is also dysregulated in subjects with emotional instability.

AN INTEGRATIVE MODEL OF ADHD AND EMOTIONAL INSTABILITY

We have presented a model in which ADHD and emotional instability disorders (such as BPD, ASPD and CD) are mechanistically related in that they all involve similar dysfunctional top-down regulation of information processing. We hypothesized that the difference between the classically defined disorders (ADHD vs. emotional instability disorders) is whether this dysfunctional regulation is related to emotional (and interoceptively associated) processing or non-emotional (and exteroceptively associated) processing (*Hypothesis 1*).

To probe this hypothesis, we have shown that it is possible to divide these two dimensions of top-down control. In summary, we have discussed that information processing in the brain is highly dependent on complex reciprocal interactions between multiple regions in large-scale networks (Mesulam, 1998, 2012; Engel et al., 2001; Dehaene and Changeux, 2011; Siegel et al., 2012) rather than isolated processes in specific regions (such as specific emotional and non-emotional regions). Moreover, emotional and non-emotional networks cannot be rigidly differentiated—since most tasks require subcomponents that include both types of processes and information interacts at every hierarchical stage. Finally, some structures may perform information processing that pertains both to emotional and non-emotional processes (Shackman et al., 2011). Nevertheless, the clinical perspective suggests that some specificity must exist, indicating that different networks focus on either emotional or non-emotional processing that can be separated to a certain degree. It is likely that each of these two putative networks has a hierarchical perception-action organization (Fuster, 2000, 2004; Fuster and Bressler, 2012), where the highest levels process more complex and temporally dispersed information. In line with this view, we have reviewed research suggesting that cACC and dlPFC perform similar types of information processing for the non-emotional (and exteroceptive) processing stream, as rACC and lOFC perform for the emotional (and interoceptive) processing stream. Both top-down systems interact with BG to choose and learn behaviors. Moreover, specific parts of the dopamine system interact with the respective system.

While it seems plausible to partially divide top-down regulatory systems that are more specifically tuned to regulate emotional and non-emotional processes, future research must better understand the degree of specificity in these systems by controlling for the other dimension—as few studies have done so far. A prediction would be that cACC and dlPFC should be more involved in top-down regulation of non-emotional processes after controlling for emotional components while rACC and lOFC should be more involved in top-down regulation of emotional processes after controlling for non-emotional components.

Similarly, we have reviewed research suggesting that ADHD involves dysfunction of cACC and dlPFC in non-emotional top-down control while emotional instability disorders involve dysfunction in rACC and lOFC in emotional regulation, in line with the predicted hypothesis. However, these studies often suffer from lack of control of the other dimension, which needs to be addressed in future studies.

A related hypothesis predicts that the classically defined phenotypes of "pure" ADHD and emotional instability disorders should be unusual if the underlying processes are mechanistically related—instead most patients will have both components in different proportions (*Hypothesis 2*). Therefore, a dimensional approach should better describe the problems of most patients. In the present article we have highlighted research suggesting that top-down regulatory capacities of the emotional and the non-emotional systems vary in their efficiency among subjects in the general population (Das et al., 2012; Petrovic et al., 2015). An extremely poor cognitive core capacity in such top-down regulation may be described as a dysregulation since it would be associated with clinical symptoms and functional loss. Dysregulation strictly encompassing the non-emotional (and exteroceptive) processes would be related to ADHD, while dysregulation strictly pertaining to the emotional (and interoceptive) processes would be related to emotional instability disorders (**Figures 11A,B**). It would therefore be possible to describe both types of disorders on a two dimensional scale where poor capacity for non-emotional regulation but normal (or at least not handicapping) emotional regulation would be associated with ADHD (**Figure 11C**). On the same scale, poor capacity for emotional regulation but normal (or at least not handicapping) non-emotional regulation would be associated with emotional instability disorders such as BPD, ASPD or CD. Comorbid states would have poor capacity for both non-emotional and emotional processing. Emotional ADHD would be explained as a disorder in which there is dysregulation of both non-emotional and emotional processes (but to a milder degree). However, these dysregulatory capacities are not independent. As we discussed previously, there is a substantial overlap between the disorders and a tight relation between degree of symptoms both in patients and in healthy individuals in line with a common underlying mechanism for all these clinical states. Possibly, the best way to describe these clinical states is with traits related to emotional dysregulation and traits related to non-emotional dysregulation that are combined to different degrees.

One possible primary candidate for a common substrate that may incorporate both dimensions is the dopamine system. This neuromodulatory system is implicated in ADHD (Swanson et al., 2007; Volkow et al., 2009) and may affect both emotional and non-emotional processing. The possibility that the dopamine system may be similarly altered in both ADHD and emotional instability disorders suggests that the same treatment, i.e., dopaminergic agonists, may be efficacious for both categories of disorders (*Hypothesis 3*). This idea is in line with initial studies, suggesting that methylphenidate also

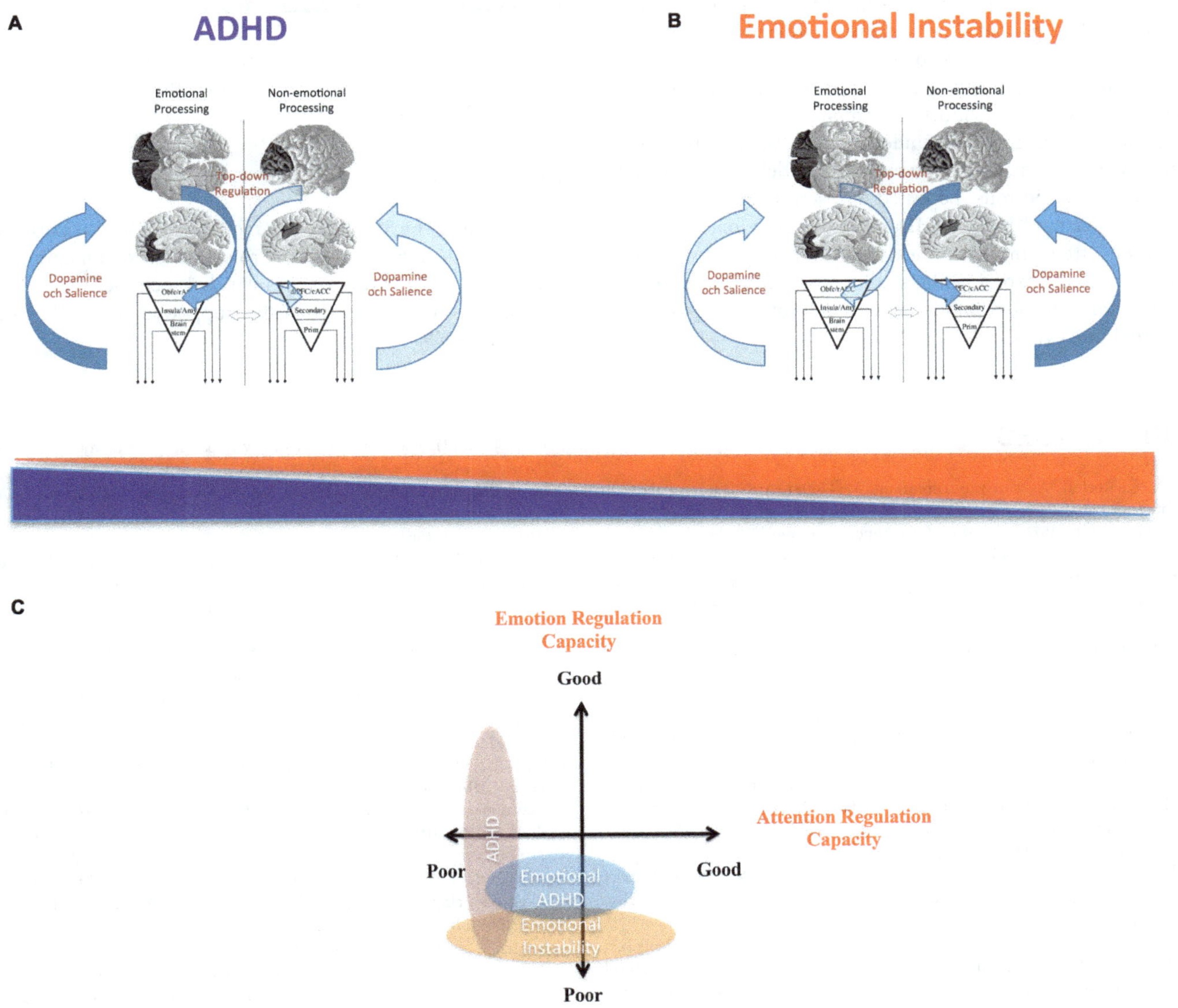

FIGURE 11 | Model of relation between emotional and non-emotional top-down regulation in ADHD and emotional instability. (A) In classical ADHD, top-down control of exteroceptive processes subserved by dlPFC and cACC and the associated dopamine system and dorsal striatum are dysfunctional (affecting "cool" executive functions)—shown in light blue. **(B)** In emotional instability disorders [such as borderline personality disorder (BPD), conduct disorder (CD) and antisocial personality disorder (ASPD)], the top-down control of interoceptive and emotional processes induced by orbitofrontal cortex OFC and rostral ACC and associated dopamine system and ventral striatum are dysfunctional (affecting "hot" executive functions and emotional regulation)—shown in light blue. Instead of representing two extreme variants, dysregulation in different individuals lies on a gradient extending from mostly non-emotional top-down control (all blue) to mainly emotional top-down control (all red). **(C)** A two-dimensional model indicating "non-emotional" attention regulation capacity on one axis and "emotional" regulation capacity on the other axis can incorporate ADHD, emotional ADHD and emotional instability disorders such as BPD, ASPD and CD.

has an impact on emotional dysregulation behaviors in ASPD and CD (Kaplan et al., 1990; Brown et al., 1991; Klein et al., 1997; Connor et al., 2000) as well as BPD (Schulz et al., 1988; Golubchik et al., 2008; Prada et al., 2015; although see Schulz et al. (1988) for possible issue with schizotypal comorbidity). Interestingly, central stimulants also reduce behaviors related to emotional impulsivity and instability in ADHD such as suicide rate (Chen et al., 2014), drug use (Chang et al., 2014) and criminal behavior (Lichtenstein et al., 2012)—possibly indicating a specific effect on emotional dysregulation in ADHD.

One possibility is that there may be graded variability in capacity of the dopamine system in the ventral vs. dorsal tiers of dopamine neurons. This would then be mirrored in and impact the whole regulatory brain network including BG, ACC and PFC processing either emotional or non-emotional related information. It would affect higher order processing and regulation as well as brain structure on a longer term.

Here, we have argued that there is a mechanistic relation between ADHD and emotional instability disorders such as

BPD, ASPD and CD. Perhaps emotional instability disorders should not be regarded as personality disorders but as emotional neuropsychiatric states. Also, using a dimensional approach, characteristics of patients may be better described than using standard categorical distinctions among psychiatric disorders. This may both improve understanding of patients' needs and their treatment. However, the model presented here is theoretical, and must be tested and scrutinized in detail. To better understand how ADHD relates to emotional instability disorders, traits must be measured in patients and healthy participants and experimental studies must be designed that can control for both non-emotional and emotional components of different processes.

AUTHOR CONTRIBUTIONS

PP and FXC wrote the article. Both authors have made substantial, direct and intellectual contribution to the work, and approved it for publication.

FUNDING

PP was funded by Swedish Research Council "Vetenskapsrådet" (K2009-61P-21306-04-4) and "Projektmedel för forskning och utveckling inom psykiatri, primärvård och geriatrik, PPG" (20140301). FXC was partially supported by NIH grant U01MH099059.

REFERENCES

Aarts, E., Roelofs, A., and van Turennout, M. (2008). Anticipatory activity in anterior cingulate cortex can be independent of conflict and error likelihood. *J. Neurosci.* 28, 4671–4678. doi: 10.1523/jneurosci.4400-07.2008

Alderson, R. M., Rapport, M. D., and Kofler, M. J. (2007). Attention-deficit/hyperactivity disorder and behavioral inhibition: a meta-analytic review of the stop-signal paradigm. *J. Abnorm. Child Psychol.* 35, 745–758. doi: 10.1007/s10802-007-9131-6

American Psychiatric Association. (1980). *Diagnostic and Statistical Manual of Mental Disorders*, 3rd Edn. Washington, DC: American Psychiatric Association.

American Psychiatric Association. (2013). *Diagnostic and Statistical Manual of Mental Disorders*, 5th Edn. Washington, DC: American Psychiatric Association.

Anckarsater, H., Stahlberg, O., Larson, T., Hakansson, C., Jutblad, S. B., Niklasson, L., et al. (2006). The impact of ADHD and autism spectrum disorders on temperament, character and personality development. *Am. J. Psychiatry* 163, 1239–1244. doi: 10.1176/appi.ajp.163.7.1239

Atlas, L. Y., and Wager, T. D. (2014). A meta-analysis of brain mechanisms of placebo analgesia: consistent findings and unanswered questions. *Handb. Exp. Pharmacol.* 225, 37–69. doi: 10.1007/978-3-662-44519-8_3

Banich, M. T., Burgess, G. C., Depue, B. E., Ruzic, L., Bidwell, L. C., Hitt-Laustsen, S., et al. (2009). The neural basis of sustained and transient attentional control in young adults with ADHD. *Neuropsychologia* 47, 3095–3104. doi: 10.1016/j.neuropsychologia.2009.07.005

Barkley, R. A. (1997). Behavioral inhibition, sustained attention, and executive functions: constructing a unifying theory of ADHD. *Psychol. Bull.* 121, 65–94. doi: 10.1037/0033-2909.121.1.65

Barkley, R. (2012). *Executive Functions - What They Are, How They Work, and Why They Evolved.* New York, NY: Guilford Publications.

Barkley, R. A., and Murphy, K. R. (2010). Impairment in occupational functioning and adult ADHD: the predictive utility of executive function (EF) ratings versus EF tests. *Arch. Clin. Neuropsychol.* 25, 157–173. doi: 10.1093/arclin/acq014

Baroni, A., and Castellanos, F. X. (2015). Stimulants, cognition and ADHD. *Current Opinion in Behavioral Sciences* 4, 109–114. doi: 10.1016/j.cobeha.2015.04.010

Bingel, U., Lorenz, J., Schoell, E., Weiller, C., and Buchel, C. (2006). Mechanisms of placebo analgesia: rACC recruitment of a subcortical antinociceptive network. *Pain* 120, 8–15. doi: 10.1016/j.pain.2005.08.027

Bishop, S. J. (2009). Trait anxiety and impoverished prefrontal control of attention. *Nat. Neurosci.* 12, 92–98. doi: 10.1038/nn.2242

Björklund, A., and Dunnett, S. B. (2007). Dopamine neuron systems in the brain: an update. *Trends Neurosci.* 30, 194–202. doi: 10.1016/j.tins.2007.03.006

Blair, R. J. (2010). Neuroimaging of psychopathy and antisocial behavior: a targeted review. *Curr. Psychiatry Rep.* 12, 76–82. doi: 10.1007/s11920-009-0086-x

Blair, R. J. (2013). The neurobiology of psychopathic traits in youths. *Nat. Rev. Neurosci.* 14, 786–799. doi: 10.1038/nrn3577

Blair, R. J., Leibenluft, E., and Pine, D. S. (2014). Conduct disorder and callous-unemotional traits in youth. *N. Engl. J. Med.* 371, 2207–2216. doi: 10.1056/nejmra1315612

Brown, R. T., Jaffe, S. L., Silverstein, J., and Magee, H. (1991). Methylphenidate and hospitalized adolescents with conduct disorder: dose effects on classroom behavior, academic performance and impulsivity. *J. Youth Adolesc.* 20, 501–518. doi: 10.1007/bf01540634

Brown, T. E. (1996). *Brown Attention-Deficit Disorder Scales (Manual).* San Antonio, TX: The Psychological Corporation.

Buchel, C., Geuter, S., Sprenger, C., and Eippert, F. (2014). Placebo analgesia: a predictive coding perspective. *Neuron* 81, 1223–1239. doi: 10.1016/j.neuron.2014.02.042

Buhle, J. T., Silvers, J. A., Wager, T. D., Lopez, R., Onyemekwu, C., Kober, H., et al. (2014). Cognitive reappraisal of emotion: a meta-analysis of human neuroimaging studies. *Cereb. Cortex* 24, 2981–2990. doi: 10.1093/cercor/bht154

Bush, G. (2010). Attention-deficit/hyperactivity disorder and attention networks. *Neuropsychopharmacology* 35, 278–300. doi: 10.1038/npp.2009.120

Bush, G., Luu, P., and Posner, M. I. (2000). Cognitive and emotional influences in anterior cingulate cortex. *Trends Cogn. Sci.* 4, 215–222. doi: 10.1016/s1364-6613(00)01483-2

Carmona, S., Hoekzema, E., Ramos-Quiroga, J. A., Richarte, V., Canals, C., Bosch, R., et al. (2012). Response inhibition and reward anticipation in medication-naive adults with attention-deficit/hyperactivity disorder: a within-subject case-control neuroimaging study. *Hum. Brain Mapp.* 33, 2350–2361. doi: 10.1002/hbm.21368

Castellanos, F. X., and Proal, E. (2012). Large-scale brain systems in ADHD: beyond the prefrontal-striatal model. *Trends Cogn. Sci.* 16, 17–26. doi: 10.1016/j.tics.2011.11.007

Castellanos, F. X., Sonuga-Barke, E. J., Milham, M. P., and Tannock, R. (2006). Characterizing cognition in ADHD: beyond executive dysfunction. *Trends Cogn. Sci.* 10, 117–123. doi: 10.1016/j.tics.2006.01.011

Chang, Z., Lichtenstein, P., Halldner, L., D'onofrio, B., Serlachius, E., Fazel, S., et al. (2014). Stimulant ADHD medication and risk for substance abuse. *J. Child Psychol. Psychiatry* 55, 878–885. doi: 10.1111/jcpp.12164

Chen, Q., Sjolander, A., Runeson, B., D'onofrio, B. M., Lichtenstein, P., and Larsson, H. (2014). Drug treatment for attention-deficit/hyperactivity disorder and suicidal behaviour: register based study. *BMJ* 348:g3769. doi: 10.1136/bmj.g3769

Cieslik, E. C., Mueller, V. I., Eickhoff, C. R., Langner, R., and Eickhoff, S. B. (2015). Three key regions for supervisory attentional control: evidence from neuroimaging meta-analyses. *Neurosci. Biobehav. Rev.* 48, 22–34. doi: 10.1016/j.neubiorev.2014.11.003

Coghill, D. R., Seth, S., and Matthews, K. (2014a). A comprehensive assessment of memory, delay aversion, timing, inhibition, decision making and variability in attention deficit hyperactivity disorder: advancing beyond the three-pathway models. *Psychol. Med.* 44, 1989–2001. doi: 10.1017/s0033291713002547

Coghill, D. R., Seth, S., Pedroso, S., Usala, T., Currie, J., and Gagliano, A. (2014b). Effects of methylphenidate on cognitive functions in children and adolescents with attention-deficit/hyperactivity disorder: evidence from a systematic review and a meta-analysis. *Biol. Psychiatry* 76, 603–615. doi: 10.1016/j.biopsych.2013.10.005

Connor, D. F., Barkley, R. A., and Davis, H. T. (2000). A pilot study of methylphenidate, clonidine, or the combination in ADHD comorbid with aggressive oppositional defiant or conduct disorder. *Clin. Pediatr. (Phila)* 39, 15–25. doi: 10.1177/000992280003900102

Cortese, S., Kelly, C., Chabernaud, C., Proal, E., Di Martino, A., Milham, M. P., et al. (2012). Toward systems neuroscience of ADHD: a meta-analysis of 55 fMRI studies. *Am. J. Psychiatry* 169, 1038–1055. doi: 10.1176/appi.ajp.2012.11101521

Craig, A. D. (2002). How do you feel? Interoception: the sense of the physiological condition of the body. *Nat. Rev. Neurosci.* 3, 655–666. doi: 10.1038/nrn894

Craig, A. D. (2009). How do you feel—now? The anterior insula and human awareness. *Nat. Rev. Neurosci.* 10, 59–70. doi: 10.1038/nrn2555

Crosbie, J., Arnold, P., Paterson, A., Swanson, J., Dupuis, A., Li, X., et al. (2013). Response inhibition and ADHD traits: correlates and heritability in a community sample. *J. Abnorm. Child Psychol.* 41, 497–507. doi: 10.1007/s10802-012-9693-9

Cuthbert, B. N., and Insel, T. R. (2013). Toward the future of psychiatric diagnosis: the seven pillars of RDoC. *BMC Med.* 11:126. doi: 10.1186/1741-7015-11-126

Damasio, A. R. (1993). *Descartes' Error: Emotion, Reason and the Human Brain.* New York, NY: Putnam.

Das, D., Cherbuin, N., Butterworth, P., Anstey, K. J., and Easteal, S. (2012). A population-based study of attention deficit/hyperactivity disorder symptoms and associated impairment in middle-aged adults. *PLoS One* 7:e31500. doi: 10.1371/journal.pone.0031500

de Araujo, I. E., Rolls, E. T., Velazco, M. I., Margot, C., and Cayeux, I. (2005). Cognitive modulation of olfactory processing. *Neuron* 46, 671–679. doi: 10.1016/j.neuron.2005.04.021

Dehaene, S., and Changeux, J. P. (2011). Experimental and theoretical approaches to conscious processing. *Neuron* 70, 200–227. doi: 10.1016/j.neuron.2011.03.018

Dickstein, S. G., Bannon, K., Castellanos, F. X., and Milham, M. P. (2006). The neural correlates of attention deficit hyperactivity disorder: an ALE meta-analysis. *J. Child Psychol. Psychiatry* 47, 1051–1062. doi: 10.1111/j.1469-7610.2006.01671.x

Distel, M. A., Carlier, A., Middeldorp, C. M., Derom, C. A., Lubke, G. H., and Boomsma, D. I. (2011). Borderline personality traits and adult attention-deficit hyperactivity disorder symptoms: a genetic analysis of comorbidity. *Am. J. Med. Genet. B Neuropsychiatr. Genet.* 156B, 817–825. doi: 10.3410/f.717952730.793458207

Dolcos, F., and McCarthy, G. (2006). Brain systems mediating cognitive interference by emotional distraction. *J. Neurosci.* 26, 2072–2079. doi: 10.1523/jneurosci.5042-05.2006

Dolcos, F., Iordan, A. D., and Dolcos, S. (2011). Neural correlates of emotion-cognition interactions: a review of evidence from brain imaging investigations. *J. Cogn. Psychol. Hove* 23, 669–694. doi: 10.1080/20445911.2011.594433

Edel, M. A., Enzi, B., Witthaus, H., Tegenthoff, M., Peters, S., Juckel, G., et al. (2013). Differential reward processing in subtypes of adult attention deficit hyperactivity disorder. *J. Psychiatr. Res.* 47, 350–356. doi: 10.1016/j.jpsychires.2012.09.026

Egner, T., Etkin, A., Gale, S., and Hirsch, J. (2008). Dissociable neural systems resolve conflict from emotional versus nonemotional distracters. *Cereb. Cortex* 18, 1475–1484. doi: 10.1093/cercor/bhm179

Eippert, F., Bingel, U., Schoell, E. D., Yacubian, J., Klinger, R., Lorenz, J., et al. (2009). Activation of the opioidergic descending pain control system underlies placebo analgesia. *Neuron* 63, 533–543. doi: 10.1016/j.neuron.2009.07.014

Eippert, F., Veit, R., Weiskopf, N., Erb, M., Birbaumer, N., and Anders, S. (2007). Regulation of emotional responses elicited by threat-related stimuli. *Hum. Brain Mapp.* 28, 409–423. doi: 10.1002/hbm.20291

Eisenberger, N. I. (2012). The pain of social disconnection: examining the shared neural underpinnings of physical and social pain. *Nat. Rev. Neurosci.* 13, 421–434. doi: 10.1038/nrn3231

Ellingsen, D. M., Wessberg, J., Eikemo, M., Liljencrantz, J., Endestad, T., Olausson, H., et al. (2013). Placebo improves pleasure and pain through opposite modulation of sensory processing. *Proc. Natl. Acad. Sci. U S A* 110, 17993–17998. doi: 10.1073/pnas.1305050110

Engel, A. K., Fries, P., and Singer, W. (2001). Dynamic predictions: oscillations and synchrony in top-down processing. *Nat. Rev. Neurosci.* 2, 704–716. doi: 10.1038/35094565

Enzi, B., Doering, S., Faber, C., Hinrichs, J., Bahmer, J., and Northoff, G. (2013). Reduced deactivation in reward circuitry and midline structures during emotion processing in borderline personality disorder. *World J. Biol. Psychiatry* 14, 45–56. doi: 10.3109/15622975.2011.579162

Ersche, K. D., Jones, P. S., Williams, G. B., Smith, D. G., Bullmore, E. T., and Robbins, T. W. (2013). Distinctive personality traits and neural correlates associated with stimulant drug use versus familial risk of stimulant dependence. *Biol. Psychiatry* 74, 137–144. doi: 10.1016/j.biopsych.2012.11.016

Ersche, K. D., Jones, P. S., Williams, G. B., Turton, A. J., Robbins, T. W., and Bullmore, E. T. (2012). Abnormal brain structure implicated in stimulant drug addiction. *Science* 335, 601–604. doi: 10.1126/science.1214463

Ersche, K. D., Turton, A. J., Pradhan, S., Bullmore, E. T., and Robbins, T. W. (2010). Drug addiction endophenotypes: impulsive versus sensation-seeking personality traits. *Biol. Psychiatry* 68, 770–773. doi: 10.1016/j.biopsych.2010.06.015

Etkin, A., Egner, T., and Kalisch, R. (2011). Emotional processing in anterior cingulate and medial prefrontal cortex. *Trends Cogn. Sci.* 15, 85–93. doi: 10.1016/j.tics.2010.11.004

Etkin, A., Egner, T., Peraza, D. M., Kandel, E. R., and Hirsch, J. (2006). Resolving emotional conflict: a role for the rostral anterior cingulate cortex in modulating activity in the amygdala. *Neuron* 51, 871–882. doi: 10.1016/j.neuron.2006.12.003

Euler, F., Sterzer, P., and Stadler, C. (2014). Cognitive control under distressing emotional stimulation in adolescents with conduct disorder. *Aggress. Behav.* 40, 109–119. doi: 10.1002/ab.21508

Fields, H. (2004). State-dependent opioid control of pain. *Nat. Rev. Neurosci.* 5, 565–575. doi: 10.1038/nrn1431

Fox, M. D., Snyder, A. Z., Vincent, J. L., Corbetta, M., Van Essen, D. C., and Raichle, M. E. (2005). The human brain is intrinsically organized into dynamic, anticorrelated functional networks. *Proc. Natl. Acad. Sci. U S A* 102, 9673–9678. doi: 10.1073/pnas.0504136102

Fransson, P. (2005). Spontaneous low-frequency BOLD signal fluctuations: an fMRI investigation of the resting-state default mode of brain function hypothesis. *Hum. Brain Mapp.* 26, 15–29. doi: 10.1002/hbm.20113

Furukawa, E., Bado, P., Tripp, G., Mattos, P., Wickens, J. R., Bramati, I. E., et al. (2014). Abnormal striatal BOLD responses to reward anticipation and reward delivery in ADHD. *PLoS One* 9:e89129. doi: 10.1371/journal.pone.0089129

Fuster, J. M. (2000). Executive frontal functions. *Exp. Brain Res.* 133, 66–70. doi: 10.1007/s002210000401

Fuster, J. M. (2004). Upper processing stages of the perception-action cycle. *Trends Cogn. Sci.* 8, 143–145. doi: 10.1016/j.tics.2004.02.004

Fuster, J. M., and Bressler, S. L. (2012). Cognit activation: a mechanism enabling temporal integration in working memory. *Trends Cogn. Sci. Regul. Ed.* 16, 207–218. doi: 10.1016/j.tics.2012.03.005

Gazzaniga, M. E. (2014). *The Cognitive Neurosciences.* Cambridge, MA: MIT Press.

Glenn, A. L., and Raine, A. (2014). Neurocriminology: implications for the punishment, prediction and prevention of criminal behaviour. *Nat. Rev. Neurosci.* 15, 54–63. doi: 10.1038/nrn3640

Goldstein, S., and Naglieri, A. (2014). *Handbook of Executive Functioning.* New York, NY: Springer-Verlag.

Golkar, A., Lonsdorf, T. B., Olsson, A., Lindstrom, K. M., Berrebi, J., Fransson, P., et al. (2012). Distinct contributions of the dorsolateral prefrontal and orbitofrontal cortex during emotion regulation. *PLoS One* 7:e48107. doi: 10.1371/journal.pone.0048107

Golubchik, P., Sever, J., Zalsman, G., and Weizman, A. (2008). Methylphenidate in the treatment of female adolescents with cooccurrence of attention deficit/hyperactivity disorder and borderline personality disorder: a preliminary open-label trial. *Int. Clin. Psychopharmacol.* 23, 228–231. doi: 10.1097/yic.0b013e3282f94ae2

Gottfried, J. A., O'Doherty, J., and Dolan, R. J. (2003). Encoding predictive reward value in human amygdala and orbitofrontal cortex. *Science* 301, 1104–1107. doi: 10.1126/science.1087919

Graybiel, A. M. (2008). Habits, rituals and the evaluative brain. *Annu. Rev. Neurosci.* 31, 359–387. doi: 10.1146/annurev.neuro.29.051605.112851

Gyurak, A., Gross, J. J., and Etkin, A. (2011). Explicit and implicit emotion regulation: a dual-process framework. *Cogn. Emot.* 25, 400–412. doi: 10.1080/02699931.2010.544160

Haber, S. N., and Behrens, T. E. (2014). The neural network underlying incentive-based learning: implications for interpreting circuit disruptions in psychiatric disorders. *Neuron* 83, 1019–1039. doi: 10.1016/j.neuron.2014.08.031

Haber, S. N., and Knutson, B. (2010). The reward circuit: linking primate anatomy and human imaging. *Neuropsychopharmacology* 35, 4–26. doi: 10.1038/npp.2009.129

Hart, H., Radua, J., Nakao, T., Mataix-Cols, D., and Rubia, K. (2013). Meta-analysis of functional magnetic resonance imaging studies of inhibition and attention in attention-deficit/hyperactivity disorder: exploring task-specific, stimulant medication and age effects. *JAMA Psychiatry* 70, 185–198. doi: 10.1001/jamapsychiatry.2013.277

Hartley, C. A., and Phelps, E. A. (2010). Changing fear: the neurocircuitry of emotion regulation. *Neuropsychopharmacology* 35, 136–146. doi: 10.1038/npp.2009.121

Holtmann, J., Herbort, M. C., Wustenberg, T., Soch, J., Richter, S., Walter, H., et al. (2013). Trait anxiety modulates fronto-limbic processing of emotional interference in borderline personality disorder. *Front. Hum. Neurosci.* 7:54. doi: 10.3389/fnhum.2013.00054

Hulvershorn, L. A., Mennes, M., Castellanos, F. X., Di Martino, A., Milham, M. P., Hummer, T. A., et al. (2014). Abnormal amygdala functional connectivity associated with emotional lability in children with attention-deficit/hyperactivity disorder. *J. Am. Acad. Child Adolesc. Psychiatry* 53, 351–361.e351. doi: 10.1016/j.jaac.2013.11.012

Indovina, I., Robbins, T. W., Nunez-Elizalde, A. O., Dunn, B. D., and Bishop, S. J. (2011). Fear-conditioning mechanisms associated with trait vulnerability to anxiety in humans. *Neuron* 69, 563–571. doi: 10.1016/j.neuron.2010.12.034

Insel, T., Cuthbert, B., Garvey, M., Heinssen, R., Pine, D. S., Quinn, K., et al. (2010). Research domain criteria (RDoC): toward a new classification framework for research on mental disorders. *Am. J. Psychiatry* 167, 748–751. doi: 10.1176/appi.ajp.2010.09091379

Jacob, G. A., Zvonik, K., Kamphausen, S., Sebastian, A., Maier, S., Philipsen, A., et al. (2013). Emotional modulation of motor response inhibition in women with borderline personality disorder: an fMRI study. *J. Psychiatry Neurosci.* 38, 164–172. doi: 10.1503/jpn.120029

James, W. (1890). *The Principles of Psychology. Classics in the History of Psychology [online].* Available online at: http://psychclassics.yorku.ca/James/Principles.

Kable, J. W., and Glimcher, P. W. (2007). The neural correlates of subjective value during intertemporal choice. *Nat Neurosci* 10, 1625–1633. doi: 10.1038/nn2007

Kanske, P., Heissler, J., Schonfelder, S., Bongers, A., and Wessa, M. (2011). How to regulate emotion? Neural networks for reappraisal and distraction. *Cereb. Cortex* 21, 1379–1388. doi: 10.1093/cercor/bhq216

Kaplan, S. L., Busner, J., Kupietz, S., Wassermann, E., and Segal, B. (1990). Effects of methylphenidate on adolescents with aggressive conduct disorder and ADDH: a preliminary report. *J. Am. Acad. Child. Adolesc. Psychiatry* 29, 719–723. doi: 10.1097/00004583-199009000-00007

Kappel, V., Lorenz, R. C., Streifling, M., Renneberg, B., Lehmkuhl, U., Strohle, A., et al. (2015). Effect of brain structure and function on reward anticipation in children and adults with attention deficit hyperactivity disorder combined subtype. *Soc. Cogn. Affect. Neurosci.* 10, 945–951. doi: 10.1093/scan/nsu135

Kerns, J. G., Cohen, J. D., MacDonald, A. W., Cho, R. Y., Stenger, V. A., and Carter, C. S. (2004). Anterior cingulate conflict monitoring and adjustments in control. *Science* 303, 1023–1026. doi: 10.1126/science.1089910

Kerr, A., and Zelazo, P. D. (2004). Development of "hot" executive function: the children's gambling task. *Brain Cogn.* 55, 148–157. doi: 10.1016/s0278-2626(03)00275-6

Klein, D. F. (1999). Harmful dysfunction, disorder, disease, illness and evolution. *J. Abnorm. Psychol.* 108, 421–429. doi: 10.1037/0021-843x.108.3.421

Klein, R. G., Abikoff, H., Klass, E., Ganeles, D., Seese, L. M., and Pollack, S. (1997). Clinical efficacy of methylphenidate in conduct disorder with and without attention deficit hyperactivity disorder. *Arch. Gen. Psychiatry* 54, 1073–1080. doi: 10.1001/archpsyc.1997.01830240023003

Krause-Utz, A., Oei, N. Y., Niedtfeld, I., Bohus, M., Spinhoven, P., Schmahl, C., et al. (2012). Influence of emotional distraction on working memory performance in borderline personality disorder. *Psychol. Med.* 42, 2181–2192. doi: 10.1017/s0033291712000153

Krause-Utz, A., Winter, D., Niedtfeld, I., and Schmahl, C. (2014). The latest neuroimaging findings in borderline personality disorder. *Curr. Psychiatry Rep.* 16:438. doi: 10.1007/s11920-014-0438-z

Kringelbach, M. L. (2005). The human orbitofrontal cortex: linking reward to hedonic experience. *Nat. Rev. Neurosci.* 6, 691–702. doi: 10.1038/nrn1747

Kringelbach, M. L., and Rolls, E. T. (2004). The functional neuroanatomy of the human orbitofrontal cortex: evidence from neuroimaging and neuropsychology. *Prog. Neurobiol.* 72, 341–372. doi: 10.1016/j.pneurobio.2004.03.006

Kringelbach, M. L., O'Doherty, J., Rolls, E. T., and Andrews, C. (2003). Activation of the human orbitofrontal cortex to a liquid food stimulus is correlated with its subjective pleasantness. *Cereb. Cortex* 13, 1064–1071. doi: 10.1093/cercor/13.10.1064

Lang, S., Kotchoubey, B., Frick, C., Spitzer, C., Grabe, H. J., and Barnow, S. (2012). Cognitive reappraisal in trauma-exposed women with borderline personality disorder. *Neuroimage* 59, 1727–1734. doi: 10.1016/j.neuroimage.2011.08.061

Lansbergen, M. M., Kenemans, J. L., and van Engeland, H. (2007). Stroop interference and attention-deficit/hyperactivity disorder: a review and meta-analysis. *Neuropsychology* 21, 251–262. doi: 10.1037/0894-4105.21.2.251

Levy, F., Hay, D. A., Mcstephen, M., Wood, C., and Waldman, I. (1997). Attention-deficit hyperactivity disorder: a category or a continuum? Genetic analysis of a large-scale twin study. *J. Am. Acad. Child Adolesc. Psychiatry* 36, 737–744. doi: 10.1097/00004583-199706000-00009

Lichtenstein, P., Halldner, L., Zetterqvist, J., Sjolander, A., Serlachius, E., Fazel, S., et al. (2012). Medication for attention deficit-hyperactivity disorder and criminality. *N. Engl. J. Med.* 367, 2006–2014. doi: 10.1056/NEJMoa1203241

Lieberman, M. D., Jarcho, J. M., Berman, S., Naliboff, B. D., Suyenobu, B. Y., Mandelkern, M., et al. (2004). The neural correlates of placebo effects: a disruption account. *Neuroimage* 22, 447–455. doi: 10.1016/j.neuroimage.2004.01.037

Lundqvist, D., Flykt, A., and Öhman, A. (1998). The karolinska directed emotional faces - KDEF, CD ROM from department of clinical neuroscience, psychology section, Karolinska Institutet. ISBN 91-630-7164-9.

Mesulam, M. (2012). The evolving landscape of human cortical connectivity: facts and inferences. *Neuroimage* 62, 2182–2189. doi: 10.1016/j.neuroimage.2011.12.033

Mesulam, M. M. (1998). From sensation to cognition. *Brain* 121, 1013–1052. doi: 10.1016/b978-0-12-178602-1.50003-8

Milad, M. R., and Quirk, G. J. (2012). Fear extinction as a model for translational neuroscience: ten years of progress. *Annu. Rev. Psychol.* 63, 129–151. doi: 10.1146/annurev.psych.121208.131631

Morein-Zamir, S., Simon Jones, P., Bullmore, E. T., Robbins, T. W., and Ersche, K. D. (2013). Prefrontal hypoactivity associated with impaired inhibition in stimulant-dependent individuals but evidence for hyperactivation in their unaffected siblings. *Neuropsychopharmacology* 38, 1945–1953. doi: 10.1038/npp.2013.90

Murray, E. A., O'Doherty, J. P., and Schoenbaum, G. (2007). What we know and do not know about the functions of the orbitofrontal cortex after 20 years of cross-species studies. *J. Neurosci.* 27, 8166–8169. doi: 10.1523/jneurosci.1556-07.2007

Nee, D. E., Wager, T. D., and Jonides, J. (2007). Interference resolution: insights from a meta-analysis of neuroimaging tasks. *Cogn. Affect. Behav. Neurosci.* 7, 1–17. doi: 10.3758/cabn.7.1.1

Nichols, S. L., and Waschbusch, D. A. (2004). A review of the validity of laboratory cognitive tasks used to assess symptoms of ADHD. *Child Psychiatry Hum. Dev.* 34, 297–315. doi: 10.1023/b:chud.0000020681.06865.97

Ochsner, K. N., Hughes, B., Robertson, E. R., Cooper, J. C., and Gabrieli, J. D. (2009). Neural systems supporting the control of affective and cognitive conflicts. *J. Cogn. Neurosci.* 21, 1842–1855. doi: 10.1162/jocn.2009.21129

Ochsner, K. N., Silvers, J. A., and Buhle, J. T. (2012). Functional imaging studies of emotion regulation: a synthetic review and evolving model of the cognitive control of emotion. *Ann. N. Y. Acad. Sci.* 1251, E1–24. doi: 10.1111/j.1749-6632.2012.06751.x

O'Doherty, J., Kringelbach, M. L., Rolls, E. T., Hornak, J., and Andrews, C. (2001). Abstract reward and punishment representations in the human orbitofrontal cortex. *Nat. Neurosci.* 4, 95–102. doi: 10.1038/82959

O'Doherty, J. P., Buchanan, T. W., Seymour, B., and Dolan, R. J. (2006). Predictive neural coding of reward preference involves dissociable responses in human ventral midbrain and ventral striatum. *Neuron* 49, 157–166. doi: 10.1016/j.neuron.2005.11.014

O'Doherty, J. P., Dayan, P., Friston, K., Critchley, H., and Dolan, R. J. (2003). Temporal difference models and reward-related learning in the human brain. *Neuron* 38, 329–337. doi: 10.1016/s0896-6273(03)00169-7

Okon-Singer, H., Hendler, T., Pessoa, L., and Shackman, A. J. (2015). The neurobiology of emotion-cognition interactions: fundamental questions and strategies for future research. *Front. Hum. Neurosci.* 9:58. doi: 10.3389/fnhum.2015.00058

Ongur, D., and Price, J. L. (2000). The organization of networks within the orbital and medial prefrontal cortex of rats, monkeys and humans. *Cereb. Cortex* 10, 206–219. doi: 10.1093/cercor/10.3.206

Ongur, D., Ferry, A. T., and Price, J. L. (2003). Architectonic subdivision of the human orbital and medial prefrontal cortex. *J. Comp. Neurol.* 460, 425–449. doi: 10.1002/cne.10609

Paulus, M. P., and Stein, M. B. (2006). An insular view of anxiety. *Biol. Psychiatry* 60, 383–387. doi: 10.1016/j.biopsych.2006.03.042

Paulus, M. P., Feinstein, J. S., Castillo, G., Simmons, A. N., and Stein, M. B. (2005). Dose-dependent decrease of activation in bilateral amygdala and insula by lorazepam during emotion processing. *Arch. Gen. Psychiatry* 62, 282–288. doi: 10.1001/archpsyc.62.3.282

Perini, I., Bergstrand, S., and Morrison, I. (2013). Where pain meets action in the human brain. *J. Neurosci.* 33, 15930–15939. doi: 10.1523/jneurosci.3135-12.2013

Pessiglione, M., Seymour, B., Flandin, G., Dolan, R. J., and Frith, C. D. (2006). Dopamine-dependent prediction errors underpin reward-seeking behaviour in humans. *Nature* 442, 1042–1045. doi: 10.1038/nature05051

Pessoa, L. (2008). On the relationship between emotion and cognition. *Nat. Rev. Neurosci.* 9, 148–158. doi: 10.1038/nrn2317

Petrovic, P., Dietrich, T., Fransson, P., Andersson, J., Carlsson, K., and Ingvar, M. (2005). Placebo in emotional processing—induced expectations of anxiety relief activate a generalized modulatory network. *Neuron* 46, 957–969. doi: 10.1016/j.neuron.2005.05.023

Petrovic, P., Ekman, C. J., Klahr, J., Tigerstrom, L., Ryden, G., Johansson, A. G., et al. (2015). Significant grey matter changes in a region of the orbitofrontal cortex in healthy participants predicts emotional dysregulation. *Soc. Cogn. Affect. Neurosci.* doi: 10.1093/scan/nsv072 [Epub ahead of print].

Petrovic, P., Kalso, E., Petersson, K. M., and Ingvar, M. (2002). Placebo and opioid analgesia—imaging a shared neuronal network. *Science* 295, 1737–1740. doi: 10.1126/science.1067176

Petrovic, P., Kalso, E., Petersson, K. M., Andersson, J., Fransson, P., and Ingvar, M. (2010). A prefrontal non-opioid mechanism in placebo analgesia. *Pain* 150, 59–65. doi: 10.1016/j.pain.2010.03.011

Petrovic, P., Pleger, B., Seymour, B., Kloppel, S., De Martino, B., Critchley, H., et al. (2008). Blocking central opiate function modulates hedonic impact and anterior cingulate response to rewards and losses. *J. Neurosci.* 28, 10509–10516. doi: 10.1523/jneurosci.2807-08.2008

Philipsen, A., Limberger, M. F., Lieb, K., Feige, B., Kleindienst, N., Ebner-Priemer, U., et al. (2008). Attention-deficit hyperactivity disorder as a potentially aggravating factor in borderline personality disorder. *Br. J. Psychiatry* 192, 118–123. doi: 10.1192/bjp.bp.107.035782

Plassmann, H., O'Doherty, J., Shiv, B., and Rangel, A. (2008). Marketing actions can modulate neural representations of experienced pleasantness. *Proc. Natl. Acad. Sci. U S A* 105, 1050–1054. doi: 10.1073/pnas.0706929105

Plichta, M. M., and Scheres, A. (2014). Ventral-striatal responsiveness during reward anticipation in ADHD and its relation to trait impulsivity in the healthy population: a meta-analytic review of the fMRI literature. *Neurosci. Biobehav. Rev.* 38, 125–134. doi: 10.1016/j.neubiorev.2013.07.012

Plichta, M. M., and Scheres, A. (2015). Measuring the neural basis of reward anticipation and reward receipt in attention-deficit/hyperactivity disorder: the importance of task design. *J. Am. Acad. Child Adolesc. Psychiatry* 54, 685–686. doi: 10.1016/j.jaac.2015.05.012

Prada, P., Nicastro, R., Zimmermann, J., Hasler, R., Aubry, J. M., and Perroud, N. (2015). Addition of methylphenidate to intensive dialectical behaviour therapy for patients suffering from comorbid borderline personality disorder and ADHD: a naturalistic study. *Atten. Defic. Hyperact. Disord.* 7, 199–209. doi: 10.1007/s12402-015-0165-2

Prehn, K., Schulze, L., Rossmann, S., Berger, C., Vohs, K., Fleischer, M., et al. (2013). Effects of emotional stimuli on working memory processes in male criminal offenders with borderline and antisocial personality disorder. *World J. Biol. Psychiatry* 14, 71–78. doi: 10.3109/15622975.2011.584906

Rahm, C., Liberg, B., Wiberg-Kristoffersen, M., Aspelin, P., and Msghina, M. (2013). Rostro-caudal and dorso-ventral gradients in medial and lateral prefrontal cortex during cognitive control of affective and cognitive interference. *Scand. J. Psychol.* 54, 66–71. doi: 10.1111/sjop.12023

Robbins, T. W., Gillan, C. M., Smith, D. G., De Wit, S., and Ersche, K. D. (2012). Neurocognitive endophenotypes of impulsivity and compulsivity: towards dimensional psychiatry. *Trends Cogn. Sci.* 16, 81–91. doi: 10.1016/j.tics.2011.11.009

Roelofs, A., van Turennout, M., and Coles, M. G. (2006). Anterior cingulate cortex activity can be independent of response conflict in Stroop-like tasks. *Proc. Natl. Acad. Sci. U S A* 103, 13884–13889. doi: 10.1073/pnas.0606265103

Rubia, K. (2011). "Cool" inferior frontostriatal dysfunction in attention-deficit/hyperactivity disorder versus "hot" ventromedial orbitofrontal-limbic dysfunction in conduct disorder: a review. *Biol. Psychiatry* 69, e69–e87. doi: 10.1016/j.biopsych.2010.09.023

Rubia, K., Halari, R., Christakou, A., and Taylor, E. (2009). Impulsiveness as a timing disturbance: neurocognitive abnormalities in attention-deficit hyperactivity disorder during temporal processes and normalization with methylphenidate. *Philos. Trans. R. Soc. Lond. B. Biol. Sci.* 364, 1919–1931. doi: 10.1098/rstb.2009.0014

Rudebeck, P. H., and Murray, E. A. (2014). The orbitofrontal oracle: cortical mechanisms for the prediction and evaluation of specific behavioral outcomes. *Neuron* 84, 1143–1156. doi: 10.1016/j.neuron.2014.10.049

Ruff, C. C., and Fehr, E. (2014). The neurobiology of rewards and values in social decision making. *Nat. Rev. Neurosci.* 15, 549–562. doi: 10.1038/nrn3776

Rutgen, M., Seidel, E. M., Silani, G., Riecansky, I., Hummer, A., Windischberger, C., et al. (2015). Placebo analgesia and its opioidergic regulation suggest that empathy for pain is grounded in self pain. *Proc. Natl. Acad. Sci. U S A* 112, E5638–5646. doi: 10.1073/pnas.1511269112

Salum, G. A., Sonuga-Barke, E., Sergeant, J., Vandekerckhove, J., Gadelha, A., Moriyama, T. S., et al. (2014). Mechanisms underpinning inattention and hyperactivity: neurocognitive support for ADHD dimensionality. *Psychol. Med.* 44, 3189–3201. doi: 10.1017/s0033291714000919

Scheres, A., Milham, M. P., Knutson, B., and Castellanos, F. X. (2007). Ventral striatal hyporesponsiveness during reward anticipation in attention-deficit/hyperactivity disorder. *Biol. Psychiatry* 61, 720–724. doi: 10.1016/j.biopsych.2006.04.042

Schiller, D., and Delgado, M. R. (2010). Overlapping neural systems mediating extinction, reversal and regulation of fear. *Trends Cogn. Sci. Regul. Ed.* 14, 268–276. doi: 10.1016/j.tics.2010.04.002

Schoenbaum, G., and Roesch, M. (2005). Orbitofrontal cortex, associative learning and expectancies. *Neuron* 47, 633–636. doi: 10.1016/j.neuron.2005.07.018

Schoenbaum, G., Roesch, M. R., Stalnaker, T. A., and Takahashi, Y. K. (2009). A new perspective on the role of the orbitofrontal cortex in adaptive behaviour. *Nat. Rev. Neurosci.* 10, 885–892. doi: 10.1038/nrn2753

Schultz, W. (2007). Behavioral dopamine signals. *Trends Neurosci.* 30, 203–210. doi: 10.1016/j.tins.2007.03.007

Schultz, W., Dayan, P., and Montague, P. R. (1997). A neural substrate of prediction and reward. *Science* 275, 1593–1599. doi: 10.1126/science.275.5306.1593

Schulz, S. C., Cornelius, J., Schulz, P. M., and Soloff, P. H. (1988). The amphetamine challenge test in patients with borderline disorder. *Am. J. Psychiatry* 145, 809–814. doi: 10.1176/ajp.145.7.809

Schulze, L., Domes, G., Kruger, A., Berger, C., Fleischer, M., Prehn, K., et al. (2011). Neuronal correlates of cognitive reappraisal in borderline patients with affective instability. *Biol. Psychiatry* 69, 564–573. doi: 10.1016/j.biopsych.2010.10.025

Schumann, G., Loth, E., Banaschewski, T., Barbot, A., Barker, G., Buchel, C., et al. (2010). The IMAGEN study: reinforcement-related behaviour in normal brain function and psychopathology. *Mol. Psychiatry* 15, 1128–1139. doi: 10.1038/mp.2010.4

Scott, D. J., Stohler, C. S., Egnatuk, C. M., Wang, H., Koeppe, R. A., and Zubieta, J. K. (2008). Placebo and nocebo effects are defined by opposite opioid and dopaminergic responses. *Arch. Gen. Psychiatry* 65, 220–231. doi: 10.1001/archgenpsychiatry.2007.34

Sebastian, A., Jung, P., Krause-Utz, A., Lieb, K., Schmahl, C., and Tuscher, O. (2014). Frontal dysfunctions of impulse control - a systematic review in borderline personality disorder and attention-deficit/hyperactivity disorder. *Front. Hum. Neurosci.* 8:698. doi: 10.3389/fnhum.2014.00698

Seidman, L. J., Biederman, J., Liang, L., Valera, E. M., Monuteaux, M. C., Brown, A., et al. (2011). Gray matter alterations in adults with attention-deficit/hyperactivity disorder identified by voxel based morphometry. *Biol. Psychiatry* 69, 857–866. doi: 10.1016/j.pscychresns.2010.08.011

Semiz, U. B., Basoglu, C., Oner, O., Munir, K. M., Ates, A., Algul, A., et al. (2008). Effects of diagnostic comorbidity and dimensional symptoms of attention-deficit-hyperactivity disorder in men with antisocial personality disorder. *Aust. N. Z. J. Psychiatry* 42, 405–413. doi: 10.1080/00048670801961099

Seymour, B., O'Doherty, J. P., Koltzenburg, M., Wiech, K., Frackowiak, R., Friston, K., et al. (2005). Opponent appetitive-aversive neural processes underlie predictive learning of pain relief. *Nat. Neurosci.* 8, 1234–1240. doi: 10.1038/nn1527

Shackman, A. J., Salomons, T. V., Slagter, H. A., Fox, A. S., Winter, J. J., and Davidson, R. J. (2011). The integration of negative affect, pain and cognitive control in the cingulate cortex. *Nat. Rev. Neurosci.* 12, 154–167. doi: 10.1038/nrn2994

Shaw, P., Eckstrand, K., Sharp, W., Blumenthal, J., Lerch, J. P., Greenstein, D., et al. (2007). Attention-deficit/hyperactivity disorder is characterized by a delay in cortical maturation. *Proc. Natl. Acad. Sci. U S A* 104, 19649–19654. doi: 10.1073/pnas.0707741104

Shaw, P., Malek, M., Watson, B., Greenstein, D., De Rossi, P., and Sharp, W. (2013). Trajectories of cerebral cortical development in childhood and adolescence and adult attention-deficit/hyperactivity disorder. *Biol. Psychiatry* 74, 599–606. doi: 10.1016/j.biopsych.2013.04.007

Shaw, P., Sharp, W. S., Morrison, M., Eckstrand, K., Greenstein, D. K., Clasen, L. S., et al. (2009). Psychostimulant treatment and the developing cortex in attention deficit hyperactivity disorder. *Am. J. Psychiatry* 166, 58–63. doi: 10.1176/appi.ajp.2008.08050781

Siegel, M., Donner, T. H., and Engel, A. K. (2012). Spectral fingerprints of large-scale neuronal interactions. *Nat. Rev. Neurosci.* 13, 121–134. doi: 10.1038/nrn3137

Silbersweig, D., Clarkin, J. F., Goldstein, M., Kernberg, O. F., Tuescher, O., Levy, K. N., et al. (2007). Failure of frontolimbic inhibitory function in the context of negative emotion in borderline personality disorder. *Am. J. Psychiatry* 164, 1832–1841.

Simpson, J. R., Ongur, D., Akbudak, E., Conturo, T. E., Ollinger, J. M., Snyder, A. Z., et al. (2000). The emotional modulation of cognitive processing: an fMRI study. *J. Cogn. Neurosci.* 12, 157–170. doi: 10.1162/089892900564019

Singer, T., Seymour, B., O'Doherty, J., Kaube, H., Dolan, R. J., and Frith, C. D. (2004). Empathy for pain involves the affective but not sensory components of pain. *Science* 303, 1157–1162. doi: 10.1126/science.1093535

Singer, T., Seymour, B., O'Doherty, J. P., Stephan, K. E., Dolan, R. J., and Frith, C. D. (2006). Empathic neural responses are modulated by the perceived fairness of others. *Nature* 439, 466–469. doi: 10.1038/nature04271

Small, D. M., Zatorre, R. J., Dagher, A., Evans, A. C., and Jones-Gotman, M. (2001). Changes in brain activity related to eating chocolate: from pleasure to aversion. *Brain* 124, 1720–1733. doi: 10.1093/brain/124.9.1720

Smoski, M. J., Salsman, N., Wang, L., Smith, V., Lynch, T. R., Dager, S. R., et al. (2011). Functional imaging of emotion reactivity in opiate-dependent borderline personality disorder. *Personal Disord.* 2, 230–241. doi: 10.1037/a0022228.supp

Soloff, P., Nutche, J., Goradia, D., and Diwadkar, V. (2008). Structural brain abnormalities in borderline personality disorder: a voxel-based morphometry study. *Psychiatry Res.* 164, 223–236. doi: 10.1016/j.pscychresns.2008.02.003

Soloff, P. H., Pruitt, P., Sharma, M., Radwan, J., White, R., and Diwadkar, V. A. (2012). Structural brain abnormalities and suicidal behavior in borderline personality disorder. *J. Psychiatr. Res.* 46, 516–525. doi: 10.1016/j.jpsychires.2012.01.003

Sonuga-Barke, E. J. (2002). Psychological heterogeneity in AD/HD—a dual pathway model of behaviour and cognition. *Behav. Brain Res.* 130, 29–36. doi: 10.1016/s0166-4328(01)00432-6

Stark, R., Bauer, E., Merz, C. J., Zimmermann, M., Reuter, M., Plichta, M. M., et al. (2011). ADHD related behaviors are associated with brain activation in the reward system. *Neuropsychologia* 49, 426–434. doi: 10.1016/j.neuropsychologia.2010.12.012

Strohle, A., Stoy, M., Wrase, J., Schwarzer, S., Schlagenhauf, F., Huss, M., et al. (2008). Reward anticipation and outcomes in adult males with attention-deficit/hyperactivity disorder. *Neuroimage* 39, 966–972. doi: 10.1016/j.neuroimage.2007.09.044

Swanson, J., Baler, R. D., and Volkow, N. D. (2011). Understanding the effects of stimulant medications on cognition in individuals with attention-deficit hyperactivity disorder: a decade of progress. *Neuropsychopharmacology* 36, 207–226. doi: 10.1038/npp.2010.160

Swanson, J. M., Kinsbourne, M., Nigg, J., Lanphear, B., Stefanatos, G. A., Volkow, N., et al. (2007). Etiologic subtypes of attention-deficit/hyperactivity disorder: brain imaging, molecular genetic and environmental factors and the dopamine hypothesis. *Neuropsychol. Rev.* 17, 39–59. doi: 10.1007/s11065-007-9019-9

Thorell, L. B. (2007). Do delay aversion and executive function deficits make distinct contributions to the functional impact of ADHD symptoms? A study of early academic skill deficits. *J. Child Psychol. Psychiatry* 48, 1061–1070. doi: 10.1111/j.1469-7610.2007.01777.x

Vogt, B., Sikes, R., and Vogt, L. (1993). "Anterior cingulate cortex and the medial pain system," in *Neurobiology of Cingulate Cortex and Limbic Thalamus: A Comprehensive Handbook*, eds B. A. Vogt and M. Gabriel (Boston, MA: Birkhaüser), 313–344.

Volkow, N. D., Wang, G. J., Kollins, S. H., Wigal, T. L., Newcorn, J. H., Telang, F., et al. (2009). Evaluating dopamine reward pathway in ADHD: clinical implications. *JAMA* 302, 1084–1091. doi: 10.1001/jama.302.13.1420-a

Vollm, B., Richardson, P., Mckie, S., Elliott, R., Dolan, M., and Deakin, B. (2007). Neuronal correlates of reward and loss in Cluster B personality disorders: a functional magnetic resonance imaging study. *Psychiatry Res.* 156, 151–167. doi: 10.1016/j.pscychresns.2007.04.008

von Rhein, D., Cools, R., Zwiers, M. P., Van Der Schaaf, M., Franke, B., Luman, M., et al. (2015). Increased neural responses to reward in adolescents and young adults with attention-deficit/hyperactivity disorder and their unaffected siblings. *J. Am. Acad. Child Adolesc. Psychiatry* 54, 394–402. doi: 10.1016/j.jaac.2015.02.012

Vuilleumier, P. (2015). Affective and motivational control of vision. *Curr. Opin. Neurol.* 28, 29–35. doi: 10.1097/wco.0000000000000159

Vuilleumier, P., and Driver, J. (2007). Modulation of visual processing by attention and emotion: windows on causal interactions between human brain regions. *Philos. Trans. R. Soc. Lond. B Biol. Sci.* 362, 837–855. doi: 10.1098/rstb.2007.2092

Wager, T. D., and Atlas, L. Y. (2015). The neuroscience of placebo effects: connecting context, learning and health. *Nat. Rev. Neurosci.* 16, 403–418. doi: 10.1038/nrn3976

Wager, T. D., Atlas, L. Y., Lindquist, M. A., Roy, M., Woo, C. W., and Kross, E. (2013). An fMRI-based neurologic signature of physical pain. *N. Engl. J. Med.* 368, 1388–1397. doi: 10.1056/NEJMoa1204471

Wager, T. D., Davidson, M. L., Hughes, B. L., Lindquist, M. A., and Ochsner, K. N. (2008). Prefrontal-subcortical pathways mediating successful emotion regulation. *Neuron* 59, 1037–1050. doi: 10.1016/j.neuron.2008.09.006

Wager, T. D., Rilling, J. K., Smith, E. E., Sokolik, A., Casey, K. L., Davidson, R. J., et al. (2004). Placebo-induced changes in FMRI in the anticipation and experience of pain. *Science* 303, 1162–1167. doi: 10.1126/science.1093065

Wager, T. D., Scott, D. J., and Zubieta, J. K. (2007). Placebo effects on human mu-opioid activity during pain. *Proc. Natl. Acad. Sci. U S A* 104, 11056–11061. doi: 10.1073/pnas.0702413104

Whalen, P. J., Bush, G., Mcnally, R. J., Wilhelm, S., Mcinerney, S. C., Jenike, M. A., et al. (1998). The emotional counting Stroop paradigm: a functional magnetic resonance imaging probe of the anterior cingulate affective division. *Biol. Psychiatry* 44, 1219–1228. doi: 10.1016/s0006-3223(98)00251-0

Whelan, R., Conrod, P. J., Poline, J. B., Lourdusamy, A., Banaschewski, T., Barker, G. J., et al. (2012). Adolescent impulsivity phenotypes characterized by distinct brain networks. *Nat. Neurosci.* 15, 920–925. doi: 10.1038/nn.3092

White, S. F., Clanton, R., Brislin, S. J., Meffert, H., Hwang, S., Sinclair, S., et al. (2014). Reward: empirical contribution. Temporal discounting and conduct disorder in adolescents. *J. Pers. Disord.* 28, 5–18. doi: 10.1521/pedi.2014.28.1.5

Willcutt, E. G., Doyle, A. E., Nigg, J. T., Faraone, S. V., and Pennington, B. F. (2005). Validity of the executive function theory of attention-deficit/hyperactivity disorder: a meta-analytic review. *Biol. Psychiatry* 57, 1336–1346. doi: 10.1016/j.biopsych.2005.02.006

Williams, S. M., and Goldman-Rakic, P. S. (1998). Widspread orgin of the primate mesofrontal dopamine system. *Cereb. Cortex* 8, 321–345. doi: 10.1093/cercor/8.4.321

Wingenfeld, K., Rullkoetter, N., Mensebach, C., Beblo, T., Mertens, M., Kreisel, S., et al. (2009). Neural correlates of the individual emotional Stroop in borderline personality disorder. *Psychoneuroendocrinology* 34, 571–586. doi: 10.1016/j.psyneuen.2008.10.024

Winter, D., Krause-Utz, A., Lis, S., Chiu, C. D., Lanius, R. A., Schriner, F., et al. (2015). Dissociation in borderline personality disorder: disturbed cognitive and emotional inhibition and its neural correlates. *Psychiatry Res.* 233, 339–351. doi: 10.1016/j.pscychresns.2015.05.018

World Health Organization. (2011). *International Statistical Classification of Diseases and Related Health Problems. - 10th Revision, Edition 2010. 3v.* Geneva: World Health Organization.

Yang, Y., and Raine, A. (2009). Prefrontal structural and functional brain imaging findings in antisocial, violent and psychopathic individuals: a meta-analysis. *Psychiatry Res.* 174, 81–88. doi: 10.1016/j.pscychresns.2009.03.012

Yu, X., Sonuga-Barke, E., and Liu, X. (2015). Preference for smaller sooner over larger later rewards in ADHD: contribution of delay duration and paradigm type. *J. Atten. Disord.* doi: 10.1177/1087054715570390 [Epub ahead of print].

Zelazo, P. D., and Mueller, U. (2002). "Executive function in typical and atypical development," in *Handbook of Childhood Cognitive Development*, ed. U. Goswami (Oxford: Blackwell), 445–469.

Zelazo, P. D., Anderson, J. E., Richler, J., Wallner-Allen, K., Beaumont, J. L., and Weintraub, S. (2013). II. NIH Toolbox Cognition Battery (CB): measuring executive function and attention. *Monogr. Soc. Res. Child Dev.* 78, 16–33. doi: 10.1111/mono.12032

Zubieta, J. K., Bueller, J. A., Jackson, L. R., Scott, D. J., Xu, Y., Koeppe, R. A., et al. (2005). Placebo effects mediated by endogenous opioid activity on μ-opioid receptors. *J. Neurosci.* 25, 7754–7762. doi: 10.1523/jneurosci.0439-05.2005

Conflict of Interest Statement: The authors declare that the research was conducted in the absence of any commercial or financial relationships that could be construed as a potential conflict of interest.

3

At Risk for Neuropsychiatric Disorders: An Affective Neuroscience Approach to Understanding the Spectrum

Edited and reviewed by:
Nuno Sousa,
University of Minho, Portugal

***Correspondence:**
Morten L. Kringelbach
morten.kringelbach@psych.ox.ac.uk

Raymond C. K. Chan[1] *and Morten L. Kringelbach*[2,3*]

[1] Neuropsychology and Applied Cognitive Neuroscience Laboratory, Key Laboratory of Mental Health, Institute of Psychology, Chinese Academy of Sciences, Beijing, China, [2] Department of Psychiatry, University of Oxford, Oxford, UK, [3] Center for Music in the Brain (MIB), Aarhus University, Aarhus, Denmark

Keywords: neuropsychiatry, neuroimaging, reward processing, affective neuroscience, pleasure

The Editorial on the Research Topic

At Risk for Neuropsychiatric Disorders: An Affective Neuroscience Approach to Understanding the Spectrum

Neuropsychiatric disorders constitute a large global burden of disease; yet the neural mechanisms of emotional and social cognitive disturbances in patients are not yet fully understood (Deco and Kringelbach, 2014). Here, we used an affective neuroscience approach to investigate the spectrum of neuropsychiatric disorders from patients to those at risk, where stress plays a major role (Sousa, 2016). This Research Topic illuminates work by leading affective neuroscience researchers on how best to understand problems with the affective processing leading to increased risk for neuropsychiatric disorders.

The 20 articles in the Research Topic can roughly be divided into five sections: 1. Overviews, 2. Methods, 3. Anxiety and Personality, 4. Social Cognition, and 5. Impulsivity/Compulsivity, although many papers will fit in multiple categories. In the following we briefly introduce each article in this context.

OVERVIEWS

Anhedonia is an underlying critical feature of neuropsychiatric disorder but has remained little understood since first being introduced by Theodore Ribot in 1896 as the "inability to experience pleasure" (Ribot, 1896). Rømer Thomsen and colleagues proposes to reconceptualize anhedonia as an impairment to the established pleasure mechanisms of wanting, liking and learning (Rømer Thomsen et al.).

Cognition interacts with emotion to play a major role in those at risk for developing neuropsychiatric disorders. In particular Petrovic and Castellanos identified the importance of the interaction between deficient cognitive top-down executive control and emotional dysregulation in neuropsychiatric patients. They develop a novel framework that can integrate attention-deficit/hyperactivity disorder (ADHD), emotional traits in ADHD, borderline and antisocial personality disorder into a related cluster of mental conditions.

Still, some neuropsychiatric disorders are not fully understood. Sallin et al. describe investigations into resignation syndrome, which is long-standing disorder predominately affecting psychologically traumatized children and adolescents in the midst of a strenuous and lengthy migration process. They evaluate several hypotheses including stress and culture-bound psychogenic catatonia, and show how models of predictive coding and in particular negative expectations could explain the down-regulation of higher order and lower order behavioral systems in vulnerable individuals.

Genetic factors are also important for the development of neuropsychiatric disorders. Xia and Yao conducted a systematic review of the genes involved in adolescent depression and found positive association between *BDNF* Val66Met genotype and adolescent depressive symptoms (Xia and Yao).

METHODS

Animal models can potentially provide new insights into the neural mechanisms of neuropsychiatric disorders. Durieux and colleagues tested the hypothesis that the known imbalance between excitatory glutamate and inhibitory GABA transmission found in some neuropsychiatric disorders can be indirectly modulated through glial mechanisms (Durieux et al.). They used mice to test that striatal glutamate levels can be shifted by N-acetylcysteine and found that the treated animals were significantly less active and more anxious in the open field test.

Still, studies on human participants are likely to be more informative and objective measurements of relevant impairments are urgently needed. In order to address this, Bland and colleagues developed a standardized test battery, comprised of existing, adapted and novel tasks, to assess four core domains of affective cognition (emotion processing, motivation, impulsivity and social cognition) in order to facilitate and enhance treatment development and evaluation in a broad range of neuropsychiatric disorders (Bland et al.).

The treatment of neuropsychiatric disorder has a long history but the development of deep brain stimulation (DBS) for the treatment of Parkinson's disease is relatively recent (Kringelbach et al., 2007). The therapeutic effects are thought to arise from a rebalancing of brain-wide networks (Kringelbach et al.) but only recent developments in methods including probabilistic tractography and whole-brain computational modeling enabled Van Hartevelt and colleagues to identify the Hebbian-like changes in structural connectivity induced by long-term deep brain stimulation (van Hartevelt et al.).

ANXIETY AND RELATED DISORDERS

Anxiety is a significant neuropsychiatric problem, especially in adolescence. Geng and colleagues investigated adolescents' susceptibility to trait anxiety (Geng et al.) and found that weaker intra- and inter-network functional connectivity of the salience network was linked to higher trait anxiety among adolescents, which may underlie altered salience processing and cognitive regulation.

Similarly, Gawda and Szepeitowska investigated the brain activity in low/high-anxious adult groups of participants based on measures of trait anxiety (Gawda and Szepietowska). They found significant differences during the performance of more complex tasks between individuals with low anxiety and those with high anxiety.

Adolescents are also prone to develop compulsive behaviors which include various forms of behavioral addictions (Blakemore and Robbins, 2012). Wang and colleagues studied the structural brains of adolescents with internet gaming disorder and found it is linked to significant alterations of gray matter volume associated with performance change in cognitive control (Wang et al.).

Borderline personality disorder is another important neuropsychiatric disorder linked with differences in brain activity. Using EEG, Van Elst and colleagues found significant intermittent rhythmic delta and theta activity in patients compared to controls (Tebartz van Elst et al).

SOCIAL COGNITION

Depression has been strongly linked to social functioning (Stroud et al., 2011). Dedovic and colleagues used neuroimaging to show that the dorsal anterior cingulate cortex responds to repeated bouts of negative personally-relevant social evaluations (Dedovic et al.). This reveals a new dimension to this brain region in processing exclusion and contributing to mental health outcomes in those vulnerable to depression.

In more evidence of how depression is linked to impaired social functioning, Young and colleagues found that depression reduces psychomotor performance and alters affective movements in caregiving interactions based on salient affective sounds (Young et al.).

More evidence of changes in social cognition was unearthed in a neuroimaging study of voice perception and handedness which showed that a polymorphism specifically affects voice-specific brain function (Koeda et al.).

Finally, Wang and colleagues used neuroimaging to examine participants with different risk for psychosis (Wang et al.). They found that different dimensions of schizotypy are correlated with brain regions involved in social cognitive abilities.

IMPULSIVITY/COMPULSIVITY

The naturally occurring behaviors of impulsivity and compulsivity can become pathological and as such are key examples of neurocognitive endophenotypes with possible cross-diagnostic significance, linked to co-morbidities and commonalities across a range of neuropsychiatic disorders (Robbins et al., 2012).

Problematic hypersexual behavior is a compulsive behavioral compulsive disorder defined as the continuous participation in sex acts with little or no control over excessive sexual compulsivity and behavior despite the awareness of the associated negative outcomes. Seok and Sohn used neuroimaging to study a group of hypersexual individuals and found significant differences compared to controls, which are consistent with other behavioral addictions (Seok and Sohn).

Hoarding disorder is another compulsive disorder, characterized by the excessive acquisition and retention of goods with limited or no value, leading to significantly cluttered living spaces, and significant associated distress and life impairment. Vickers and colleagues used behavioral methods to investigate hoarding disorder and found that individuals in the high hoarding group were more impatient for consumables than for monetary reward, which suggest a specific, potent desire for consumable rewards (Vickers et al.).

Tahmasian and colleagues used positron emission tomography to investigate correlations between glucose metabolism and impulsivity in patients with Parkinson's disease (Tahmasian et al.). They found that high impulsivity is associated with increased metabolism within the fronto-insular network.

The anticipation of reward is an important component of the pleasure system which can become unbalanced in neuropsychiatric disorders, especially in adolescence. Li and colleagues used neuroimaging to investigate anticipatory pleasure in healthy adolescents and found that activity in the mesolimbic pathway during the anticipation of monetary reward could to some extent be predicted by subjective anticipatory pleasure (Li et al.).

Anticipation of reward has been studied in the context of delayed discounting and intertemporal decision-making. Ludwig and colleagues used neuroimaging to uncover the neural correlates of delay discounting during reward delivery and found that impulsivity and subclinical anxious-depressive traits are related to stronger neural responses for winning immediate relative to delayed rewards (Ludwig et al.).

CONCLUSION

Overall, this collection of 20 works of original research and reviews provides both novel ideas and a novel foundation upon which to build future research into the functional neuroanatomy of the spectrum of neuropsychiatric disorders. Drawing upon a wide variety of fields and using a diverse set of methods, techniques, and populations, this body of work points to some exciting future avenues of research.

AUTHOR CONTRIBUTIONS

All authors listed, have made substantial, direct and intellectual contribution to the work, and approved it for publication.

FUNDING

RC is supported by a grant from the "Strategic Priority Research Program (B)" of the Chinese Academy of Sciences (XDB02030002), the National Science Fund China (81088001, 91132701), the Beijing Training Project for Leading Talents in S&T (Z151100000315020). MK is supported by an ERC Consolidator Grant CAREGIVING (n.615539).

REFERENCES

Blakemore, S. J., and Robbins, T. W. (2012). Decision-making in the adolescent brain. *Nat. Neurosci.* 15, 1184–1191. doi: 10.1038/nn.3177

Deco, G., and Kringelbach, M. L. (2014). Great expectations: using whole-brain computational connectomics for understanding neuropsychiatric disorders. *Neuron* 84, 892–905. doi: 10.1016/j.neuron.2014.08.034

Kringelbach, M. L., Jenkinson, N., Owen, S. L. F., and Aziz, T. Z. (2007). Translational principles of deep brain stimulation. *Nat. Rev. Neurosci.* 8, 623–635. doi: 10.1038/nrn2196

Ribot, T. (1896). *La Psychologie des Sentiment [The Psychology of Feelings]*. Paris: Felix Alcan.

towards dimensional psychiatry. *Trends Cogn. Sci.* 16, 81–91. doi: 10.1016/j.tics.2011.11.009

Sousa, N. (2016). The dynamics of the stress neuromatrix. *Mol. Psychiatry* 21, 302–312. doi: 10.1038/mp.2015.196

Stroud, C. B., Davila, J., Hammen, C., and Vrshek-Schallhorn, S. (2011). Severe and nonsevere events in first onsets versus recurrences of depression: evidence for stress sensitization. *J. Abnorm. Psychol.* 120, 142–154. doi: 10.1037/a0021659

Conflict of Interest Statement: The authors declare that the research was conducted in the absence of any commercial or financial relationships that could be construed as a potential conflict of interest.

4

The Involvement of Genes in Adolescent Depression

*Liangwei Xia[1] and Shuqiao Yao[1,2]**

[1] *Medical Psychological Institute, Second Xiangya Hospital, Central South University, Changsha, Hunan, China,* [2] *National Technology Institute of Psychiatry, Changsha, Hunan, China*

Edited by:
Morten L. Kringelbach, University of Oxford, UK; University of Aarhus, Denmark

***Correspondence:**
Shuqiao Yao
shuqiaoyao@163.com

Numerous studies have reported on the roles of genetic factors in the development of depression in adolescents and young adults. However, there are few systematic reviews that update our understanding of adolescent depression with the biological findings identifying the roles of gene expression and/or polymorphism(s). This review systematically summarized the findings that clearly identified the contribution of a gene to the risk of depression in adolescents between the ages of 10 and 19 years old and young adults between the ages of 20 and 25 years old. Data were obtained through searching PubMed, Embase, and Web of Science. A total of 47 studies on early adolescence and three studies on young adults were included in the current review. Most articles studied genes in the serotonergic system (n = 26), dopaminergic system (n = 3), and the Brain-derived neurotropic factor (BDNF) gene (n = 12). 92.3% of studies (24/26) identified positive associations of 5-HTTLPR polymorphism with depressive illness or depressive symptoms. 83.3% of studies (10/12) found positive association between *BDNF* Val66Met genotype and adolescent depressive symptoms. More studies should be conducted on the 18 genes reported in a few studies to clarify their roles in the risk for adolescent depression.

Keywords: adolescent, depression, gene, genetics, polymorphism, single nucleotide

INTRODUCTION

Depression is a common disorder affecting an estimated 350 million people worldwide. Long-lasting depression with moderate or severe intensity is a serious medical condition that can lead to suicide. An estimated 1 million deaths each year are related to suicide. Although treatments for depression are effective, fewer than half of all individuals with depression around the world (in some countries, fewer than 10%) take anti-depressants (WHO, 2014a). Barriers to effective care include a lack of resources, a lack of trained health care providers, and social stigma associated with mental disorders (WHO EMRO, 2014). Inaccurate assessment and incorrect diagnosis of depression in its early stages can also prevent the effective care of individuals with depression. It is commonly believed that depression is a result of the complex interaction of social, psychological, and biological factors. Numerous studies have reported the involvement of abnormal gene expression or single nucleotide polymorphisms (SNPs) of genes in the development of depression (Bufalino et al., 2013).

Depression is also the leading cause of disability in young people worldwide. An estimated nine percent of children and adolescents in the US are affected by depression (Dunn et al., 2011). Although the diagnostic criteria for children and adolescent depression are no different from those for adults, one epidemiological study showed that there are different risk factors for the onset of depression in young people and in adults (Jaffee et al., 2002). For example, depressive adolescents experienced more perinatal insults, caretaker instability, and criminality than adult-onset depressive patients. Also, depressive adolescents have more behavioral and socioemotional problems than the adult-onset patients. In contrast, the adult-onset patients experienced more sexual abuse in their childhood than depressive adolescents (Jaffee et al., 2002).

Moreover, studies in neuroscience have demonstrated that adolescence is a special period of development characterized by significant changes in the structure and connectivity of the brain, as well as changes in cognition and behavior (Cousins and Goodyer, 2015). These neurological changes may interplay between genes and the environment (Paus, 2013). Results from several family and twin studies suggest that etiologic genetics do exist in depression during adolescence (Rice, 2009). A few reviews or meta-analyses have also summarized the gene × environment interaction in adolescents with depression (Franić et al., 2010; Rice, 2010; Dunn et al., 2011). However, the age range for adolescence was not accurately defined. Heterogeneity within a group of depressive patients may be problematic for the development of theory, research, and treatment of depressive patients (Jaffee et al., 2002). It is therefore necessary to summarize the findings in adolescents with an accurately defined age range: (1) to update the findings on gene expression or polymorphism in adolescent depression and (2) to evaluate the value of all genes as a biomarker of adolescent depression. The WHO defines adolescence as having an age range of 10–19 years old and as a dynamic period with biological, social, and psychological changes (WHO, 2014b). In this study, the age range of 10–19 years was defined as adolescence while an age range of 20–25 years was defined as young adult for analysis.

The goal of the current review is to systematically analyze studies that tested the role of a gene in the development of depression or as a risk factor of depression in adolescents. We focused specifically on the findings and ultimately provide substantive conclusions on which gene expression or polymorphism could be a biomarker of depression in adolescents.

METHODS

Eligibility Criteria

A systematic review of original studies on gene expression or genetic polymorphisms in adolescents with depression was conducted. Reports on gene expression or polymorphisms measured in peripheral blood or postmortem studies in adolescents were eligible for review. A study was included in the analysis when: (1) adolescents with depression or depressive symptoms fell into the range of 10–19 years old (WHO, 2014b) or young adult at an age of 20–25 years and (2) original research with the age range and gene being clearly identified. Studies were excluded if: (1) a study had subjects with age not in the two age ranges; (2) a study only provided a mean age; (3) A study contained anxious adolescents only; (4) studies that were conducted in animals or *in vitro*; or (5) review or studies that were not written in English.

Information Sources

Studies were pulled from the electronic databases of PubMed, Embase, and Web of Science.

Search Strategy

The primary search strategy was carried out using both the keywords and test words: "depression" and "adolescent" and "gene"; "depression" and "adolescent" and "polymorphism"; "depression" and "adolescent" and "genetics"; "depression" and "adolescent" and "genetic variants"; and "depression" and "adolescent" and "genotype".

Data Collection Process

The abstract of each study was screened and the full-text articles of potentially relevant studies were then retrieved and assessed. Data were extracted from the retrieved papers by two authors (LX and SY) independently. Disagreements were resolved by discussion in a meeting that included several experts from within the Department. The study selection process was presented in a flow diagram (**Figure 1**).

Data Items

Data on age range, study design, demographic characteristics of patients, and control individuals, gene expression or polymorphism, tissue type, and the results were extracted.

Outcomes

The association of gene expression or polymorphisms with disease risk, severity of depressive symptoms, and treatment outcomes.

Risk of Bias in Individual Studies

Risk of bias was assessed by evaluating choice of study design, selection of study population, allocation of control individuals, and quality of assay used.

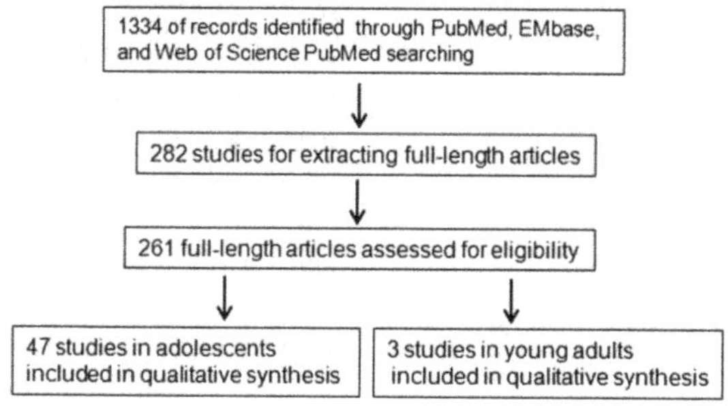

FIGURE 1 | A flowchart of literature search strategy. A flowchart of the inclusions and exclusions of studies in the current study.

Data Synthesis

Data was summarized for each gene including the main outcomes or conclusion, positive and negative association with depression.

RESULTS

The literature search identified 1334 articles from PubMed, EMbase, and Web of Science using the keywords mentioned above after the removal of duplicates. The end date for the search is August 29, 2015. The abstracts of the 1334 articles were screened one by one and articles not written in English, review articles not for depression in adolescents, comments, and articles for animal or *in vitro* studies were excluded from this study. The studies where the gene name could not be identified in the abstract were also excluded from further analysis. A total of 282 studies were finally used for extracting full-length articles. However, only 261 full-length articles were downloaded for careful identification. Full-length articles of screening studies, studies in non-adolescents or with a mixed sample with the age beyond the range of 10–19 years for adolescents or 20–25 years for young adults, studies with only the mean age, studies without clearly identified gene expression or polymorphism, or others was excluded from the analysis. Finally, 47 full-length articles (Eley et al., 2004; Mamalakis et al., 2004; Burcescu et al., 2005; Miraglia del Giudice et al., 2006; Sjöberg et al., 2006; Geng et al., 2007; Hilt et al., 2007; Pandey et al., 2007, 2012; Feng et al., 2008; Aslund et al., 2009; Duncan et al., 2009; Goodyer et al., 2009, 2010; Guo and Tillman, 2009; Laucht et al., 2009; Nilsson et al., 2009; Nobile et al., 2009; Benjet et al., 2010; Brent et al., 2010; Mata et al., 2010; Nederhof et al., 2010; Uddin et al., 2010, 2011; Bouma et al., 2011; Hankin et al., 2011; Jenness et al., 2011; Mata and Gotlib, 2011; Thompson et al., 2011; Chen et al., 2012, 2013; Petersen et al., 2012; Buchmann et al., 2013; Bobadilla et al., 2013; Comasco et al., 2013; Cutuli et al., 2013; Kohen et al., 2013; Otten and Engels, 2013; Oppenheimer et al., 2013; Priess-Groben and Hyde, 2013; Stavrakakis et al., 2013; Banducci et al., 2014; Cicchetti and Rogosch, 2014; Cruz-Fuentes et al., 2014; Little et al., 2014; Zhang et al., 2015) in adolescents and three studies (Hammen et al., 2010; Starr et al., 2013; Thompson et al., 2014) in young adults were included in this study (**Figure 1**). The 47 studies in adolescence included 20 genes or gene families while the three studies in young adults included three genes (**Table 1**).

Among the studies in early adolescence, only three articles reported the association between gene expression and depression in adolescents (Mamalakis et al., 2004; Pandey et al., 2007, 2012) and one study reported a linkage analysis (Feng et al., 2008). 91.5% (43/47) of articles reported the results of nucleotide polymorphism analysis of a gene in adolescents with depressive disease or depressive symptoms (**Table 1**). Most studies were related to neurotransmitter receptors and their associated metabolic enzymes, including the dopaminergic system (*DRD2, DRD4,* and *COMT*) and serotonergic system (serotonin 2A, *5-HTT, MAOA,* and *TPH*). *5-HTT* (*5-HTTLPR* polymorphism) is the most frequently examined gene (26 articles) followed by Brain-derived neurotropic factor (BNDF; 12 articles). Thirteen genes were only reported in one article. Seven genes (*COMT*, serotonin 2A, *MAOA*, estrogen receptor α and β, *AR*, glucocorticoid receptor, and adipose polyunsaturated fatty acid gene) showed no association with depression in adolescents. Four genes (*DRD2, DRD4, TPH1/2,* and *CREB/CREB1*) were reported by two or three articles with inconsistencies. The 26 studies on *5-HTTLPR* contained a total of 14,616 samples, and the 12 studies on *BDNF* contained a total of 7646 samples.

Approximately 92.3% (24/26) of studies for the association between *5-HTTLPR* polymorphism and depression in adolescents yielded a positive outcome (**Table 2**). Among the 26 studies for *5-HTTLPR* polymorphism, 22 studies analyzed the association between polymorphism and depressive symptoms (two studies showed negative findings), while four studies analyzed the role of *5-HTTLPR* polymorphism in depression. Only one study analyzed the association between *5-HTTLPR* polymorphism and the severity of depressive symptoms. It appears that *5-HTTLPR* polymorphism is associated with both the risk and severity of depression in adolescents. There was no study to compare the role of *5-HTTLPR* polymorphism in anxiety and depression. The association between *5-HTTLPR* polymorphism and different types of depression (i.e., anxiety vs. irritability vs. cognitive dysfunction) was not analyzed in this study because only a few studies analyzed the association between *5-HTTLPR* polymorphism and the cognitive dysfunction and the irritability.

BDNF was the second most frequently studied gene in adolescents. All 12 studies analyzed the association between *BDNF* Val66Met genotype/gene plasticity index and depressive symptoms. Among them, one study investigated the *BDNF* gene plasticity index in adolescents with depressive symptoms without observing any association. Eleven studies (Hilt et al., 2007; Duncan et al., 2009; Goodyer et al., 2010; Mata et al., 2010; Chen et al., 2012, 2013; Buchmann et al., 2013; Comasco et al., 2013; Stavrakakis et al., 2013; Cicchetti and Rogosch, 2014; Cruz-Fuentes et al., 2014) investigated the association between the *BDNF* Val66Met genotype and adolescent depressive symptoms with only one study showing no association (Nederhof et al., 2010; **Table 3**). However, no study analyzed the association between *BDNF* Val66Met genotype and severity of depressive symptoms. No study compared the role of *BDNF* Val66Met genotype in anxiety and depression. The association between *BDNF* Val66Met genotype and different types of depression was not analyzed in this study because no studies analyzed the *BDNF* Val66Met genotypes and irritability. Only one study investigated the association of *BDNF* Val66Met genotypes with cognitive dysfunction. Two studies reported the association of genetic variants in the dopaminergic system with adolescent depression (Bobadilla et al., 2013; Stavrakakis et al., 2013; **Table 3**).

Only three studies investigated the gene polymorphism and the risk of depression in young adults at an age range of 20–25 years. Thompson et al. (2014) study found that OXTR (oxytocin receptor gene) polymorphism influences the development of depressive symptoms. Starr et al. (2013) study showed that *5-HTTLPR* S-allele can predict relative increases in probability of depression among boys. Hammen et al. (2010) study revealed that chronic family stress at age 15 predicted

TABLE 1 | Summary of literature and outcomes in adolescents.

Gene	Reference	Measurement	Association with depression
DRD2	Guo and Tillman (2009), Stavrakakis et al. (2013) and Zhang et al. (2015)	Polymorphism	1 no/2 yes
DRD4	Guo and Tillman (2009), Bobadilla et al. (2013) and Stavrakakis et al. (2013)	Polymorphism	1 no/2 yes
Catechol-O-methyltransferase (COMT)	Stavrakakis et al. (2013)	Polymorphism	no
Serotonin 2A	Stavrakakis et al. (2013)	Polymorphism	no
Monoamine oxidase A (MAOA)	Eley et al. (2004) and Stavrakakis et al. (2013)	Polymorphism	no
Tryptophan hydroxylase gene (TPH1/2)	Nobile et al. (2009), Stavrakakis et al. (2013) and Eley et al. (2004)	Polymorphism	1 no/2 yes
Serotonin transporter gene (5-HTT)	Eley et al. (2004), Sjöberg et al. (2006), Aslund et al. (2009), Goodyer et al. (2009, 2010), Laucht et al. (2009), Nobile et al. (2009), Benjet et al. (2010), Uddin et al. (2010, 2011), Hankin et al. (2011), Jenness et al. (2011), Mata and Gotlib (2011), Petersen et al. (2012), Buchmann et al. (2013), Comasco et al. (2013), Cutuli et al. (2013), Kohen et al. (2013), Oppenheimer et al. (2013), Otten and Engels (2013), Priess-Groben and Hyde (2013), Stavrakakis et al. (2013), Banducci et al. (2014), Cicchetti and Rogosch (2014) and Little et al. (2014)	Polymorphism	24 yes/2 no
BDNF	Hilt et al. (2007), Duncan et al. (2009), Goodyer et al. (2010), Mata et al. (2010), Nederhof et al. (2010), Chen et al. (2012, 2013), Buchmann et al. (2013), Comasco et al. (2013), Stavrakakis et al. (2013), Cicchetti and Rogosch (2014) and Cruz-Fuentes et al. (2014).		
FK506 binding protein 5 (FKBP5) gene	Brent et al. (2010)	Polymorphism	yes
Estrogen receptor α, β	Geng et al. (2007)	Polymorphism	no
Androgen receptor (AR)	Geng et al. (2007)	Polymorphism	no
Glucocorticoid receptor	Bouma et al. (2011)	Polymorphism	no
IL-1β/IL-6/TNF-α	Pandey et al. (2012)	Expression	yes
Neurotrophic tyrosine kinase receptor	Feng et al. (2008)	Linkage analysis	yes
CREB/CREB1	Burcescu et al. (2005) and Pandey et al. (2007)	Expression/Polymorphism	yes/no
Adipose polyunsaturated fatty acid gene	Mamalakis et al. (2004)	Expression	no
CART	Miraglia del Giudice et al. (2006)	Polymorphism	yes
OXTR	Thompson et al. (2011)	Polymorphism	yes
AP-2β	Nilsson et al. (2009)	Polymorphism	yes
HTR2A/2C	Eley et al. (2004)	Polymorphism	yes

higher depression scores at age 20 among females with one or two S alleles of *5-HTT* gene (**Table 4**).

Risk of bias was evaluated for the study design, allocation of control individuals, and quality of assay methods. There was a wide variation in methods and analysis. Most studies did not include age or gender-matched control individuals. Most studies did not provide detailed information about current medical treatment in the full study sample. Most studies did not provide observer-based rating scores of depressive symptom severity.

DISCUSSION

Studies in twins, families, and populations have revealed the genetic influences on depression (Rice, 2009). Deregulated gene expression and specific functional genetic polymorphisms have been demonstrated to be risk factors of depression or to be associated with the severity of depressive symptoms (Dunn et al., 2011). Numerous studies have confirmed the existence of biological etiology in the development and progression of depression during childhood and adolescence (Dunn et al., 2011; Paus, 2013; Cousins and Goodyer, 2015). However, the published reviews did not summarize the up to date biological findings in only adolescents with defined age ranges. Heterogeneity within study subjects is a main concern for the research in depressive patients because the risk factors for the onset of depression in adolescents and in adults are different. Moreover, the depressive adolescents may experience more psychopathology, behavioral and socioemotional problems than adult-depressive patients (Jaffee et al., 2002). It is therefore important to summarize the biological findings in depressive patients with a defined age range. This study updated the genetic findings in adolescent depression with an age range of 10–19 years defined by WHO as adolescence and 20–25 years as young adult. This study demonstrated that genetic polymorphism or expression of 13 genes was associated, but seven tested genes were not associated with the risk or severity of depression in early adolescence, while the polymorphism of three genes was associated with the risk of depression in late adolesence. This review highlighted the role of several genes or gene families as risk factors

TABLE 2 | Outcomes of studies on the relationship between 5-HTTLPR and depression in adolescents.

Reference	Sample size	Main outcomes or conclusion
Stavrakakis et al. (2013)	1196	Adolescents' depressive symptoms are not modified by 5-HTTLPR
Nobile et al. (2009)	607	Short alleles were associated with higher affective problems scores
Kohen et al. (2013)	192	The s/l vs. l/l genotype showed greater reduction in depression symptoms
Comasco et al. (2013)	1393	5-HTTLPR interacted with unfavorable environment in relation to depressive symptoms
Cutuli et al. (2013)	267	Positive G × E effects on depression were found
Priess-Groben and Hyde (2013)	309	Short allele confers susceptibility to stress for females with depression
Jenness et al. (2011)	200	5-HTTLPR predict depressive symptoms
Otten and Engels (2013)	310	Cannabis use increases the risk of depression only in the presence of 5-HTTLPR short allele genotype
Uddin et al. (2011)	2574	The sl genotype carriers had *less* higher depressive symptom score
Goodyer et al. (2010)	401	5-HTTLPR short allele modify the risk of a new depressive episode associated with elevated morning salivary cortisol
Benjet et al. (2010)	78	Short alleles confers vulnerability to depressive symptoms in girls
Goodyer et al. (2009)	403	Episode of depression was increased in those with the "s" allele
Laucht et al. (2009)	309	LL genotype of 5-HTTLPR displayed significantly higher rates of depressive disorders and more depressive symptoms
Sjöberg et al. (2006)	200	Females carrying the short 5-HTTLPR allele tend to develop depressive symptoms
Nederhof et al. (2010)	1096	Interaction between 5-HTTLPR polymorphism and childhood adversities did not predict depression score
Cicchetti and Rogosch (2014)	1096	G × E interaction of 5-HTTLPR and maltreatment on depression symptoms
Little et al. (2014)	174	Structural abnormalities in the left hippocampus may be partly responsible for an indirect association between 5-HTTLPR genotype and depressive illness
Banducci et al. (2014)	222	Among girls, but not boys, each copy of the s allele of the 5-HTTLPR was related to increased depressive symptoms
Buchmann et al. (2013)	259	The carriers of the BDNF Met and 5-HTTLPR s allele are susceptible to depressive symptoms
Oppenheimer et al. (2013)	241	Youth with SS genotype of 5-HTTLPR experienced greatest increases in depressive symptoms when exposed to elevations in materal symptoms
Petersen et al. (2012)	436	Stress affect adolescents' likelihood of experiencing depressed symptoms when they have a low serotonin TE (A/Gmodified5-HTTLPR) genotype
Mata et al. (2010)	50	Girls with homozygous for short 5-HTTLPR allele showed stronger association between depressive and bulimic symptoms the long allele
Hankin et al. (2011)	220	5-HTTLPR confers susceptibility to depression via stress reactivity
Uddin et al. (2010)	524	5-HTTLPR sl genotype is a risk of depressive symptom in adolescent male
Aslund et al. (2009)	1482	A GxE interaction effect of 5HTTLPR ss allele was found among girls, not boys
Eley et al. (2004)	377	A significant genotype-environmental risk interaction for 5HTTLPR in the risk of depression in girls only

for the development of depression in adolescents. This study improved our understanding of the etiology of adolescent depression, and also identified *5-HTTLPR* and *BDNF* Val66Met polymorphisms as the most studied biomarkers in adolescent depression.

Low serotonin-receptor levels in the brain have been widely recognized to be a key cause of depression. Polymorphisms of the 5-hydroxytryptamine (serotonin) transporter gene-linked polymorphic region (*5-HTTLPR*) have been widely demonstrated to be a risk factor for depression

TABLE 3 | Outcomes of studies on the relationship between BDNF and dopaminergic pathway and depression in adolescents.

Reference	Sample size	Main outcomes or conclusion
Stavrakakis et al. (2013)	1196	Adolescents' depressive symptoms are not modified by BDNF
Comasco et al. (2013)	1393	Depressive symptoms and depression were more common among carriers of either the Val/Val or Met genotypes
Goodyer et al. (2010)	401	*BDNF* (Val66Met) modify the risk of a new depressive episode associated with elevated morning salivary cortisol
Chen et al. (2012)	780	Interaction between *BDNF* Val66Met polymorphism and environmental stress on depression was observed
Nederhof et al. (2010)	1096	Depression score was not significantly predicted by interaction between BDNF Val66Met polymorphism and childhood adversities
Mata et al. (2010)	82	BDNF met allele moderate the relation between exercise and depressive symptoms
Duncan et al. (2009)	217	Val/Val genotype correlated with higher levels of depression symptoms
Hilt et al. (2007)	100	Val/Val genotype was associated with more depressive symptoms
Cicchetti and Rogosch (2014)	1096	G × G × E interaction of BDNF, *5-HTTLPR/CRHR1* and maltreatment on depression symptoms
Cruz-Fuentes et al. (2014)	246	Possession of BDNF Met allele was statistically linked with a resilient phenotype of major depression disorder
Buchmann et al. (2013)	259	The carriers of the BDNF Met and *5-HTTLPR* s allele are susceptible to depressive symptoms
Chen et al. (2013)	780	*BDNF* Val allele modulates the influence of environmental stress on depression
Stavrakakis et al. (2013)	1196	Adolescents' depressive symptoms are not modified by COMT
Guo and Tillman (2009)	2286	DRD2*304/178 and DRD4*379/379 genotype are associated with a level of depressive symptoms
Bobadilla et al. (2013)	1882	DRD4 polymorphism is linked to comorbid marijuana use and depression

TABLE 4 | Summary of literature and outcomes in young adult.

Gene	Reference	Measurement	Association with depression
OXTR	Thompson et al. (2014)	Polymorphism, $n = 441$	OXTR influences the development of depressive symptoms
5HTTLRP	Starr et al. (2013)	Polymorphism, $n = 354$	S-allele predicts relative increases in probability of depression among boys with low security
5HTT	Hammen et al. (2010)	Polymorphism, $n = 346$	Chronic family stress at age 15 predicted higher depression scores at 20 among those females with one or two S alleles

following adverse life experiences. In this review, a total of 26 articles reported an association between *5-HTTLPR* variations and depression in adolescents. About 92.3% of studies ($n = 24$) identified positive associations of 5-HTTLPR polymorphism with the risk for or susceptibility to depression, new depressive episodes, and more severe depressive symptoms. The most commonly examined polymorphism was the *5-HTTLPR* variable number tandem repeat (VNTR), which consists of the s/s, s/l, and l/l genotypes. In most studies, the short (S) allele or heterozygote genotype carriers (s/l) of 5-HTTLPR might experience a greater reduction in depressive symptoms over time compared with adolescents with the *5-HTTLPR* l/l genotype (**Table 2**). A recent meta-analysis of the association between the *5-HTTLPR*, stress, and the development of depression contained 81 studies with a mean age from 9–77 years. A significant relationship between the short form of the *5-HTTLPR* and depression was confirmed ($p = 0.0000009$). However, nearly 26% of the 81 studies failed to show any significant association, and four studies even showed opposite results (Sharpley et al., 2014). Only two studies investigated the *5-HTTLPR* polymorphism and the risk of depression in young adults at an age range of 20–25 years. These two studies showed a positive association between *5-HTTLPR* S-allele and the increased probability of depression in adolescents (Hammen et al., 2010; Starr et al., 2013). These findings suggest that *5-HTTLPR* polymorphism is a risk factor for both early onset and late onset depression.

Tryptophan hydroxylase-2 (*TPH2*) gene has been acknowledged for many years as the only form of tryptophan hydroxylase (TPH) responsible for the synthesis of serotonin in the brain and peripheral tissues. A recent report suggested that *TPH2* gene expression in the dorsal raphe nuclei of depressed suicidal patients is upregulated [14]. This review included 2 studies on *TPH2* in adolescents (Nobile et al., 2009; Stavrakakis et al., 2013). However, adolescents' depressive symptoms are not associated with the gene plasticity index of *TPH2* (Stavrakakis et al., 2013). Monoamine oxidase A is a monoamine oxidase encoded by the *MAOA* gene that preferentially deaminates norepinephrine, epinephrine, serotonin, and dopamine. Studies in adolescents demonstrated that depressive symptoms are not associated with gene plasticity index of the *MAOA* gene (Stavrakakis et al., 2013), whereas gene × environment interaction of the *5-HTTLPR* was further moderated by *MAOA* activity level (Nobile et al., 2009).

BDNF is the most abundant neurotrophin in the mammalian central nervous system, and reduced BDNF level in the hippocampus has been revealed to be related to the onset of depression (Bai et al., 2012). A single nucleotide polymorphism (SNP) in the *BDNF* gene (Val66Met) has been shown to influence the activity of the BDNF protein and cause subsequent memory impairment and harm avoidance (Jiang et al., 2005). A significant interaction between *BDNF* Val66Met and life stress in depression was widely observed in adults (Hosang et al., 2014). In this review, the *BDNF* gene is the second most frequently studied gene in adolescents with depression. Two studies on the *BDNF* gene plasticity index and BDNF level showed controversial outcomes. The depressive symptoms were not associated with gene plasticity index of the *BDNF* gene in adolescents (Stavrakakis et al., 2013), whereas *BDNF* mRNA level correlated with symptom improvement in adult patients with depression (Cattaneo et al., 2010). Seven studies investigated the association between *BDNF* Val66Met polymorphism and adolescent depression. Two studies showed no association between *BDNF* Val66Met polymorphism and depression score, but 10 studies found significant correlations between BDNF polymorphism and adolescent depression. A recent meta-analysis of the interaction between the *BDNF* Val66Met polymorphism and stress in depression contained 22 studies with a mean age range from 8.85–65 years. Results showed that the Met allele of *BDNF* Val66Met significantly moderates the relationship between life stress and depression ($p = 0.03$; Hosang et al., 2014). This review only contained three studies with an age range from 9–19 years. Moreover, a meta analysis of genes and suicide in 16 studies showed that hypermethylation of *BDNF* is associated with individuals that died of suicide (Lockwood et al., 2015). The involvement of genetic polymorphisms in the *BDNF* gene in peripheral tissues of patients with depression may reflect changes in the BDNF level in their brain. The Val66Met polymorphism has been demonstrated to impair the packaging and secretion of BDNF and subsequently reduces hippocampal volume and impairs memory (Kimpton, 2012; Harrisberger et al., 2015).

Dopamine is a major neurotransmitter in the central nervous system, and dysregulation of the dopaminergic-system is widely reported in people with depression. The hypofunction of the mesolimbic dopaminergic pathway has been linked to anhedonia, one of the major symptoms of depression (Leggio et al., 2013). Studies that directly link genetic polymorphisms in the dopaminergic pathway to depression are abundant but show inconsistent findings (Lawford et al., 2006). For example, Lawford et al study demonstrated that patients with *DRD2**A1/A2 genotype had significantly higher depression scores compared to those with the *DRD2**A2/A2 genotype (Lawford et al., 2006). An interaction between *DAT1* polymorphism and perceived maternal rejection can influence the onset of depressive disorder and suicidal ideation (Haeffel et al., 2008). A significant association between the 48 bp repeat polymorphism of *DRD4* and depression was reported (Manki et al., 1996). In contrast, Frisch et al. (1999) found no association of polymorphisms in *DRD4, DAT1*, and *COMT* with depression. Kirov et al. (1999) found that six dopaminergic genes (*DBH, DAT1, COMT, DRD2, DRD3*, and *DRD5*) played no role in bipolar disorder. However, the roles of genetic polymorphisms in the dopaminergic pathway in adolescent depression have not been summarized. In this study, three studies reported associations between genetic variants in the dopaminergic system and adolescent depression (Bobadilla et al., 2013; Stavrakakis et al., 2013). Significant associations between *DRD2, DRD4*, and *COMT* polymorphisms and the risk of depression, as well as the severity of depressive symptoms, were reported.

Selective serotonin reuptake inhibitors (SSRIs) are the first line treatment for depression in the clinic. These inhibitors work by increasing serotonin levels in the brain to counteract the low serotonin-receptor levels. A meta-analysis has demonstrated that the *5-HTTLPR* long-allele carriers had higher probability of response than patients with short-allele homozygotes of *5-HTTLPR* with heterogeneity effect (Serretti et al., 2007). No study investigated the effect of *5-HTTLPR* polymorphism on the efficacy of SSRIs treatment at an age range from 9–19 years. Rotberg et al. (2013) study in 83 children and adolescents aged 7–18 years showed that the *5-HTTLPR* ss genotype was associated with a poorer clinical response to citalopram with regards to depressive symptoms. A recent meta analysis showed that the BDNF Met carriers had a better response rate to SSRI than Val/Val, while Met/Val carriers had a weak effect of response to SSRIs than Val/Val carriers (Yan et al., 2014). Based on the report from Hammen et al. (2010) study that patients younger than 18 years old have an increased risk of suicidal thoughts or behaviors (4% with SSRIs vs. 2% with placebo) with an antidepressant (Gordon and Melvin, 2013), FDA suggests that adolescents taking SSRIs must be closely monitored to reduce the risk for suicide. However, the risk is small and the risk hasn't been replicated very well in studies of adolescent depression treated with SSRIs. For example, Hetrick et al. (2012) study showed that no significant increase in suicide-related outcomes was observed in children and adolescents after using individual SSRIs, such as paroxetine, fluoxetine, sertraline, citalopram, and escitalopram.

In conclusion, there are more published positive associations between the genetic polymorphisms in the serotoninergic system, dopaminergic system, and the Val66Met polymorphism of BDNF with adolescent depression. However, some biases should be considered: (1) the publication bias for positive findings; (2) numerous negative findings may be unpublished; (3) a bias for investigations of these three polymorphisms first because of the high profile papers that brought them to attention; and (4) the polymorphisms can be easily genotyped. Although the expression or polymorphism of 18 genes has been reported to be or not be associated with the risk of depression, they were reported by only a few studies. Therefore, further studies are needed to accurately identify their roles in depression in adolescents.

AUTHOR CONTRIBUTIONS

LX: data extraction, data analysis, and manuscript writing. SY: study design, data extraction, data analysis, critical revision of manuscript, and a guarantor of the review.

FUNDING

This study is supported by grants from the National Natural Science Foundation of China (81471384 to SY).

REFERENCES

Aslund, C., Leppert, J., Comasco, E., Nordquist, N., Oreland, L., and Nilsson, K. W. (2009). Impact of the interaction between the 5HTTLPR polymorphism and maltreatment on adolescent depression. A population-based study. *Behav. Genet.* 39, 524–531. doi: 10.1007/s10519-009-9285-9

Bai, M., Zhu, X., Zhang, Y., Zhang, S., Zhang, L., Xue, L., et al. (2012). Abnormal hippocampal BDNF and miR-16 expression is associated with depression-like behaviors induced by stress during early life. *PLoS One* 7:e46921. doi: 10.1371/journal.pone.0046921

Banducci, A. N., Gomes, M., MacPherson, L., Lejuez, C. W., Potenza, M. N., Gelernter, J., et al. (2014). A preliminary examination of the relationship between the 5-HTTLPR and childhood emotional abuse on depressive symptoms in 10–12-year-old youth. *Psychol. Trauma* 6, 1–7. doi: 10.1037/a0031121

Benjet, C., Thompson, R. J., and Gotlib, I. H. (2010). 5-HTTLPR moderates the effect of relational peer victimization on depressive symptoms in adolescent girls. *J. Child Psychol. Psychiatry* 51, 173–179. doi: 10.1111/j.1469-7610.2009.02149.x

Bobadilla, L., Vaske, J., and Asberg, K. (2013). Dopamine receptor (D4) polymorphism is related to comorbidity between marijuana abuse and depression. *Addict. Behav.* 38, 2555–2562. doi: 10.1016/j.addbeh.2013.05.014

Bouma, E. M., Riese, H., Nolte, I. M., Oosterom, E., Verhulst, F. C., Ormel, J., et al. (2011). No associations between single nucleotide polymorphisms in corticoid receptor genes and heart rate and cortisol responses to a standardized social stress test in adolescents: the TRAILS study. *Behav. Genet.* 41, 253–261. doi: 10.1007/s10519-010-9385-6

Brent, D., Melhem, N., Ferrell, R., Emslie, G., Wagner, K. D., Ryan, N., et al. (2010). Association of FKBP5 polymorphisms with suicidal events in the Treatment of Resistant Depression in Adolescents (TORDIA) study. *Am. J. Psychiatry* 167, 190–197. doi: 10.1176/appi.ajp.2009.09040576

Buchmann, A. F., Hellweg, R., Rietschel, M., Treutlein, J., Witt, S. H., Zimmermann, U. S., et al. (2013). BDNF Val 66 Met and 5-HTTLPR genotype moderate the impact of early psychosocial adversity on plasma brain-derived neurotrophic factor and depressive symptoms: a prospective study. *Eur. Neuropsychopharmacol.* 23, 902–929. doi: 10.1016/j.euroneuro.2012.09.003

Bufalino, C., Hepgul, N., Aguglia, E., and Pariante, C. M. (2013). The role of immune genes in the association between depression and inflammation: a review of recent clinical studies. *Brain Behav. Immun.* 31, 31–47. doi: 10.1016/j.bbi.2012.04.009

Burcescu, I., Wigg, K., King, N., Vetró, A., Kiss, E., Katay, L., et al. (2005). Association study of CREB1 and childhood-onset mood disorders. *Am. J. Med. Genet. B Neuropsychiatr. Genet.* 137B, 45–50. doi: 10.1002/ajmg.b.30201

Cattaneo, A., Bocchio-Chiavetto, L., Zanardini, R., Milanesi, E., Placentino, A., and Gennarelli, M. (2010). Reduced peripheral brain-derived neurotrophic factor mRNA levels are normalized by antidepressant treatment. *Int. J. Neuropsychopharmacol.* 13, 103–108. doi: 10.1017/S1461145709990812

Chen, J., Li, X., and McGue, M. (2012). Interacting effect of BDNF Val66Met polymorphism and stressful life events on adolescent depression. *Genes Brain Behav.* 11, 958–965. doi: 10.1111/j.1601-183x.2012.00843.x

Chen, J., Li, X., and McGue, M. (2013). The interacting effect of the BDNF Val66Met polymorphism and stressful life events on adolescent depression is not an artifact of gene-environment correlation: evidence from a longitudinal twin study. *J. Child Psychol. Psychiatry* 54, 1066–1073. doi: 10.1111/jcpp.12099

Cicchetti, D., and Rogosch, F. A. (2014). Genetic moderation of child maltreatment effects on depression and internalizing symptoms by serotonin transporter linked polymorphic region (5-HTTLPR), brain-derived neurotrophic factor (BDNF), norepinephrine transporter (NET) and corticotropin releasing hormone receptor 1 (CRHR1) genes in African American children. *Dev. Psychopathol.* 26, 1219–1239. doi: 10.1017/s0954579414000984

Comasco, E., Åslund, C., Oreland, L., and Nilsson, K. W. (2013). Three-way interaction effect of 5-HTTLPR, BDNF Val66Met and childhood adversity on depression: a replication study. *Eur. Neuropsychopharmacol.* 23, 1300–1306. doi: 10.1016/j.euroneuro.2013.01.010

Cousins, L., and Goodyer, I. M. (2015). Antidepressants and the adolescent brain. *J. Psychopharmacol.* 29, 545–555. doi: 10.1177/0269881115573542

Cruz-Fuentes, C. S., Benjet, C., Martínez-Levy, G. A., Pérez-Molina, A., Briones-Velasco, M., and Suárez-González, J. (2014). BDNF Met66 modulates the cumulative effect of psychosocial childhood adversities on major depression in adolescents. *Brain Behav.* 4, 290–297. doi: 10.1002/brb3.220

Cutuli, J. J., Raby, K. L., Cicchetti, D., Englund, M. M., and Egeland, B. (2013). Contributions of maltreatment and serotonin transporter genotype to depression in childhood, adolescence and early adulthood. *J. Affect. Disord.* 149, 30–37. doi: 10.1016/j.jad.2012.08.011

Duncan, L. E., Hutchison, K. E., Carey, G., and Craighead, W. E. (2009). Variation in brain-derived neurotrophic factor (BDNF) gene is associated with symptoms of depression. *J. Affect. Disord.* 115, 215–219. doi: 10.1016/j.jad.2008.08.016

Dunn, E. C., Uddin, M., Subramanian, S. V., Smoller, J. W., Galea, S., and Koen, K. C. (2011). Research review: gene-environment interaction research in youth depression—a systematic review with recommendations for future research. *J. Child Psychol. Psychiatry* 52, 1223–1238. doi: 10.1111/j.1469-7610.2011.02466.x

Eley, T. C., Sugden, K., Corsico, A., Gregory, A. M., Sham, P., McGuffin, P., et al. (2004). Gene-environment interaction analysis of serotonin system markers with adolescent depression. *Mol. Psychiatry* 9, 908–915. doi: 10.1038/sj.mp.4001546

Feng, Y., Vetró, A., Kiss, E., Kapornai, K., Daróczi, G., Mayer, L., et al. (2008). Association of the neurotrophic tyrosine kinase receptor 3 (NTRK3) gene and childhood-onset mood disorders. *Am. J. Psychiatry* 165, 610–616. doi: 10.1176/appi.ajp.2007.07050805

Franić, S., Middeldorp, C. M., Dolan, C. V., Ligthart, L., and Boomsma, D. I. (2010). Childhood and adolescent anxiety and depression: beyond heritability. *J. Am. Acad. Child Adolesc. Psychiatry* 49, 820–829. doi: 10.1016/j.jaac.2010.05.013

Frisch, A., Postilnick, D., Rockah, R., Michaelovsky, E., Postilnick, S., Birman, E., et al. (1999). Association of unipolar major depressive disorder with genes of the serotonergic and dopaminergic pathways. *Mol. Psychiatry* 4, 389–392. doi: 10.1038/sj.mp.4000536

Geng, Y. G., Su, Q. R., Su, L. Y., Chen, Q., Ren, G. Y., Shen, S. Q., et al. (2007). Comparison of the polymorphisms of androgen receptor gene and estrogen alpha and beta gene between adolescent females with first-onset major depressive disorder and controls. *Int. J. Neurosci.* 117, 539–547. doi: 10.1080/00207450600773640

Goodyer, I. M., Bacon, A., Ban, M., Croudace, T., and Herbert, J. (2009). Serotonin transporter genotype, morning cortisol and subsequent depression in adolescents. *Br. J. Psychiatry* 195, 39–45. doi: 10.1192/bjp.bp.108.054775

Goodyer, I. M., Croudace, T., Dudbridge, F., Ban, M., and Herbert, J. (2010). Polymorphisms in BDNF (Val66Met) and 5-HTTLPR, morning cortisol and subsequent depression in at-risk adolescents. *Br. J. Psychiatry* 197, 365–371. doi: 10.1192/bjp.bp.110.077750

Gordon, M., and Melvin, G. (2013). Selective serotonin re-uptake inhibitors-a review of the side effects in adolescents. *Aust. Fam. Physician* 42, 620–623.

Guo, G., and Tillman, K. H. (2009). Trajectories of depressive symptoms, dopamine D2 and D4 receptors, family socioeconomic status and social support in adolescence and young adulthood. *Psychiatr. Genet.* 19, 14–26. doi: 10.1097/YPG.0b013e32831219b6

Haeffel, G. J., Getchell, M., Koposov, R. A., Yrigollen, C. M., DeYoung, C. G., Klinteberg, B., et al. (2008). Association between polymorphisms in the dopamine transporter gene and depression: evidence for a gene-environment interaction in a sample of juvenile detainees. *Psychol. Sci.* 19, 62–69. doi: 10.1111/j.1467-9280.2008.02047.x

Hammen, C., Brennan, P. A., Keenan-Miller, D., Hazel, N. A., and Najman, J. M. (2010). Chronic and acute stress, gender and serotonin transporter gene-environment interactions predicting depression symptoms in youth. *J. Child Psychol. Psychiatry* 51, 180–187. doi: 10.1111/j.1469-7610.2009.02177.x

Hankin, B. L., Jenness, J., Abela, J. R., and Smolen, A. (2011). Interaction of 5-HTTLPR and idiographic stressors predicts prospective depressive symptoms specifically among youth in a multiwave design. *J. Clin. Child Adolesc. Psychol.* 40, 572–585. doi: 10.1080/15374416.2011.581613

Harrisberger, F., Smieskova, R., Schmidt, A., Lenz, C., Walter, A., Wittfeld, K., et al. (2015). BDNF Val66Met polymorphism and hippocampal volume in neuropsychiatric disorders: a systematic review and meta-analysis. *Neurosci. Biobehav. Rev.* 55, 107–118. doi: 10.1016/j.neubiorev.2015.04.017

Hetrick, S. E., McKenzie, J. E., Cox, G. R., Simmons, M. B., and Merry, S. N. (2012). Newer generation antidepressants for depressive disorders in children and adolescents. *Cochrane Database Syst. Rev.* 11:CD004851. doi: 10.1002/14651858.CD004851

Hilt, L. M., Sander, L. C., Nolen-Hoeksema, S., and Simen, A. A. (2007). The BDNF Val66Met polymorphism predicts rumination and depression differently in young adolescent girls and their mothers. *Neurosci. Lett.* 429, 12–16. doi: 10.1016/j.neulet.2007.09.053

Hosang, G. M., Shiles, C., Tansey, K. E., McGuffin, P., and Uher, R. (2014). Interaction between stress and the BDNF Val66Met polymorphism in depression: a systematic review and meta-analysis. *BMC Med.* 12:7. doi: 10.1186/1741-7015-12-7

Jaffee, S. R., Moffitt, T. E., Caspi, A., Fombonne, E., Poulton, R., and Martin, J. (2002). Differences in early childhood risk factors for juvenile-onset and adult-onset depression. *Arch. Gen. Psychiatry* 59, 215–222. doi: 10.1001/archpsyc.59.3.215

Jenness, J. L., Hankin, B. L., Abela, J. R., Young, J. F., and Smolen, A. (2011). Chronic family stress interacts with 5-HTTLPR to predict prospective depressive symptoms among youth. *Depress. Anxiety* 28, 1074–1080. doi: 10.1002/da.20904

Jiang, X., Xu, K., Hoberman, J., Tian, F., Marko, A. J., Waheed, J. F., et al. (2005). BDNF variation and mood disorders: a novel functional promoter polymorphism and Val66Met are associated with anxiety but have opposing effects. *Neuropsychopharmacology* 30, 1353–1361. doi: 10.1038/sj.npp.1300703

Kimpton, J. (2012). The brain derived neurotrophic factor and influences of stress in depression. *Psychiatr. Danub.* 24, S169–S171.

Kirov, G., Jones, I., McCandless, F., Craddock, N., and Owen, M. J. (1999). Family-based association studies of bipolar disorder with candidate genes involved in dopamine neurotransmission: DBH, DAT1, COMT, DRD2, DRD3 and DRD5. *Mol. Psychiatry* 4, 558–565. doi: 10.1038/sj.mp.4000565

Kohen, R., Myaing, M. T., Richards, J., Zhou, C., McCauley, E. A., Katon, W., et al. (2013). Depression persistence and serotonin transporter genotype in adolescents under usual care conditions. *J. Child Adolesc. Psychopharmacol.* 23, 290–294. doi: 10.1089/cap.2011.0137

Laucht, M., Treutlein, J., Blomeyer, D., Buchmann, A. F., Schmid, B., Becker, K., et al. (2009). Interaction between the 5-HTTLPR serotonin transporter polymorphism and environmental adversity for mood and anxiety psychopathology: evidence from a high-risk community sample of young adults. *Int. J. Neuropsychopharmacol.* 12, 737–747. doi: 10.1017/s1461145708009875

Lawford, B. R., Young, R., Noble, E. P., Kann, B., and Ritchie, T. (2006). The D-2 dopamine receptor (DRD2) gene is associated with co-morbid depression, anxiety and social dysfunction in untreated veterans with post-traumatic stress disorder. *Eur. Psychiatry* 21, 180–185. doi: 10.1016/j.eurpsy.2005.01.006

Leggio, G. M., Salomone, S., Bucolo, C., Platania, C., Micale, V., Caraci, F., et al. (2013). Dopamine D(3) receptor as a new pharmacological target for the treatment of depression. *Eur. J. Pharmacol.* 719, 25–33. doi: 10.1016/j.ejphar.2013.07.022

Little, K., Olsson, C. A., Whittle, S., Youssef, G. J., Byrne, M. L., Simmons, J. G., et al. (2014). Association between serotonin transporter genotype, brain structure and adolescent-onset major depressive disorder: a longitudinal prospective study. *Transl. Psychiatry* 4:e445. doi: 10.1038/tp.2014.85

Lockwood, L. E., Su, S., and Youssef, N. A. (2015). The role of epigenetics in depression and suicide: a platform for gene-environment interactions. *Psychiatry Res.* 228, 235–242. doi: 10.1016/j.psychres.2015.05.071

Mamalakis, G., Kiriakakis, M., Tsibinos, G., and Kafatos, A. (2004). Depression and adipose polyunsaturated fatty acids in an adolescent group. *Prostaglandins Leukot. Essent. Fatty Acids* 71, 289–294. doi: 10.1016/j.plefa.2004.04.002

Manki, H., Kanba, S., Muramatsu, T., Higuchi, S., Suzuki, E., Matsushita, S., et al. (1996). Dopamine D2, D3 and D4 receptor and transporter gene polymorphisms and mood disorders. *J. Affect. Disord.* 40, 7–13. doi: 10.1016/0165-0327(96)00035-3

Mata, J., and Gotlib, I. H. (2011). 5-HTTLPR moderates the relation between changes in depressive and bulimic symptoms in adolescent girls: a longitudinal study. *Int. J. Eat. Disord.* 44, 383–388. doi: 10.1002/eat.20850

Mata, J., Thompson, R. J., and Gotlib, I. H. (2010). BDNF genotype moderates the relation between physical activity and depressive symptoms. *Health Psychol.* 29, 130–133. doi: 10.1037/a0017261

Miraglia del Giudice, E., Santoro, N., Fiumani, P., Dominguez, G., Kuhar, M. J., and Perrone, L. (2006). Adolescents carrying a missense mutation in the CART gene exhibit increased anxiety and depression. *Depress. Anxiety* 23, 90–92. doi: 10.1002/da.20156

Nederhof, E., Bouma, E. M., Oldehinkel, A. J., and Ormel, J. (2010). Interaction between childhood adversity, brain-derived neurotrophic factor val/met and serotonin transporter promoter polymorphism on depression: the TRAILS study. *Biol. Psychiatry* 68, 209–212. doi: 10.1016/j.biopsych.2010.04.006

Nilsson, K. W., Sjöberg, R. L., Leppert, J., Oreland, L., and Damberg, M. (2009). Transcription factor AP-2 beta genotype and psychosocial adversity in relation to adolescent depressive symptomatology. *J. Neural Transm. Vienna* 116, 363–370. doi: 10.1007/s00702-009-0183-3

Nobile, M., Rusconi, M., Bellina, M., Marino, C., Giorda, R., Carlet, O., et al. (2009). The influence of family structure, the TPH2 G-703T and the 5-HTTLPR serotonergic genes upon affective problems in children aged 10–14 years. *J. Child Psychol. Psychiatry* 50, 317–325. doi: 10.1111/j.1469-7610.2008.01958.x

Otten, R., and Engels, R. C. (2013). Testing bidirectional effects between cannabis use and depressive symptoms: moderation by the serotonin transporter gene. *Addict. Biol.* 18, 826–835. doi: 10.1111/j.1369-1600.2011.00380.x

Pandey, G. N., Dwivedi, Y., Ren, X., Rizavi, H. S., Roberts, R. C., and Conley, R. R. (2007). Cyclic AMP response element-binding protein in post-mortem brain of teenage suicide victims: specific decrease in the prefrontal cortex but not the hippocampus. *Int. J. Neuropsychopharmacol.* 10, 621–629. doi: 10.1017/s1461145706007231

Pandey, G. N., Rizavi, H. S., Ren, X., Fareed, J., Hoppensteadt, D. A., Roberts, R. C., et al. (2012). Proinflammatory cytokines in the prefrontal cortex of teenage suicide victims. *J. Psychiatr. Res.* 46, 57–63. doi: 10.1016/j.jpsychires.2011.08.006

Paus, T. (2013). How environment and genes shape the adolescent brain. *Horm. Behav.* 64, 195–202. doi: 10.1016/j.yhbeh.2013.04.004

Petersen, I. T., Bates, J. E., Goodnight, J. A., Dodge, K. A., Lansford, J. E., and Pettit, G. S. (2012). Interaction between serotonin transporter polymorphism (5-HTTLPR) and stressful life events in adolescents' trajectories of anxious/depressed symptoms. *Dev. Psychol.* 48, 1463–1475. doi: 10.1037/a0027471

Priess-Groben, H. A., and Hyde, J. S. (2013). 5-HTTLPR X stress in adolescent depression: moderation by MAOA and gender. *J. Abnorm. Child Psychol.* 41, 281–294. doi: 10.1007/s10802-012-9672-1

Rice, F. (2009). The genetics of depression in childhood and adolescence. *Curr. Psychiatry Rep.* 11, 167–173. doi: 10.1007/s11920-009-0026-9

Rice, F. (2010). Genetics of childhood and adolescent depression: insights into etiological heterogeneity and challenges for future genomic research. *Genome Med.* 2:68. doi: 10.1186/gm189

Rotberg, B., Kronenberg, S., Carmel, M., Frisch, A., Brent, D., Zalsman, G.,

5

EMOTICOM: A Neuropsychological Test Battery to Evaluate Emotion, Motivation, Impulsivity and Social Cognition

Edited by:
Raymond C. K. Chan,
Chinese Academy of Sciences, China

***Correspondence:**
Rebecca Elliott
rebecca.elliott@manchester.ac.uk

Amy R. Bland[1], *Jonathan P. Roiser*[2], *Mitul A. Mehta*[3], *Thea Schei*[4], *Heather Boland*[1], *Daniel K. Campbell-Meiklejohn*[5], *Richard A. Emsley*[6], *Marcus R. Munafo*[7], *Ian S. Penton-Voak*[7], *Ana Seara-Cardoso*[8, 9], *Essi Viding*[8], *Valerie Voon*[10, 11], *Barbara J. Sahakian*[10, 11], *Trevor W. Robbins*[4, 11] *and Rebecca Elliott*[1]*

[1] Neuroscience and Psychiatry Unit, University of Manchester, Manchester, UK, [2] Institute of Cognitive Neuroscience, University College London, London, UK, [3] Institute of Psychiatry, Psychology and Neuroscience, Kings College London, London, UK, [4] Department of Psychology, University of Cambridge, Cambridge, UK, [5] School of Psychology, University of Sussex, Brighton, UK, [6] Institute of Population Health, University of Manchester, Manchester, UK, [7] School of Experimental Psychology, University of Bristol, Bristol, UK, [8] Psychology and Language Sciences, University College London, London, UK, [9] School of Psychology, University of Minho, Guimaraes, Portugal, [10] Department of Psychiatry, University of Cambridge, Cambridge, UK, [11] Behavioural and Clinical Neuroscience Institute, University of Cambridge, Cambridge, UK

In mental health practice, both pharmacological and non-pharmacological treatments are aimed at improving neuropsychological symptoms, including cognitive and emotional impairments. However, at present there is no established neuropsychological test battery that comprehensively covers multiple affective domains relevant in a range of disorders. Our objective was to generate a standardized test battery, comprised of existing, adapted and novel tasks, to assess four core domains of affective cognition (emotion processing, motivation, impulsivity and social cognition) in order to facilitate and enhance treatment development and evaluation in a broad range of neuropsychiatric disorders. The battery was administered to 200 participants aged 18–50 years (50% female), 42 of whom were retested in order to assess reliability. An exploratory factor analysis identified 11 factors with eigenvalues greater than 1, which accounted for over 70% of the variance. Tasks showed moderate to excellent test-retest reliability and were not strongly correlated with demographic factors such as age or IQ. The EMOTICOM test battery is therefore a promising tool for the assessment of affective cognitive function in a range of contexts.

Keywords: EMOTICOM, neuropsychological tests, social cognition, motivation and emotion, implusivity, neuropsychiatry, mental health

INTRODUCTION

Mental health problems represent an extremely significant health burden, with global costs estimated at $2.5 trillion, projected to increase to $6.5 trillion by 2030, more than any other form of disease (Bloom et al., 2012; Fineberg et al., 2013). Impairments of emotional, motivational and social function are increasingly thought to be fundamental to the neurobehavioral pathology of psychiatric disorders and are becoming important targets for therapeutic intervention (Roiser et al., 2012). Major advances in treatment development will therefore be facilitated by well-designed, carefully validated measures of a comprehensive range of emotional, motivational, and social functions. This is critically important in clinical trials, of both of pharmacological and psychological interventions, which specifically aim to target emotional, motivational, and social processes. Currently, the outcome measures used in trials of such interventions are typically changes in clinical symptoms, and there is a pressing need for new outcome measures that quantitatively measure the effects of these treatments. A validated affective battery would also have important implications in other research contexts; for example, investigating cognitive profiles relevant to the NIMH Research Domain Criteria (RDoC) initiative that aims to create a new framework for mental health research (Insel et al., 2010; Sanislow et al., 2010) focusing on dimensions that cut across DSM diagnostic categories, investigating endophenotypes for genetic studies' or identifying biomarkers for high-risk individuals. However, at present there is no established neuropsychological test battery that offers a comprehensive assessment of "hot" cognitive functions.

Various individual tests have been developed and validated to test specific cognitive hypotheses. However, without standardization, it is difficult to make progress, replicate results, or identify gaps that need to be addressed (Elliott et al., 2011). Multi-center studies and clinical trials would benefit from a comprehensive, validated battery probing emotional, motivational, and social functions. The success of existing, standardized cognitive batteries highlights their recognized importance for assessing cognitive function. For example, the Cambridge Automated Neuropsychological Test Battery (CANTAB; Cambridge Cognition Ltd) has become a widely used battery in both academic research and clinical trials (Robbins et al., 1994, 1998; Cambridge Cognition Ltd). However, the focus is primarily on "cold" cognitive functions (Roiser and Sahakian, 2013) such as executive function, visuospatial memory and various types of attention. Here we generate normative data for a battery of neuropsychological tasks, which assesses a comprehensive range of processes relevant to affective cognition.

Affective Cognition

Affective cognition is a term used to describe aspects of cognitive function where stimuli have affective salience; the term "hot" cognition has been coined to distinguish these aspects of cognition from non-emotive "cold" cognitions (Roiser and Sahakian, 2013). Affective cognition, can be defined as reflecting an interface at which emotional and cognitive processes are integrated to generate behavior (Elliott et al., 2011).

Disrupted affective cognition is a core feature of many mental health disorders and cuts across DSM diagnostic categories. For example, biases in processing emotional stimuli have been observed in depression (Surguladze et al., 2004), anxiety (Mogg and Bradley, 2002), schizophrenia (Pomarol-Clotet et al., 2010), substance abuse (Ersche and Sahakian, 2007), eating disorders (Lovell et al., 1997), ADHD (Seymour et al., 2015), and phobic anxiety (Watts et al., 1986). Reward learning and motivation have been shown to be impaired in schizophrenia (Murray et al., 2007; Waltz et al., 2010), Parkinson's Disease (Voon et al., 2010), substance abuse (Park et al., 2010), affective disorders (Murphy et al., 2003), and ADHD (Thomas et al., 2015). Impulsivity has been in described in substance abuse (Voon et al., 2014), eating disorders (Mobbs et al., 2011), and ADHD (Malloy-Diniz et al., 2007). Finally, social cognition impairments have been demonstrated in autism (Happé and Frith, 1996), depression (Zahn et al., 2015), and schizophrenia (Fett et al., 2011). Social, emotional, and motivational aspects of cognition are thought to be key predictors of functional outcomes. Therefore, novel interventions targeting affective cognition may be effective for improving functional outcomes, as well as reducing symptoms. Examples include cognitive bias modification in depression (Baert et al., 2010; Roiser et al., 2012), social cognition training in schizophrenia (Combs et al., 2007), or pharmacological agents to promote social function such as oxytocin (Feifel et al., 2012).

A number of studies have explored the potential factor structure of affective cognition in mental health disorders. For example, the MATRICS project identified five sub-processes relevant to schizophrenia including, theory of mind, social perception, social knowledge, attributional bias, and emotional processing (Green et al., 2008). Others have identified four factors including perceiving emotions, facilitating thought, understanding emotions, and managing emotions (Mayer and Salovey, 1997; Mayer et al., 2003); or two factors including an emotional perception and understanding factor and an emotional facilitation and management factor (Eack et al., 2010).

However, despite a clear consensus that "hot" cognitive function is a multidimensional construct with many underlying sub-processes, no comprehensive battery assessing affective function is currently available. There are a number of batteries that include a limited number of affective tasks in predominately "cold" cognitive test batteries (e.g., CANTAB; www.cambridgecognition.com, MATRICS; www.matricsinc.org, CogState; www.cogstate.com, WebNeuro; www.brainresource.com). A recently developed explicit hot cognition battery, the Emotional Test Battery (ETB; www.p1vital.com), focuses on emotion processing tasks of particular relevance to depression.

In developing the test battery described here we chose to focus on four distinct domains of affective cognition: *emotion processing*, the ability to process and respond to affective stimuli, including emotional faces; *motivation*, the ability to learn, apply effort and make decisions driven by incentives; *impulsivity*, premature or risky responding; and *social cognition*, the ability to process information about situations involving interpersonal interactions. For each of these domains we piloted in 30 individuals a combination of novel, adapted and existing tasks designed to probe key underlying affective functions. We selected for inclusion in the final battery those tasks that were feasible in brief versions, readily understood and well-tolerated by participants and (for existing or adapted tasks) that elicited robust replication of previously observed effects. Further details of excluded tasks are available from the authors on request.

Emotional Processing

Emotion recognition/categorization

Recognition of facial expressions is a widely-used paradigm in neuropsychiatry, particularly in studies of depressed patients who tend to rate ambiguous expressions as more negative

(Bouhuys et al., 1999; Surguladze et al., 2004). Harmer et al. (2011) argues that emotional face recognition may be a sensitive biomarker for effective antidepressant treatment. We therefore aimed to develop a task that effectively probed emotional facial recognition. The Emotion Recognition Task (ERT) included in the CANTAB battery (Cambridge Cognition Ltd) has proven to be a promising task examining emotion recognition in clinical populations. However, in order to include an ERT in EMOTICOM with limited time available, we opted to focus on basic emotions; happy, sad, anger and fear and chose to exclude more complex emotions such as surprise and disgust. We also adapted the task to include two versions; one that assessed facial recognition, similarly to the original CANTAB ERT and one that more specifically assessed eye recognition. Including emotional eyes recognition was motivated by evidence supporting the "reading the mind from the eyes" test (Baron-Cohen et al., 2001) as an effective assessment of the ability to recognize the emotional state of others using just the expressions around the eyes. We further adapted the task to include control conditions, i.e., identifying the age of a face and eyes, to provide baseline measurement in neuroimaging investigations.

Attentional bias

Biased emotional attention can be effectively measured using the affective go/no-go test (Cambridge Cognition Ltd). Attentional biases have been observed in depression (Murphy et al., 1999; Erickson et al., 2005), mania (Murphy et al., 1999), anxiety disorders (Watts et al., 1986; Mogg et al., 1995), substance abuse (Ersche and Sahakian, 2007), and eating disorders (Lovell et al., 1997). Negative biases in processing emotional stimuli have been suggested as an important biomarker for antidepressant efficacy and may predict responses to both psychological and pharmacological interventions (Harmer et al., 2009; Roiser et al., 2012). We therefore adapted two versions of the Affective Go No-Go task: one similar to the CANTAB with word stimuli and one with face stimuli. The motivation for adapting the AGN to include faces was to potentially improve any cross-cultural, educational, and age influences on the word version. For example, emotionally salient word stimuli may require a minimum reading level that may not be suitable for use in children. Indeed, a facial version of the AGN has shown to be a promising tool in pediatric anxiety and depression (Ladouceur et al., 2006). Additionally, an emotionally cued Posner task (Posner, 1980) using eye gaze in emotional facial expressions was piloted as part of the development of the EMOTICOM battery but did not show significant condition effects.

Emotional memory

Biased emotional memory for personal experiences has been suggested as an important trait marker for depression (Brittlebank et al., 1993). Depressed patients also show a more general bias toward remembering negative information (Hamilton and Gotlib, 2008) and patients with schizophrenia show deficits in remembering positive stimuli (Herbener et al., 2008) suggesting a possible double dissociation between the two disorders. We therefore developed an emotional memory task that required an encoding phase presented at the start of the EMOTICOM battery and a retrieval phase presented at the end in order to assess biases in emotional memory. We also piloted an emotional working memory task using a spatial n-back (for review see Owen et al., 2005) with emotional faces, however this did not produce sufficient significant condition effects.

Motivation and Reward

Reinforcement learning

Behavioral tests assessing reinforcement learning (RL) in humans are directly comparable to operant conditioning tasks used in animals (Roberts et al., 1988; Birrell and Brown, 2000). Human reinforcement learning tests typically involve learning which abstract stimuli predict winning or losing points or money (Owen et al., 1991; Pessiglione et al., 2006). Reinforcement learning, and corresponding responses in the brain's reward system, are reliably disrupted in several neuropsychiatric diseases, including schizophrenia (Murray et al., 2007; Waltz et al., 2010), Parkinson's Disease (Voon et al., 2010), alcohol dependence (Park et al., 2010), and depression (Murphy et al., 2003). One weakness of several tests is the conflation of reward and punishment learning (Cools et al., 2002). This is important, since reward and punishment may be subserved by separable, opponent processes in the brain (Daw et al., 2006). We therefore aimed to develop a novel reinforcement learning task that separated reward and punishment feedback in order to assess sensitivity to these independently.

Incentive motivation

Tests of incentive motivation measure how much effort an individual is prepared to exert to gain reward. The monetary incentive delay (MID) functional neuroimaging task features a speeded response to obtain a reward or avoid a loss (Knutson et al., 2001). However, the behavioral measure arising from this paradigm has seldom been shown to be altered by diagnosis or pharmacological manipulation (Knutson et al., 2004; Scheres et al., 2007). Indeed, the MID continually updates the threshold for success, which might reduce behavioral differences between conditions. Hence we aimed to develop an incentive motivation task that produced reliable behavioral differences that have the potential to provide important biomarkers for assessment and treatment interventions. We adapted the Salience Attribution Task (Roiser et al., 2009a) which has previously shown robust behavioral markers of adaptive motivational salience in Schizophrenia and developed a version that specifically evaluated motivation relating to reward and punishment separately.

Value-based choice

Tests of value-based choice investigate how subjects use different types of information (e.g., probability, reward, punishment) in order to guide economic decision-making. In contrast to tests of reinforcement learning, there is typically no learning component in tests of value-based choice. As such, the widely-used Iowa Gambling Task (Bechara et al., 1994) is not a specific test of value-based choice, since it also involves learning. The Cambridge Gamble Task (CGT: Rogers et al., 1999), part of the CANTAB suite of tests, asks subjects to decide on which of two options to bet, and to stake a certain percentage of their points on this bet. The CGT is sensitive to unipolar (Murphy, et al., 2001) and bipolar depression (Roiser et al., 2009b), schizophrenia (Hutton et al., 2002), and psychopharmacological manipulation (Rogers et al., 1999). However, it cannot determine whether decision-making is influenced by reward seeking or punishment avoidance. A later development (Rogers et al., 2003) can distinguish between these and is sensitive to several neuropsychiatric conditions (Roiser et al., 2006; Chandler et al., 2009) and psychopharmacological manipulations (Scarna et al., 2005), but includes a very restricted set of probabilities. We therefore adapted the CANTAB CGT (Cambridge Cognition Ltd) to investigate reward seeking and punishment avoidance separately.

Impulsivity

Waiting impulsivity

Coordination between initiation and inhibition of actions is required for successful behavior. Patients with ADHD (Aron and Poldrack, 2005), obsessive compulsive disorder (Malloy-Diniz et al., 2007), and schizophrenia (Kaladjian et al., 2007) show impairments in impulsivity. The four choice serial reaction time task (4-CSRTT) is a novel translation from the widely used 5-choice serial reaction time rodent task (5-CSRTT; Robbins, 2002). It has demonstrated clear deficits in substance abuse (Voon et al., 2014) and is sensitive to effects of dietary tryptophan depletion which is thought to reduce central 5-HT (Worbe et al., 2014). We therefore decided to incorporate the 4CSRTT (Voon et al., 2014) into the EMOTICOM battery which measures incentive motivation to rewards and premature responses elicited by anticipated reward.

Delay and probability discounting

Another aspect of impulsivity is the preference for immediate gratification, even when waiting longer might lead to higher absolute gain. Delay discounting is the progressive reduction in subjective value of a reinforcer with time. It can be assessed using two types of task—hypothetical or experiential. Hypothetical discounting tasks require choices between immediate (e.g., £1 now) and delayed (e.g., £5 in 1 month) rewards (Mazur, 1987; Green et al., 1996; Kirby, 2009). The experiential discounting tasks differs from hypothetical in that respondents directly experience the delay and receive the reward during the task (Reynolds and Schiffbauer, 2004). Patients with ADHD and substance use disorders show steeper discounting rates in such tasks, which also show good temporal stability similar to personality traits (Ohmura et al., 2006; Kirby, 2009). We therefore developed a computerized delay discounting task based on Richards et al.'s (1999) adjustment procedure.

Social Cognition

Moral emotion

Moral emotions can be experimentally induced either in response to verbal descriptions or pictures of specific interpersonal behavior (Moll and de Oliveira-Souza, 2007) or behavior contravening normal social values (Zahn et al., 2009). Patients with ventromedial prefrontal (VMPFC) lesions show abnormal responses to hypothetical moral dilemmas (Ciaramelli et al., 2007; Koenigs et al., 2007) and patients with antisocial personality disorder (Blair, 1995) and Autism (Moran et al., 2011) show deficits in moral judgment. We developed a novel computerized Moral Emotions task that comprising of cartoon scenarios rather than lengthy vignettes that are more likely to be affected by reading ability, intelligence and age.

Theory of mind

Theory of Mind (TOM) refers to the ability to infer the mental states of others (Frith and Frith, 2003). A number of paradigms have been proposed to probe this function including false belief tasks (Frith and Corcoran, 1996), "faux pas" tests, visual jokes, understanding irony and the "Reading the Mind in the Eyes" test (Baron-Cohen et al., 2001; although note that this is most similar to an emotional recognition task—see above). Patients with autism typically show impaired TOM (Happé and Frith, 1996) and it is also sensitive to schizophrenia (Frith and Corcoran, 1996; Bora et al., 2009; Fett et al., 2011). While valuable in populations with overt impairment, existing TOM tasks are typically insensitive to variation in normal adult performance as most participants perform at ceiling. Therefore, we developed a complementary task that depicted ambiguous social situations with no right or wrong answer, thus allowing greater variation of responses in healthy volunteers. Rather than assessing whether participants have TOM ability, this task assesses the extent to which people choose to use TOM information.

Social economic exchange games

Economic games, such as the Ultimatum Game and Prisoners' Dilemma are popular tasks for exploring the neurobiology of social decision-making (King-Casas et al., 2005; Miller, 2005; Fehr and Camerer, 2007; Crockett, 2009). A number of patient groups have been studied using these games, including psychopathy (Koenigs et al., 2010; Rilling et al., 2015), schizophrenia (Agay et al., 2008), autism (Andari et al., 2010), depression (Pulcu et al., 2015), and borderline personality

TABLE 1 | Demographic characteristics of sample ($N = 200$), stratified by age, IQ, gender, and ethnicity for the standardization of the EMOTICOM neuropsychological test battery.

	Mean	SD
Age	26.66	9.81
Years in Education	14.40	2.01
WTAR IQ	112.18	6.29
Gender	**N**	**%**
Female	100	50
White	157	78.5
ETHNICITY		
Afro Caribbean	7	3.5
Asian-Indian	10	5
East-Asian	9	4.5
Mixed	9	4.5
Other	8	4

TABLE 2 | Full list of neuropsychological tasks with outcome measures which are included in the EMOTICOM neuropsychological test battery.

EMOTION PROCESSING	
Emotion recognition/categorization	**Task 1: Emotional Recognition Task (ERT)** We developed two versions of an ERT; one with full faces, and one with eyes only. In these tasks, the participant is shown a series of faces or eyes that appear on the screen briefly, and is asked to identify the emotion (happiness, sadness, anger or fear). In the control condition, participants are asked to identify the age of a face (child, young adult, middle aged, elderly). **Time to administer:** 12 min **Outcome Measures:** Accuracy scores were calculated for each facial emotion (happiness, sadness, anger, and fear). *Average accuracy* refers to average accuracy across all four emotions. *Affective bias* scores were calculated by subtracting accuracy for sad faces from accuracy from happy faces. This analysis was also performed for the eyes emotional recognition test.
	Task 2: Emotional Intensity Morphing Task This task assesses the point of emotional intensity at which participants can recognize a facial emotion. Participants view faces that either increase or decrease in emotional intensity and are instructed to respond when they either (a) detect the presence of emotion or (b) no longer detect the presence of emotion. The emotion that they were detecting was made explicit to participants. The task includes five different emotions: happiness, sadness, anger, fear, and disgust. **Time to administer:** 5 min **Outcome Measures:** The point of detection was calculated by taking the level of intensity in the facial expression needed in order to detect (increasing) or no longer detect (decreasing) each emotion. The *Average point of detection* refers to average point of detection across all five emotions. *Affective bias* scores were calculated by subtracting the point of detection for sad faces from point of detection from happy faces.
Attentional bias	**Task 3: Face Affective Go No-Go Task** This task assesses information processing biases for positive and negative facial expressions. The participant is told a target emotion (happy, sad, neutral), and asked to press a button only when the target emotion is present. The task consists of six blocks, each of which presents a series of faces: (1) happy target/sad distractor, (2) happy target/neutral distractor, (3) neutral target/happy distract, (4) neutral target/sad distract, (5) sad target/happy distract, and (6) sad target/neutral distract. **Time to administer:** 6 min **Outcome Measures:** Reaction times (RT) were calculated for all "hit" responses for each of the six conditions. *Affective bias* scores were calculated by subtracting the sad target/happy distract condition RT from the happy target/sad distractor condition RT.
	Task 4: Word Affective Go No-Go This task assesses information processing biases for positive, negative and neutral emotional words. Words were chosen based on their ratings in a pilot study in an independent cohort of 30 volunteers and were matched for valence, arousal, frequency and word length. Participants are given a target emotion (happy, sad, neutral), and asked to press a button only when the target emotion is present. Similarly to the faces affective go no go, the task consists of six blocks, each of which presents a series of words: (1) happy target/sad distractor, (2) happy target/neutral distractor, (3) neutral target/happy distractor, (4) neutral target/sad distractor, (5) sad target/happy distractor, and (6) sad target/neutral distractor. Note that this task is not the same as the Cambridge Cognition (www.cambridgecognition.com) word affective go no-go task. **Time to administer:** 6 min **Outcome Measures:** Reaction times (RT) were calculated for all "hit" responses for each of the six conditions. *Affective bias* scores were calculated by subtracting the sad target/happy distract condition RT from the happy target/sad distractor condition RT.
Emotional memory	**Task 5: The Emotional Memory Recognition Task** This task assesses biases in the recognition of emotional stimuli. During the *encoding* stage, participants are asked to rate images displaying positive, negative or neutral scenes, on valence and arousal intensity. Images were of scenes without people and were validated as positive, negative or neutral on the basis of pilot testing in an independent cohort of 30 volunteers. During the *retrieval* stage, images from the encoding phase are paired with new images. Participants are asked to indicate which image they saw previously. The encoding phase consists of 30 images (10 positive, 10 negative and 10 neutral) whilst the retrieval phase consists of 60 images (20 positive, 20 negative and 20 neutral), half of which were previously seen in the encoding phase. **Time to administer:** 5 min **Outcome Measures:** Valence and intensity ratings from the encoding phase were calculated for each valence condition; positive, negative and neutral. Retrieval affective bias was calculated by subtracting accuracy for negative stimuli from accuracy for positive stimuli.

(Continued)

TABLE 2 | Continued

MOTIVATION AND REWARD	
Reinforcement learning	**Task 6: Reinforcement Learning Task** This task separately assesses reward and punishment learning. Participants are shown colored circles, and asked to make a choice between the two based on which one they thought was more likely to win money and not lose money. Participants receive feedback and are continually updated on their total score. There are two conditions; one condition is a *no lose* condition whereby participants either win (£0.50 presented as 50p) or fail to win (0p). The second condition is a *no win* in condition whereby they lose (50p) or avoid losing (0p). Participants must learn, through sampling the circles, which of the two is the better option, with probabilities (unknown to participants) set at 70%/30%. In the *transfer* phase, all possible pairs of circles are presented and participants choose their preferred option. In this phase, no feedback is given. **Time to administer:** 12 min **Outcome Measures:** A reinforcement learning model was applied to the data. Learning rate (alpha) refers to how fast the participant learns new information. A high learning rate indicates that the participant incorporates new information more quickly. Alpha was calculated for win and loss conditions separately.
Incentive motivation	**Task 7: The Monetary Incentive Reward (MIR) Task** This task assesses effort to avoid punishments and gain rewards. Participants see a pair of identical circles displayed on the screen, shortly followed by a black box. Participants are instructed to make a response as soon as the black box appears. The circles contain colored lines, which indicate that on that trial they will either gain or lose money. The distance between the lines indicates the size of loss/gain. The faster they respond the more money they win or the less money they lose, and this relationship remains constant throughout the task. **Time to administer:** 10 min **Outcome Measures:** Reaction times were calculated for each condition; high win, low win, low loss and high loss. These reaction times were further standardized by subtracting each of the four conditions from the neutral "baseline" reaction time. High and low win reaction times were combined to produce the *average reaction time for wins*. Likewise high and low loss reaction times were combined to produce the *average reaction time for loss.*
	Task 8: The Progressive Ratio Task Progressive ratio tasks have been widely used to examine motivation in non-human subjects (Hodos, 1961; Bradshaw and Killeen, 2012). More recently, progressive ratio tasks have been adapted for use in humans using a variety of rewards (e.g., money, stimulants, food) to assess self-control and identify participants' motivational "breakpoint," i.e., the maximum effort that a participant will expend in order to receive a reward (Roane, 2008). In this task participants are presented with four red squares on the screen and are instructed to select the square that differs in size to the other three. Participants are paid progressively less per trial as they continue with the task. They are also told that they can stop their participation in the task at any point, but that they still have to sit facing the screen for the remaining time (20 min minus the time they performed the task). **Time to administer:** 20 min **Outcome Measures:** The progressive Ratio task was adapted part way through the study therefore data is only presented for the adapted task (participant $n = 78$). The total number of trials was calculated in order to estimate the *breakpoint,* i.e., the point at which participants did not wish to continue with the task. *Running rate* was calculated as the time taken to complete the block of trials. The *post reinforcement pause* was the average time taken to initiate the next trial following a reward. Approximately 57% of participants completed the task therefore only allowing us to calculate a breakpoint for the remaining participants. Consequently, the progressive ratio task was not included in the factor analysis and test-retest reliability determinations.
Value-based choice	**Task 9: The adapted Cambridge Gambling Task** This task was developed to assess decision-making and risk-taking behavior, with reward and loss trials administered separately. On each trial, the participant is presented with a roulette wheel; a proportion of which is colored purple and a proportion of which is orange. There are 5 different proportions ranging from very certain to very uncertain. Participants must place a bet on the outcome they expect. A spinning pointer is then displayed, which lands on one of the colors, providing feedback for the participant. There are two conditions; a loss condition and a win condition which allows the separation of reward and punishment. **Time to administer:** 10 min **Outcome Measures:** The average value of chips placed on each level of probability was calculated separately for the win and loss conditions. Only choices of the most likely outcome were included. This was used to compute a *risk adjustment* (RA) score using the formula: *Risk adjustment = (2*bet at 90%) + (1*bet at 80%) + (0*bet at 70%) - (1*bet at 60%) - (2*bet at 50%)/Average bet*. RA was calculated for win and loss conditions separately.

(Continued)

TABLE 2 | Continued

IMPULSIVITY	
Waiting impulsivity	**Task 10: The four-choice serial reaction time task** This task (Voon et al., 2014) assesses visual attention, and ability to monitor and respond to unpredictable targets. Participants have to indicate a box, from 4 choices, in which a target has appeared. **Time to administer:** 25 min **Outcome Measures:** Data from 175 participants was utilized in the analyses due to initial technical problems. The motivational index was calculated by using the following formula: *motivational index = (baseline reaction time−post baseline reaction time)/ baseline reaction time.* The number of premature events was calculated as the combination of the number of premature releases (releasing the spacebar prematurely) and the number of premature responses (releasing the space bar prematurely and touching the screen).
Delay and probability discounting	**Task 11: The Discounting Task** This task assesses the rate of discounting across delays and probabilities. There are ten conditions; five levels of delay (0, 30, 90, 180, 365 days) and five levels of probability (100, 90, 75, 50, 25%). Participants must decide whether they would prefer a standard fixed amount (always £20) associated with a particular delay or probability, compared to an alternative amount definitely available immediately. **Time to administer:** 7 min **Outcome Measures:** Indifference points were calculated for each length of delay or degree of uncertainty. These indifference points refer to the amount of immediately available money that the participant considered to be equivalent to the delayed or uncertain reward. For delay discounting, the area under the curve was used to calculate the level of discounting using the following formula: *Area under the curve = [(2-0)*((indifference point at 0 days + indifference point at 2 days)/2)]+[(30-2)*((indifference point at 2 days + indifference point at 30 days)/2)+[(180-30)*((indifference point at 3 days + indifference point at 180 days)/2)]+ [(365 -180)*((indifference point at 180 days+ indifference point at 365)/2)].* A smaller AUC, indicates more severe discounting of the delayed reward and thus greater impulsivity. A similar analysis was conducted for probability discounting, whereby smaller AUC indicates greater risk aversion.
SOCIAL COGNITION	
Moral emotion	**Task 12: The Moral Emotions task** This task uses cartoon figures to depict moral scenarios. Half of the scenarios depicted a deliberate harm whereas the remaining half depicted an accidental harm in order to explore the effect of intention upon moral emotions. Participants were asked to imagine how they would feel in the situation as either the actor or the victim, and rated the following emotions; guilt, shame, anger and feeling "bad." **Time to administer:** 13 min **Outcome Measures:** The average rating for feeling bad was calculated across all conditions: victim vs. agent and intentional vs. unintentional. Agent ratings for guilt were also calculated.
Theory of Mind	**Task 13: Social Information Preference Test** This task assesses information sampling in socially ambiguous situations. Participants are shown a scene, with three faces (feelings), three thoughts and three facts about the scene hidden from view. Participants are able to select only four out of nine pieces of information to help resolve ambiguity. They then choose between three possible outcomes of the situation (negative, positive or neutral), which provides a measure of interpretational bias. **Time to administer:** 10 min **Outcome Measures:** The proportion of thoughts selected and the valence of the chosen outcome, positive, negative or neutral was calculated. The *affective bias* in interpretation was calculated by subtracting the proportion of negative outcomes chosen from the proportion of positive outcomes chosen.
Social economic exchange games	**Task 14: Prisoners' Dilemma** This task assesses cooperation with a computerized opponent. On each trial, participants must repeatedly press the space bar as fast as they can in order to fill a jar with coins. Each trial is manipulated so that the participant wins more coins, the opponent wins more coins, or they both win equal amounts. The coin totals are then combined and participants are instructed that they may either split or steal the total sum. Participants are told that if they both choose to split, they get half the money each, and if they both steal, they each get nothing. If they split and the opponent steals they get nothing and the opponent gets everything. Alternatively, if they steal and their opponent splits, they get everything and the opponent nothing. Participants are faced with three different opponents each with a different strategy: aggressive (tit for tat, but starts with steal), tit for two tats (starts with split, then changes behavior after the player has stolen two times consecutively) and a cooperative player who always splits. **Time to administer:** 10 min **Outcome Measures:** The average steal proportion was calculated as the proportion of trials that participants chose to steal from their opponent from the total number of trials across each type of opponent (aggressive, tit for two tats and cooperative).

(Continued)

TABLE 2 | Continued

Task 15: Ultimatum Game

This task assesses sensitivity to fairness and tendency to inflict punishment. Similarly to the Prisoner's Dilemma, participants initially complete a task in which they can win money. Here they can select 3 balls from a choice of 9 and depending on what colors are revealed behind the balls, participants can win money. Each trial is manipulated so that the participant wins more money, the opponent wins more money, or they both win equal amounts. This money is then combined with the opponent's total. Next, participants are informed whether they get to decide how the money is split or whether it is up to the opponent. If the opponent divides the money, the participant gets the choice to either accept or reject their offer. These offers have seven levels ranging from fair (50:50) to increasingly unfair (10:90). If the participant accepts, they each get the allotted amount, and if they reject, they both get nothing. When the participant divides, they can choose from four divisions differing in fairness (50:50, 40:60, 30:70, 20:80, and 10:90).

Time to administer: 12 min

Outcome Measures: The proportion of offers accepted was calculated as the number of trials that participants chose to accept the offer from their opponent from the total number of trials. Risk adjustment was further calculated by using the following formula: *Risk adjustment = (2*acceptance at 50% offer) + (1* acceptance at 40% offer) + (0* acceptance at 30% offer) – (1* acceptance at 20% offer) – (2* acceptance at 10% offer)/Average offer.* The average offer proposed refers to proportion of times participants chose each of the four levels of offer available.

Task 16: Inference Task

Participants initially view a series of face pairs and are instructed to touch the more confident of each pair. This confirms that they are able to read confidence in faces. Participants are then asked to guess the contents of a series of buckets (mostly red or mostly blue jellybeans), based on a combination of information sources. On each trial, the subject and the honest computer (who never lies) each take a sample from the bucket. The participant is provided with: a sample of eight jellybeans, the *answer* of the honest computer (based on its own sample; it does not know the participant's) and the *confidence* of the honest computer in the answer it provided. This confidence is expressed with a human facial expression, either positive or skeptical. Each bucket is different from the rest, and independently numbered. The sample, answer of the computer and computer confidence are independently manipulated. Optimally, the subject will be able to increase the computer's influence when it expresses confidence and decrease its influence when it is apparently unsure of its decision. Information inferred from the choice and confidence of the computer must also be combined with information directly observed in one's own

Time to administer: 16 min

Outcome Measures: The proportion of red and blue buckets chosen was calculated for each level of probability (i.e., number of red jellies in participants hand 1/8, 2/8, 3/8, 4/8, 5/8, 6/8, 7/8) and for each condition of computer choice (red or blue) and confidence (confident and unconfident). Area under the curve was calculated for each. The effect of probability refers to the area under the curve collapsed across all computer choice and confidence conditions. The effect of computer choice was calculated by subtracting the AUC when the computer chose blue from AUC then the computer chose red.

disorder (King-Casas et al., 2008; Seres et al., 2009; Unoka et al., 2009). It has been argued that these games may provide specific and sensitive biomarkers for social pathologies (Kishida et al., 2010). Traditionally, these games are long and involve a complex set-up with multiple players, which are unsuitable for neuropsychological testing. Therefore, we developed a simple one-player game of the Ultimatum Game and Prisoners' Dilemma, which probe social interaction within the context of a test battery.

Social decision making

Optimal decision-making in social contexts recruits a combination of associative and inferential computations. For example, one may have first-hand experience, one may observe choices of other people (or receive a recommendation), and one may infer the knowledge or intentions of the others to weight the influence of their decision. Therefore, we included the Inference Task which approximates the contribution of each of these processes to decision-making. Specifically, it employs the useful heuristic of confidence which can be used to infer the certainty of an agent's information and weight the influence of his/her endorsement on privately held beliefs (Thomas and McFadyen, 1995). The effects of such inferences on value computation are hypothesized to underlie the reassuring influence of another's confidence and generate distinct representations of value in the subject. Successful task performance requires cue combination, the integration of value computations, and theoretically, social inferences of other people's knowledge.

Aims and Objectives

The specific aims of the project were to: (a) generate a computerized test battery assessing multiple aspects of "hot" cognition; (b) demonstrate ease of administration, feasibility, and tolerability; (c) standardize the test battery in a large cohort of healthy volunteers, including an exploratory factor analysis to identify important, independent constructs; and (d) establish measurement stability in a smaller sample of healthy volunteers.

Hypotheses

We hypothesized a factor analysis would reveal that the tasks would probe affective function best explained by a four factor model mapping onto *emotion processing*, *motivation*, *impulsivity*, and *social cognition*. We further hypothesized that tasks without a learning component would show at least moderate test-retest reliability.

MATERIALS AND METHODS

Participants

Two hundred healthy volunteers were assessed (see **Table 1** for demographic characteristics), 42 of whom were re-tested within 5–10 days in order to assess test re-test reliability. This will furnish sufficient power to detect test-retest reliability of >0.35 ($p = 0.05$, 80% power). Potential participants were recruited via advertisements in the local community and on social media. Following telephone screening, participants were included if they met the following criteria: 18–50 years old; no self-reported previous or current psychiatric disorders, including depression, anxiety, eating disorders, and drug/alcohol dependence; no neurological disorders; no significant head injury resulting in unconsciousness; no current use of medication known to affect mood or cognition; no first-degree relatives suffering from any psychiatric disorders; smoked fewer than five cigarettes per day; drank less than the government guidelines for weekly alcohol intake (www.drinkaware.co.uk); and fluent in English. Participants completed the Brief Symptom

TABLE 3 | Summary of the means and standard deviations.

Domain and task	Test score used	Mean	SD
EMOTION			
Facial recognition	Face: affective bias	9.48	19.76
	Eyes: affective bias	5.03	26.33
Emotional intensity	Increasing affective bias	−16.21	15.65
	Decreasing affective bias	3.18	14.51
Face affective go/no-go	Affective bias RT (ms)	−30.27	66.93
Word affective go/no-go	Affective bias RT (ms)	−3.30	195.10
Emotional memory	Retrieval affective bias	−4.05	10.66
	Average retrieval accuracy	93.67	7.83
REWARD/MOTIVATION			
Reinforcement learning	Win Learning rate	0.23	0.33
	Loss Learning rate	0.27	0.34
Monetary incentive reward	Win−neutral RT (ms)	34.50	34.42
	Loss−neutral RT (ms)	28.60	33.44
Adapted Cambridge gambling	Win risk adjustment	1.61	1.34
	Loss risk adjustment	1.94	1.17
Progressive ratio[a]	Breakpoint	78.12	32.35
	Post reinforcement pause (seconds)	2.00	0.74
IMPULSIVITY			
4CSRTT[b]	Motivational Index	0.16	0.15
Delay discounting	Delay discounting	3308.95	1928.79
	Probability discounting	989.71	255.20
SOCIAL COGNITION			
Moral emotions	Agent guilt ratings	79.68	12.22
	Feeling bad ratings	22.98	9.16
Information preference	Thoughts chosen	54.10	14.86
	Affective bias in outcome	10.59	20.57
Prisoners' dilemma	Average steal	39.63	28.39
Ultimatum game	Risk adjustment	2.06	1.80
	Value of offers proposed	36.80	10.07
Inference task	Effect of probability	388.00	65.84
	Effect of computer choice	177.75	129.37

[a] *Only 78 participants were included in the analyses for the Progressive ratio task due to an update to the task part way through the study.*
[b] *Only 175 participants were included in the correlation analyses for the 4CSRTT due to technical failure.*

Inventory (Derogatis and Melisaratos, 1983), meeting the criteria for adult non-patients across nine symptom dimensions; somatisation, obsessive compulsive, interpersonal sensitivity, depression, anxiety, hostility, phobic anxiety, paranoid ideation, and psychoticism. Participants were further interviewed using the Mini International Neuropsychiatric Interview (Sheehan et al., 1998) to exclude any psychopathology.

Eligible participants were invited to attend a 3.5-h appointment at the Neuroscience and Psychiatry Unit, University of Manchester or the Behavioral and Clinical Neuroscience Institute, University of Cambridge. Participants provided written informed consent after the study procedures were explained, and their IQ was estimated using the WTAR (Wechsler, 2008). This study was approved by the University of Manchester and the University of Cambridge Research Ethics Committees.

Design

Participants completed 16 neuropsychological tests programmed in PsychoPy (Peirce, 2007) on a touchscreen laptop (Dell XT3).

TABLE 4 | Summary of the factor loadings for EMOTICOM tests on factors 1–11.

Test	Factors										
	1	2	3	4	5	6	7	8	9	10	11
EMOTIONAL RECOGNITION											
Eyes affective bias	0.63										
Face affective bias	0.74										
INTENSITY MORPHING											
Increasing affective bias	−0.66										
Decreasing affective bias	0.62										
WORDS AFFECTIVE GO/NO-GO											
Affective bias (RT)		0.49									
REINFORCEMENT LEARNING											
Loss learning rate		−0.77									
Win learning rate			0.66								
FACES AFFECTIVE GO/NO-GO											
Affective bias (RT)			−0.74								
ULTIMATUM GAME											
Risk adjustment				0.78							
DELAY DISCOUNTING											
Delay discounting				−0.60							
Probability discounting					−0.49						
EMOTIONAL MEMORY											
Retrieval affective bias					0.75						
CAMBRIDGE GAMBLING TASK											
Win RA						0.79					
Loss RA						0.82					
MONETARY INCENTIVE REWARD											
Win-neutral RT							0.87				
Loss-neutral RT							0.83				
MORAL EMOTIONS											
Guilt rating (agent)								−0.87			
Feeling "bad" rating								0.89			
INFORMATION PREFERENCE											
Proportion thoughts									−0.70		
Outcome affective bias									0.65		
PRISONERS DILEMMA											
Steal rate (%)										−0.82	
ULTIMATUM GAME											
Value of offers proposed										0.83	
INFERENCE TASK											
Effect of probability											0.96
Effect of computer choice											0.95

The tasks were administered in a quiet testing room over 3 h. Some participants chose to complete the tasks over two sessions no longer than 1 week apart. The tests were administered in a randomized sequence to eliminate systematic effects of fatigue. Participants were reimbursed for their time and travel expenses, they also received an additional bonus of up to £10, calculated on the basis of the average money won on tasks that involved a monetary incentive.

Neuropsychological Tasks

Analysis

All analyses were performed with SPSS statistical software (IBM SPSS Statistics Version 20.0).

Factor Analysis

The measures thought to be most reflective of the constructs investigated were standardized using *z*-scores (after transformation if appropriate) and entered into a factor analysis to determine the underlying latent variable structure of the data. Here, we conducted an exploratory factor analysis to identify the number of factors needed to maximize the amount of variance explained. An eigenvalue cut-off of 1 was used to determine whether a factor explained sufficient variability in the data. The method employed utilized varimax rotation with Kaiser normalization.

Reliability Analysis

The reliability and stability of the tasks was assessed by comparing performance in 42 volunteers who competed the battery on two occasions, 5–10 days apart. Test-retest was assessed by calculating the average-measures intraclass correlation coefficient using a two-way mixed effects model, which controls for overall changes in performance between sessions (i.e., repetition effects). Different guidelines exist for the interpretation of the ICC. Here we take an ICC value of less than 0.40 to be poor, 0.41–0.59 as fair, 0.60–0.74 as good and values exceeding 0.75 as excellent (Fleis et al., 2003). These terms should be interpreted with caution as they do not take into account the confidence intervals of the ICC measure.

Correlation Analysis

In an exploratory supplemental analysis, two tailed Pearson's correlations were used to correlate task performance with demographic measures such as age, IQ and years of education. Gender differences were examined using independent samples *t*-tests. The statistical significance of all correlations were corrected for multiple comparisons (*0.05/n; n = number of task variables*).

Task Variables

For each task there are a number of possible outcome measures. For the factor analysis, test-retest analysis and correlations with demographic variables, which are the focus of the present publication, we chose the primary outcome measures outlined in **Table 2**.

RESULTS

Standardization

A summary of the means and standard deviations can be found in **Table 3**.

Factor Analysis

Data from all participants were entered into the factor analysis. The results of the varimax rotation for the tasks are shown in **Table 4**. An eleven-factor solution was derived based on eigenvalues greater than 1, which cumulatively accounted for 70% of the variance (see **Figure 1**). Only factor loadings greater than 0.40 are shown. Data were assessed for the adequacy of factor analytic methods. Bartlett's test was highly significant [$\chi^2_{(276)} = 1071.72$, $p < 0.001$], suggesting that variable correlations did not form an identity matrix. Measures of sampling adequacy were also sufficient (KMO = 0.54).

Factor 1 represents affective biases in emotional recognition whereas Factors 2 and 3 capture affective biases in reaction times. Factor 4 contains tasks that have an element of value adjustment. Bias in emotional memory and probability discounting load onto Factor 5. Factor 6 represents measures of probabilistic decision making. Factor 7 represents latency measures of incentive motivation. Factor 8 represents social cognition, specifically moral emotions. Factor 9 represents social information preference and Factor 10 captures cooperation in social exchange games. Finally, Factor 11 loads onto social decision making. The 4CSRTT was omitted from the analysis in order to retain the full sample of participants; however, when running the factor analysis with the motivational index included, this variable loads onto factors 2 and 3 (affective biases in RTs).

Test-Retest Reliability

Test-retest reliability results are summarized in **Table 5**.

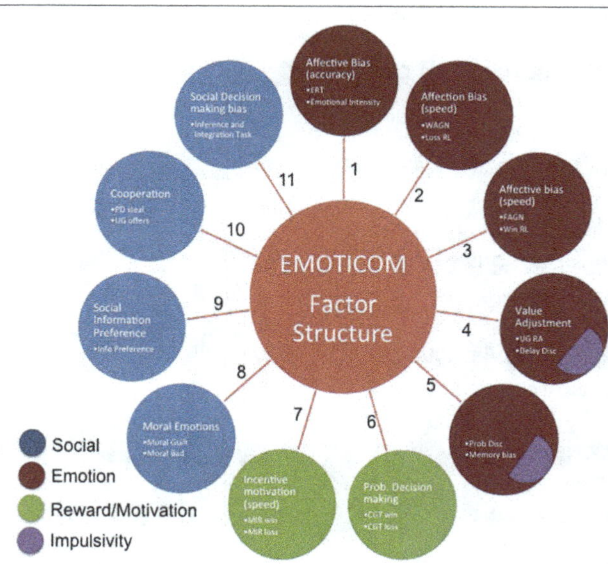

FIGURE 1 | Eleven-factor solution derived from an exploratory factor analysis.

TABLE 5 | Test re-test reliability.

Domain and task ($N = 200$)	Test score used	Intraclass correlation coefficient
EMOTION		
Facial recognition	Face: affective bias	0.86
	Eyes: affective bias	0.74
Emotional Intensity	Increasing affective bias	0.80
	Decreasing affective bias	0.73
Face affective go/no-go	Affective bias (RT)	0.34
Word affective go/no-go	Affective bias (RT)	0.44
Emotional memory	Retrieval affective bias	0.41
	Average retrieval accuracy	0.64
REWARD/MOTIVATION		
Reinforcement learning	Win learning rate	0.15
	Loss learning rate	−0.27
Monetary incentive reward	Win−neutral RT	0.37
	Loss−neutral RT	0.31
Adapted Cambridge gambling	Win risk adjustment	0.75
	Loss risk adjustment	0.75
IMPULSIVITY		
4CSRTT[a]	Motivational index	0.54
Delay discounting	Delay discounting	0.70
	Probability discounting	0.58
SOCIAL COGNITION		
Moral emotions	Agent guilt ratings	0.94
	Feeling bad ratings	0.87
Information preference	Proportion thoughts	0.62
	Affective bias in outcome	0.66
Prisoners' dilemma	Average steal rate	0.64
Ultimatum game	Risk adjustment	0.58
	Value of offers proposed	0.71
Inference task	Effect of probability	0.65
	Effect of computer choice	0.77

[a]*Only 32 participants were included into the reliability analyses for the 4CSRTT.*

Associations with Demographic Factors

Demographic factors associated with test performance are listed in **Table 6**.

DISCUSSION

Neuropsychological test batteries are vital tools for assessing the efficacy of treatment in neuropsychiatric disorders. In order to provide valid assessments of cognitive function, a neuropsychological test battery must possess good test retest reliability and examine a variety of cognitive functions with little redundancy. A further requirement of a test battery specifically assessing emotional and social function is that it should be (at least to some extent) independent of cognitive ability or IQ. In this paper we have presented data from 200 participants' performance to demonstrate that these requirements are met by the EMOTICOM neuropsychological test battery. This battery draws upon adaptations of pre-existing tasks as well as novel tasks in order to provide a comprehensive assessment of emotion processing, rewards and motivation, impulsivity and social cognition.

An exploratory factor analysis identified 11 factors, many of them loading onto a single task. Not all the factors are readily explicable and factors including variables with poor reliability should be viewed with considerable caution. We therefore do not attempt to draw conclusions about the meaning of individual factors. Rather we suggest that the central conclusion is simply that the tasks measure multiple constructs and therefore the battery has little redundancy. Our hypothesis of a four factor solution was categorially disproved suggesting that our prior operational concept of four domains was an over-simplification. This highlights the importance of administering multiple tests in order to assess these "hot" cognitive processes. Various reviews and meta-analyses have identified multiple domains of social cognition (Green and Leitman, 2008; Savla et al., 2012), however existing standardized batteries such as the MATRICS Consensus Cognitive Battery (MCCB; www.matricsinc.org) and CANTAB contain only one task targeting social cognition. The results presented here clearly indicate that there are different components of "hot" cognition that load onto multiple factors and therefore cannot be captured by a single test. Therefore, the EMOTICOM test battery provides a more comprehensive assessment of performance in a variety of affective processes and represents a significant advance over batteries including only a single test.

The majority of EMOTICOM tasks also showed moderate to excellent test-retest reliability. This is extremely important for assessing the efficacy of treatments and interventions, where it is important that differences in task performance can be attributed to effects of the interventions rather than methodological issues or random fluctuations. Furthermore, we demonstrate that our "hot" cognitive tasks have comparable retest reliability to traditional "cold" cognitive tasks (e.g., Lowe and Rabbitt, 1998). However, reliability of the reinforcement learning outcome variable was poor, consistent with previous observations that learning and memory tasks often do not exhibit good re-test reliability (Lowe and Rabbitt, 1998; Dikmen et al., 1999). Learning on these tasks transfers from the first session to the second. Such learning transfer results in significantly improved scores and lower variability at session 2, as we observed here. Given this poor reliability, the EMOTICOM reinforcement learning task could potentially be improved by creating parallel versions using different stimuli, although participants are still likely to be able to generalize rule-learning from the first session. Reliability of bias measures in the Affective Go No Go and Monetary Incentive Reward tasks were also poor. Bias reliability scores in reaction times are often reported to be much lower than mean RTs from each condition (Eide et al., 2002; Strauss et al., 2005; Brown et al., 2014) and our results are therefore comparable with previous studies. Poor test-retest reliability on specific tasks suggests caution in using these measures in longitudinal contexts with healthy volunteers, however it does not preclude the use of these tasks in between-group studies with patient populations.

TABLE 6 | Association between tasks and demographic characteristics.

Domain and task ($N = 200$)	Test score used	Age (r)	IQ (r)	Years in education (r)	Gender (t)
EMOTION					
Facial recognition	Face: affective bias	0.27*	−0.16	−0.08	0.52
	Eyes: affective bias	0.37*	−0.09	−0.01	2.29
Emotional intensity	Increasing affective bias	−0.01	−0.01	−0.03	−1.30
	Decreasing affective bias	0.05	−0.05	−0.03	2.43
Face affective go/no-go	Affective bias (RT)	−0.01	−0.06	−0.09	−0.19
Word affective go/no-go	Affective bias (RT)	−0.11	−0.01	−0.01	1.23
Emotional memory	Retrieval affective bias	−0.01	0.04	0.04	−0.33
REWARD/MOTIVATION					
Reinforcement learning	Win learning rate	−0.02	0.02	0.13	−1.69
	Loss learning rate	−0.07	−0.04	0.03	−0.64
Monetary incentive reward	Win-neutral RT	0.01	−0.12	−0.04	−1.83
	Loss-neutral RT	0.02	−0.00	−0.04	−1.74
Cambridge gambling task	Win risk adjustment	−0.12	0.16	0.08	0.42
	Loss risk adjustment	−0.25*	0.27*	0.18	1.21
Progressive ratio[a]	Breakpoint	0.07	−0.07	−0.09	−0.35
	Post reinforcement pause	0.23	−0.32	−0.03	−0.67
IMPULSIVITY					
4 CSRTT[b]	Motivational index	−0.14	0.01	0.14	0.31
Delay discounting	Delay discounting	−0.16	0.27*	0.24*	1.28
	Probability discounting	0.03	−0.05	0.11	0.69
SOCIAL COGNITION					
Moral emotions	Agent guilt ratings	0.05	−0.02	−0.04	−4.02*$
	Feeling bad ratings	−0.12	0.11	0.14	1.96
Information preference	Proportion thoughts	−0.08	−0.05	−0.13	0.84
	Affective bias in outcome	0.07	0.01	0.07	−0.54
Prisoners dilemma	Average steal rate	−0.02	0.04	0.06	0.57
Ultimatum game	Risk adjustment	−0.13	0.13	0.09	−0.66
	Average value of offers proposed	0.19	−0.08	−0.09	0.22
Inference task	Effect of jelly probability	−0.16	0.15	0.18	−0.38
	Effect of computer choice	−0.19	0.15	0.18	−0.70

Results show Pearson correlations (r) or t-statistics (t) from independent t-test.

$^{*}p < 0.002$; $N = 200$.

[a]Only 78 participants were included in the correlation analyses for the Progressive ratio task due to an update to the task part way through the study.

[b]Only 175 participants were included in the correlation analyses for the 4CSRTT due to technical failure.

[$]Females showed greater guilt ratings.

The majority of EMOTICOM tasks were not strongly correlated with demographic factors such as age, years in education or IQ suggesting that performance of these tasks is not dependent upon general intellectual function. There are a few exceptions: the risk adjustment measure from the loss condition in the adapted Cambridge Gambling Task and the delay discounting measures were correlated with IQ, with delay discounting also being correlated with years in education. Previous studies have also suggested that gambling (Demaree et al., 2010; Webb et al., 2014) and delay discounting (Shamosh and Gray, 2008) correlate with intelligence. Therefore, it is recommended that studies using these measures take particular care to control for IQ and years of education. Interestingly we observed emotional bias measures in the face and eyes emotional recognition task to be significantly correlated with age, such that biases became more positive with increasing age. This finding supports a line of research that has recently gathered momentum, with many recent studies demonstrating that people attend to and remember positive information more as they get older (e.g., Mather and Carstensen, 2003; Reed and Carstensen, 2012). In spite of a prevailing view that hot cognitive tests are dependent on gender, we only observed a significant effect of gender in the Moral Emotions Task, whereby females show greater guilt ratings compared to males. This is in line with existing meta-analyses showing that women tend to experience negative emotions, such as guilt, more intensely than men (Else-Quest et al., 2012). This task may therefore be useful in understanding gender differences in treatment outcomes, particularly in terms of self-blame biases and their suggested link to a vulnerability to depression (Green et al., 2013).

Limitations

The ethnic characteristics of our sample of 200 participants was representative of the UK demographic (Office for National Statistics, 2011). Nevertheless, caution is recommended in generalizing these findings across cultures. Evidence suggests that cultural variations are evident in affective cognition. For example cultural variations have been observed in emotional facial recognition (Prado et al., 2014) economical games such as the Ultimatum Game and Prisoners' Dilemma (Oosterbeek et al., 2004; Wong and Hong, 2005) and arguably moral judgment (Gibbs et al., 2007). Such differences observed in performance across cultures suggest care in generalizing performance on UK validated and standardized tasks to other cultures. Another limitation is that we were not able to enter all the task variables into the factor analysis due to the reduced number of participants who completed some of the tasks. For instance, the progressive ratio parameters were improved part way through the study and so data were only available from 78 participants. Similarly, only a subset of participants completed the 4CSRTT. Therefore, in order to increase power and retain the full participant sample, the decision was made to omit these measures from factor analysis. A limitation of the test-retest reliability component was that we only assessed reliability over a short duration; in future it will important to assess longer durations to determine the potential value of the tasks in different intervention contexts.

In summary, we have demonstrated the potential power of the EMOTICOM test battery for the assessment of affective cognitive function. We have shown that affective cognition is far from a unitary construct, implying that assessment of multiple aspects of affective cognition is required. Our 16 task battery has little redundancy from the 11 factor underlying structure. We have also demonstrated that the majority of tasks have moderate to excellent test-retest reliability and are not strongly correlated with demographic factors such as IQ. We therefore conclude that the EMOTICOM test battery meets certain key criteria for a useful and valid tool with potential utility in clinical trials and studies investigating psychiatric disorders and relevant treatment interventions.

Important future directions include validation in patients and validation in intervention studies in both healthy controls and patients in order to further investigate the utility of EMOTICOM test battery, and diagnosis-appropriate subsets of tasks, as an investigative tool in mental health research. This will enable us assess which tasks are most valid, sensitive and reliable for use in particular patient populations and which can be used as outcome measures in intervention trials.

FUNDING

This work was supported by the MRC under Grant MR/J011894/1.

ACKNOWLEDGMENTS

We thank our colleagues at the University of Manchester, University of Cambridge, University College London and Kings College London for their contribution to discussions. In particular we thank Dr Vincent Valton (UCL) and Dr Sanja Abbott (University of Cambridge) for assistance with analyses. We also thank Dr Jonathan Peirce (University of Nottingham) and Dr Martyn McFarquar (University of Manchester) for their guidance and expertise in PsychoPy.

REFERENCES

Agay, N., Kron, S., Carmel, Z., Mendlovic, S., and Levkovitz, Y. (2008). Ultimatum bargaining behavior of people affected by schizophrenia. *Psychiatry Res.* 157, 39–46. doi: 10.1016/j.psychres.2006.03.026

Andari, E., Duhamel, J.-R., Zalla, T., Herbrecht, E., Leboyer, M., and Sirigu, A. (2010). Promoting social behavior with oxytocin in high-functioning autism spectrum disorders. *Proc. Natl. Acad. Sci. U.S.A.* 107, 4389–4394. doi: 10.1073/pnas.0910249107

Aron, A. R., and Poldrack, R. A. (2005). The cognitive neuroscience of response inhibition: relevance for genetic research in attention-deficit/hyperactivity disorder. *Biol. Psychiatry* 57, 1285–1292. doi: 10.1016/j.biopsych.2004.10.026

Baert, S., De Raedt Schacht, R. R., and Koster, E. H. W. (2010). Attentional bias training in depression: therapeutic effects depend on depression severity. *J. Behav. Ther. Exp. Psychiatry* 41, 265–274. doi: 10.1016/j.jbtep.2010.02.004

Baron-Cohen, S., Wheelwright, S., Hill, J., Raste, Y., and Plumb, I. (2001). The 'reading the mind in the eyes' test revised version: a study with normal adults, and adults with asperger syndrome or high-functioning autism. *J. Child Psychol. Psychiatry* 42, 241–251. doi: 10.1111/1469-7610.00715

Bechara, A., Damasio, A. R., Damasio, H., and Anderson, S. W. (1994). Insensitivity to future consequences following damage to human prefrontal cortex. *Cognition* 50, 7–15. doi: 10.1016/0010-0277(94)90018-3

Birrell, J. M., and Brown, V. J. (2000). Medial frontal cortex mediates perceptual attentional set shifting in the rat. *J. Neurosci.* 20, 4320–4324.

Blair, R. J. (1995). A cognitive developmental approach to mortality: investigating the psychopath. *Cognition* 57, 1–29. doi: 10.1016/0010-0277(95)00676-P

Bloom, D. E., Cafiero, E., Jané-Llopis, E., Abrahams-Gessel, S., Bloom, L. R., Fathima, S., et al. (2012). *The Global Economic Burden of Noncommunicable Diseases (No. 8712)*. Program on the Global Demography of Aging. Available online at: https://ideas.repec.org/p/gdm/wpaper/8712.html

Bora, E., Yucel, M., and Pantelis, C. (2009). Theory of mind impairment in schizophrenia: meta-analysis. *Schizophr. Res.* 109, 1–9. doi: 10.1016/j.schres.2008.12.020

Bouhuys, A. L., Geerts, E., and Gordijn, M. (1999). Gender-specific mechanisms associated with outcome of depression: perception of emotions, coping and interpersonal functioning. *Psychiatry Res.* 85, 247–261. doi: 10.1016/S0165-1781(99)00003-7

Bradshaw, C. M., and Killeen, P. R. (2012). A theory of behaviour on progressive ratio schedules, with applications in behavioural pharmacology. *Psychopharmacology* 222, 549–564. doi: 10.1007/s00213-012-2771-4

Brittlebank, A. D., Scott, J., Williams, J. M., and Ferrier, I. N. (1993). Autobiographical memory in depression: state or trait marker? *Br. J. Psychiatry* 162, 118–121. doi: 10.1192/bjp.162.1.118

Brown, H. M., Eley, T. C., Broeren, S., MacLeod, C., Rinck, M., Hadwin, J. A., et al. (2014). Psychometric properties of reaction time based experimental paradigms measuring anxiety-related information-processing biases in children. *J. Anxiety Disord.* 28, 97–107. doi: 10.1016/j.janxdis.2013.11.004

Chandler, R. A., Wakeley, J., Goodwin, G. M., and Rogers, R. D. (2009). Altered risk-aversion and risk-seeking behavior in bipolar disorder. *Biol. Psychiatry* 66, 840–846. doi: 10.1016/j.biopsych.2009.05.011

Ciaramelli, E., Muccioli, M., Ladavas, E., and di Pellegrino, G. (2007). Selective deficit in personal moral judgment following damage to ventromedial prefrontal cortex. *Soc. Cogn. Affect. Neurosci.* 2, 84–92. doi: 10.1093/scan/nsm001

Combs, D. R., Adams, S. D., Penn, D. L., Roberts, D., Tiegreen, J., and Stem, P. (2007). Social cognition and interaction training (SCIT) for inpatients with schizophrenia spectrum disorders. *Prelim. Find.* 91, 112–116. doi: 10.1016/j.schres.2006.12.010

Cools, R., Clark, L., Owen, A. M., and Robbins, T. W. (2002). Defining the neural mechanisms of probabilistic reversal learning using event-related functional magnetic resonance imaging. *J. Neurosci.* 22, 4563–4567.

Crockett, M. J. (2009). The neurochemistry of fairness. *Ann. N.Y. Acad. Sci.* 1167, 76–86. doi: 10.1111/j.1749-6632.2009.04506.x

Daw, N. D., O'Doherty, J. P., Dayan, P., Seymour, B., and Dolan, R. J. (2006). Cortical substrates for exploratory decisions in humans. *Nature* 441, 876–879. doi: 10.1038/nature04766

Demaree, H. A., Burns, K. J., and DeDonno, M. A. (2010). Intelligence, but not emotional intelligence, predicts iowa gambling task performance. *Intelligence* 38, 249–254. doi: 10.1016/j.intell.2009.12.004

Derogatis, L. R., and Melisaratos, N. (1983). The brief symptom inventory: an introductory report. *Psychol. Med.* 13, 595–605. doi: 10.1017/S0033291700048017

Dikmen, S. S., Heaton, R. K., Grant, I., and Temkin, N. R. (1999). TestReitan neuropsychological test battery. *J. Inter. Neuropsychol. Soc.* 5, 346–356.

Eack, S. M., Greeno, C. G., Pogue-Geile, M. F., Newhill, C. E., Hogarty, G. E., and Keshavan, M. S. (2010). Assessing social-cognitive deficits in schizophrenia with the mayer-salovey-caruso emotional intelligence test. *Schizophr. Bull.* 36, 370–380. doi: 10.1093/schbul/sbn091

Eide, P., Kemp, A., Silberstein, R. B., Nathan, P. J., and Stough, C. (2002). Test-Retest reliability of the emotional stroop task: examining the paradox of measurement change. *J. Psychol.* 136, 514–520. doi: 10.1080/00223980209605547

Elliott, R., Zahn, R., William Deakin, J. F., and Anderson, I. M. (2011). Affective cognition and its disruption in mood disorders. *Neuropsychopharmacology* 36, 153–182. doi: 10.1038/npp.2010.77

Else-Quest, N. M., Higgins, A., Allison, C., and Morton, L. C. (2012). Gender differences in self-conscious emotional experience: a meta-analysis. *Psychol. Bull.* 138, 947–981. doi: 10.1037/a0027930

Erickson, K., Drevets, W. C., Clark, L., Cannon, D. M., Bain, E. E., Zarate, C. A., et al. (2005). Mood-congruent bias in affective go/no-go performance of unmedicated patients with major depressive disorder. *Am. J. Psychiatry* 162, 2171–2173. doi: 10.1176/appi.ajp.162.11.2171

Ersche, K. D., and Sahakian, B. J. (2007). The neuropsychology of amphetamine and opiate dependence: implications for treatment. *Neuropsychol. Rev.* 17, 317–336. doi: 10.1007/s11065-007-9033-y

Fehr, E., and Camerer, C. F. (2007). Social neuroeconomics: the neural circuitry of social preferences. *Trends Cogn. Sci.* 11, 419–427. doi: 10.1016/j.tics.2007.09.002

Feifel, D., Macdonald, K., Cobb, P., and Minassian, A. (2012). adjunctive intranasal oxytocin improves verbal memory in people with schizophrenia. *Schizophr. Res.* 139, 207–210. doi: 10.1016/j.schres.2012.05.018

Fett, A.-K. J., Viechtbauer, W., Dominguez, M. G., Penn, D. L., van Os, J., and Krabbendam, L. (2011). The relationship between neurocognition and social cognition with functional outcomes in schizophrenia: a meta-analysis. *Neurosci. Biobehav. Rev.* 35, 573–588. doi: 10.1016/j.neubiorev.2010.07.001

Fineberg, N. A., Haddad, P. M., Carpenter, L., Gannon, B., Sharpe, R., Young, A. H., et al. (2013). The size, burden and cost of disorders of the brain in the UK. *J. Psychopharmacol. (Oxford).* 27, 761–770. doi: 10.1177/0269881113495118

Fleis, J. L., Levin, B., and Paik, M. C. (2003). *Statistical Methods for Rates and Proportions.* Hoboken, NJ: John Wiley & Sons.

Frith, C. D., and Corcoran, R. (1996). Exploring'theory of mind'in people with schizophrenia. *Psychol. Med.* 26, 521–530. doi: 10.1017/S0033291700035601

Frith, U., and Frith, C. D. (2003). Development and neurophysiology of mentalizing. *Philos. Trans. R. Soc. Lond. Ser. B* 358, 459–473. doi: 10.1098/rstb.2002.1218

Gibbs, J. C., Basinger, K. S., Grime, R. L., and Snarey, J. R. (2007). Moral judgment development across cultures: revisiting kohlberg's universality claims. *Dev. Rev.* 27, 443–500. doi: 10.1016/j.dr.2007.04.001

Green, L., Myerson, J., Lichtman, D., Rosen, S., and Fry, A. (1996). Temporal discounting in choice between delayed rewards: the role of age and income. *Psychol. Aging* 11, 79–84. doi: 10.1037/0882-7974.11.1.79

Green, M. F., and Leitman, D. I. (2008). Social cognition in schizophrenia. *Schizophr. Bull.* 34, 670–672. doi: 10.1093/schbul/sbn045

Green, M. F., Penn, D. L., Bentall, R., Carpenter, W. T., Gaebel, W., Gur, R. C., et al. (2008). Social cognition in schizophrenia: an nimh workshop on definitions, assessment, and research opportunities. *Schizophr. Bull.* 34, 1211–1220. doi: 10.1093/schbul/sbm145

Green, S., Lambon Ralph, M. A., Moll, J., Zakrzewski, J., William Deakin, J. F., Grafman, J., et al. (2013). The neural basis of conceptual-emotional integration and its role in major depressive disorder. *Soc. Neurosci.* 8, 417–433. doi: 10.1080/17470919.2013.810171

Hamilton, J. P., and Gotlib, I. H. (2008). Neural substrates of increased memory sensitivity for negative stimuli in major depression. *Biol. Psychiatry* 63, 1155–1162. doi: 10.1016/j.biopsych.2007.12.015

Happé, F., and Frith, U. (1996). The neuropsychology of autism. *Brain* 119, 1377–1400. doi: 10.1093/brain/119.4.1377

Harmer, C. J., Goodwin, G. M., and Cowen, P. J. (2009). Why do antidepressants take so long to work? a cognitive neuropsychological model of antidepressant drug action. *Br. J. Psychiatry* 195, 102–108. doi: 10.1192/bjp.bp.108.051193

Harmer, C. J., Cowen, P. J., and Goodwin, G. M. (2011). Efficacy markers in depression. *J. Psychopharmacol.* 25, 1148–1158. doi: 10.1177/0269881110367722

Herbener, E. S., Song, W., Khine, T. T., and Sweeney, J. A. (2008). What aspects of emotional functioning are impaired in schizophrenia? *Schizophr. Res.* 98, 239–246. doi: 10.1016/j.schres.2007.06.025

Hodos, W. (1961). Progressive ratio as a measure of reward strength. *Science* 134, 943–944. doi: 10.1126/science.134.3483.943

Hutton, S. B., Murphy, F. C., Joyce, E. M., Rogers, R. D., Cuthbert, I. T., Robbins, T. W., et al. (2002). Decision making deficits in patients with first-episode and chronic schizophrenia. *Schizophr. Res.* 55, 249–257. doi: 10.1016/S0920-9964(01)00216-X

Insel, T., Cuthbert, B., Garvey, M., Heinssen, R., Pine, D. S., Quinn, K., et al. (2010). Research domain criteria (RDoC): toward a new classification framework for research on mental disorders. *Am. J. Psychiatry* 167, 748–751. doi: 10.1176/appi.ajp.2010.09091379

Kaladjian, A., Jeanningros, R., Azorin, J.-M., Grimault, S., Anton, J.-L., and Mazzola-Pomietto, P. (2007). Blunted activation in right ventrolateral prefrontal cortex during motor response inhibition in schizophrenia. *Schizophr. Res.* 97, 184–193. doi: 10.1016/j.schres.2007.07.033

King-Casas, B., Sharp, C., Lomax-Bream, L., Lohrenz, T., Fonagy, P., and Montague, P. R. (2008). The rupture and repair of cooperation in borderline personality disorder. *Science (N.Y.)* 321, 806–810. doi: 10.1126/science.1156902

King-Casas, B., Tomlin, D., Anen, C., Camerer, C. F., Quartz, S. R., and Montague, P. R. (2005). Getting to know you: reputation and trust in a two-person economic exchange. *Science* 308, 78–83. doi: 10.1126/science.1108062

Kirby, K. N. (2009). One-year temporal stability of delay-discount rates. *Psychon. Bull. Rev.* 16, 457–462. doi: 10.3758/PBR.16.3.457

Kishida, K. T., King-Casas, B., and Montague, P. R. (2010). Neuroeconomic approaches to mental disorders. *Neuron* 67, 543–554. doi: 10.1016/j.neuron.2010.07.021

Knutson, B., Adams, C. M., Fong, G. W., and Hommer, D. (2001). Anticipation of increasing monetary reward selectively recruits nucleus accumbens. *J. Neurosci.* 21, RC159.

Knutson, B., Bjork, J. M., Fong, G. W., Hommer, D., Mattay, V. S., and Weinberger, D. R. (2004). Amphetamine modulates human incentive processing. *Neuron* 43, 261–269. doi: 10.1016/j.neuron.2004.06.030

Koenigs, M., Kruepke, M., and Newman, J. P. (2010). Economic decision-making in psychopathy: a comparison with ventromedial prefrontal lesion patients. *Neuropsychologia* 48, 2198–2204. doi: 10.1016/j.neuropsychologia.2010.04.012

Koenigs, M., Young, L., Adolphs, R., Tranel, D., Cushman, F., Hauser, M., et al. (2007). Damage to the prefrontal cortex increases utilitarian moral judgements. *Nature* 446, 908–911. doi: 10.1038/nature05631

Ladouceur, C. D., Dahl, R. E., Williamson, D. E., Birmaher, B., Axelson, D. A., Ryan, N. D., et al. (2006). Processing emotional facial expressions influences performance on a Go/NoGo task in pediatric anxiety and depression. *J. Child Psychol. Psychiatry* 47, 1107–1115. doi: 10.1111/j.1469-7610.2006.01640.x

Lovell, D. M., Mark, J., Williams, G., and Hill, A. B. (1997). Selective processing of shape–related words in women with eating disorders, and those who have recovered. *Br. J. Clin. Psychol.* 36, 421–432. doi: 10.1111/j.2044-8260.1997.tb01249.x

Lowe, C., and Rabbitt, P. (1998). Test\re-Test reliability of the CANTAB and ISPOCD neuropsychological batteries: theoretical and practical issues. *Neuropsychologia* 36, 915–923. doi: 10.1016/S0028-3932(98)00036-0

Malloy-Diniz, L., Fuentes, D., Borges Leite, W., Correa, H., and Bechara, A. (2007). Impulsive behavior in adults with attention deficit/hyperactivity disorder: characterization of attentional, motor and cognitive impulsiveness. *J. Inter. Neuropsychol. Soc.* 13, 693–698. doi: 10.1017/s1355617707070889

Mather, M., and Carstensen, L. L. (2003). Aging and attentional biases for emotional faces. *Psychol. Sci.* 14, 409–415. doi: 10.1111/1467-9280.01455

Mayer, J. D., and Salovey, P. (1997). "What is emotional intelligence?," in *Emotional Development and Emotional Intelligence: Educational Implications*, eds P. Salovey and D. J. Sluyter (New York, NY: Harper Collins), 3–34.

Mayer, J. D., Salovey, P., Caruso, D. R., and Sitarenios, G. (2003). Measuring emotional intelligence with the MSCEIT V2.0. *Emotion* 3, 97–105.

Mazur, J. E. (1987). An adjusting procedure for studying delayed reinforcement. *Qt. Analys. Behav.* 5, 55–73.

Miller, G. (2005). Economic game shows how the brain builds trust. *Science* 308:36. doi: 10.1126/science.308.5718.36a

Mobbs, O., Iglesias, K., Golay, A., and Van der Linden, M. (2011). Cognitive deficits in obese persons with and without binge eating disorder. Investigation using a mental flexibility task. *Appetite* 57, 263–271. doi: 10.1016/j.appet.2011.04.023

Mogg, K., and Bradley, B. P. (2002). Selective orienting of attention to masked threat faces in social anxiety. *Behav. Res. Ther.* 40, 1403–1414. doi: 10.1016/S0005-7967(02)00017-7

Mogg, K., Bradley, B. P., and Williams, R. (1995). Attentional bias in anxiety and depression: the role of awareness. *Br. J. Clin. Psychol.* 34, 17–36. doi: 10.1111/j.2044-8260.1995.tb01434.x

Moll, J., and de Oliveira-Souza, R. (2007). Moral judgments, emotions and the utilitarian brain. *Trends Cogn. Sci.* 11, 319–321. doi: 10.1016/j.tics.2007.06.001

Moran, J. M., Young, L. L., Saxe, R., Lee, S. M., O'Young, D., Mavros, P. L., et al. (2011). Impaired theory of mind for moral judgment in high-functioning autism. *Proc. Natl. Acad. Sci. U.S.A.* 108, 2688–2692. doi: 10.1073/pnas.1011734108

Murphy, F. C., Michael, A., Robbins, T. W., and Sahakian, B. J. (2003). Neuropsychological impairment in patients with major depressive disorder: the effects of feedback on task performance. *Psychol. Med.* 33, 455–467. doi: 10.1017/S0033291702007018

Murphy, F. C., Sahakian, B. J., Rubinsztein, J. S., Michael, A., Rogers, R. D., Robbins, T. W., et al. (1999). Emotional bias and inhibitory control processes in mania and depression. *Psychol. Med.* 29, 1307–1321. doi: 10.1017/S0033291799001233

Murphy, F. C., Rubinsztein, J. S., Michael, A., Rogers, R. D., Robbins, T. W., Paykel, E. S., et al. (2001). Decision-making cognition in mania and depression. *Psychol. Med.* 31, 679–693. doi: 10.1017/S0033291701003804

Murray, G. K., Corlett, P. R., Clark, L., Pessiglione, M., Blackwell, A. D., Honey, G., et al. (2007). Substantia nigra/ventral tegmental reward prediction error disruption in psychosis. *Mol. Psychiatry* 13, 267–276. doi: 10.1038/sj.mp.4002058

Office for National Statistics (2011). *Census: Ethnic Group, Local Authorities in England and Wales.*

Ohmura, Y., Takahashi, T., Kitamura, N., and Wehr, P. (2006). Three-month stability of delay and probability discounting measures. *Exp. Clin. Psychopharmacol.* 14, 318. doi: 10.1037/1064-1297.14.3.318

Oosterbeek, H., Sloof, R., and van de Kuilen, G. (2004). Cultural differences in ultimatum game experiments: evidence from a meta-analysis. *Exp. Econ.* 7, 171–188. doi: 10.1023/B:EXEC.0000026978.14316.74

Owen, A. M., McMillan, K. M., Laird, A. R., and Bullmore, E. D. (2005). N-Back working memory paradigm: a meta-analysis of normative functional neuroimaging studies. *Hum. Brain Mapp.* 25, 46–59. doi: 10.1002/hbm.20131

Owen, A. M., Roberts, A. C., Polkey, C. E., Sahakian, B. J., and Robbins, T. W. (1991). Extra-dimensional versus intra-dimensional set shifting performance following frontal lobe excisions, temporal lobe excisions or amygdalo-hippocampectomy in man. *Neuropsychologia* 29, 993–1006. doi: 10.1016/0028-3932(91)90063-E

Park, S. Q., Kahnt, T., Beck, A., Cohen, M. X., Dolan, R. J., Wrase, J., et al. (2010). Prefrontal cortex fails to learn from reward prediction errors in alcohol dependence. *J. Neurosci.* 30, 7749–7753. doi: 10.1523/JNEUROSCI.5587-09.2010

Peirce, J. W. (2007). PsychoPy—psychophysics software in python. *J. Neurosci. Methods* 162, 8–13. doi: 10.1016/j.jneumeth.2006.11.017

Pessiglione, M., Seymour, B., Flandin, G., Dolan, R. J., and Frith, C. D. (2006). Dopamine-dependent prediction errors underpin reward-seeking behaviour in humans. *Nature* 442, 1042–1045. doi: 10.1038/nature05051

Pomarol-Clotet, E., Hynes, F., Ashwin, C., Bullmore, E. T., McKenna, P. J., and Laws, K. R. (2010). Facial emotion processing in schizophrenia: a non-specific neuropsychological deficit? *Psychol. Med.* 40, 911–919. doi: 10.1017/S0033291709991309

Posner, M. I. (1980). Orienting of attention. *Q. J. Exp. Psychol.* 32, 3–25. doi: 10.1080/00335558008248231

Prado, C., Mellor, D., Linda Byrne, K., Wilson, C., Xu, X., and Liu, H. (2014). Facial emotion recognition: a cross-cultural comparison of chinese, chinese living in Australia, and Anglo-Australians. *Motiv. Emot.* 38, 420–428. doi: 10.1007/s11031-013-9383-0

Pulcu, E., Thomas, E. J., Trotter, P. D., McFarquhar, M., Juhasz, G., Sahakian, B. J., et al. (2015). Social-economical decision making in current and remitted major depression. *Psychol. Med.* 45, 1301–1313. doi: 10.1017/S003329171400 2414

Reed, A. E., and Carstensen, L. L. (2012). The Theory behind the age-related positivity effect. *Front. Psychol.* 3:339. doi: 10.3389/fpsyg.2012.00339

Reynolds, B., and Schiffbauer, R. (2004). Measuring state changes in human delay discounting: an experiential discounting task. *Behav. Processes* 67, 343–356. doi: 10.1016/S0376-6357(04)00140-8

Richards, J. B., Zhang, L., Mitchell, S. H., and de Wit, H. (1999). Delay or probability discounting in a model of impulsive behavior: effect of alcohol. *J. Exp. Anal. Behav.* 71, 121–143. doi: 10.1901/jeab.1999.71-121

Rilling, J. K., Glenn, A. L., Jairam, M. R., Pagnoni, G., Goldsmith, D. R., Elfenbein, H. A., et al. (2015). Neural correlates of social cooperation and non-cooperation as a function of psychopathy. *Biol. Psychiatry* 61, 1260–1271. doi: 10.1016/j.biopsych.2006.07.021

Roane, H. S. (2008). On the applied use of progressive-ratio schedules of reinforcement. *J. Appl. Behav. Anal.* 41, 155–161. doi: 10.1901/jaba.2008.41-155

Robbins, T. W. (2002). The 5-choice serial reaction time task: behavioural pharmacology and functional neurochemistry. *Psychopharmacology (Berl).* 163, 362–380. doi: 10.1007/s00213-002-1154-7

Robbins, T. W., James, M., Owen, A. M., Sahakian, B. J., Lawrence, A. D., McInnes, L., et al. (1998). A study of performance on tests from the CANTAB battery sensitive to frontal lobe dysfunction in a large sample of normal volunteers: implications for theories of executive functioning and cognitive aging. Cambridge neuropsychological test automated batte. *J. Int. Neuropsychol. Soc.* 4, 474–490. doi: 10.1017/S1355617798455073

Robbins, T. W., James, M., Owen, A. M., Sahakian, B. J., McInnes, L., and Rabbitt, P. (1994). Cambridge neuropsychological test automated battery (CANTAB): a factor analytic study of a large sample of normal elderly volunteers. PG - 266-81. *Dementia* 5, 266–81. doi: 10.1159/000106735

Roberts, A. C., Robbins, T. W., and Everitt, B. J. (1988). The effects of intradimensional and extradimensional shifts on visual discrimination learning in humans and non-human primates. *Q. J. Exp. Psychol.* 40, 321–341.

Rogers, R. D., Blackshaw, A. J., Middleton, H. C., Matthews, K., Hawtin, K., Crowley, C., et al. (1999). Tryptophan Depletion impairs stimulus-reward learning while methylphenidate disrupts attentional control in healthy young adults: implications for the monoaminergic basis of impulsive behaviour. *Psychopharmacology (Berl).* 146, 482–491. doi: 10.1007/PL00005494

Rogers, R. D., Tunbridge, E. M., Bhagwagar, Z., Drevets, W. C., Sahakian, B. J., and Carter, C. S. (2003). Tryptophan depletion alters the decision-making of healthy volunteers through altered processing of reward cues. *Neuropsychopharmacology* 28, 153–162. doi: 10.1038/sj.npp.1300001

Roiser, J. P., Elliott, R., and Sahakian, B. J. (2012). Cognitive mechanisms of treatment in depression. *Neuropsychopharmacology* 37, 117–136. doi: 10.1038/npp.2011.183

Roiser, J. P., Stephan, K. E., Den Ouden, H. E. M., Barnes, T. R. E., Friston, K. J., and Joyce, E. M. (2009a). Do patients with schizophrenia exhibit aberrant salience? *Psychol. Med.* 39, 199. doi: 10.1017/S0033291708003863

Roiser, J. P., Blackwell, A. D., Cools, R., Clark, L., Rubinsztein, D. C., Robbins, T. W., et al. (2006). Serotonin transporter polymorphism mediates vulnerability to loss of incentive motivation following acute tryptophan depletion. *Neuropsychopharmacology* 31, 2264–2272. doi: 10.1038/sj.npp.1301084

Roiser, J. P., Cannon, D. M., Gandhi, S. K., Tavares, J. T., Erickson, K., Wood, S., et al.. (2009b). Hot and cold cognition in unmedicated depressed subjects with bipolar disorder. *Bipolar Disord.* 11, 178–189. doi: 10.1111/j.1399-5618.2009.00669.x

Roiser, J. P., and Sahakian, B. J. (2013). Hot and cold cognition in depression. *CNS Spectr.* 18, 139–149. doi: 10.1017/S1092852913000072

Sanislow, C. A., Pine, D. S., Quinn, K. J., Kozak, M. J., Garvey, M. A., Heinssen, R. K., et al. (2010). Developing constructs for psychopathology research: research domain criteria. *J. Abnorm. Psychol.* 119, 631–639. doi: 10.1037/a0020909

Savla, G. N., Vella, L., Armstrong, C. C., Penn, D. L., and Twamley, E. W. (2012). Deficits in domains of social cognition in schizophrenia: a meta-analysis of the empirical evidence. *Schizophr. Bull.* 39, 979–992. doi: 10.1093/schbul/sbs080

Scarna, A. S., McTavish, F. B., Cowen, P. J., Goodwin, G. M., and Rogers, R. D. (2005). The effects of a branched chain amino acid mixture supplemented with tryptophan on biochemical indices of neurotransmitter function and decision-making. *Psychopharmacology (Berl).* 179, 761–768. doi: 10.1007/s00213-004-2105-2

Scheres, A., Milham, M. P., Knutson, B., and Castellanos, F. X. (2007). Ventral striatal hyporesponsiveness during reward anticipation in attention-deficit/hyperactivity disorder. *Biol. Psychiatry* 61, 720–724. doi: 10.1016/j.biopsych.2006.04.042

Seres, I., Unoka, Z., and Keri, S. (2009). The broken trust and cooperation in borderline personality disorder. *Neuroreport* 20, 388–392. doi: 10.1097/WNR.0b013e328324eb4d

Seymour, K. E., Reinblatt, S. P., Benson, L., and Carnell, S. (2015). Overlapping neurobehavioral circuits in adhd, obesity, and binge eating: evidence from neuroimaging research. *CNS Spectr.* 20, 401–411. doi: 10.1017/S1092852915000383

Shamosh, N. A., and Gray, J. R. (2008). Delay discounting and intelligence: a meta-analysis. *Intelligence* 36, 289–305. doi: 10.1016/j.intell.2007.09.004

Sheehan, D. V., Lecrubier, Y., Sheehan, K. H., Amorim, P., Janavs, J., Weiller, E., et al. (1998). The mini-international neuropsychiatric interview (M.I.N.I.): the development and validation of a structured diagnostic psychiatric interview for DSM-IV and ICD-10. *J. Clin. Psychiatry* 20, 22–33.

Strauss, G. P., Allen, D. N., Jorgensen, M. L., and Cramer, S. L. (2005). Test-retest reliability of standard and emotional stroop tasks: an investigation of color-word and picture-word versions. *Assessment* 12, 330–337. doi: 10.1177/1073191105276375

Surguladze, S. A., Young, A. W., Senior, C., Brébion, G., Travis, M. J., and Phillips, M. L. (2004). Recognition accuracy and response bias to happy and sad facial expressions in patients with major depression. *Neuropsychology* 18:212. doi: 10.1037/0894-4105.18.2.212

Thomas, J. P., and McFadyen, R. G. (1995). The confidence heuristic: a game-theoretic analysis. *J. Econ. Psychol.* 16, 97–113. doi: 10.1016/0167-4870(94)00032-6

Thomas, R., Sanders, S., Doust, J., Beller, E., and Glasziou, P. (2015). Prevalence of attention-deficit/hyperactivity disorder: a systematic review and meta-analysis. *Pediatrics* 135, 994–1001. doi: 10.1542/peds.2014-3482

Unoka, Z., Seres, I., Aspan, N., Bodi, N., and Keri, S. (2009). Trust game reveals restricted interpersonal transactions in patients with borderline personality disorder. *J. Pers. Disord.* 23, 399–409. doi: 10.1521/pedi.2009.23.4.399

Voon, V., Irvine, M. A., Derbyshire, K., Worbe, Y., Lange, I., Abbott, S., et al. (2014). Measuring 'waiting' impulsivity in substance addictions and binge eating disorder in a novel analogue of rodent serial reaction time task. *Biol. Psychiatry* 75, 148–155. doi: 10.1016/j.biopsych.2013.05.013

Voon, V., Pessiglione, M., Brezing, C., Gallea, C., Fernandez, H. H., Dolan, R. J., et al. (2010). Mechanisms underlying dopamine-mediated reward bias in compulsive behaviors. *Neuron* 65, 135–142. doi: 10.1016/j.neuron.2009.12.027

Waltz, J. A., Schweitzer, J. B., Ross, T. J., Kurup, P. K., Salmeron, B. J., Rose, E. J., et al. (2010). Abnormal responses to monetary outcomes in cortex, but not in the basal ganglia, in schizophrenia. *Neuropsychopharmacology* 35, 2427–2439. doi: 10.1038/npp.2010.126

Watts, F. N., McKenna, F. P., Sharrock, R., and Trezise, L. (1986). Colour naming of phobia-related words. *Br. J. Psychol.* 77, 97–108. doi: 10.1111/j.2044-8295.1986.tb01985.x

Webb, C. A., DelDonno, S., and Killgore, W. D. S. (2014). The role of cognitive versus emotional intelligence in iowa gambling task performance: what's emotion got to do with it? *Intelligence* 44, 112–119. doi: 10.1016/j.intell.2014.03.008

Wechsler, D. (2008). *Wechsler Adult Intelligence scale–Fourth Edition (WAIS-IV).* San Antonio, TX: NCS Pearson.

Wong, R. Y.-M., and Hong, Y. (2005). Dynamic influences of culture on cooperation in the prisoner's dilemma. *Psychol. Sci.* 16, 429–434. doi: 10.1111/j.0956-7976.2005.01552.x

Worbe, Y., Savulich, G., Voon, V., Fernandez-Egea, E., and Robbins, T. W. (2014). Serotonin depletion induces 'waiting impulsivity' on the human four-choice serial reaction time task: cross-species translational significance. *Neuropsychopharmacology* 39, 1519–1526. doi: 10.1038/npp.2013.351

Zahn, R., Lythe, K. E., Gethin, J. A., Green, S., Deakin, J. F. W., Workman, C., et al. (2015). Negative emotions towards others are diminished in remitted major depression. *Eur. Psychiatry* 30, 448–453. doi: 10.1016/j.eurpsy.2015.02.005

Zahn, R., Moll, J., Paiva, M., Garrido, G., Krueger, F., Huey, E. D., et al. (2009). The neural basis of human social values: evidence from functional MRI. *Cereb. Cortex (N.Y.)* 19, 276–283. doi: 10.1093/cercor/bhn080

Conflict of Interest Statement: The authors declare that the research was conducted in the absence of any commercial or financial relationships that could be construed as a potential conflict of interest.

Targeting Glia with N-Acetylcysteine Modulates Brain Glutamate and Behaviors Relevant to Neurodevelopmental Disorders in C57BL/6J Mice

Edited by:
Raymond C. K. Chan,
Chinese Academy of Sciences, China

***Correspondence:**
Po-Wah So
po-wah.so@kcl.ac.uk;
Grainne McAlonan
grainne.mcalonan@kcl.ac.uk

†These authors have contributed equally to this work.
‡Both authors are joined senior authors.

Alice M. S. Durieux[1†], Cathy Fernandes[2†], Declan Murphy[1], Marie Anais Labouesse[3], Sandra Giovanoli[3,4], Urs Meyer[3,4], Qi Li[5], Po-Wah So[6‡] and Grainne McAlonan[1*‡]*

[1] Department of Forensic and Neurodevelopmental Sciences, Institute of Psychiatry, Psychology and Neuroscience, King's College London, London, UK, [2] Social, Genetic and Developmental Psychiatry Centre, Institute of Psychiatry, Psychology and Neuroscience, King's College London, London, UK, [3] Physiology and Behaviour Laboratory, Swiss Federal Institute of Technology, Schwerzenbach, Switzerland, [4] Institute of Pharmacology and Toxicology, University of Zurich-Vetsuisse, Zurich, Switzerland, [5] Department of Psychiatry, Li Ka Shing Faculty of Medicine, The University of Hong Kong, Hong Kong, China, [6] Department of Neuroimaging, Institute of Psychiatry, Psychology and Neuroscience, King's College London, London, UK

An imbalance between excitatory (E) glutamate and inhibitory (I) GABA transmission may underlie neurodevelopmental conditions such as autism spectrum disorder (ASD) and schizophrenia. This may be direct, through alterations in synaptic genes, but there is increasing evidence for the importance of indirect modulation of E/I balance through glial mechanisms. Here, we used C57BL/6J mice to test the hypothesis that striatal glutamate levels can be shifted by N-acetylcysteine (NAC), which acts at the cystine-glutamate antiporter of glial cells. Striatal glutamate was quantified *in vivo* using proton magnetic resonance spectroscopy. The effect of NAC on behaviors relevant to ASD was examined in a separate cohort. NAC induced a time-dependent decrease in striatal glutamate, which recapitulated findings of lower striatal glutamate reported in ASD. NAC-treated animals were significantly less active and more anxious in the open field test; and NAC-treated females had significantly impaired prepulse inhibition of startle response. This at least partly mimics greater anxiety and impaired sensorimotor gating reported in neurodevelopmental disorders. Thus glial mechanisms regulate glutamate acutely and have functional consequences even in adulthood. Glial cells may be a potential drug target for the development of new therapies for neurodevelopmental disorders across the life-span.

Keywords: N-acetylcysteine, magnetic resonance spectroscopy, glutamate, neurodevelopmental disorders, anxiety, prepulse inhibition

INTRODUCTION

Neurodevelopmental disorders such as autism spectrum disorder (ASD) and schizophrenia affect about 1% of the population (Saha et al., 2005; Baron-Cohen et al., 2009). Their etiology is poorly understood, and treatments are limited. However, recent advances in research suggest an imbalance between excitatory (E) glutamate and inhibitory (I) GABA is a key pathophysiological feature that may explain both core and common comorbid symptoms such as anxiety (Rubenstein and Merzenich, 2003; Cortese and Phan, 2005; Lewis and Kim, 2009; Coghlan et al., 2012; Moghaddam and Javitt, 2012).

E/I imbalance in neurodevelopmental conditions can arise directly via alteration in genes encoding glutamatergic receptors or synaptic adhesion proteins (Silverman et al., 2012, 2015; Spooren et al., 2012). For example, the synapse organizers Neurexins and their binding partner Neuroligins are crucial to the formation and maintenance of excitatory and inhibitory synapses. Abnormalities in the genes encoding these proteins have been reported in both ASD and schizophrenia (Bang and Owczarek, 2013), and animal models have confirmed their role in synaptic transmission and behaviors relevant to neurodevelopmental disorders (Graf et al., 2004; Dahlhaus and El-Husseini, 2010; Grayton et al., 2013).

However, synaptic gene abnormalities account for only a relatively small proportion of the neurodevelopmental spectrum (Devlin and Scherer, 2012); and there is increasing evidence that E/I balance can also be modulated by glial mechanisms (Di Benedetto and Rupprecht, 2013). The brain's glial support system includes astrocytes, which support and protect neurons; and microglia, the resident macrophages of the central nervous system. These cells are now appreciated to have a critical role in synapse development, maintenance and remodelling (Koyama and Ikegama), but can also influence excitatory and inhibitory synaptic transmission (Auld and Robitaille, 2003). For instance, astrocytes regulate brain levels of glutamate and GABA through the glutamate/glutamine cycle (Liang et al., 2006); and activated microglia release glutamate (Domercq et al., 2013). A role for glial cells in neurodevelopmental disorders is supported by reports of abnormalities in astrocyte gene expression in both ASD and schizophrenia (Fatemi et al., 2008; Bernstein et al., 2009); and an increased number of activated microglia in adults with ASD (Onore et al., 2012).

System x_c-, the cysteine-glutamate antiporter found on the cell membrane of glia, is central to their influence on synaptic transmission. It can be stimulated by the compound N-Acetylcysteine (NAC, an FDA approved drug) to increase glutamate in the extrasynaptic space, thereby activating presynaptic mGluR2/3, which in turn inhibit the synaptic release of glutamate (Baker et al., 2003; Moran et al., 2005; Dean et al., 2011; Kupchik et al., 2012). Therefore, in this study we administered NAC to standard "wild-type" laboratory C57BL/6J mice to provide proof-of-concept evidence that acute modulation of glia alters glutamate levels *in vivo*; and has functional (behavioral) consequences. We used proton magnetic resonance spectroscopy (^{1}H-MRS) to quantify glutamate in the left striatum, as both structural and functional abnormalities in this area are well documented in neurodevelopmental disorders (Haznedar et al., 2006; Scott-Van Zeeland et al., 2010; Simpson et al., 2010; De La Fuente-Sandoval et al., 2011; Baez-Mendoza and Schultz, 2013; Naaijen et al., 2015). In a separate cohort we assessed prepulse inhibition of startle response (PPI), a measure of sensorimotor gating which is impaired in ASD and schizophrenia (Braff et al., 2001; McAlonan et al., 2002; Kumari et al., 2003; Perry et al., 2007). We also measured anxiety in the open field arena, as this is a common comorbidity of neurodevelopmental disorders (Braga et al., 2013; Joshi et al., 2013; Matson and Cervantes, 2014).

MATERIALS AND METHODS

Animals

Two cohorts of C57BL/6J mice (Charles River, Margate, Kent, UK) aged 7–8 weeks were used in the study. Animals were acclimatized to our facilities for a week before beginning the experimental procedures, during which they were group housed (2–4 per cage) in Tecniplast cages (32 cm × 16 cm × 14 cm) with sawdust (Litaspen premium, Datesand Ltd, Manchester), a cardboard shelter and additional bedding material (Sizzlenest, Datesand Ltd, Manchester) and maintained on a 12h/12 h light/dark cycle (07:00–19:00 h) at constant room temperature (21°C) and humidity (45%). The mice were fed a standard diet (Rat and Mouse #1 Diet, Special Diet Services, Essex, UK) and provided with water *ad libitum*. Both sexes were used in this study to avoid sex specific confounds. The oestrous phase of the female mice was not checked in this study. However, it is unlikely that this affected results because there were no major effects in the variance between males and females. All housing and experimental procedures were performed in compliance with the local ethical review panel of King's College London, and the UK Home Office Animals Scientific Procedures Act 1986. The work was carried out under license (PPL: 70/7184) and all efforts were made to minimize animal suffering and to reduce the number of animals used.

Drug Treatment

NAC was purchased from Sigma-Aldrich (UK), and dissolved in saline. Prior to experimental procedures, mice were injected (i.p.) with either 150 mg/kg NAC solution (30 g/L); injection volume approximately 100 microL or vehicle (saline).

Proton Magnetic Resonance Spectroscopy of the Brain

In cohort I, 32 animals (16/sex) were treated with either NAC or vehicle, 115–175 min before data acquisition began. Animals were anaesthetized throughout the scan using an isofluorane/oxygen mix (5% induction, 2% maintenance). Body temperature and respiratory frequency were monitored and carefully regulated throughout the procedure.

Data were acquired on a 7T horizontal bore scanner (Agilent Technologies Inc., Walnut Creek, CA, USA) using a 33 mm internal diameter quadrature volume coil (Rapid Biomedical, Rimpar, Germany). The field was shimmed to <14 MHz, width at half height of the water peak. Pilot MR images for voxel positioning were acquired using a fast spin-echo sequence with repetition $time_{(TR)}$ = 1000 ms, effective echo $time_{(TE)}$ = 60 ms, field of view 20 × 20 mm, 27 contiguous axial slices of 0.5 mm thickness, and two averages. These MR images were used for placement of a voxel (2.2 × 1.3 × 1.9 mm) in the left striatum for localized ^{1}H-MRS as shown in **Figure 1A**. Point-RESolved Spectroscopy (PRESS; Bottomley, 1987) was used to acquire ^{1}H-MRS data from the voxel with acquisition parameters: TR, 3000 ms; TE, 24 ms; 2048 data points; spectral width, 5208 Hz and 1000 averages. Water suppression was achieved using VAriable Pulse Power and Optimized Relaxation delays (VAPOR; Griffey and Flamig, 1990). PRESS was performed again but without water suppression with the same parameter values except collecting only eight averages from the same voxel.

Each spectrum was visually reviewed to ensure adequate signal to noise ratio, as well as the absence of artifacts. Spectra were analyzed using LCModel version 6.3-0I (Provencher, 1993) using a basis set of 21 metabolites including creatine (Cr) and glutamate (Glu). Model metabolites and concentrations used in the basis set are fully detailed in the LCModel manual (http://s-provencher.com/pages/lcm-manual.shtml). Poorly fitted metabolite peaks (Cramer-Rao minimum variance bounds of >20% as reported by LCModel) were excluded from further analysis.

Behavioral Testing

In cohort II, 42 animals (20 males and 22 females) were treated with either NAC or vehicle 130 min prior to the assessment of open field locomotor activity. Animals were brought back to their home-cage for 10–15 min, and then PPI was performed 155 min post-treatment. Behavioral testing was carried out under stringent environmental control of housing and husbandry as well as the handling of the mice, balance and uniformity in testing, the experimenter, test location and standardized test procedures. Behavioral testing was conducted in the light phase of the light/dark cycle. After each individual test, boli and urine were removed from the test arena which was cleaned with 1% Anistel® solution (high level surface disinfectant, Trisel Solution Ltd, Cambridgeshire, UK) to remove any odors. Experimenters were blind to experimental treatment group during the testing.

Open Field Locomotor Activity

Locomotor activity in a novel open field area was assessed as a measure of anxiety as previously published (Grayton et al., 2013). Animals were placed in a square 40 × 40 cm arena under white light (8 lux) for 10 min and video recorded. The central (20 × 20 cm) and peripheral outer (remaining) areas of the arena were defined and movements in each zone were tracked with Ethovision software version 3.1 (Noldus Information Technologies bv, Wageningen, Netherlands). Time spent in the central zone was used as measure of anxiety, and distance travelled in the arena was used as measure of locomotor activity.

Prepulse Inhibition of the Acoustic Startle Response

PPI was assessed using a chamber for mice which recorded startle response amplitude (San Diego Instruments, San Diego, CA, USA), following a previously well-validated protocol (Vuillermot et al., 2011; Labouesse et al., 2013). Animals were placed in the Plexiglas enclosure and presented with a series of discrete trials. Four different trial types were used, including pulse alone trials, prepulse alone trials, prepulse-pulse trials and no-stimulus trials (where no sound was played other than the constant background noise). The pulse and prepulse stimuli consisted of a sudden elevation of the broadband white noise from the background level of 65 dB_A with a rise time of 0.2–1 ms, for 40 and 20 ms respectively. Three pulse intensities (100, 110 and 120 dB_A), and three prepulse intensities (71, 77 and 83 dB_A—which corresponded to 6, 12 and 18 dB_A above the background noise respectively) were used. The onset of the pulse was presented 100 ms after the onset of the prepulse, for all prepulse-pulse trials.

Animals were allowed to adapt to the enclosure for 2 min before the beginning of the first trial. They were presented with six pulse only trials (two trials of each intensity) for habituation, which were not included in the analysis. The test phase consisted of 10 blocks of 16 discrete trials. Each block included three pulse alone trials (100, 110 and 120 dB_A), three prepulse alone

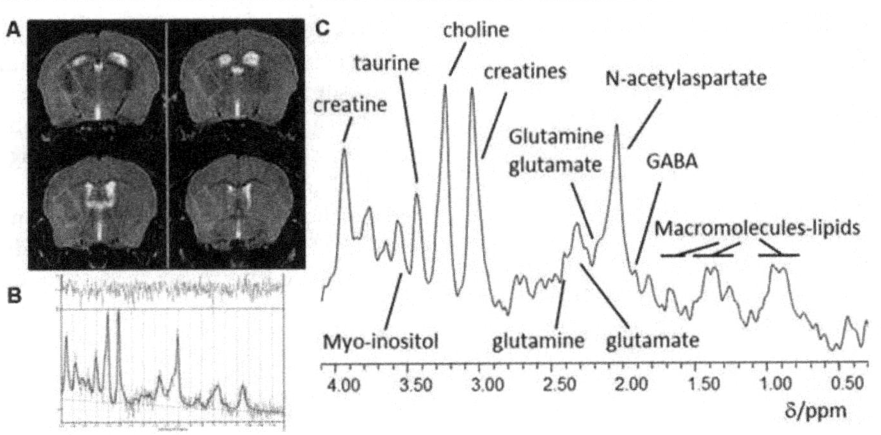

FIGURE 1 | (A) Typical placement of a striatal voxel on T2-weighted pilot MR images of the mouse brain; **(B)** *In vivo* localized ^{1}H-MR spectrum from a striatal voxel and **(C)** LCModel analysis of a ^{1}H MR spectrum.

trials (71, 77 and 83 dB_A), nine prepulse-pulse trials (all possible prepulse-pulse combinations), and one no-stimulus trial. Within each block, the 16 trials were presented in pseudorandom order and separated by a variable interval of 10–20 s (average 15 s).

For each trial type, average reactivity was calculated over the whole experiment, excluding the first six pulse alone trials. PPI was measured as the percent inhibition of startle response (%PPI) in pulse only trials. For each animal, it was calculated as follows: [(mean reactivity on pulse alone trials) − (mean reactivity on prepulse-pulse trials)/(mean reactivity on pulse alone trials)] * 100; for each pulse intensity (100, 110 and 120 dB_A), and each prepulse intensity (71, 77 and 83 dB_A).

STATISTICAL ANALYSIS

^{1}H-MRS and open field data were analyzed using a general linear model (IBM SPSS Statistics version 21) including group and sex as between subject factors. The time post-dose, $t_{post-dose}$ was included as covariate in the analysis of metabolite concentrations, and correlations between metabolite concentrations and $t_{post-dose}$ were explored using Pearson correlation coefficients.

For PPI analysis, reactivity to pulse alone trials were analyzed in a 3 × 2 × 2 repeated measures ANOVA (pulse level × group × sex). %PPI data were analyzed in 3 × 3 × 2 × 2 repeated measure ANOVA (prepulse level × pulse level × group × sex). Where there was a significant interaction between sex and another factor on %PPI, data were re-analyzed separately for each sex.

RESULTS

Localized ^{1}H-MRS of the Brain

Creatine (Cr)

A representative ^{1}H-MRS spectrum of the left striatum is shown in **Figures 1B,C**. There was no main effect of treatment or sex on creatine (from creatine and phosphocreatine; all $F_{(1,26)} < 0.3$, all $p > 0.6$). All subsequent metabolite concentrations were therefore calculated in reference to Cr to account for potential inter-individual differences in voxel composition (Gussew et al., 2012).

Glutamate (Glu)

Glu/Cr concentrations were significantly lower in the NAC treated group, as indicated by a main effect of treatment ($F_{(1,26)} = 5.77, p = 0.02$). There was also a main effect of $t_{post-dose}$ on Glu/Cr ($F_{(1,26)} = 10.2$, $p = 0.004$). Furthermore Glu/Cr was negatively correlated with $t_{post-dose}$ in the NAC group ($r = -0.657$, $p = 0.008$), but not in the vehicle group ($r = -0.417$, $p = 0.108$); as there was no main effect of sex on Glu/Cr, both sexes were examined together for the correlation analysis. Please refer to **Figure 2**.

Open Field Locomotor Activity

Distance Travelled

There were main effects of treatment ($F_{(1,38)} = 4.90$, $p = 0.033$) and sex ($F_{(1,38)} = 17.98$, $p < 0.001$) on distance travelled in the arena of the open field, and no sex × treatment interaction. NAC treated mice travelled significantly less than their saline treated counterparts. Overall females travelled less distance than males (please refer to **Figure 3A**).

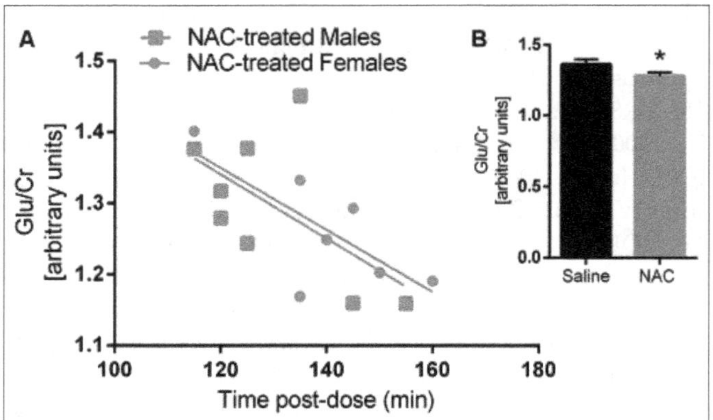

FIGURE 2 | Glutamate/Creatine was negatively correlated with time post-dose in the N-acetylcysteine (NAC)-treated group (A) but not in the saline group. Glutamate/Creatine levels were significantly lower in NAC treated animals **(B)**, $^*p < 0.05$.

Time in Central Zone

As shown in **Figure 3B**, there was a main effect of treatment on time spent in central zone ($F_{(1,38)} = 8.22$, $p = 0.007$), but no main effect of sex and no sex × treatment interaction. NAC treated animals spent significantly less time in the central zone. This treatment main effect remained significant when co-varying for distance travelled ($F_{(1,37)} = 8.39$, $p = 0.006$), which indicates that the difference was not likely to be due to a change in locomotor activity.

Prepulse Inhibition (PPI) of the Acoustic Startle Response

Mean reactivity was higher at higher pulse intensity in pulse alone trials, as indicated by a mains effect of pulse intensity ($F_{(1.8,67.7)} = 689.4$, $p < 0.001$). There was also a main effect of sex on reactivity to pulse alone trials ($F_{(1,38)} = 66.23$, $p < 0.001$), as well as a pulse × sex interaction ($F_{(1.8,67.7)} = 41.4$, $p < 0.001$).

There was no main effect of treatment or sex on %PPI. The treatment × sex interaction approached significance ($F_{(1,38)} = 3.11$, $p = 0.086$), therefore the analysis was repeated in each sex separately (please refer to **Figure 3C**). There was no effect of treatment on %PPI in males. However NAC treated females displayed a significant reduction in %PPI compared with controls ($F_{(1,20)} = 5.29$, $p = 0.032$). The disruption of PPI by NAC emerged independently of specific pulse and prepulse intensities, as shown by non-significant interactions of pulse and prepulse with treatment.

DISCUSSION

This study provided proof-of-concept evidence that glutamate levels and behavior can be altered acutely by extra-synaptic mechanisms targeting glial cells. Activation of system x_c- by

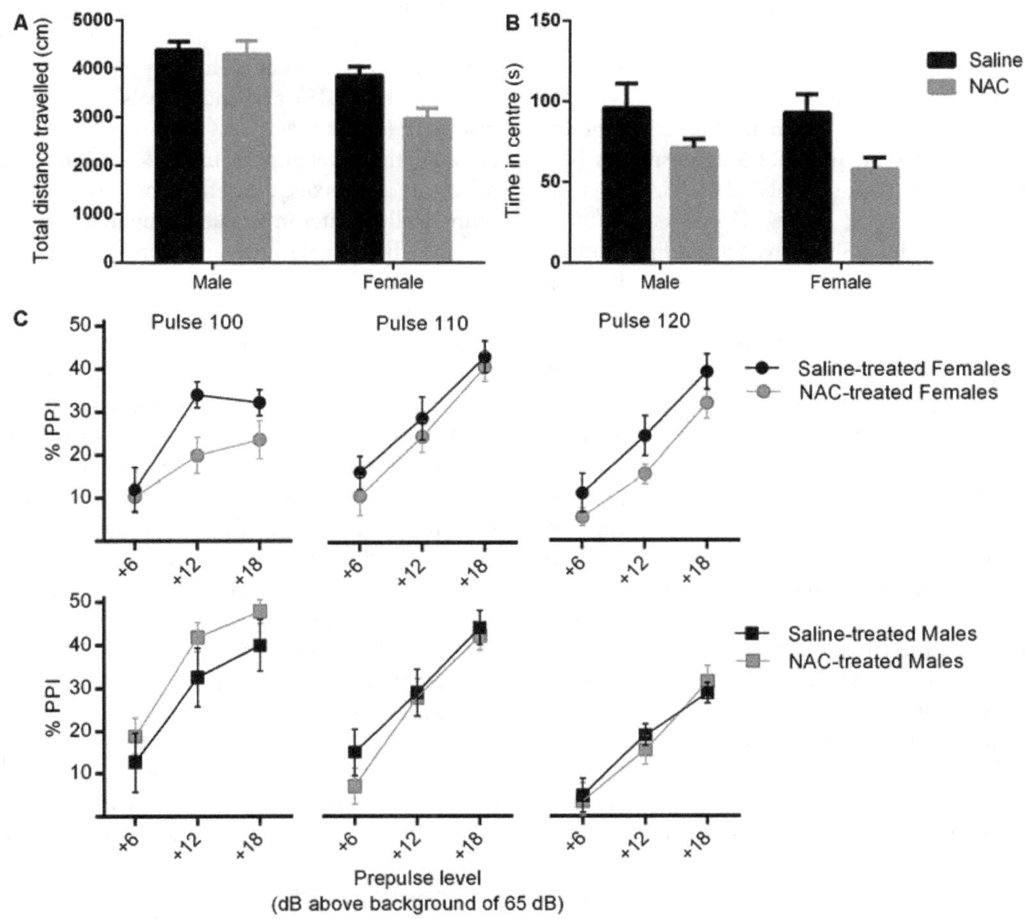

FIGURE 3 | NAC treatment reduced locomotor activity (main effect of treatment, $p = 0.033$) (A) and increased anxiety (main effect of treatment, $p = 0.007$) (B), in females more than males. In **(C)**, percent prepulse inhibition (%PPI) is shown as a function of the three pulse levels (100, 110 or 120 dB_A), and the three prepulse levels (6, 12 or 18 dB_A above background level of 65 dB_A). %PPI was reduced by NAC treatment in females only (main effect of treatment, $p = 0.032$).

NAC lowered glutamate concentrations in the striatum in a time-dependent fashion. NAC-treated animals displayed reduced locomotor activity in the open field as well as increased anxiety, which was independent from general activity levels. NAC treatment reduced the prepulse inhibition of startle response in females exclusively.

The acute glutamatergic effects of NAC observed in this study are consistent with, and extend previous findings. For example previous studies showed that NAC reduces excitatory currents in an mGluR2/3 dependent fashion (Moran et al., 2005; Kupchik et al., 2012). One ^{1}H-MRS study in a mouse model of schizophrenia found that chronic NAC treatment reduces cortical glutamate levels in developing animals (Das Neves Duarte et al., 2012). Here, we show that one dose of NAC is sufficient to lower striatal glutamate in a time-dependent fashion; the lowest glutamate levels are evident 120 min post-dose and continue to decrease for at least 60 min. We report that a single dose of NAC also disrupts behavior from 120 min post-administration. We interpret the behavioral differences as likely due to a glutamate decrease, but acknowledge the evidence is indirect. These findings may have translational importance as they suggest that targeting glia can shift glutamate levels; and this is relevant to neurodevelopmental disorders such as ASD and schizophrenia, where glial abnormalities and E/I imbalance are prominent features.

Our finding of reduced striatal glutamate is analogous to the decrease of glutamate and its metabolite glutamine observed in the striatum of adult males with ASD (Horder et al., 2013). Our observations of greater anxiety and impaired sensorimotor gating in NAC-treated animals also mimics impairments commonly found in ASD and related neurodevelopmental disorders (McAlonan et al., 2002; Perry et al., 2007; Braga et al., 2013; Joshi et al., 2013; Matson and Cervantes, 2014). Thus, although our design did not make it possible to assess glutamate levels and behavior in the same animals, behavioral findings may well relate to a change in glutamate concentrations.

For example, locomotor activity, anxiety and PPI at least partly depend on glutamatergic transmission (Takeuchi et al.,

2001; O'Neill et al., 2003; Wieronska and Pilc, 2013; Saitoh et al., 2014). Here, we report that indirect mGluR2/3 agonism via NAC causes lower activity. This is consistent with a role for mGluR2/3 in the tonic inhibition of locomotion; and the observation that mGluR2/3 antagonism increases locomotion (O'Neill et al., 2003). However, mGluR2/3 agonism has been reported to both increase (Imre et al., 2006; Satow et al., 2008) and decrease (Imre et al., 2006; Grivas et al., 2013) anxiety, depending on the dose. Similarly, acute administration of mGluR2/3 agonists has been reported to have either no effect (intra-peritoneal administration of LY379268; Hikichi et al., 2010), or impair (intracerebral administration of *L*-CCG-I; Grauer and Marquis, 1999), PPI. Thus, the mGluR2/3 response is likely to be complex and depend on the dose and administration regime of compounds targeting these receptors.

Although we show here that NAC administration mimics lower striatal glutamate and causes behavioral abnormalities similar to those found in ASD, paradoxically, NAC has shown clinical benefits in small scale double blind trials in this condition (Hardan et al., 2012; Ghanizadeh and Moghimi-Sarani, 2013). However, the latter study examined NAC as an adjunct alongside risperidone, and a recently completed Clinical Trial of NAC in ASD did not find evidence of efficacy (K. Gray, personal communication). There are a number of possible explanations for these inconsistencies. First, the acute effects of NAC may be quite distinct from the effects of repeated administration in clinical settings. Arguably, the glutamate system responds differently to chronic modulation compared to acute challenge. Secondly, the developmental stage studied may be critical, as glutamate levels in humans are known to vary with age (Segovia et al., 2001; Kaiser et al., 2005). The clinical trials of NAC in ASD were mostly completed in children (Hardan et al., 2012; Ghanizadeh and Moghimi-Sarani, 2013), while we used adult animals. Third, the effects of NAC may be different in a "disordered" system. We used standard in-bred laboratory mice in this study; it is possible that the effects of NAC would be different in a mouse model showing baseline E/I imbalance. Some support for this latter suggestion comes from preliminary work in schizophrenia. NAC has shown benefits in adults with schizophrenia (Zavodnick and Ali, 2014), but a study in healthy volunteers found that NAC pretreatment worsened auditory mismatch negativity following ketamine administration (Gunduz-Bruce et al., 2012), a paradigm thought to mimic psychosis. Finally, it is possible that the clinical benefits of chronic administration of NAC are in fact mediated by its antioxidant actions, rather than its glutamatergic action (Dean et al., 2009; Rushworth and Megson, 2013). Thus, we emphasize that our findings do not speak to the therapeutic use of NAC in neurodevelopmental disorders, for which there is no clear consensus. Rather, we suggest that our finding shows that modulating glutamate and behavior via glial mechanisms is possible, and suggests that glial mechanisms may be a tractable target for drugs which aim to modulate E/I.

We acknowledge some unexpected findings in this study. We elected to study NAC in both female and male animals and found sex-differences in the PPI response following NAC administration. PPI is particularly sensitive to sex-differences in both laboratory animals (Lehmann et al., 1999; Ralph et al., 2001; Zhang et al., 2015) and individuals with neurodevelopmental disorders (Kumari et al., 2004; Gogos et al., 2009). Moreover, although there were no treatment × sex interactions in measures of activity and anxiety, the effects of NAC on these measures was numerically greater in females compared to males. It is therefore possible that female mice are more sensitive to the behavioral consequences of the change in glutamate, however larger sample sizes would be needed to explore this in more detail. It would also be valuable to determine whether there are any sex differences in glial mechanisms. We echo the call for more research into sex differences in neurodevelopmental disorders, particularly as it becomes apparent that their prevalence in females may be higher than thought previously (Brix et al., 2015). We also acknowledge that an important limitation of this study was that we did not measure glutamate levels and assess behavior in the same animals. The current design was chosen to avoid confounds related to putting the same animals through several experimental procedures sequentially. Previous work has shown that invasive behavioral testing could induce changes in neural activity patterns (Xu et al., 2012), and brain metabolite levels (Zhou et al., 2012). On the other hand, the imaging procedure, which required 2 h of anaesthesia, is a significant exposure and could impact upon subsequent behavioral testing. Therefore we chose to use a naïve cohort of mice animals for the behavioral and the imaging experiments. Future research will aim to correlate E/I and behavioral measures in the same animals, possibly using *ex vivo* methods. Finally, the PRESS spectroscopy acquisition protocol we used did not allow for estimation of GABA concentration. Glutamate and GABA are constantly in flux and measuring the other side of the E/I ratio would be useful to obtain a fuller picture in the future.

In summary, this work confirms that glial mechanisms regulate glutamate acutely and have functional consequences in adult animals. Glial cells may therefore be a potential drug target for the development of new therapies for neurodevelopmental disorders even in the adult system.

AUTHOR CONTRIBUTIONS

AMSD, GM, P-WS, CF, DM, QL, ML, SG and UM designed the research. AMSD, P-WS, CF, ML, SG and UM acquired the data. AMSD, GM, P-WS, CF, ML, QL, SG and UM analyzed the data. AMSD, GM, P-WS, CF, DM, ML, QL, SG and UM critically interpreted the data. AMSD and GM drafted the manuscript. AMSD, GM, P-WS, CF, DM, ML, QL, SG and UM approved the final version.

FUNDING

AMSD is supported by a PhD studentship from the National Institute for Health Research (NIHR) Biomedical Research Center at South London and Maudsley NHS Foundation Trust and King's College London. The views expressed are those of the author(s) and not necessarily those of the NHS, the NIHR or the Department of Health. This work was funded by the Sackler Institute for Translational Development.

ACKNOWLEDGMENT

Thanks to the British Heart Foundation for funding the purchase of the 7T MRI scanner used in the study.

REFERENCES

Auld, D. S., and Robitaille, R. (2003). Glial cells and neurotransmission: an inclusive view of synaptic function. *Neuron* 40, 389–400. doi: 10.1016/S0896-6273(03)00607-X

Baez-Mendoza, R., and Schultz, W. (2013). The role of the striatum in social behavior. *Front. Neurosci.* 7:233. doi: 10.3389/fnins.2013.00233

Baker, D. A., Mcfarland, K., Lake, R. W., Shen, H., Toda, S., and Kalivas, P. W. (2003). N-acetyl cysteine-induced blockade of cocaine-induced reinstatement. *Ann. N. Y. Acad. Sci.* 1003, 349–351. doi: 10.1196/annals.1300.023

Bang, M. L., and Owczarek, S. (2013). A matter of balance: role of neurexin and neuroligin at the synapse. *Neurochem. Res.* 38, 1174–1189. doi: 10.1007/s11064-013-1029-9

Baron-Cohen, S., Scott, F. J., Allison, C., Williams, J., Bolton, P., Matthews, F. E., et al. (2009). Prevalence of autism-spectrum conditions: UK school-based population study. *Br. J. Psychiatry.* 194, 500–509. doi: 10.1192/bjp.bp.108.059345

Bernstein, H. G., Steiner, J., and Bogerts, B. (2009). Glial cells in schizophrenia: pathophysiological significance and possible consequences for therapy. *Expert Rev. Neurother.* 9, 1059–1071. doi: 10.1586/ern.09.59

Bottomley, P. A. (1987). Spatial localization in NMR spectroscopy *in vivo*. *Ann. N. Y. Acad. Sci.* 508, 333–348. doi: 10.1111/j.1749-6632.1987.tb32915.x

Braff, D. L., Geyer, M. A., and Swerdlow, N. R. (2001). Human studies of prepulse inhibition of startle: normal subjects, patient groups and pharmacological studies. *Psychopharmacology Berl.* 156, 234–258. doi: 10.1007/s00213010 0810

Braga, R. J., Reynolds, G. P., and Siris, S. G. (2013). Anxiety comorbidity in schizophrenia. *Psychiatry. Res.* 210, 1–7. doi: 10.1016/j.psychres.2013.07.030

Brix, M. K., Ersland, L., Hugdahl, K., Gruner, R., Posserud, M. B., Hammar, A., et al. (2015). "Brain MR spectroscopy in autism spectrum disorder-the GABA excitatory/inhibitory imbalance theory revisited". *Front. Hum. Neurosci.*9: 365. doi: 10.3389/fnhum.2015.00365

Coghlan, S., Horder, J., Inkster, B., Mendez, M. A., Murphy, D. G., and Nutt, D. J. (2012). GABA system dysfunction in autism and related disorders: from synapse to symptoms. *Neurosci. Biobehav. Rev.* 36, 2044–2055. doi: 10.1016/j.neubiorev.2012.07.005

Cortese, B. M., and Phan, K. L. (2005). The role of glutamate in anxiety and related disorders. *CNS Spectr.* 10, 820–830. doi: 10.1017/S10928529000 10427

Dahlhaus, R., and El-Husseini, A. (2010). Altered neuroligin expression is involved in social deficits in a mouse model of the fragile X syndrome. *Behav. Brain Res.* 208, 96–105. doi: 10.1016/j.bbr.2009.11.019

Das Neves Duarte, J. M., Kulak, A., Gholam-Razaee, M. M., Cuenod, M., Gruetter, R., and Do, K. Q. (2012). N-acetylcysteine normalizes neurochemical changes in the glutathione-deficient schizophrenia mouse model during development. *Biol. Psychiatry.* 71, 1006–1014. doi: 10.1016/s0920-9964(12)70162-7

De La Fuente-Sandoval, C., Leon-Ortiz, P., Favila, R., Stephano, S., Mamo, D., Ramirez-Bermudez, J., et al. (2011). Higher levels of glutamate in the associative-striatum of subjects with prodromal symptoms of schizophrenia and patients with first-episode psychosis. *Neuropsychopharmacology* 36, 1781–1791. doi: 10.1038/npp.2011.65

Dean, O., Giorlando, F., and Berk, M. (2011). N-acetylcysteine in psychiatry: current therapeutic evidence and potential mechanisms of action. *J. Psychiatry. Neurosci.* 36, 78–86. doi: 10.1503/jpn.100057

Dean, O. M., Van Den Buuse, M., Bush, A. I., Copolov, D. L., Ng, F., Dodd, S., et al. (2009). A role for glutathione in the pathophysiology of bipolar disorder and schizophrenia? Animal models and relevance to clinical practice. *Curr. Med. Chem.* 16, 2965–2976. doi: 10.2174/092986709788803060

Devlin, B., and Scherer, S. W. (2012). Genetic architecture in autism spectrum disorder. *Curr. Opin. Genet. Dev.* 22, 229–237. doi: 10.1016/j.gde.2012.03.002

Di Benedetto, B., and Rupprecht, R. (2013). Targeting glia cells: novel perspectives for the treatment of neuropsychiatric diseases. *Curr. Neuropharmacol.* 11, 171–185. doi: 10.2174/1570159x11311020004

Domercq, M., Vazquez-Villoldo, N., and Matute, C. (2013). Neurotransmitter signaling in the pathophysiology of microglia. *Front. Cell. Neurosci.* 7:49. doi: 10.3389/fncel.2013.00107

Fatemi, S. H., Folsom, T. D., Reutiman, T. J., and Lee, S. (2008). Expression of astrocytic markers aquaporin 4 and connexin 43 is altered in brains of subjects with autism. *Synapse* 62, 501–507. doi: 10.1002/syn.20519

Ghanizadeh, A., and Moghimi-Sarani, E. (2013). A randomized double blind placebo controlled clinical trial of N-Acetylcysteine added to risperidone for treating autistic disorders. *BMC Psychiatry.* 13:196. doi: 10.1186/1471-244x-13-196

Gogos, A., Van Den Buuse, M., and Rossell, S. (2009). Gender differences in prepulse inhibition (PPI) in bipolar disorder: men have reduced PPI, women have increased PPI. *Int. J. Neuropsychopharmacol.* 12, 1249–1259. doi: 10.1017/s1461145709000480

Graf, E. R., Zhang, X., Jin, S. X., Linhoff, M. W., and Craig, A. M. (2004). Neurexins induce differentiation of GABA and glutamate postsynaptic specializations via neuroligins. *Cell* 119, 1013–1026. doi: 10.1016/j.cell.2004.11.035

Grauer, S. M., and Marquis, K. L. (1999). Intracerebral administration of metabotropic glutamate receptor agonists disrupts prepulse inhibition of acoustic startle in Sprague-Dawley rats. *Psychopharmacology (Berl)* 141, 405–412. doi: 10.1007/s002130050850

Grayton, H. M., Missler, M., Collier, D. A., and Fernandes, C. (2013). Altered social behaviours in neurexin 1alpha knockout mice resemble core symptoms in neurodevelopmental disorders. *PLoS One* 8:e67114. doi: 10.1371/journal.pone.0067114

Griffey, R., and Flamig, D. (1990). VAPOR for solvent-suppressed, short echo, volume-localized spectroscopy. *J. Mag. Res.* 88, 161–166. doi: 10.1016/0022-2364(90)90120-x

Grivas, V., Markou, A., and Pitsikas, N. (2013). The metabotropic glutamate 2/3 receptor agonist LY379268 induces anxiety-like behavior at the highest dose tested in two rat models of anxiety. *Eur. J. Pharmacol.* 715, 105–110. doi: 10.1016/j.ejphar.2013.05.048

Gunduz-Bruce, H., Reinhart, R. M., Roach, B. J., Gueorguieva, R., Oliver, S., D'souza, D. C., et al. (2012). Glutamatergic modulation of auditory information processing in the human brain. *Biol. Psychiatry.* 71, 969–977. doi: 10.1016/j.biopsych.2011.09.031

Gussew, A., Erdtel, M., Hiepe, P., Rzanny, R., and Reichenbach, J. R. (2012). Absolute quantitation of brain metabolites with respect to heterogeneous tissue compositions in (1)H-MR spectroscopic volumes. *MAGMA* 25, 321–333. doi: 10.1007/s10334-012-0305-z

Hardan, A. Y., Fung, L. K., Libove, R. A., Obukhanych, T. V., Nair, S., Herzenberg, L. A., et al. (2012). A randomized controlled pilot trial of oral N-acetylcysteine in children with autism. *Biol. Psychiatry.* 71, 956–961. doi: 10.1016/j.biopsych.2012.01.014

Haznedar, M. M., Buchsbaum, M. S., Hazlett, E. A., Licalzi, E. M., Cartwright, C., and Hollander, E. (2006). Volumetric analysis and three-dimensional glucose metabolic mapping of the striatum and thalamus in patients with autism spectrum disorders. *Am. J. Psychiatry.* 163, 1252–1263. doi: 10.1176/appi.ajp.163.7.1252

Hikichi, H., Nishino, M., Fukushima, M., Satow, A., Maehara, S., Kawamoto, H., et al. (2010). Pharmacological effects of metabotropic glutamate receptor ligands on prepulse inhibition in DBA/2J mice. *Eur. J. Pharmacol.* 639, 99–105. doi: 10.1016/j.ejphar.2010.03.046

Horder, J., Lavender, T., Mendez, M. A., O'gorman, R., Daly, E., Craig, M. C., et al. (2013). Reduced subcortical glutamate/glutamine in adults with autism spectrum disorders: a [(1)H]MRS study. *Transl. Psychiatry.* 3:e279. doi: 10.1038/tp.2013.53

Imre, G., Salomons, A., Jongsma, M., Fokkema, D. S., Den Boer, J. A., and Ter Horst, G. J. (2006). Effects of the mGluR2/3 agonist LY379268 on ketamine-evoked behaviours and neurochemical changes in the dentate gyrus of the rat. *Pharmacol. Biochem. Behav.* 84, 392–399. doi: 10.1016/j.pbb.2006.05.021

Joshi, G., Wozniak, J., Petty, C., Martelon, M. K., Fried, R., Bolfek, A., et al. (2013). Psychiatric comorbidity and functioning in a clinically referred population of adults with autism spectrum disorders: a comparative study. *J. Autism. Dev. Disord.* 43, 1314–1325. doi: 10.1007/s10803-012-1679-5

Kaiser, L. G., Schuff, N., Cashdollar, N., and Weiner, M. W. (2005). Age-related glutamate and glutamine concentration changes in normal human brain: 1H MR spectroscopy study at 4 T. *Neurobiol. Aging.* 26, 665–672. doi: 10.1016/j.neurobiolaging.2004.07.001

Kumari, V., Aasen, I., and Sharma, T. (2004). Sex differences in prepulse inhibition deficits in chronic schizophrenia. *Schizophr. Res.* 69, 219–235. doi: 10.1016/j.schres.2003.09.010

Kumari, V., Gray, J. A., Geyer, M. A., Ffytche, D., Soni, W., Mitterschiffthaler, M. T., et al. (2003). Neural correlates of tactile prepulse inhibition: a functional MRI study in normal and schizophrenic subjects. *Psychiatry. Res.* 122, 99–113. doi: 10.1016/s0925-4927(02)00123-3

Kupchik, Y. M., Moussawi, K., Tang, X. C., Wang, X., Kalivas, B. C., Kolokithas, R., et al. (2012). The effect of N-acetylcysteine in the nucleus accumbens on neurotransmission and relapse to cocaine. *Biol. Psychiatry.* 71, 978–986. doi: 10.1016/j.biopsych.2011.10.024

Labouesse, M. A., Stadlbauer, U., Langhans, W., and Meyer, U. (2013). Chronic high fat diet consumption impairs sensorimotor gating in mice. *Psychoneuroendocrinology* 38, 2562–2574. doi: 10.1016/j.psyneuen.2013.06.003

Lehmann, J., Pryce, C. R., and Feldon, J. (1999). Sex differences in the acoustic startle response and prepulse inhibition in Wistar rats. *Behav. Brain Res.* 104, 113–117. doi: 10.1016/s0166-4328(99)00058-3

Lewis, M., and Kim, S. J. (2009). The pathophysiology of restricted repetitive behavior. *J. Neurodev. Disord.* 1, 114–132. doi: 10.1007/s11689-009-9019-6

Liang, S. L., Carlson, G. C., and Coulter, D. A. (2006). Dynamic regulation of synaptic GABA release by the glutamate-glutamine cycle in hippocampal area CA1. *J. Neurosci.* 26, 8537–8548. doi: 10.1523/jneurosci.0329-06.2006

Matson, J. L., and Cervantes, P. E. (2014). Commonly studied comorbid psychopathologies among persons with autism spectrum disorder. *Res. Dev. Disabil.* 35, 952–962. doi: 10.1016/j.ridd.2014.02.012

McAlonan, G. M., Daly, E., Kumari, V., Critchley, H. D., Van Amelsvoort, T., Suckling, J., et al. (2002). Brain anatomy and sensorimotor gating in Asperger's syndrome. *Brain* 125, 1594–1606. doi: 10.1093/brain/awf150

Moghaddam, B., and Javitt, D. (2012). From revolution to evolution: the glutamate hypothesis of schizophrenia and its implication for treatment. *Neuropsychopharmacology* 37, 4–15. doi: 10.1038/npp.2011.181

Moran, M. M., Mcfarland, K., Melendez, R. I., Kalivas, P. W., and Seamans, J. K. (2005). Cystine/glutamate exchange regulates metabotropic glutamate receptor presynaptic inhibition of excitatory transmission and vulnerability to cocaine seeking. *J. Neurosci.* 25, 6389–6393. doi: 10.1523/jneurosci.1007-05.2005

Naaijen, J., Lythgoe, D. J., Amiri, H., Buitelaar, J. K., and Glennon, J. C. (2015). Fronto-striatal glutamatergic compounds in compulsive and impulsive syndromes: a review of magnetic resonance spectroscopy studies. *Neurosci. Biobehav. Rev.* 52, 74–88. doi: 10.1016/j.neubiorev.2015.02.009

O'Neill, M. F., Heron-Maxwell, C., Conway, M. W., Monn, J. A., and Ornstein, P. (2003). Group II metabotropic glutamate receptor antagonists LY341495 and LY366457 increase locomotor activity in mice. *Neuropharmacology* 45, 565–574. doi: 10.1016/s0028-3908(03)00232-6

Onore, C., Careaga, M., and Ashwood, P. (2012). The role of immune dysfunction in the pathophysiology of autism. *Brain Behav. Immun.* 26, 383–392. doi: 10.1016/j.bbi.2011.08.007

Perry, W., Minassian, A., Lopez, B., Maron, L., and Lincoln, A. (2007). Sensorimotor gating deficits in adults with autism. *Biol. Psychiatry.* 61, 482–486. doi: 10.1016/j.biopsych.2005.09.025

Provencher, S. W. (1993). Estimation of metabolite concentrations from localized *in vivo* proton NMR spectra. *Mag. Res. Med.* 30, 672–679. doi: 10.1002/mrm.1910300604

Ralph, R. J., Paulus, M. P., and Geyer, M. A. (2001). Strain-specific effects of amphetamine on prepulse inhibition and patterns of locomotor behavior in mice. *J. Pharmacol. Exp. Ther.* 298, 148–155.

Rubenstein, J. L., and Merzenich, M. M. (2003). Model of autism: increased ratio of excitation/inhibition in key neural systems. *Genes. Brain Behav.* 2, 255–267. doi: 10.1034/j.1601-183x.2003.00037.x

Rushworth, G. F., and Megson, I. L. (2013). Existing and potential therapeutic uses for N-acetylcysteine: the need for conversion to intracellular glutathione for antioxidant benefits. *Pharmacol. Ther.* 141, 150–159. doi: 10.1016/j.pharmthera.2013.09.006

Saha, S., Chant, D., Welham, J., and Mcgrath, J. (2005). A systematic review of the prevalence of schizophrenia. *PLoS Med* 2:e141. doi: 10.1016/s0920-9964(14)70102-1

Saitoh, A., Ohashi, M., Suzuki, S., Tsukagoshi, M., Sugiyama, A., Yamada, M., et al. (2014). Activation of the prelimbic medial prefrontal cortex induces anxiety-like behaviors via N-Methyl-D-aspartate receptor-mediated glutamatergic neurotransmission in mice. *J. Neurosci. Res.* 92, 1044–1053. doi: 10.1002/jnr.23391

Satow, A., Maehara, S., Ise, S., Hikichi, H., Fukushima, M., Suzuki, G., et al. (2008). Pharmacological effects of the metabotropic glutamate receptor 1 antagonist compared with those of the metabotropic glutamate receptor 5 antagonist and metabotropic glutamate receptor 2/3 agonist in rodents: detailed investigations with a selective allosteric metabotropic glutamate receptor 1 antagonist, FTIDC [4-[1-(2-fluoropyridine-3-yl)-5-methyl-1H-1,2,3-triazol-4-yl]-N-isopropyl-N-methy l-3,6-dihydropyridine-1(2H)-carboxamide]. *J. Pharmacol. Exp. Ther.* 326, 577–586. doi: 10.1124/jpet.108.138107

Scott-Van Zeeland, A. A., Dapretto, M., Ghahremani, D. G., Poldrack, R. A., and Bookheimer, S. Y. (2010). Reward processing in autism. *Autism. Res.* 3, 53–67. doi: 10.1186/2040-2392-3-7

Segovia, G., Porras, A., Del Arco, A., and Mora, F. (2001). Glutamatergic neurotransmission in aging: a critical perspective. *Mech. Ageing Dev.* 122, 1–29. doi: 10.1016/s0047-6374(00)00225-6

Silverman, J. L., Pride, M. C., Hayes, J. E., Puhger, K. R., Butler-Struben, H. M., Baker, S., et al. (2015). GABAB receptor agonist r-baclofen reverses social deficits and reduces repetitive behavior in two mouse models of autism. *Neuropsychopharmacology* 40, 2228–2239. doi: 10.1038/npp.2015.66

Silverman, J. L., Smith, D. G., Rizzo, S. J., Karras, M. N., Turner, S. M., Tolu, S. S., et al. (2012). Negative allosteric modulation of the mGluR5 receptor reduces repetitive behaviors and rescues social deficits in mouse models of autism. *Sci. Transl. Med.* 4, 131ra151. doi: 10.1126/scitranslmed.3003501

Simpson, E. H., Kellendonk, C., and Kandel, E. (2010). A possible role for the striatum in the pathogenesis of the cognitive symptoms of schizophrenia. *Neuron* 65, 585–596. doi: 10.1016/j.neuron.2010.02.014

Spooren, W., Lindemann, L., Ghosh, A., and Santarelli, L. (2012). Synapse dysfunction in autism: a molecular medicine approach to drug discovery in neurodevelopmental disorders. *Trends Pharmacol. Sci.* 33, 669–684. doi: 10.1016/j.tips.2012.09.004

Takeuchi, T., Kiyama, Y., Nakamura, K., Tsujita, M., Matsuda, I., Mori, H., et al. (2001). Roles of the glutamate receptor epsilon2 and delta2 subunits in the potentiation and prepulse inhibition of the acoustic startle reflex. *Eur. J. Neurosci.* 14, 153–160. doi: 10.1046/j.0953-816x.2001.01620.x

Vuillermot, S., Feldon, J., and Meyer, U. (2011). Nurr1 is not essential for the development of prepulse inhibition deficits induced by prenatal immune activation. *Brain Behav. Immun.* 25, 1316–1321. doi: 10.1016/j.bbi.2011.06.012

Wieronska, J. M., and Pilc, A. (2013). Glutamate-based anxiolytic ligands in clinical trials. *Expert Opin. Investig. Drugs* 22, 1007–1022. doi: 10.1517/13543784.2013.803066

Xu, J. Y., Xia, Q. Q., and Xia, J. (2012). A review on the current neuroligin mouse models. *Sheng. Li. Xue. Bao.* 64, 550–562.

Zavodnick, A. D., and Ali, R. (2014). N-Acetylcysteine and metabotropic glutamate receptors: implications for the treatment of schizophrenia: a literature review. *Psychiatr. Q.* 85, 177–185. doi: 10.1007/s11126-013-9281-3

Zhang, X., Li, Q., Wong, N., Zhang, M., Wang, W., Bu, B., et al. (2015). Behaviour and prefrontal protein differences in C57BL/6N and 129 X1/SvJ mice. *Brain Res. Bull.* 116, 16–24. doi: 10.1016/j.brainresbull.2015.05.003

Zhou, I. Y., Ding, A. Y., Li, Q., McAlonan, G. M., and Wu, E. X. (2012). Magnetic resonance spectroscopy reveals N-acetylaspartate reduction in hippocampus and cingulate cortex after fear conditioning. *Psychiatry. Res.* 204, 178–183. doi: 10.1016/j.pscychresns.2012.09.010

Conflict of Interest Statement: The authors declare that the research was conducted in the absence of any commercial or financial relationships that could be construed as a potential conflict of interest.

7

Evidence from a Rare Case Study for Hebbian-like Changes in Structural Connectivity Induced by Long-term Deep Brain Stimulation

Edited by:
Raymond C. K. Chan, Institute of Psychology, Chinese Academy of Sciences, China

***Correspondence:**
Morten L. Kringelbach, Department of Psychiatry, University of Oxford, Warneford Hospital, Oxford OX3 7JX, UK
morten.kringelbach@psych.ox.ac.uk

Tim J. van Hartevelt[1,2]*, Joana Cabral*[1,3]*, Arne Møller*[2]*, James J. FitzGerald*[4]*, Alexander L. Green*[4]*, Tipu Z. Aziz*[1,4]*, Gustavo Deco*[3,5] *and Morten L. Kringelbach*[1,2,4]*

[1] Department of Psychiatry, University of Oxford, Oxford, UK, [2] Center of Functionally Integrative Neuroscience (CFIN), Aarhus University, Aarhus, Denmark, [3] Center of Brain and Cognition, Theoretical and Computational Neuroscience Group, Universitat Pompeu Fabra, Barcelona, Spain, [4] Nuffield Department of Surgical Sciences, John Radcliffe Hospital, Oxford, UK, [5] Institució Catalana de la Recerca i Estudis Avançats (ICREA), Universitat Pompeu Fabra, Barcelona, Spain

It is unclear whether Hebbian-like learning occurs at the level of long-range white matter connections in humans, i.e., where measurable changes in structural connectivity (SC) are correlated with changes in functional connectivity. However, the behavioral changes observed after deep brain stimulation (DBS) suggest the existence of such Hebbian-like mechanisms occurring at the structural level with functional consequences. In this rare case study, we obtained the full network of white matter connections of one patient with Parkinson's disease (PD) before and after long-term DBS and combined it with a computational model of ongoing activity to investigate the effects of DBS-induced long-term structural changes. The results show that the long-term effects of DBS on resting-state functional connectivity is best obtained in the computational model by changing the structural weights from the subthalamic nucleus (STN) to the putamen and the thalamus in a Hebbian-like manner. Moreover, long-term DBS also significantly changed the SC towards normality in terms of model-based measures of segregation and integration of information processing, two key concepts of brain organization. This novel approach using computational models to model the effects of Hebbian-like changes in SC allowed us to causally identify the possible underlying neural mechanisms of long-term DBS using rare case study data. In time, this could help predict the efficacy of individual DBS targeting and identify novel DBS targets.

Keywords: deep brain stimulation, Hebbian-like learning, Parkinson's disease, DTI, subthalamic nucleus

Introduction

Deep brain stimulation (DBS) is a well-established treatment for several neurological conditions including Parkinson's disease (PD; Benabid et al., 2009; Lozano and Lipsman, 2013). However, the underlying neural mechanisms of DBS and its long-term effects on brain connectivity remain unclear. This limitation restricts the efficacy of DBS since the identification of individual DBS targets and the settings of stimulation parameters cannot be optimally performed beforehand.

Uncovering these aspects will improve the clinical benefits of DBS in the treatment of such diseases.

In general terms, the effects of DBS must be closely linked to at least three factors: (1) the stimulation parameters such as frequency, amplitude, pulse width and duration; (2) the physiological properties of the neural tissue (which may be dependent on disease state); and (3) the interactions between the electrode and the surrounding neural tissue and specific anatomy of the targeted region (Kringelbach et al., 2007, 2010). This third factor includes the extended brain-wide connectivity pattern from the electrode where this specific structural "fingerprint" of connectivity is an important factor for the efficacy (Fernandes et al., 2015). Thus rather than solely acting locally, the evidence clearly shows that DBS affects a network of neural elements; foremost myelinated axons,and to a lesser degree cell bodies. Thus the most likely mechanism of DBS is through stimulation-induced modulation of the activity of macroscopic brain networks (Montgomery and Baker, 2000; Vitek, 2002; McIntyre and Hahn, 2010; Kringelbach et al., 2011). This has been confirmed by optogenetic experiments in rodents which show that the therapeutic effects within the subthalamic nucleus (STN) can be accounted for by direct selective stimulation of afferent axons projecting to this region (Gradinaru et al., 2009). It is not clear, however, which of the many connections from a given DBS target are most influential in providing a clinical benefit and whether DBS creates long-term changes in brain connectivity.

In this case study, we exploit the unique opportunity of having preoperative and five-month postoperative diffusion tensor imaging (DTI) data from a single patient with DBS in the STN for the treatment of PD. This allowed us to reconstruct the three-dimensional networks of white-matter connections—or structural connectivity (SC)—before and after long-term DBS, which we used to simulate the corresponding spontaneous dynamics using a whole-brain computational model (Deco et al., 2013b).

We hypothesized that computational modeling of the effects of changes in SC following DBS would allow us to identify the significant, causal neural mechanisms of DBS compared to not applying DBS. In order to do this, we calculated the change of brain activity induced by the DBS by simulating resting state activity before and after DBS. We analyzed under which conditions the predicted change of neuronal activity correlates with the changes in the SC observed 5 months after operation, i.e., assuming the existence of Hebbian-like learning, where the weights in the model were changed in a Hebbian-like manner. We were able to test this by systematically changing the weight of the structural connections from the STN to itself and its known projections in the putamen, caudate and thalamus. We thus used established principles of Hebbian-like learning to change the functional dynamics between STN and its projections to find the optimal weights that best describe the long-term changes in SC induced by DBS.

Finally, we calculated the overall impact of long-term DBS on measures of integration and segregation, representing two fundamental aspects of brain organization and information processing (Deco et al., 2015).

Materials and Methods

Brief Description of Analysis Pipeline

In this case study, we investigated the underlying neural mechanisms of long-term DBS in terms of connectivity changes by using a computational dynamic mean field (DMF) model (Deco and Jirsa, 2012; Deco et al., 2013b) on pre- and post-operative DTI data. Briefly, we analyzed the data as follows (and further described in details below):

1. *Structural connectivity.* Structural connectomes were constructed for the pre- and post-operative data. We also computed the difference between pre- to post-operative connectomes (SC*). In addition, we generated a group-averaged connectome from healthy participants to optimize the DMF model (see **Figures 1**, **2A** and "Structural Brain Networks" Section).
2. *Computational dynamical mean field model.* The DMF model was optimized in the same way as described in our previous case-study (van Hartevelt et al., 2014), i.e., by fitting the FC and SC from healthy individuals [see **Figure 2B** and "Model of Spontaneous Functional Connectivity (FC)" Section]. As shown in previous studies (Cabral et al., 2014), this model accurately captures many features of the resting-state dynamics of FC.
3. *Finding optimal fit of model.* The DMF model was applied to the pre-operative structural connectome (SC_pre) to generate the pre-operative functional resting-state activity (FC_pre). Crucially, we then added the four established targets of the DBS electrode in STN (itself, thalamus, caudate and putamen) (I*), and used the DMF model on FC_pre with I* to generate the putative post-operative functional resting-state activity (FC_pos). This allowed us to compute the difference between the pre- and post-operative FC matrices (FC*). We then systematically optimized the parameters of I* to find the best possible fit, i.e., we compared the effects of changing I* to get the maximal correlation between each of the SC* and FC* pairs (see **Figure 2C**).
4. *Determine the causal contribution of each STN projection.* Once we had found the optimal fit of weights for STN projections (I*), we systematically varied each of the four structural weights while holding the other weights constant (see **Figure 3A**). This allowed us to determine which of these projections best predict the effects of STN DBS on postoperative FC.
5. *Determine the global influence of long-term Hebbian-like changes in SC following DBS.* We used the DMF model to compute measures of integration and segregation of information processing in the pre- and post-operative brain compared to the healthy brain (see "Functional Measures" Section).

Patient and Healthy Participants

We acquired DTI data preoperatively and 5 months postoperatively after continuous DBS in a 45-year-old female PD patient. The patient's main symptoms included on/off fluctuations and dyskinesias. The patient received continuous

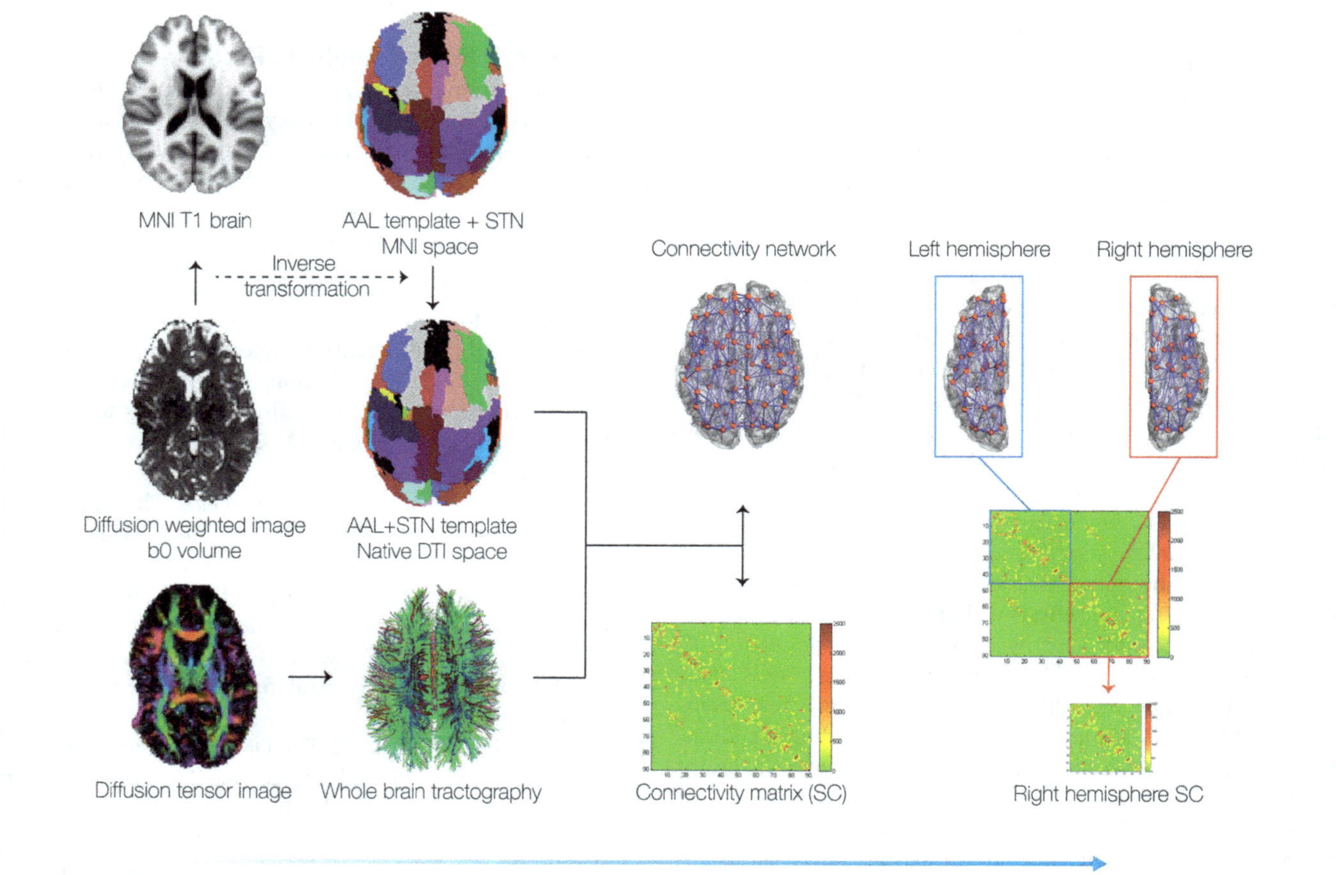

FIGURE 1 | Pipeline for generating the connectivity matrices. We collected pre and post diffusion tensor imaging (DTI) data from a patient and then generated the whole-brain tractography for all voxels (bottom left). In addition to the 90 cortical and subcortical regions in the automated anatomical labeling (AAL) template, we incorporated the subthalamic nucleus (STN), based on the binarised version of a probabilistic mask (Forstmann et al., 2012). This resulted in a total of 92 cortical and subcortical regions (46 per hemisphere). We reconstructed the whole-brain connectivity matrix between these 92 brain regions using the methods described in van Hartevelt et al. (2014). Due to the electrode artifact in the left hemisphere (see bottom left), in the subsequent analyses we only used the right hemisphere connectivity matrices.

DBS *on* and *off* over 5 months during stimulation optimization. In order to plan a lead revision (warranted by adverse side effects including emotional lability) post DBS DTI data were acquired. The new target for the lead revisions was the internal Globus Pallidus. Following DBS surgery, the medication was continued with Pramipexole 0.7 one and a half tablets thrice daily. Stalevo was reduced to 50 mg thrice daily (from 150 mg in the morning, 50 mg twice daily and 100 mg in the evening) and Amantadine was stopped completely (from 100 mg twice daily). During the periods when the DBS was turned *off*, the patient was advised to return to her preoperative medication regime. Whereas right DBS lead titration resulted in symptom reduction, left DBS lead titration was more problematic and resulted in adverse side effects. A possible explanation for this is the suboptimal positioning of the electrode. During the 5 months between DTI acquisitions the stimulation parameters changed due to fine tuning and titration of the DBS electrodes. Additional DTI data were acquired for nine healthy participants (three females, age range 22–40 years). This study was approved by the National Research Ethics Service (NRES) committee South Central—Berkshire in Bristol.

Surgical Procedure

The DBS electrodes were implanted in the bilateral STN. Prior to surgery, anatomical T1 and T2 MRI scans with 1 × 1 × 1 mm voxel size were acquired for electrode implant protocol planning. The surgery was performed under local anesthesia using a Cosman–Roberts–Wells stereotactic. See Kringelbach et al. (2009) for more details on the surgical procedure.

Image Acquisition

All DTI data for the patient and healthy participants were acquired on a Philips Achieva 1.5 Tesla MR scanner in Oxford. Whole brain diffusion weighted imaging was performed using a single-shot echo planar sequence. The scanning parameters were echo *time* (TE) = 65 ms, repetition *time* (TR) = 9390 ms, reconstructed matrix 176 × 176 and reconstructed voxel size of 1.8 × 1.8 mm and slice thickness of 2 mm. We used 33 optimal nonlinear diffusion gradient directions ($b = 1200$ s/mm^2) and one

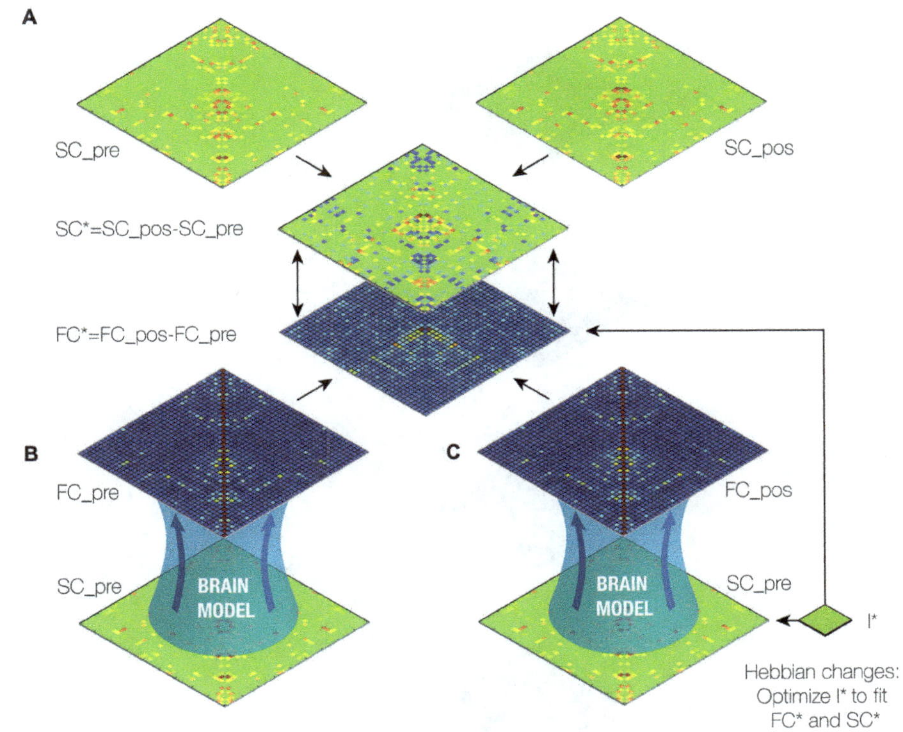

FIGURE 2 | Outline of brain model analysis and optimization. (A) First, we created the difference (SC*) between the pre- and post-operative structural connectivity (SC) matrices (SC_pos-SC_pre; see **Figure 1**) (van Hartevelt et al., 2014). **(B)** The functional connectivity matrix (FC_pre) was generated with a dynamic mean-field (DMF) model using SC_pre. **(C)** We then iteratively generated the functional connectivity post-DBS (FC_pos) using the computational model with SC_pre and the I*, the weights of the known connections from the STN. We subsequently optimized I* such that the difference between FC_pre and FC_pos (FC*) was made to fit SC*. In this way, we estimated the optimal working weights from the STN. Finally, we calculated the contribution of each of the connections from the STN to the changes in functional connectivity caused by DBS by varying the weights of each of the connections and measuring the impact on the fit (see **Figure 3**).

non-diffusion weighted volume ($b = 0$) for the DTI acquisition. The post-DBS DTI data was acquired with DBS turned off.

Structural Brain Networks

The whole-brain structural networks were constructed in a two-step process used successfully in previous published studies (Cabral et al., 2013; van Hartevelt et al., 2014; Fernandes et al., 2015). First, the brain was parcellated into different regions or nodes. Secondly, the edges, or connections between nodes, were estimated using probabilistic tractography (**Figure 1**). Each of these two steps is described in detail in the following.

Parcellation of the Brain

The brain was parcellated into 90 cortical and subcortical regions (45 for each hemisphere) using the automated anatomical labeling (AAL) template (Tzourio-Mazoyer et al., 2002). Additionally a mask of the STN from Forstmann et al. (2012) was incorporated to get a total of 92 cortical and subcortical regions (46 per hemisphere). In order to preserve as much information as possible, the parcellation of the brain was done in DTI native space.

We used the Flirt tool (FMRIB, Oxford; Jenkinson et al., 2002) for linearly coregistration of the b0 image in DTI space to the T1 structural image. The T1 image was in turn coregistered to the T1 template of ICBM152 in MNI space (Collins et al., 1994). The resulting transformations were concatenated and inversed and subsequently applied to transform the AAL template (Tzourio-Mazoyer et al., 2002) and the STN masks (Forstmann et al., 2012) from MNI space to DTI native space. This transformation of the template was conducted using a nearest-neighbor interpolation method to ensure that the discrete labeling values were preserved.

To minimize the effects of the DBS electrode artifact, a binary mask of the electrode lead in the post-DBS DTI data was created. This mask was subtracted from the brain masks and data of the pre-DBS DTI data as well as from the DTI data of the healthy controls.

Whole-brain Network Connectivity

We used FMRIB's Diffusion Toolbox (FDT), which is a part of FSL (version 5.0, FMRIB, Oxford)[1] to process the DTI data. The preprocessing involved coregistering the diffusion-weighted images to a reference volume using an affine transformation for the correction of head motion. This step also includes an eddy current correction. Next, the local probability distribution

[1] http://www.fmrib.ox.ac.uk/fsl/

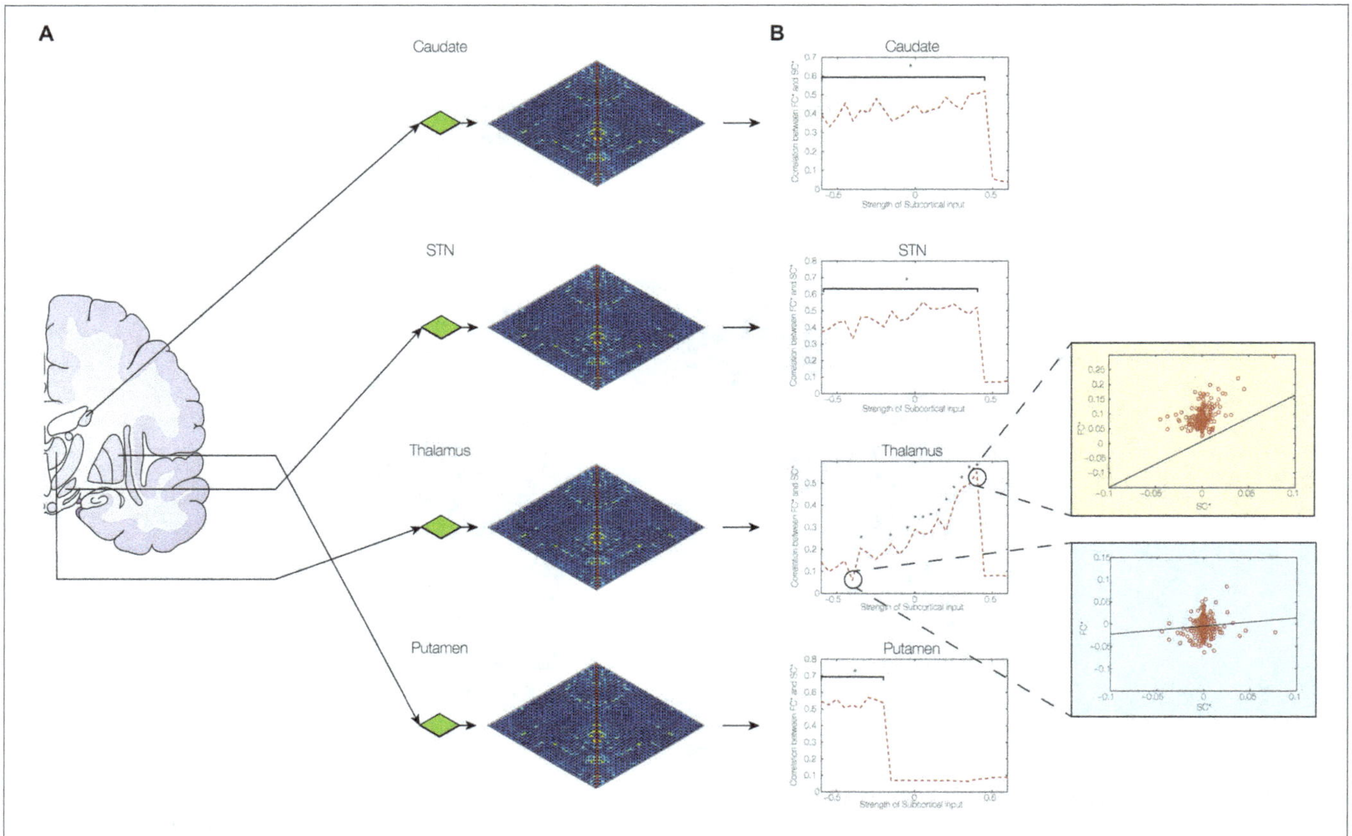

FIGURE 3 | Determining the contribution of subcortical connections of STN. (A) We found the optimum fit of I* and then varied each of the model parameters of the connections from the STN to the putamen, caudate, thalamus and STN itself to estimate their contributions to the changes in functional connectivity caused by DBS. Compared to no DBS, the optimum fit was highly significant ($p < 10^{-7}$). **(B)** The figure clearly demonstrates the importance of the changes in connectivity weights to the thalamus and the putamen with the consequences of the best fit in thalamic connectivity shown in top right (light yellow) and poorest fit shown in bottom right (light blue) (with a star indicating significance levels of $p < 0.05$).

of fiber direction was estimated at each voxel using the default bedpostx parameters of FSL v5.0 (Behrens et al., 2003). Using the parameter estimation from bedpostx, the probtrackx algorithm (allowing for automatic estimation of two fiber directions within each voxel) was used, improving the tracking sensitivity of non-dominant fibers in the brain (Behrens et al., 2007).

We estimated the connectivity probability by applying probabilistic tractography using the default sampling settings of 5000 streamline fibers per voxel. The connectivity from a seed voxel i to another voxel j was defined by the proportion of fibers passing through voxel i that reach voxel j (Behrens et al., 2007). In a brain region, or node, consisting of n voxels, 5000*n fibers were sampled. The connectivity C_{ij} from region i to region j is calculated as the number of sampled fibers connecting the voxels in region i to the voxels in region j divided by n, with n being the number of voxels in the seed region i.

The connectivity value for a given region to each of the 91 other regions was calculated. As probabilistic tractography depends on the seeding location, the connectivity from i to j is not necessarily equivalent to that from j to i. The connectivity values are highly correlated though across the brain for all participants (the least Pearson $r = 0.70$, $p < 10–50$). The symmetrical, undirectional connectivity C_{ij} between regions i and j was calculated by averaging the two connectivity values. Therefore, we considered the SC between the two areas, where $C_{ij} = C_{ji}$. The connectivity values were calculated using in-house Perl scripts and were normalized for the regions' volume with n voxels. The connectivity matrices were created for the preoperative condition (*SC_pre*), the postoperative condition (*SC_pos*) and one average connectivity matrix for the healthy subjects (*SC_normal*).

Due to the artifact of the DBS lead in the left hemisphere in the postoperative DTI data (see bottom left of **Figure 1**), only the sub-network corresponding to the right hemisphere was considered. In other words, we only used the 46 × 46 matrix corresponding to the right hemisphere (without inter-hemispheric connections) and not the full 92 × 92 connectivity matrix as shown in **Figure 1**. All further analyses and simulations were done using the right hemisphere only for preoperative, postoperative and healthy connectivity matrices.

Model of Spontaneous Functional Connectivity

To illuminate the impact of DBS induces local structural changes on whole-brain activity, we used a DMF model to simulate the spontaneous dynamics of each brain area in the structural connectome (Deco and Jirsa, 2012; Deco et al., 2013b). The model is a reduction of the spiking network model, which includes the whole dynamics of excitatory and inhibitory populations of spiking neurons interconnected by AMPA, GABA and NMDA receptors and their respective equations (Wong and Wang, 2006). It describes the mean field activity of each brain area with a single one-dimensional equation and the level of excitation/inhibition of each node is balanced in order to maintain negligible short-range correlations and long-range functional correlations are introduced by excitatory inputs received from coupled brain regions according to the structural connectome. Thus the global dynamics of coupled brain areas can be simply and consistently described by the following set of coupled differential equations:

$$\frac{dS_i(t)}{dt} = -\frac{S_i}{\tau_S} + (1 - S_i)\gamma H(x_i) + \sigma \upsilon_i(t), \quad (1)$$

$$H(x_i) = \frac{ax_i - b}{1 - \exp\left(-d(ax_i - b)\right)}, \quad (2)$$

$$x_i = wJ_N S_i + GJ_N \sum_j C_{ij} S_j + I_0, \quad (3)$$

where $H(x_i)$ and S_i denote the population rate and the average synaptic gating variable at the local cortical area i (from 1 to N = 46 areas in our case), respectively. $w = 0.9$ is the local excitatory recurrence and C_{ij} corresponds to the coupling weight between the areas i and j. Note that C_{ij} is estimated from the SC, i.e., in proportion to the number of connections (or connectivity value) detected between areas i and j, and therefore this parameter is changed between pre-DBS, post-DBS and control data. G is the global coupling weight that scales all couplings uniformly. Parameter values for the input–output function (2) are a =270 VnC, b = 108 Hz, and d =0.154 s. The kinetic parameters are γ = 0.641/1000 (the factor 1000 is for expressing everything in ms), and τ_s =100 ms. The synaptic couplings are $J_N = 0.2609$ nA and the overall effective external input is $I_0 = 0.3$ nA. In equation (1) υ_i is uncorrelated standard Gaussian noise and the noise amplitude at each node is $\sigma = 0.001$ nA.

We used the Balloon-Windkessel hemodynamic model to transform the mean field activity into (simulated) BOLD signal, This model describes the transduction of neuronal activity into BOLD signal (Friston et al., 2003). The level of synaptic activity in each brain region represented by the synaptic variable S_i, is used to compute the BOLD-signal estimation in that specific brain region as in (Deco and Jirsa, 2012; Cabral et al., 2013; van Hartevelt et al., 2014). The simulated BOLD signal was down-sampled at 2 s to have the same temporal resolution typically used in fMRI. The simulated FC between all brain areas is obtained by computing the temporal correlation matrix of the simulated BOLD signals.

The optimal fit of the model was calculated using an exhaustive search, i.e., we fitted all combinations of inputs (STN, thalamus, putamen and caudate) scanning them from values of −0.6 to 0.6 in steps of 0.05. From this search, we found the optimal working point of the model which is where the strengths of inputs from those subcortical areas yielded a maximal correlation between the differences in FC (FC*) and SC (SC*), i.e., where there is a maximal Hebbian-like correlation.

In order to determine the contribution of each individual connection on this fit, one of each of the four individual inputs from these subcortical areas were systematically changed while the other points were fixed at the optimal fit. Thus to determine the influence of the STN, for example, we systematically changed the values of the STN from −0.6 to 0.6, while keeping the values of the other three regions for the optimal fit. This process was then repeated for the putamen, caudate and thalamus, while keeping all other inputs fixed at the values of the optimal fit.

Functional Measures

Two fundamental aspects of brain organization are the segregation of brain areas (that differ in terms of local functional specialization) and their global integration during perception and behavior (Tononi et al., 1994; Deco et al., 2015). As such, we investigated how these properties were affected before the surgery and to what extent DBS helped recover them towards normal values.

Segregation

To measure the segregation, we first estimate the mutual information between BOLD signals, which can be easily calculated—assuming Gaussianity of the mean BOLD responses—using the following equation:

$$I(\chi_1; \chi_2; \ldots; \chi_N) = -\log\left(det(C)\right), \quad (4)$$

where x_i refers to the BOLD signal of the i = 1, N nodes (brain areas) of the brain network and C is the correlation matrix between them, which corresponds to the FC.

The input segregation is then simply defined by

$$S = 1 - \frac{I}{I_{\max}}, \quad (5)$$

where $I_{\max}$ is an appropriate normalization specifying the maximal mutual information condition.

Integration

We measure the integration of FC based on a measure of the size of the largest connected component. More specifically, for a given absolute threshold θ between 0 and 1, the functional connectivity matrix FC can be binarized (using the criteria $|FC_{ij}| < \theta$; which determines if it will be given a value of 0 and 1) and the largest component extracted as a measure of integration. The largest component is the length (number of nodes) of the connected sub-graph of the undirected graph defined by the binarized matrix (which itself is considered as an adjacency matrix). This is the largest sub-graph in which any two vertices are connected to each other by paths, and which connects to no additional vertices in the super-graph. Finally, to get a measure that is independent of the threshold, this curve can be integrated in the range of the threshold between 0 and 1. This integration measure is normalized by the maximal number of connected brain areas (that is, all N areas) for each integration step and by the number of integration steps such that the maximal integration is normalized to one.

Network Measures from Graph Theory

The analyses of the DTI data resulted in three 46 × 46 matrices, *SC_pre*, *SC_pos* and *SC_normal*, which can be analyzed as graphs. The brain networks were characterized using common measures from graph theory, namely the connection density, global efficiency, clustering coefficient, small-world index and hierarchy. We used the Brain Connectivity Toolbox to calculate all these global graph measures (Rubinov and Sporns, 2010; Sporns, 2011). These graph measures have been used and described in a previous study of brain connectivity in DBS (van Hartevelt et al., 2014).

These global graph measures were calculated for all three different anatomical brain networks, i.e., *SC_pre*, *SC_pos* and *SC_normal*. The average and standard deviation of the individual outcomes were then calculated and reported.

Results

We investigated the consequences of having a DBS electrode implanted in the STN using the SC matrices, *SC_pre* and *SC_pos*, arising from the DTI of a PD patient before and 5 months after DBS surgery. Since the SC remains mostly unchanged over relatively short periods of time in healthy subjects (Cheng et al., 2012), we considered the difference between these matrices, *SC**, as alterations induced by DBS in the patient's structural connectome (see **Figure 2A**).

A DMF model was used to run simulations (see "Materials and Methods" Section) first using the SC *SC_pre*, from which we obtained the resulting *FC_pre* (see **Figure 2B**). We then iteratively optimized the weights of the known connections from the STN, namely to the putamen, the thalamus, the caudate and the STN itself, to estimate *FC_pos* such that the difference between *FC_pre* and *FC_pos*, *FC**, optimally fitted *SC** (see **Figure 2C**). This step is based on the assumption that the global network dynamics of a brain working at the critical instability border amplifies the underlying structure of anatomical connections (Deco et al., 2013a). In other words, at the optimal working point, the FC maximally reflects the underlying SC and hence, FC* maximally reflects SC*.

Once the optimum fit was found, we investigated the contribution of each of these brain regions to the changes in FC caused by DBS (see **Figure 3**). We found that the optimal connection strengths were −0.5 for the putamen, 0.4 for the thalamus, 0.4 for the caudate and 0.3 for the STN. Using this optimal fit with these connection strength values, show how individual variation of the coupling strength values influences the level of Hebbian-like learning induced (**Figure 3**), i.e., the correlation between the change in SC (SC, SC_pos-SC_pre) and the change predicted by the simulation according to the FC (functional connectivity, DBS—no DBS). The figure shows the correlation as a function of connection strength, indicating with a star those with a significance value of $p < 0.05$. Only the connection weights to the thalamus show a sensitive influence on the induction or not of the overall plasticity (i.e., of inducing high correlations between changes in SC and predicted changes in FC), while the other subcortical nuclei are inducing the same level of plasticity if the weights are within the right range (e.g., putamen below −0.2). Thus the thalamus would appear to be the most critical location for the DBS to induce optimum changes.

To further investigate the structural changes induced by DBS in the functional networks in terms of segregation and integration of information processing, we estimated these two measures in FC_pre, FC_pos and FC_normal (the latter obtained with the model from SC_normal). As expected, we found that both the segregation and integration measures improved after 5 months of DBS, although not to the level found in the normal population (see **Figure 4**).

Finally, we used measures from graph theory to investigate the effects of long-term DBS on global network SC. The results that are reported in **Table 1** show that there was no effect of DBS on global measures of connection density, average clustering coefficient, global efficiency, small-world index or hierarchy.

Discussion

The results in this unique case study show that the changes in SC following long-term DBS can be used together with advanced computational modeling to uncover the underlying neural mechanisms of DBS. Using the rare opportunity of having pre- and post-DBS DTI in a patient with PD, we investigated the functional consequences of changes in SC after long-term DBS. We mapped the optimum changes in connectivity weights from the implanted electrode in the STN and demonstrated that the optimal fit of connectivity weights from the STN to the putamen, caudate, STN itself and the thalamus was significantly changed the fit of the model, i.e., was significantly better than using no DBS. Importantly, we were also able to show that the functional changes induced by DBS not only led to clinical improvements but also significantly recovered the measures of segregation and integration towards normality. Specifically, our results show that DBS exerts its effects on network-wide brain functional connectivity through local Hebbian-like changes in specific connections from the STN.

We have previously shown significant structural changes following long-term DBS suggestive of a global change (van Hartevelt et al., 2014). The present results significantly extend these findings by showing that the STN. DBS is causing specific changes in the connectivity from the STN and that there is an optimum connection weighting of connections to the thalamus, caudate, putamen and STN. This is important as it

TABLE 1 | Graph theoretical measures for pre, post and normal connectomes.

	SC_pre	SC_pos	SC_normal
Connection density (%)	45.09	45.94	46.51 (SD 8.35)
Average clustering coefficient	0.6680	0.6955	0.6924 (SD 0.0432)
Global efficiency	0.7295	0.7341	0.7336 (SD 0.0520)
Small-world index	1.191	1.212	1.2634 (SD 0.2809)
Hierarchy	0.1369	0.1233	0.1271 (SD 0.0355)

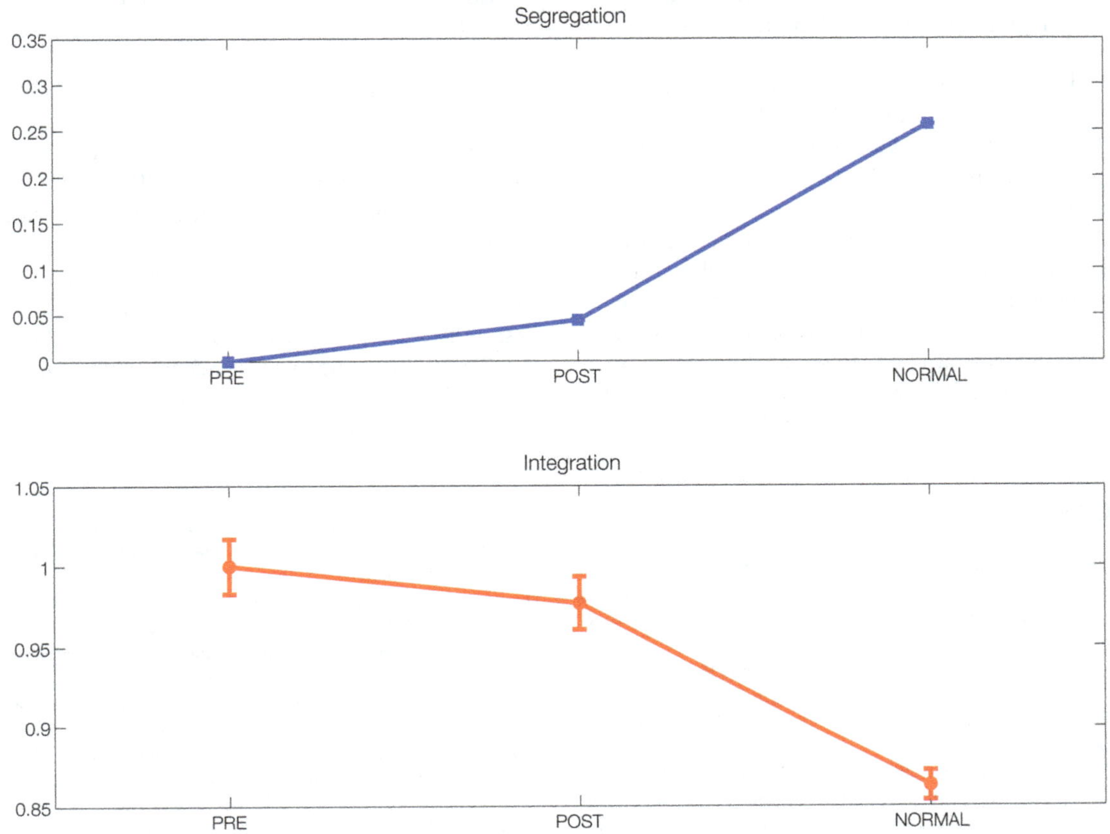

FIGURE 4 | Segregation and integration. Segregation and integration measures in the simulated functional networks before and after DBS (FC_pre and FC_pos) compared to the ones found in the simulated functional network obtained using the connectivity from the healthy population (FC_normal). Both measures improved after 5 months of DBS, although not to the level found in the normal population.

offers novel evidence on the underlying neural mechanisms of DBS.

The present findings offer new insights into how DBS reaches its efficacy and could potentially be combined with the findings of a specific connectivity fingerprint for successful DBS cases (Fernandes et al., 2015). This might open up new possibility for future studies and might allow us to further elucidate the exact underlying mechanisms of DBS. Among other things, this might improve pre-surgical targeting as this would allow us determine which areas are important to be connected to the target for DBS in order to achieve a successful outcome.

Using the whole-brain computational modeling approach, as described in this paper, might also be applicable in other disorders. It could be a possibility to investigate how unbalanced functional connectivity networks might be restored, or rebalanced, to a healthy regime by altering specific weights or connections in order to find the optimal fit with a healthy functional connectome (Kringelbach et al., 2011). The potential benefits of this technique would not only be limited to neurodegenerative disorders but would be possible to extend to neuropsychiatric disorders (Deco and Kringelbach, 2014).

This is the first study investigating the underlying mechanisms of previously shown long-term structural changes (van Hartevelt et al., 2014) related to long-term DBS for PD. Although this data is unique and has allowed for the first time to investigate the underlying mechanisms of DBS *in vivo* using advanced whole-brain computational modeling, it should be emphasized that this is a case study. Due to the unique nature of DBS and the complications it brings forth, it is, at this point in time, extremely difficult to obtain more neuroimaging data for this particular patient group. Despite this being a case study, the results obtained from this data with the advanced graph analysis and whole-brain computational modeling has given us a unique insight into the potential underlying mechanisms of long-term DBS.

While the results of this unique case study using novel methods are exciting there is one important limitation linked to the imaging artifact introduced by DBS. The externalized lead on the left side of the brain causes a significant dropout in MRI signal leading to the limited use of only the right hemisphere. Although this is a limitation, it should be noted here that titration of the right electrode resulted in significant symptom improvement in the patient, whereas titration of the left electrode was more bothersome and was accompanied by adverse side effects. In addition, this case study also carries further potential limitations linked the course of medication typically found in advanced PD and especially changes in the medication regime during the long-term DBS period investigated.

It should also be noted that we did not specifically test different learning algorithms. Thus it is possible that the causal changes in STN connectivity could be achieved by other learning rules, which are not Hebbian-like. This would be of considerable interest to test in future studies.

Overall, this unique case study provides the first indication that DBS selectively changes the connectivity weights from the region where the electrode is implanted with consequences at the level of macroscopic functional networks. This is highly suggestive of neural Hebbian-like changes in white matter tracts induced by long-term DBS. This novel approach opens the possibility for computational models to predict the efficacy of individual DBS targeting pre-surgery and may even help identify novel DBS targets.

Acknowledgments

MLK is supported by the TrygFonden Charitable Foundation and ERC Consolidator Grant: CAREGIVING (n. 615539). TZ is supported by the Medical Research Council, Norman Collisson Foundation, Charles Wolfson Charitable Trust, and NIHR Biomedical Research Centre. GD is supported by the ERC Advanced Grant: DYSTRUCTURE (n. 295129), by the Spanish Research Project SAF2010-16085, by the CONSOLIDER-INGENIO 2010 Programme CSD2007-00012, by the FP7-ICT BrainScales and by the Brain Network Recovery Group through the James S. McDonnell Foundation.

References

Behrens, T. E., Berg, H. J., Jbabdi, S., Rushworth, M. F., and Woolrich, M. W. (2007). Probabilistic diffusion tractography with multiple fibre orientations: what can we gain? *Neuroimage* 34, 144–155. doi: 10.1016/j.neuroimage.2006.09.018

Behrens, T. E., Woolrich, M. W., Jenkinson, M., Johansen-Berg, H., Nunes, R. G., Clare, S., et al. (2003). Characterization and propagation of uncertainty in diffusion-weighted MR imaging. *Magn. Reson. Med.* 50, 1077–1088. doi: 10.1002/mrm.10609

Benabid, A. L., Chabardes, S., Mitrofanis, J., and Pollak, P. (2009). Deep brain stimulation of the subthalamic nucleus for the treatment of Parkinson's disease. *Lancet Neurol.* 8, 67–81. doi: 10.1016/S1474-4422(08)70291-6

Cabral, J., Fernandes, H. M., Van Hartevelt, T. J., James, A. C., Kringelbach, M. L., and Deco, G. (2013). Structural connectivity in schizophrenia and its impact on the dynamics of spontaneous functional networks. *Chaos* 23:046111. doi: 10.1063/1.4851117

Cabral, J., Kringelbach, M. L., and Deco, G. (2014). Exploring the network dynamics underlying brain activity during rest. *Prog. Neurobiol.* 114, 102–131. doi: 10.1016/j.pneurobio.2013.12.005

Cheng, H., Wang, Y., Sheng, J., Kronenberger, W. G., Mathews, V. P., Hummer, T. A., et al. (2012). Characteristics and variability of structural networks derived from diffusion tensor imaging. *Neuroimage* 61, 1153–1164. doi: 10.1016/j.neuroimage.2012.03.036

Collins, D., Neelin, P., Peters, T., and Evans, A. C. (1994). Automatic 3D intersubject registration of MR volumetric data in standardized Talairach space. *J. Comput. Assist. Tomogr.* 18, 192–205. doi: 10.1097/00004728-199403000-00005

Deco, G., and Jirsa, V. K. (2012). Ongoing cortical activity at rest: criticality, multistability and ghost attractors. *J. Neurosci.* 32, 3366–3375. doi: 10.1523/JNEUROSCI.2523-11.2012

Deco, G., Jirsa, V. K., and McIntosh, A. R. (2013a). Resting brains never rest: computational insights into potential cognitive architectures. *Trends Neurosci.* 36, 268–274. doi: 10.1016/j.tins.2013.03.001

Deco, G., Ponce-Alvarez, A., Mantini, D., Romani, G. L., Hagmann, P., and Corbetta, M. (2013b). Resting-state functional connectivity emerges from structurally and dynamically shaped slow linear fluctuations. *J. Neurosci.* 33, 11239–11252. doi: 10.1523/JNEUROSCI.1091-13.2013

Deco, G., and Kringelbach, M. L. (2014). Great expectations: using whole-brain computational connectomics for understanding neuropsychiatric disorders. *Neuron* 84, 892–905. doi: 10.1016/j.neuron.2014.08.034

Deco, G., Tononi, G., Boly, M., and Kringelbach, M. L. (2015). Rethinking segregation and integration: contributions of whole-brain modelling. *Nat. Rev. Neurosci.* 16. doi: 10.1038/nrn3963

Fernandes, H. M., Van Hartevelt, T. J., Boccard, S. G. J., Owen, S. L. F., Cabral, J., Deco, G., et al. (2015). Novel fingerprinting method characterises the necessary and sufficient structural connectivity from deep brain stimulation electrodes for a successful outcome. *New J. Phys.* 17:015001. doi: 10.1088/1367-2630/17/1/015001

Forstmann, B. U., Keuken, M. C., Jahfari, S., Bazin, P. L., Neumann, J., Schäfer, A., et al. (2012). Cortico-subthalamic white matter tract strength predicts interindividual efficacy in stopping a motor response. *Neuroimage* 60, 370–375. doi: 10.1016/j.neuroimage.2011.12.044

Friston, K. J., Harrison, L., and Penny, W. (2003). Dynamic causal modelling. *Neuroimage* 19, 1273–1302. doi: 10.1016/s1053-8119(03)00202-7

Gradinaru, V., Mogri, M., Thompson, K. R., Henderson, J. M., and Deisseroth, K. (2009). Optical deconstruction of parkinsonian neural circuitry. *Science* 324, 354–359. doi: 10.1126/science.1167093

Jenkinson, M., Bannister, P., Brady, M., and Smith, S. (2002). Improved optimization for the robust and accurate linear registration and motion correction of brain images. *Neuroimage* 17, 825–841. doi: 10.1006/nimg.2002.1132

Kringelbach, M. L., Green, A. L., and Aziz, T. Z. (2011). Balancing the brain: resting state networks and deep brain stimulation. *Front. Integr. Neurosci.* 5:8. doi: 10.3389/fnint.2011.00008

Kringelbach, M. L., Green, A. L., Owen, S. L., Schweder, P. M., and Aziz, T. Z. (2010). Sing the mind electric-principles of deep brain stimulation. *Eur. J. Neurosci.* 32, 1070–1079. doi: 10.1111/j.1460-9568.2010.07419.x

Kringelbach, M. L., Jenkinson, N., Owen, S. L. F., and Aziz, T. Z. (2007). Translational principles of deep brain stimulation. *Nat. Rev. Neurosci.* 8, 623–635. doi: 10.1038/nrn2196

Kringelbach, M. L., Pereira, E. A. C., Green, A. L., Owen, S. L. F., and Aziz, T. Z. (2009). Deep brain stimulation for chronic pain. *J. Pain Manage.* 2, 301–314.

Lozano, A. M., and Lipsman, N. (2013). Probing and regulating dysfunctional circuits using deep brain stimulation. *Neuron* 77, 406–424. doi: 10.1016/j.neuron.2013.01.020

McIntyre, C. C., and Hahn, P. J. (2010). Network perspectives on the mechanisms of deep brain stimulation. *Neurobiol. Dis.* 38, 329–337. doi: 10.1016/j.nbd.2009.09.022

Montgomery, E. B. Jr., and Baker, K. B. (2000). Mechanisms of deep brain stimulation and future technical developments. *Neurol. Res.* 22, 259–266.

Rubinov, M., and Sporns, O. (2010). Complex network measures of brain connectivity: uses and interpretations. *Neuroimage* 52, 1059–1069. doi: 10.1016/j.neuroimage.2009.10.003

Sporns, O. (2011). The human connectome: a complex network. *Ann. N Y Acad. Sci.* 1224, 109–125. doi: 10.1111/j.1749-6632.2010.05888.x

Tononi, G., Sporns, O., and Edelman, G. M. (1994). A measure for brain complexity: relating functional segregation and integration in the nervous system. *Proc. Natl. Acad. Sci. U S A* 91, 5033–5037. doi: 10.1073/pnas.91.11.5033

Tzourio-Mazoyer, N., Landeau, B., Papathanassiou, D., Crivello, F., Etard, O., Delcroix, N., et al. (2002). Automated anatomical labeling of activations in SPM using a macroscopic anatomical parcellation of the MNI MRI single-subject brain. *Neuroimage* 15, 273–289. doi: 10.1006/nimg.2001.0978

van Hartevelt, T. J., Cabral, J., Deco, G., Møller, A., Green, A. L., Aziz, T. Z., et al. (2014). Neural plasticity in human brain connectivity: the effects of long term deep brain stimulation of the subthalamic nucleus in Parkinson's disease. *PLoS One* 9:e86496. doi: 10.1371/journal.pone.0086496

Vitek, J. L. (2002). Mechanisms of deep brain stimulation: excitation or inhibition. *Mov. Disord.* 17, S69–S72. doi: 10.1002/mds.10144

Wong, K. F., and Wang, X. J. (2006). A recurrent network mechanism of time integration in perceptual decisions. *J. Neurosci.* 26, 1314–1328. doi: 10.1523/jneurosci.3733-05.2006

Conflict of Interest Statement: The authors declare that the research was conducted in the absence of any commercial or financial relationships that could be construed as a potential conflict of interest.

8

Decreased Intra- and Inter-Salience Network Functional Connectivity is Related to Trait Anxiety in Adolescents

Edited by:
Morten L. Kringelbach, University of Oxford, UK and Aarhus University, Denmark

***Correspondence:**
Xuebing Li
lixb@psych.ac.cn

***Haiyang Geng*[1,2]*, Xuebing Li*[1*]*, Jie Chen*[1]*, Xinying Li*[1] *and Ruolei Gu*[3]**

[1] Key Laboratory of Mental Health, Institute of Psychology, Chinese Academy of Sciences, Beijing, China, [2] State Key Laboratory of Cognitive Neuroscience and Learning, Beijing Normal University, Beijing, China, [3] Key Laboratory of Behavioral Science, Institute of Psychology, Chinese Academy of Sciences, Beijing, China

Objective: Adolescence is a critical period for the vulnerability of anxiety. Imaging studies focusing on adolescents' susceptibility to anxiety suggest that the different development trajectories between the limbic system and the executive control system may play important roles in this phenomenon. However, few studies have explored the brain basis of this susceptibility from the perspective of functional networks. The salience network (SN) consists of a series of key limbic and prefrontal regions that are engaged in the development of anxiety, such as the amygdala, anterior insula (AI), and dorsal anterior cingulate cortex (dACC). Intra- and inter-network connections in this system play essential roles in bottom-up attention and top-down regulation of anxiety, nevertheless, little is known about whether the SN-centered connections are associated with trait anxiety (i.e., susceptibility to anxiety) in adolescents.

Method: Here, we applied resting-state functional magnetic resonance imaging (fMRI) to explore the relationship between intra- and inter-network functional connectivity (FC) of the SN and trait anxiety in adolescents using the amygdala, AI and dACC as the regions of interest (ROI).

Results: We found that trait anxiety levels were inversely associated with both characteristic AI-dACC FC in the SN and distributed inter-network FC between the SN and multiple functional systems, which included the default mode network and the executive control network.

Conclusions: Our results indicate that weaker intra- and inter-network FC of the SN was linked to higher trait anxiety among adolescents, and it may underlie altered salience processing and cognitive regulation.

Keywords: anxiety, salience network (SN), anterior insula (AI), dorsal anterior cingulate cortex (dACC), resting-state fMRI

INTRODUCTION

The classical neurocognitive model of anxiety proposes that the disruption of the amygdala-prefrontal circuitry in anxiety, which represents deficient recruitment of prefrontal control and amygdala hyper-responsivity to threat, leads to alterations in salience processing, and cognitive control (Bishop, 2007). These mechanisms are implicated in the maintenance and possibly even the etiology of anxiety (Bishop, 2007). Specific to the adolescent stage, adolescents experience persistent negative, and labile mood states (e.g., anxiety; Somerville et al., 2010). Sustained high anxiety during this period can result in increased vulnerability to anxiety-related disorders (Paus et al., 2008). Although adolescents are highly vulnerable to anxiety (Crone and Dahl, 2012), the neurocognitive underpinning of this vulnerability remains poorly understood.

A neurodevelopmental theory examining this susceptibility, which combines the classical model of anxiety and neurodevelopment evidences, suggests that different developmental trajectories of the amygdala and prefrontal cortex may underlie adolescents' heightened responsiveness to threat and immature engagement of cognitive regulation (Somerville et al., 2010). Aside from the amygdala and prefrontal cortex, the anterior insula (AI) and dorsal anterior cingulate cortex (dACC) are also heavily involved in the core mechanisms of anxiety, such as appraising and regulating emotional salience (Craig, 2009; Etkin et al., 2011; Uddin et al., 2011). The activation of these structures plays a crucial role in the threat-related processing bias found in anxious individuals. However, it is unclear whether interactions between these core regions are related to anxiety.

In our opinion, the salience network (SN), which mainly consists of the amygdala, AI and dACC, may be a candidate for examining the neural basis underlying the vulnerability of anxiety in adolescents. Many brain-imaging studies suggest that the SN plays a central role in detecting emotional salience and triggering cognitive control via its functional connectivity with several distributed brain systems, including the limbic system, primary cortices and the cognitive control network (Seeley et al., 2007; Bressler and Menon, 2010). Moreover, these three regions in this network are individually involved in salience processing and cognitive control, and intra-connections in this network may play distinct roles in these two processes. Amygdala-related circuits are more involved in salience processing (Kim et al., 2011; Baur et al., 2013); in contrast, the AI-dACC circuit mainly triggers dorsal lateral prefrontal cortex (dlPFC)-involved cognitive control (Sridharan et al., 2008; Bressler and Menon, 2010). The amygdala is known to react to emotional and novel stimuli via its connectivity with polymodal associative cortices (LeDoux, 1995), which suggests a crucial role in bottom-up salience processing (Santos et al., 2011). The AI is linked to emotional awareness and subjective feelings generated from the body (Craig, 2010). Signals received from polymodal associative cortices can converge with a higher-order interoceptive representation in the amygdala-AI circuit, which was found to represent state anxiety (Baur et al., 2013). Additionally, activation of the dACC was also found in different types of threat appraisal (Etkin et al., 2011). Two resting-state fMRI studies found that the amygdala-AI and the amygdala-dACC circuits were positively related to state anxiety (Kim et al., 2011; Baur et al., 2013). The authors suggested that stronger connections between these regions reflected an increased sensitivity to salient events, which biased attentional and perceptual processing (Kim et al., 2011; Baur et al., 2013).

Conversely, the AI-dACC circuit in the SN may play a major role in cognitive control instead of simple salience processing. Firstly, the AI and dACC showed reliable activation at the beginning and through sustained periods across multiple tasks, which indicated that the system that includes these two regions may select and modulate the goal-related information at hand (Dosenbach et al., 2006). Furthermore, one Granger causality and latency analysis study found that the AI-dACC network showed directed connectivity to the dlPFC and earlier activation compared to the dlPFC across task paradigms and stimulus modalities. This suggested that the AI-dACC network plays a critical and causal role in triggering the executive control network that includes dlPFC (Sridharan et al., 2008). Critically, two important reviews proposed a central role of dACC in dlPFC-involved cognitive control mechanisms triggered by salience (motivation, conflict, and error) evaluation (Botvinick et al., 2001). In an anxiety-related context, Bishop (2009) proposed that the weaker cognitive control that is indicated by dlPFC activation is a core feature of trait anxiety. Although the activation of the dACC was not found to be involved in Bishop's study, the author suggests that the connection between the dACC and the dlPFC probability plays a role in triggering cognitive control of anxiety (Bishop, 2009). Taken together, the AI-dACC circuit is proposed to be strongly involved in dlPFC-related cognitive control triggered by salience evaluation (Mathews and MacLeod, 1994; Desimone and Duncan, 1995; Mathews and Mackintosh, 1998; Bressler and Menon, 2010), which may be impaired in individuals with anxiety. However, no study has examined the relationship between anxiety and the AI-dACC circuit.

The current study focuses on linking trait anxiety at the individual level with the SN. Trait anxiety is often used as an index of vulnerability to anxiety disorders (Kim and Whalen, 2009; Indovina et al., 2011). Theoretical models and empirical evidence suggest that high trait anxiety and anxiety disorders share common altered activations and connections of SN-related regions (Etkin and Wager, 2007; Sylvester et al., 2012), which are involved in fear, conflict salience, and cognitive control. Therefore, we suggest that trait anxiety be regarded as a candidate to investigate SN-centered networks that underlies the vulnerability to anxiety disorders without the confounding effects of psychotropic medication or chronic illness.

In this experiment, we collected the resting-state imaging data and used the basolateral amygdala (BLA), AI and dACC as regions of interest (ROI) to examine the relationship between the intra-network functional connectivity (FC) of the SN and individual levels of trait anxiety in 60 adolescents. The trait anxiety levels were measured using the trait anxiety scale of Spielberger's State and Trait Anxiety Inventory (STAI-T; Spielberger et al., 1983; Shek, 1993). Voxel-wise resting-state functional connectivity (rsFC) analysis using the same ROIs was employed to detect whether the inter-network FC of the SN with other regions in the whole brain is related to trait anxiety in adolescents. Most importantly, considering the AI-dACC circuit is involved in cognitive control triggered by salience evaluation, we hypothesized that higher levels of trait anxiety in adolescents would be associated with weaker AI-dACC FC, which would indicate impaired cognitive control in trait anxiety. Moreover, considering the amygdala-AI and amygdala-dACC circuits may underlie salience and vigilance in a particular situation, we hypothesized that the FC of these connections would be positively associated with state anxiety compared to trait anxiety. Finally, the SN may have altered inter-network FC with distributed brain regions engaged in emotional processing and cognitive control.

METHODS

Emotional Measurements

Sixty-three healthy participants (Mean ± SD: 15.67 ± 1.00 years, 35 Male/28 Female) were recruited from the local community via media advertisements. They had no history of substance abuse, brain injury, or neurological diseases and no personal or family history of mental disorders, which were measured by an in-house questionnaire. Non-clinical samples were of interest for the questions in the current study because the neural underpinnings of non-psychiatric individuals with trait anxiety may predict those individuals' risk of psychopathology, and they are less likely to be confounded with a disease state. All participants (right-hand) completed the Chinese version of the trait form of Spielberger's State and Trait Anxiety Inventory (STAI-T; Spielberger et al., 1983; Shek, 1993). The STAI-T has been used in multiple studies that investigated anxious characteristics in non-clinical samples, largely due to its sensitivity as a marker of one's risk for anxiety disorders (Grupe and Nitschke, 2013). Many studies suggest that the STAI state scale is highly related to the trait scale and so it is not good enough to dissociate from the trait scale (Spielberger et al., 1983; Shek, 1993); therefore, the Negative Affect subschedule (NAS) of the Positive and Negative Affect Schedule (PANAS) was used to estimate the emotional states of participants before scanning (Watson and Clark, 1999). To control for the effect of depression during analysis, the Children's Depression Inventory (CDI) was used to assess self-reported symptoms of depression (Kovacs, 1985). One participant was excluded because his STAI-T score (25) was lower than the mean value of the sample (M ± SD: 39.63 ± 6.12) minus two standard deviations. This study has been approved by the Ethics Committee of the Institute of Psychology, Chinese Academy of Sciences, and has therefore been performed in accordance with the ethical standards laid down in the 1964 Declaration of Helsinki.

MRI Data Acquisition and Preprocessing

Experiments were performed in a 3 Tesla SIEMENS MRI scanner (Beijing, China). Functional images were acquired with single-shot gradient-recalled echo planar imaging (GR-EPI) sequences (TR = 2000 ms, TE = 30 ms, FA = 90°, matrix = 64 × 64, FOV = 22 cm, 3-mm slice thickness, 1 mm spacing between slices, 32 transverse slices), aligned along the anterior commissure-posterior commissure (AC-PC) line, and they lasted for 450 s. Subjects were instructed to keep their eyes closed and think of nothing, but to not fall asleep. For spatial normalization, T1-weighted anatomical images were acquired in an axial orientation using a 3D gradient-recalled sequence (TR = 2530 ms, TE = 3.37 ms, FA = 7°, matrix = 256 × 192, 1.33-mm slice thickness) for each subject.

Data preprocessing was performed using DPARSF software (Yan and Zang, 2010, http://www.restfmri.net). The first 10 volumes were discarded to guarantee steady-state longitudinal magnetization. The remaining volumes were then realigned to correct for head motion. Two subjects were excluded because their head movement exceeded ± 3 mm in translation or ± 3° in rotation. Subsequently, realigned volumes were corrected for slice acquisition timing, and then were normalized into a standard stereotaxic space with a resolution of 3 × 3 × 3 mm^3 using the Montreal Neurological Institute (MNI) echo-planar imaging template in Statistical Parametric Mapping 8 (SPM8; Wellcome Trust Centre for Neuroimaging), which is a free and open source software written in MATLAB (The MathWorks, Inc.). Functional images were spatially smoothed by convolution with an isotropic Gaussian kernel (FWHM = 4 mm). Linear detrend and filtering (0.01–0.08 Hz) were applied. Nuisance signals involving six head motion parameters, cerebrospinal fluid signals, and white matter signals were regressed out.

Functional ROI Definition

Left and right BLA ROIs in the current study were obtained as the result masks from a previous study in the Montreal Neurological Institute (MNI) space (Baur et al., 2013). The authors used maximum probability maps (the threshold is 40%), which allow for the construction of non-overlapping ROIs where each voxel of the amygdala was assigned to one specific subregion on the basis of the maximum probability of belonging to a subgroup (SPM8; Wellcome Trust Centre for Neuroimaging). Furthermore, two AI ROIs (left AI, right AI) were also obtained from Baur's study (2013). Baur et al. (2013) performed a seed-based rsFC approach to map functionally defined AI based on previous finding that the AI and posterior insula (PI) were respectively connected to the dACC and secondary somatosensory cortex (Cauda et al., 2011). Additionally, we created 6-mm-radius spherical dACC ROIs centered on the respective coordinates (MNI; 5, 26, 31 for right dACC; −5, 26, 31 for left dACC) from the study of Baur et al. (2013) with DPARSF software.

Association Between Anxiety and ROI-Wise Functional Connectivity and Second Level Analysis of the Functional Connectivity

To exclude the effects arising from micro-motion, the "scrubbing" procedure described by Power et al. (2012) was used. The framewise displacement (FD) of head position was calculated as the sum of the absolute values of the six translational and rotational realignment parameters. In the current study, FDs were first computed on a frame-by-frame basis for each participant. Frames with FDs larger than 0.5 were removed from subsequent intrinsic functional connectivity analysis. After this "scrubbing" procedure, an average of 90.9% (7.6% standard deviation) of the frames remained. In other words, only about 9.1% of the data were removed from the statistical analysis. With DPARSF, for each BLA, AI, and dACC subregion ROI, mean time courses were extracted from the data after being scrubbed using the before-described procedure and cross-correlated. Next, correlations were r-to-z transformed for group-level statistics. Firstly, we examined whether the connections (z-value) between six nodes in the SN exist by using one sample T-test. Secondly, we used Pearson correlations to investigate whether the rsFC magnitudes between BLA, AI and dACC (z-value) were correlated with trait anxiety. All p-values were two-tailed. Correlations were evaluated with IBM SPSS16 (IBM, Armonk, New York). Moreover, to examine whether intra-salience network FC are influenced by the participants' emotional states before scanning, we found the Pearson correlation between the NAS and the same rsFC in the SN.

Voxel-Wise Functional Connectivity Analyses and Associations with Anxiety

We used the same ROIs from the ROI-wise analysis when we extracted time courses to make the voxel-wise functional connectivity analysis. Furthermore, the correlations between the trait anxiety score and the whole brain functional connectivity were calculated with the REST toolbox (Song et al., 2011). Finally, we achieved six related whole brain maps by setting the threshold at a significance level of $p < 0.05$ and correcting for multiple comparisons using the AlphaSim correction in REST. Briefly, the statistical threshold was set at $p < 0.005$ and the cluster size was set at $>324\ mm^3$, which corresponded to a corrected $p < 0.05$. This correction was confined within whole-brain mask (size: $1912437\ mm^3$) and was determined by Monte Carlo simulations (Ledberg et al., 1998) using the AFNI AlphaSim program (http://afni.nimh.nih.gov/pub/dist/doc/program_help/AlphaSim.html). Depression score was entered into the analysis as a covariable, and partial correction results were achieved (AlphaSim corrected $p < 0.05$).

RESULTS

Emotional Measurements

Emotional measurements of the remaining 60 participants (15.68 ± 1.00 years, 35 Male/25 Female, 15.65 ± 1.01 years for female, 15.73 ± 1.00 years for male) were acquired see **Table 1** for TAI and CDI scores in the sample.

TABLE 1 | Demographics and emotional measurements.

	M ± SD ($N = 60$)
Gender(n: male/female)	35M/25F
Age(years)	15.68 ± 1.00
TAI	39.63 ± 6.12
CDI	11.13 ± 2.65
NAS	19.98 ± 5.01

Correlations Between Intra-Network Functional Connectivity of the SN and Anxiety Level

We firstly examined the 12 functional connections between the six nodes in the SN. The finding showed that all 12 connections were significantly more than zero (shown in Supplementary Table 1 in the Supplemental Material). Furthermore, we tested the correlation between BLA, AI, and dACC rsFC (left/right sides) and trait anxiety in the whole sample. Significant negative correlations were observed between the left AI-right dACC, right AI-right dACC FC and trait anxiety (uncorrected:$r = -0.336$, $p = 0.009$; $r = -0.337$, $p = 0.008$; **Figure 1**). In addition, depression and trait anxiety were significantly correlated ($r = 0.525$, $p < 0.001$); after controlling for depression, the left AI-right dACC and right AI-right dACC FC correlations with anxiety were marginally significant ($r = -0.219$, $p = 0.095$; $r = -0.224$, $p = 0.087$). Furthermore, no correlation was observed between the AI-BLA or dACC-BLA functional connections and anxiety or depression. Additionally, the NAS score was correlated with trait anxiety ($r = 0.333$, $p = 0.009$), and no correlation between the FC in the SN and the NAS was found (**Table 2**).

Correlations Between Inter-Network Functional Connectivity of the SN and Anxiety Level

The voxel-wise FC analysis showed that higher levels of trait anxiety in adolescents were related to weaker functional connectivity of the SN with a number of brain systems outside this network (**Figure 2**, **Table 3**, Supplementary Figures 1–6 in the Supplemental Material). The regions involved included the following: (1) the left and right precuneus, which are part of the DMN, (2) the superior temporal gyrus, superior occipital gyrus and fusiform in the sensory and perceptual processing system, (3) the limbic (parahippocampal gyrus) and cerebellum system, including the pons and declive, and (4) the emotional and cognitive regulation regions, including the inferior frontal gyrus and the superior frontal gyrus. There was no region that showed a larger connectivity with the SN. When depression was entered in the analysis of the whole brain functional connectivity, control analyses revealed that the findings above remained seldom changed in the whole brain (**Table 4**).

DISCUSSION

By linking the intra- and inter-salience network functional connectivity to trait anxiety in adolescents, we found that the intra-network FC of the SN, particularly the AI-dACC circuit, was associated with trait anxiety in adolescents. This pathway has been suggested to play a critical role in cognitive control according to previous studies (Sridharan et al., 2008; Uddin et al., 2011). Furthermore, we found that the distributed inter-network FC between the SN and multiple brain systems (including DMN and CEN) were also related to a vulnerability to anxiety in adolescents. In short, the current study provides direct evidence of resting-state functional connectivity and how it aids in the understanding of the relationship between intra-

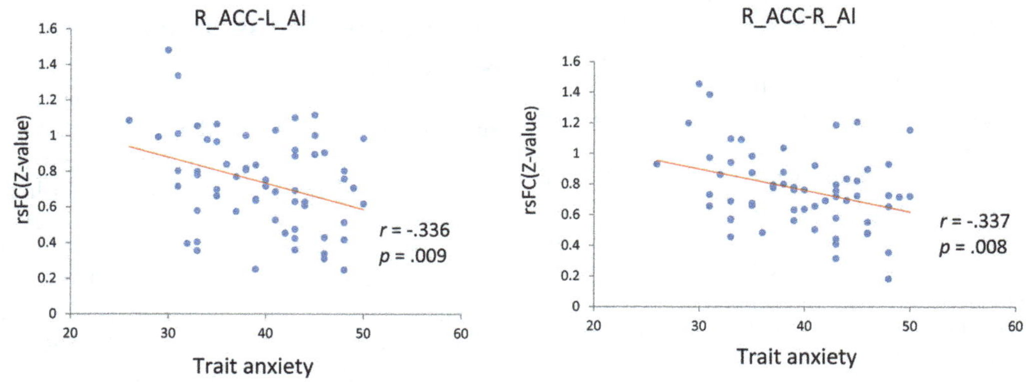

FIGURE 1 | Correlations of AI-dACC resting-state functional connectivity with trait anxiety. L, Left; R, Right; ACC, anterior cingulate cortex; AI, anterior insula; rsFC, resting-state functional connectivity.

TABLE 2 | Correlations of intra-salience network FC with NAS.

Resting-state connectivity	NAS	
	r	*p*
left AI-left BLA	−0.031	0.811
left AI–right BLA	−0.096	0.463
left AI–left dACC	−0.108	0.409
left AI–right dACC	−0.138	0.291
right AI–left BLA	−0.069	0.599
right AI–right BLA	−0.081	0.541
right AI–left dACC	−0.088	0.502
right AI–right dACC	−0.072	0.583
left BLA–left dACC	0.062	0.634
left BLA–right dACC	0.003	0.981
righ BLA–left dACC	−0.014	0.913
right BLA–right dACC	−0.034	0.793

and inter-network connections of the SN and trait components of vulnerability to anxiety in adolescents.

We found that decreased AI-dACC FC in the SN was associated with higher anxiety in adolescents, which may indicate the altered cognitive control function of the SN in anxiety. This issue has been highlighted by other studies in adults (Menon and Uddin, 2010). Previous studies have revealed that there are functional and structural connections between the two regions (Critchley et al., 2004), which provide a rapid relay of information between the distributed brain systems (Allman et al., 2010). Menon (2011) suggest that this feature of this circuit is fundamental for detecting salience signals and triggering executive control, both of which play central roles in the pathology of anxiety. Our finding extends previous knowledge and indicates that the AI-dACC FC also contributes to trait anxiety in adolescents. Specifically, we found that the connectivity of this neural circuit was negatively correlated with anxiety characteristics. Our result provides initial and direct evidence for understanding the relationship between this pathway in the SN and the anxiety disposition in adolescents. A previous resting-state and structural fMRI study indicated that weaker connections in SN might underlie less flexible cognitive control during childhood compared to adulthood (Uddin et al., 2011). In the present study, the decreased AI-dACC FC in anxious adolescents may be associated with weaker cognitive control, which is consistent with an anxiety theory that suggests that trait anxiety includes an impoverished recruitment of prefrontal attentional mechanisms to trigger the allocation of attentional resource (Bishop, 2009). This model is supported by the discovery that weaker AI-ACC connections in adults were associated with general social anxiety disorder, which indicates problems in attention control and emotion regulation (Klumpp et al., 2012). It is also in line with another study that reported a weaker correlation between the ventromedial prefrontal cortex (including Brodmann 32, dACC) and the bilateral insula, which represents a weaker control function in anxiety-prone adults (Stein et al., 2007). Our finding about the association between the AI-dACC circuit and trait anxiety in adolescents encourages further research into the roles of the SN in the cognitive control involved in the pathology of anxiety.

In the current study, both the BLA-AI and BLA-dACC FC were found in adolescents, but neither the BLA-AI nor the BLA-dACC circuit showed any association with trait anxiety or state emotional level when measured by the NAS in adolescents. However, two recent resting-state fMRI studies in adults found that these two circuits were positively correlated with state anxiety (Kim et al., 2011; Baur et al., 2013). In those studies, the BLA-AI and BLA-AI FC were suggested to underlie the temporal anxiety state. This type of state anxiety reflects a larger sensitivity to salient events, which may be related to the MRI environment considering an MRI scanner can function as a stressor. Conversely, anxiety proneness as a trait, which the current study focuses on, may rely more on the ability to recruit the prefrontal cortex, which is strongly associated with the AI-dACC circuit rather than the BLA-related circuits. In addition, unexpectedly, a correlation between the BLA-AI or the BLA-dACC and the NAS was not found, possibly because the NAS was not sensitive enough to the anxiety state in specific situations,

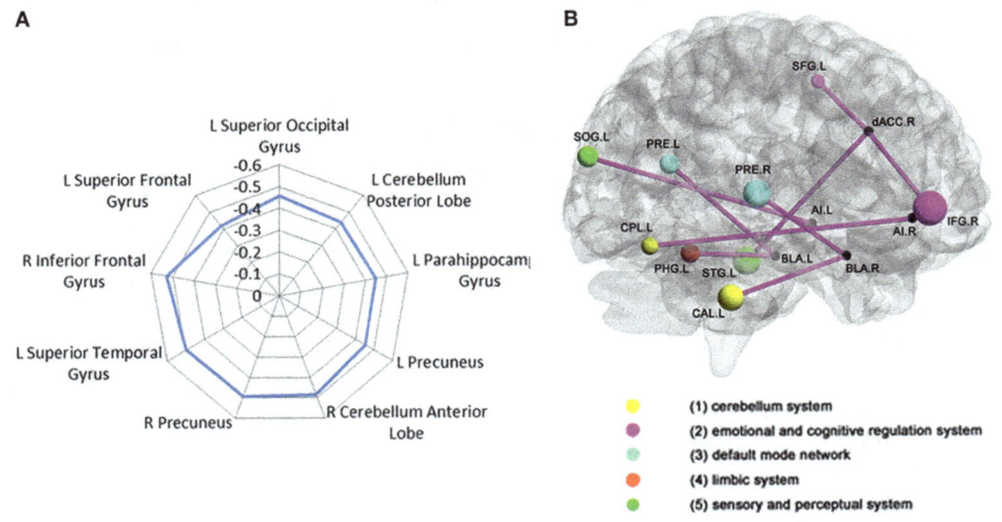

FIGURE 2 | Correlation between adolescent anxiety and inter-SN functional connectivity. (A) Radar plot showing the correlation between anxiety and inter-salience network connectivity with multiple regions broadly classified into five functional brain systems: (1) cerebellum system (2) emotional and cognitive regulation system (3) DMN (4) limbic system (5) sensory and perceptual system. **(B)** Brain regions (represented by different color-coded nodes) that showed a significant correlation between anxiety and inter-salience network functional connectivity. CAL, CerebellumAnteriorLobe; CPL, CerebellumPosteriorLobe; IFG, InferiorFrontalGyrust; SFG, SuperiorFrontalGyrus; PRE, precuneuns; PHPG, parahippocampalgyrus; IOG, InferiorOccipitalGyrus; STG, SuperiorTemporalGyrus; L, left; R, right.

so it could not capture the immediate stressful feeling of an MRI environment. In future studies, we suggest that biological measurements (such as skin conductance response) be used to illustrate the relationship between state anxiety levels and BLA-related connections.

Aside from intra-network connectivity, we also found that decreased connectivity between the key nodes in the SN and the distributed brain areas was associated with higher trait anxiety. These regions can be grouped into several functional systems, which are involved in salience processing and cognitive control (Uddin et al., 2011), as follows: (1) the sensory and perceptual processing network including the fusiform, occipital lobe, and temporal lobe; (2) the DMN including the left and right precuneus; (3) the cerebellum system and limbic system including the parahippocampal gyrus; (4) the emotional and cognitive control system including the inferior frontal gyrus and superior frontal gyrus. Studies in healthy adults with high anxiety and patients who suffered from anxiety disorders have found an abnormality in the connectivity between key nodes in the SN and these systems (Etkin et al., 2009; Liao et al., 2010a,b; Kim et al., 2011). Below, we discuss the potential relationships between these systems and trait anxiety in a point-by-point manner.

First, the functional connectivity between the SN and sensory and perceptual networks decreased as a function of trait anxiety, which is consistent with the resting-state study that found that the adult patients with social anxiety disorder showed weaker FC in somato-motor and visual networks. The weaker connection may be explained by the vigilance and alertness involved in anxiety (Liao et al., 2010a).

Additionally, the SN, particularly the AI, plays a pivot role in switching between the CEN and DMN across task paradigms and stimulus modalities (Menon and Uddin, 2010). Our result is in line with the resting-state study, which found a correlation between insula-DMN FC and self-report anxiety in youths (Dennis et al., 2011). Seeing that the DMN underlies the representation of negative and self-referential information in anxiety and depression (Dennis et al., 2011), the connection between the SN and DMN may help allocate cognitive sources to self-related information processing during the task state, which is highly involved in anxiety (Menon and Uddin, 2010).

The parahippocampal gyrus within the limbic system plays an important role in the encoding and recognition of environmental scenes and faces (Aguirre et al., 1998). The SN-parahippocampal gyrus connection may be related to attentiveness to face and environmental stimuli, but this requires verification from future studies. Additionally, weaker functional connections between the SN and the cerebellum were found in highly anxious adolescents. This result is in line with a previous resting-state study, which found weaker FC in adolescents with GAD compared with the healthy controls (Roy et al., 2013). The SN and cerebellum are involved in detecting errors and conflicts to adjust future performance (Dosenbach et al., 2006; Buckner, 2013). Given that errors and conflicts are both perceived as threats along the dimension of biological salience (Etkin et al., 2011), we suggest that the SN-cerebellum FC may be associated with bottom–up salience detection of errors and conflicts. Briefly, adolescents experience huge changes in social context when salient stimuli and events are involved (Crone and Dahl, 2012). Our results, combined with previous resting-state fMRI studies of

TABLE 3 | Results of correlation of two sides of BLA, AI, and dACC voxel-wise functional connectivity with trait anxiety.

Region of interest	Region	Cluster size (# voxels)	Maximum intensity voxel coordinates			*r*-value
LEFT BLA						
	L Middle Temporal Gyrus	13	−51	−15	−18	−0.561
	L Parahippocampa Gyrus	13	−36	−33	−18	−0.479
	L Precuneus	64	−12	−60	18	−0.468
RIGHT BLA						
	R Cerebellum Anterior Lobe	69	18	−51	−36	−0.479
	L Cerebellum Posterior Lobe	17	−21	−78	−30	−0.425
	R Precuneus	32	15	−36	6	−0.446
LEFT AI						
	L Cerebellum Posterior Lobe	27	−24	−84	−33	−0.444
	R Cerebellum Posterior Lobe	13	27	−81	−33	−0.454
	L Fusiform	29	−36	−57	−21	−0.488
	R Cerebellum Anterior Lobe	17	6	−66	−12	−0.437
	L Occipital Lobe	15	−30	−75	−6	−0.476
	R Inferior Frontal Gyrus	12	57	30	9	−0.426
	L Superior Occipital Gyrus	16	−18	−96	21	−0.453
	R Cingulate Gyrus	17	15	−15	39	−0.495
	R Middle Frontal Gyrus	33	36	−3	48	−0.486
	R Parietal Lobe	13	51	−18	60	−0.444
RIGHT AI						
	L Cerebellum Posterior Lobe	22	−9	−72	−15	−0.478
	R Anterior Cingulate	25	12	27	27	−0.458
	R Cingulate Gyrus	16	15	6	39	−0.510
Left dACC						
	R Cingulate Gyrus	12	12	9	36	−0.458
	L Frontal Lobe	15	−18	−21	36	−0.426
	R Postcentral Gyrus	13	54	−18	57	−0.436
RIGHT DACC						
	L Superior Temporal Gyrus	31	−48	3	−21	−0.471
	R Insula	14	33	9	0	−0.431
	R Inferior Frontal Gyrus	70	51	24	0	−0.536
	R Cingulate Gyrus	29	15	12	33	−0.499
	L Superior Temporal Gyrus	14	−42	−27	6	−0.470
	L Superior Frontal Gyrus	13	−6	9	51	−0.449

anxious individuals, suggest that multiple SN-related functional connections may be involved in salience processing in this particular period.

Finally, decreased functional connections between the SN and both the superior frontal gyrus and the inferior frontal gyrus were observed. Our results may be implied by the resting-state study of adults with a panic disorder, which found weaker FC between the dACC and both the bilateral frontal pole and the right superior parietal lobule (Pannekoek et al., 2013). Those connections have been postulated to have core roles in salience signal transmission to the CEN for cognitive control (Sylvester et al., 2012). The negative correlation between those functional connections and trait anxiety may be related to the weak cognitive control in anxiety, which is supported by the following studies. As Campbell-Sills et al. (2011) suggested, emotionally salient stimuli are more difficult for anxious individuals to engage effective emotional control. Furthermore, Bishop (2007) argued that the ability to recruit the prefrontal control mechanisms should be seen as the key locus of anxiety-related individual differences. Crone and Dahl (2012) suggest that the degree to which cognitive control is engaged in adolescence is strongly influenced by the motivational salience of the context. These arguments are highly consistent with the model that proposes that the SN-centered connection profile detects salience and triggers cognitive control, which plays a key role in anxiety (Menon and Uddin, 2010). The convergence of the current results and previous models suggests that the attenuated inter-network connectivity of the SN is associated with a vulnerability to anxiety in adolescents, which may underlie the salience-related engagement of cognitive control.

TABLE 4 | Voxel-wise functional connectivity in the whole brain correlation with anxiety controlling cdi as covariable.

Region of interest	Region	Cluster size (# voxels)	Maximum intensity voxel coordinates			*r*-value
LEFT BLA	**None**					
RIGHT BLA						
	L Cerebellum Posterior Lobe	13	−24	−78	−30	−0.457
	R Thalamus	13	21	−15	15	−0.465
LEFT AI						
	L Cerebellum Posterior Lobe	25	−24	−81	−30	−0.486
	L Medial Frontal Gyrus	13	−3	51	0	−0.432
	L L Superior Occipital Gyrus	13	−21	−93	24	−0.414
	L Superior Frontal Gyrus	12	−12	54	36	−0.401
	L Middle Frontal Gyrus	13	−42	−3	45	−0.422
	R Middle Frontal Gyrus	12	36	0	45	−0.446
RIGHT AI						
	L Medial Frontal Gyrus	14	−9	51	3	−0.409
LEFT dACC						
	R Cingulate Gyrus	18	15	15	33	−0.531
RIGHT dACC						
	R Inferior Frontal Gyrus	15	51	24	0	−0.475
	R Cingulate Gyrus	13	15	15	30	−0.461
	L Superior Frontal Gyrus	16	−15	57	33	−0.466

MNI, Montreal Neurologic Institute, coordinates of most significant voxels in cluster; L, left; R, right.

Adolescents experience rapid cognitive and emotional changes compared to adults (Crone and Dahl, 2012). The interaction between the environment and the development of the brain may lead to dysfunctions of emotional processing and cognitive control (Paus et al., 2008). Our study makes an important first step in depicting the association between SN-centered brain networks and trait anxiety in adolescents, and it provides some reasonable explanations for the association, which need to be verified by future studies that illustrate the neurocognitive mechanisms underlying these links. Furthermore, longitudinal studies would be necessary to examine the causal correlation between trait anxiety and brain network development.

A few limitations of the current study should be addressed. First, the NAS scale was used to assess the participants' instant emotional states, which was different from other studies that used self-report or the STAI state anxiety scale. Thus, we could not determine the roles of the amygdala-AI and amygdala-dACC rsFC in state anxiety, which have been reported in other resting-state studies (Kim et al., 2011; Baur et al., 2013). Second, although trait anxiety is often used as an index for vulnerability to an anxiety disorder, and high trait anxiety shares common psychological and neural factors with all anxiety disorders, it would be better to directly choose clinical individuals to investigate the role of the SN on the pathology of anxiety disorders. Thirdly, this study only used resting-state MRI data, and it remains unclear whether the SN would also show abnormal intra- and inter-SN connectivity when highly anxious individuals were participating in cognitive tasks that involved salience processing and cognitive control. Thus, our interpretation of the current findings is only supposed and needs future studies to be clarified.

CONCLUSION

In the present study, we found the association between trait anxiety in adolescents and characteristic intra-SN (AI-dACC circuit) and distributed inter-SN connections, which are considered to play important roles in salience processing and cognitive control. Our preliminary findings provide implications for and encourage further understanding of the neural network profile involved in the engagement of cognitive control modulated by emotional salience, which has been proposed as the core mechanism underlying anxiety in adolescents.

ACKNOWLEDGMENTS

This research was supported by National Nature Science Foundation of China [NSFC 31530031, 30900441, 31300841]; Key Laboratory of Mental Health, Institute of Psychology, Chinese Academy of Sciences; Open Research Fund of the State Key Laboratory of Cognitive Neuroscience and Learning.

SUPPLEMENTARY MATERIAL

The Supplementary Material for this article can be found online at: http://journal.frontiersin.org/article/10.3389/fnbeh.2015.00350

REFERENCES

Aguirre, G. K., Zarahn, E., and D'Esposito, M. (1998). An area within human ventral cortex sensitive to "building" stimuli: evidence and implications. *Neuron* 21, 373–383.

Allman, J. M., Tetreault, N. A., Hakeem, A. Y., Manaye, K. F., Semendeferi, K., Erwin, J. M., et al. (2010). The von Economo neurons in frontoinsular and anterior cingulate cortex in great apes and humans. *Brain Struct. Funct.* 214, 495–517. doi: 10.1007/s00429-010-0254-0

Baur, V., Hanggi, J., Langer, N., and Jancke, L. (2013). Resting-state functional and structural connectivity within an insula-amygdala route specifically index state and trait anxiety. *Biol. Psychiatry* 73, 85–92. doi: 10.1016/j.biopsych.2012.06.003

Bishop, S. J. (2007). Neurocognitive mechanisms of anxiety: an integrative account. *Trends Cogn. Sci.* 11, 307–316. doi: 10.1016/j.tics.2007.05.008

Bishop, S. J. (2009). Trait anxiety and impoverished prefrontal control of attention. *Nat. Neurosci.* 12, 92–98. doi: 10.1038/nn.2242

Botvinick, M. M., Braver, T. S., Barch, D. M., Carter, C. S., and Cohen, J. D. (2001). Conflict monitoring and cognitive control. *Psychol. Rev.* 108, 624–652. doi: 10.1037/0033-295X.108.3.624

Bressler, S. L., and Menon, V. (2010). Large-scale brain networks in cognition: emerging methods and principles. *Trends Cogn. Sci.* 14, 277–290. doi: 10.1016/j.tics.2010.04.004

Buckner, R. L. (2013). The cerebellum and cognitive function: 25 years of insight from anatomy and neuroimaging. *Neuron* 80, 807–815. doi: 10.1016/j.neuron.2013.10.044

Campbell-Sills, L., Simmons, A. N., Lovero, K. L., Rochlin, A. A., Paulus, M. P., and Stein, M. B. (2011). Functioning of neural systems supporting emotion regulation in anxiety-prone individuals. *Neuroimage* 54, 689–696. doi: 10.1016/j.neuroimage.2010.07.041

Cauda, F., D'Agata, F., Sacco, K., Duca, S., Geminiani, G., and Vercelli, A. (2011). Functional connectivity of the insula in the resting brain. *Neuroimage* 55, 8–23. doi: 10.1016/j.neuroimage.2010.11.049

Craig, A. D., (Bud). (2009). How do you feel—now? The anterior insula and human awareness. *Nat. Rev. Neurosci.* 10, 59–70. doi: 10.1038/nrn2555

Craig, A. D., (Bud). (2010). The sentient self. *Brain Struct. Funct.* 214, 563–577.

Critchley, H. D., Wiens, S., Rotshtein, P., Öhman, A., and Dolan, R. J. (2004). Neural systems supporting interoceptive awareness. *Nat. Neurosci.* 7, 189–195. doi: 10.1038/nn1176

Crone, E. A., and Dahl, R. E. (2012). Understanding adolescence as a period of social-affective engagement and goal flexibility. *Nat. Rev. Neurosci.* 13, 636–650. doi: 10.1038/nrn3313

Dennis, E. L., Gotlib, I. H., Thompson, P. M., and Thomason, M. E. (2011). Anxiety modulates insula recruitment in resting-state functional magnetic resonance imaging in youth and adults. *Brain Connect.* 1, 245–254. doi: 10.1089/brain.2011.0030

Desimone, R., and Duncan, J. (1995). Neural mechanisms of selective visual attention. *Ann. Rev. Neurosci.* 18, 193–222. doi: 10.1146/annurev.ne.18.030195.001205

Dosenbach, N. U., Visscher, K. M., Palmer, E. D., Miezin, F. M., Wenger, K. K., Kang, H. C., et al. (2006). A core system for the implementation of task sets. *Neuron* 50, 799–812. doi: 10.1016/j.neuron.2006.04.031

Etkin, A., Egner, T., and Kalisch, R. (2011). Emotional processing in anterior cingulate and medial prefrontal cortex. *Trends Cogn. Sci.* 15, 85–93. doi: 10.1016/j.tics.2010.11.004

Etkin, A., Prater, K. E., Schatzberg, A. F., Menon, V., and Greicius, M. D. (2009). Disrupted amygdalar subregion functional connectivity and evidence of a compensatory network in generalized anxiety disorder. *Arch. Gen. Psychiatry* 66, 1361–1372. doi: 10.1001/archgenpsychiatry.2009.104

Etkin, A., and Wager, T. D. (2007). Functional neuroimaging of anxiety: a meta-analysis of emotional processing in PTSD, social anxiety disorder, and specific phobia. *Am. J. Psychiatry* 164, 1476–1488. doi: 10.1176/appi.ajp.2007.07030504

Grupe, D. W., and Nitschke, J. B. (2013). Uncertainty and anticipation in anxiety: an integrated neurobiological and psychological perspective. *Nat. Rev. Neurosci.* 14, 488–501. doi: 10.1038/nrn3524

Indovina, I., Robbins, T. W., Núñez-Elizalde, A. O., Dunn, B. D., and Bishop, S. J. (2011). Fear-conditioning mechanisms associated with trait vulnerability to anxiety in humans. *Neuron* 69, 563–571. doi: 10.1016/j.neuron.2010.12.034

Kim, M. J., Gee, D. G., Loucks, R. A., Davis, F. C., and Whalen, P. J. (2011). Anxiety dissociates dorsal and ventral medial prefrontal cortex functional connectivity with the amygdala at rest. *Cereb. Cortex* 21, 1667–1673. doi: 10.1093/cercor/bhq237

Kim, M. J., and Whalen, P. J. (2009). The structural integrity of an amygdala–prefrontal pathway predicts trait anxiety. *J. Neurosci.* 29, 11614–11618. doi: 10.1523/JNEUROSCI.2335-09.2009

Klumpp, H., Angstadt, M., and Phan, K. L. (2012). Insula reactivity and connectivity to anterior cingulate cortex when processing threat in generalized social anxiety disorder. *Biol. Psychol.* 89, 273–276. doi: 10.1016/j.biopsycho.2011.10.010

Kovacs, M. (1985). The Children's Depression Inventory (CDI). *Psychopharmacol. Bull.* 21, 995–998

Ledberg, A., Åkerman, S., and Roland, P. E. (1998). Estimation of the probabilities of 3D clusters in functional brain images. *Neuroimage* 8, 113–128.

LeDoux, J. E. (1995). Emotion: clues from the brain. *Annu. Rev. Psychol.* 46, 209–235.

Liao, W., Chen, H., Feng, Y., Mantini, D., Gentili, C., Pan, Z., et al. (2010a). Selective aberrant functional connectivity of resting state networks in social anxiety disorder. *Neuroimage* 52, 1549–1558. doi: 10.1016/j.neuroimage.2010.05.010

Liao, W., Qiu, C., Gentili, C., Walter, M., Pan, Z., Ding, J., et al. (2010b). Altered effective connectivity network of the amygdala in social anxiety disorder: a resting-state fMRI study. *PLoS ONE* 5:e15238. doi: 10.1371/journal.pone.0015238

Mathews, A., and Mackintosh, B. (1998). A cognitive model of selective processing in anxiety. *Cogn. Ther. Res.* 22, 539–560. doi: 10.1023/A:1018738019346

Mathews, A., and MacLeod, C. (1994). Cognitive approaches to emotion and emotional disorders. *Ann. Rev. Psychol.* 45, 25–50. doi: 10.1146/annurev.ps.45.020194.000325

Menon, V., and Uddin, L. Q. (2010). Saliency, switching, attention and control: a network model of insula function. *Brain Struct. Funct.* 214, 655–667. doi: 10.1007/s00429-010-0262-0

Menon, V. (2011). Large-scale brain networks and psychopathology: a unifying triple network model. *Trends Cogn. Sci.* 15, 483–506. doi: 10.1016/j.tics.2011.08.003

Pannekoek, J. N., Veer, I. M., van Tol, M.-J., van der Werff, S. J. A., Demenescu, L. R., Aleman, A., et al. (2013). Aberrant limbic and salience network resting-state functional connectivity in panic disorder without comorbidity. *J. Affect. Disord.* 145, 29–35. doi: 10.1016/j.jad.2012.07.006

Paus, T., Keshavan, M., and Giedd, J. N. (2008). Why do many psychiatric disorders emerge during adolescence? *Nat. Rev. Neurosci.* 9, 947–957. doi: 10.1038/nrn2513

Power, J. D., Barnes, K. A., Snyder, A. Z., Schlaggar, B. L., and Petersen, S. E. (2012). Spurious but systematic correlations in functional connectivity MRI networks arise from subject motion. *Neuroimage* 59, 2142–2154. doi: 10.1016/j.neuroimage.2011.10.018

Roy, A. K., Fudge, J. L., Kelly, C., Perry, J. S. A., Daniele, T., Carlisi, C., et al. (2013). Intrinsic functional connectivity of amygdala-based networks in adolescent generalized anxiety disorder. *J. Am. Acad. Child Adolesc. Psychiatry* 52, 290–299. doi: 10.1016/j.jaac.2012.12.010

Santos, A., Mier, D., Kirsch, P., and Meyer-Lindenberg, A. (2011). Evidence for a general face salience signal in human amygdala. *Neuroimage* 54, 3111–3116. doi: 10.1016/j.neuroimage.2010.11.024

Seeley, W. W., Menon, V., Schatzberg, A. F., Keller, J., Glover, G. H., Kenna, H., et al. (2007). Dissociable intrinsic connectivity networks for salience processing and executive control. *J. Neurosci.* 27, 2349–2356. doi: 10.1523/JNEUROSCI.5587-06.2007

Shek, D. T. (1993). The Chinese version of the State-Trait Anxiety Inventory: its relationship to different measures of psychological well-being. *J. Clin. Psychol.* 49, 349–358.

Somerville, L. H., Jones, R. M., and Casey, B. (2010). A time of change: Behavioral and neural correlates of adolescent sensitivity to appetitive and aversive environmental cues. *Brain Cogn.* 72, 124. doi: 10.1016/j.bandc.2009.07.003

Song, X.-W., Dong, Z.-Y., Long, X.-Y., Li, S.-F., Zuo, X.-N., Zhu, C.-Z., et al. (2011). REST: a toolkit for resting-state functional magnetic resonance imaging data processing. *PLoS ONE* 6:e25031. doi: 10.1371/journal.pone.0025031

Spielberger, C. D., Gorsuch, R. L., Lushene, R., Vagg, P. R., and Jacobs, G. A. (1983). *Manual for the State-Trait Anxiety Inventory.* Palo Alto, CA: Consulting Psychologists Press.

Sridharan, D., Levitin, D. J., and Menon, V. (2008). A critical role for the right fronto-insular cortex in switching between central-executive and default-mode networks. *Proc. Natl. Acad. Sci. U.S.A.* 105, 12569–12574. doi: 10.1073/pnas.0800005105

Stein, M. B., Simmons, A. N., Feinstein, J. S., and Paulus, M. P. (2007). Increased amygdala and insula activation during emotion processing in anxiety-prone subjects. *Am. J. Psychiatry* 164, 318–327. doi: 10.1176/ajp.2007.164.2.318

Sylvester, C. M., Corbetta, M., Raichle, M. E., Rodebaugh, T. L., Schlaggar, B. L., Sheline, Y. I., et al. (2012). Functional network dysfunction in anxiety and anxiety disorders. *Trends Neurosci.* 35, 527–535. doi: 10.1016/j.tins.2012.04.012

Uddin, L. Q., Supekar, K. S., Ryali, S., and Menon, V. (2011). Dynamic reconfiguration of structural and functional connectivity across core neurocognitive brain networks with development. *J. Neurosci.* 31, 18578–18589. doi: 10.1523/JNEUROSCI.4465-11.2011

Watson, D., and Clark, L. A. (1999). *The PANAS-X: Manual for the Positive and Negative Affect Schedule - Expanded Form.* Iowa City: Department of Psychology Publications.

Yan, C., and Zang, Y. (2010). DPARSF: a MATLAB toolbox for "pipeline" data analysis of resting state fMRI. *Front. Syst. Neurosci.* 4:13. doi: 10.3389/fnsys.2010.00013

Conflict of Interest Statement: The authors declare that the research was conducted in the absence of any commercial or financial relationships that could be construed as a potential conflict of interest.

9

Trait Anxiety Modulates Brain Activity during Performance of Verbal Fluency Tasks

Edited by:
Morten L. Kringelbach, University of Oxford, UK and Aarhus University, Denmark

***Correspondence:**
Barbara Gawda

Barbara Gawda [1]* and Ewa Szepietowska [2]

[1] Department of Psychology of Emotion and Cognition, University of Maria Curie Sklodowska, Lublin, Poland, [2] Department of Clinical Psychology and Neuropsychology, University of Maria Curie-Sklodowska, Lublin, Poland

Trait anxiety is thought to be associated with pathological anxiety, and a risk factor for psychiatric disorders. The present study examines the brain mechanisms associated with trait anxiety during the performing of verbal fluency tasks. The aim is to show how trait anxiety modulates executive functions as measured by verbal fluency, and to explore the link between verbal fluency and anxiety due to the putative negative biases in high-anxious individuals. Seven tasks of verbal fluency were used: letter "k," "f," verbs, "animals," "vehicles," "joy," and "fear." The results of 35 subjects (whole sample), and 17 subjects (nine men, eight women) selected from the whole sample for the low/high-anxious groups on the basis of Trait Anxiety scores were analyzed. The subjects were healthy, Polish speaking, right-handed and aged from 20 to 35 years old. fMRI (whole-brain analysis with FWE corrections) was used to show the neural signals under active participation in verbal fluency tasks. The results confirm that trait anxiety slightly modulates neural activation during the performance of verbal fluency tasks, especially in the more difficult tasks. Significant differences were found in brain activation during the performance of more complex tasks between individuals with low anxiety and those with high anxiety. Greater activation in the right hemisphere, frontal gyri, and cerebellum was found in people with low anxiety. The results reflect better integration of cognitive and affective capacities in individuals with low anxiety.

Keywords: trait anxiety, verbal fluency, neuroimaging, executive functions

INTRODUCTION

Trait anxiety is a stable personality trait describing one's tendency to respond fearfully to a wide variety of stimuli (Spielberger et al., 1970). This is a general disposition to experiencing anxiety-relevant feelings or thoughts, or exhibiting anxiety-related behaviors (Spielberger, 1979). Highly trait-anxious people tend to perceive situations as more threatening, and they experience anxious states more frequently. They modify their perception of reality in such a way that they attribute a variety of stimuli with negative valence, and concentrate on these negatively perceived stimuli [the mechanism of attention inhibition (Öhman et al., 2000)]. Trait anxiety as a personality factor is associated with biological predispositions (e.g., Most et al., 2006; Öhman, 2008), pathological anxiety (Schmidt et al., 2008), and a risk factor for psychiatric disorders (Bienvenu et al., 2001). Anxiety and fear share many common physiological and cognitive properties, but may be distinguishable (Hartley and Phelps, 2012). Fear is a reaction to specific and short-term stimuli, while anxiety may be experienced in the absence of a direct threat, and lasts a longer period of time.

Trait anxiety is a relatively consistent individual trait which is thought to be formed as a result of interaction between stress in early life and dispositional emotional arousal, which moderates the neuroplasticity of fear learning and memory (Kindt, 2014).

While the neurobiological bases of fear conditioning are well documented, the neural mechanisms of trait anxiety are not fully understood. However, these two topics are related because the development of trait anxiety is linked to the processes of facilitated fear conditioning and reduced fear extinction. People who are at risk of developing fear/anxiety disorders display impairments in extinction learning and reduced extinction memory (Kindt, 2014). The neural circuitry of fear conditioning has been extensively investigated in humans (Myers and Davis, 2002). Interestingly, the social fear learned through observation has similar neural mechanisms to those underlying classical fear conditioning (Olsson et al., 2007). The amygdala plays a central role in fear acquisition, storage, and expression. The amygdala is thought to be the site of association and storage of fear, with projections to the brainstem, the hypothalamus which mediates autonomic fear expression, and the ventral striatum which mediates coping with fear. In addition, the hippocampus and insula are important in the contextual modulation of fear. Then, the dorsal anterior cingulate cortex is thought to be involved in the modulation of fear acquisition. Fear circuitry also comprises some motor areas such as the primary motor cortex and dorsal basal ganglia (Butler et al., 2007). Cognitive-based fear engages motor control networks including the cortico-striato-thalamic loops. It reflects a state of motor readiness in response to danger (Butler et al., 2007). Control and/or extinction of fear is associated with the activity of the ventromedial prefrontal cortex (Peters et al., 2009; Sehlmeyer et al., 2009).

Although fear and anxiety can be distinguished, several theories propose that dysregulation of the neurocircuitry associated with fear conditioning are critically involved in the etiology and maintenance of anxiety (Mineka and Zinbarg, 2006). Trait anxiety is associated with increased amygdala activation and with elevated fear expression during fear acquisition (Lissek et al., 2005; Indovina et al., 2011). Anxiety also impairs extinction learning and emotional regulation of fear (Indovina et al., 2011; Sehlmeyer et al., 2011). In particular, this manifests in an inability to consistently inhibit fearful memories following extinction, and it results in a maladaptive expression of fear (Steinfurth et al., 2014). The role of the amygdala and the hippocampal formation in fear memory consolidation has been demonstrated (Albrecht et al., 2010), and amygdala activation is thought to be essential in selective attention to threat, as well as threat interpretation (Knight et al., 2009). In order to explain this process, researchers have considered the functional connectivity between the amygdala and prefrontal cortical regions (see Bishop, 2007). The medial prefrontal cortex, the dorsal ACC, and hippocampal areas comprise a part of the extinction circuitry (Hartley and Phelps, 2012). It is believed that these regions control the expression of fear by inhibiting amygdala activity. Anxious individuals show reduced response in both the rostral anterior cingulate region, implicated in detecting conflict from emotional stimuli, and in lateral prefrontal regions implicated in augmenting attentional control (Bremner et al., 2005; Rauch et al., 2005). Hyporesponsivity of the prefrontal regions and hyperresponsivity of the amygdala result in a disruption of the frontal-amygdala circuitry that, in turn, can influence attention, control, and interpretive mechanisms in highly anxious individuals (Morgan et al., 1993; Phelps et al., 2004). Trait anxiety associated with enhanced activation of the amygdala and decreased activity of dACC during late extinction learning was interpreted as delayed and reduced extinction of fear. This suggests that highly anxious subjects are not able to maintain inhibitory activation of dACC during the extinction process, this results in a failure to adapt to altering circumstances (Sehlmeyer et al., 2011).

Similar findings were shown for people who exhibited anxiety disorders: the hypo-activation of ACC during emotional processing (Etkin and Wager, 2007). Trait anxiety correlates inversely with the structural integrity of the vmPCF-amygdala pathway, suggesting an anatomical basis for heightened reactivity and impaired emotional regulation in anxiety (Kim and Wallen, 2009). The role of vmPFC in selective fear inhibition was shown; it inhibits fear response to one stimulus by facilitating the transference of this response on the currently predictive stimulus (Schiller et al., 2008). In addition, atrophy of the hippocampus in clinically anxious patients suggests that contextual modulation of fear may also be impaired. Thus, anxious individuals show an increased generalization of conditioned fear to similar stimuli (Lissek et al., 2010). A simple learned fear association may easily transfer to an overgeneralization of fear, however, trait anxiety is related to a generalization of fear responding only after an unpredictable aversive event (Kindt, 2014). Furthermore, a more sustained arousal and vigilance typical for anxious people is supported by the activation of the bed nucleus of the stria terminalis, which is a region in the ventral basal forebrain (Somerville et al., 2010). Moreover, the heightened perception of bodily sensation and interoception in anxious individuals appears to be associated with the role of altered insula which is thought to contribute to the maintenance of anxiety (Paulus and Stein, 2010).

The above mentioned results illustrate that the neural mechanisms of trait anxiety play an essential role for fear expression, sustained arousal, vigilance, heightened interoception, heightened reactivity, and impaired emotional regulation in anxious individuals. All these findings show that anxiety and trait anxiety may have an impact not only on emotional information processing, but also on cognitive processes. Recent neuroimaging studies suggest that the dysregulation of the fear conditioning circuitry and alterations in cognitive functioning in anxiety are based on the same neural mechanisms (Bishop, 2007). Two principal characteristics of information processing in anxious people were highlighted: a bias to pay attention to threat-related information, and a bias toward negative interpretation of ambiguous stimuli (Hartley and Phelps, 2012). Studies indicate that anxious people exhibit a tendency to facilitate the detection of threat-related stimuli, and a difficulty in disengaging attention from negative stimuli (Cisler and Kostner, 2010). In particular, when stimuli are more complex anxiety is related to a more negative interpretation (Bar-Haim et al., 2007). Likewise, differences in brain activity during positive vs. negative information processing were shown. During positive emotion processing, trait anxiety was found to modify neural activity in the right caudate head, and in the left superior temporal gyrus during the processing of negative emotion (Lemche et al., 2013). This biased attention in trait anxious people reflects increased amygdala activity to attended to threatening stimuli, as well as to unattended threat stimuli, and a decreased prefrontal activation under a condition of attention competition (Bishop, 2009). This altered threat sensitivity was documented by many studies (Bishop et al., 2004; Etkin et al., 2004; Haas et al., 2007). The threat-related biases, which are key-mechanisms of trait anxiety may develop as a result of abnormal safety learning in childhood, and they may be related to attention, appraisal, learning, memory, and threat sensitivity in adulthood. It is worth noting that these threat-biases are observed in anxious individuals at multiple levels of information processing (Britton et al., 2011).

Trait anxiety involves impaired attention and working memory. It involves perturbed attention allocation in the appraisal of potentially dangerous situations. This is supported by evidence of amygdala hyper-activation in anxiety disorders, and greater amygdala activation to negative stimuli, e.g., fearful faces (Britton et al., 2011). Associations between anxiety and memory were also documented. Appraisal processes are linked to cortical regions; activation of vmPFC during threat appraisal reflects the ability to discriminate between safety and threat; perturbations found in vmPFC activation during threat appraisal may reflect fear overgeneralization; finally a reduction in vmPFC activation is associated with poor long-term outcomes (Britton et al., 2011). Decreased positive amygdala-prefrontal functional connectivity was reported for young individuals with emotional dysregulation (Bertocci et al., 2014). Likewise, a large body of research suggests that anxiety may alter decision making, because uncertainty (associated with decision process) evokes threat-related information processing biases, and results in altered decision making (Hartley and Phelps, 2012). Anxious individuals are biased toward interpreting ambiguous contexts negatively (Grillon et al., 2004). Studies examining the neural substrates of processing ambiguity highlight the roles of the amygdala and the PFC; risk processing is more dependent on activity in the orbital prefrontal regions, whereas ambiguity processing recruits dlPFC (Krain et al., 2006). Ambiguity and risk processing are particularly aversive in anxious individuals. Studies also suggest that an increased level of anxiety is associated with greater loss aversion, because the above-mentioned pattern of brain activation seems to have a common underlying mechanism with an expression of fear and anxiety-related attentional biases (Hartley and Phelps, 2010, 2012). That is why anxiety increases the attention given to a negative choice option, negative interpretation of ambiguity, and the tendency to avoid potential negative outcomes which may inhibit flexibility of behavior (Hartley and Phelps, 2012).

Examining verbal fluency in anxious people may provide important information on their cognitive functioning; how they retrieve information, how they represent it, and organize it in memory. Verbal fluency tests are a measure of executive functions. The concept of executive functions refers to the top-down control of cognitive processes. The central executive component of the working memory model is characterized by an attentional control system (Larsson et al., 2007). Shimamura's (2000) dynamic filtering theory defines executive control as the monitoring, selection, and control of cognitive processes. Selection refers to the ability to direct attention toward a perceptual stimulus or a representation in memory. Maintenance refers to the ability to hold selected information active. Updating refers to the ability to modulate and reorganize information in working memory, and rerouting is associated with the ability to shift attention between different response sets. In a verbal fluency task, a participant is to generate words beginning with a specific letter (letter fluency), or belonging to a specific category (semantic fluency). Verbal fluency is dependent on both the ability to retrieve words from long-term storage and on executive functions. Shimamura (2002) pointed out that verbal fluency requires the ability to selectively focus attention on a semantic category, the ability to "on-line monitor" previously recalled words, and continuously update the words that have been used. Verbal fluency tests require an adequate mental set-shifting ability which guides the strategic search of words (Rende et al., 2002). Thus, the retrieval of semantic knowledge is dependent upon all domains of cognitive control because these domains are closely referring to attention and memory. Some data are particularly valuable, studies report close relationships between anxiety and cognitive functions, among them a relationship between anxiety and verbal information processing. For instance, verbal instruction may modify extinction processing which supports the idea that cognitive process is the primary mechanism of change during exposure therapy (Phelps et al., 2001). Hofmann (2008) reviewed empirical data and theoretical models suggesting that fear conditioning, fear extinction, and psychotherapy involve high-order cognitive processes. Thus, links between anxiety and cognitive processes are evident. First, because anxiety is conceptualized as a cognitive association of basic emotions, meanings, and responses (Barlow, 2002). Second, the neuroscience literature shows that cognitive process are critically important even in primitive forms of learning, thus it is not surprising that they are important in the acquisition and extinction of fear (Hofmann, 2008).

Due to verbal fluency's dependence upon executive control it seems to be reasonable to assume that the ability to retrieve semantic knowledge, as measured by verbal fluency, can be used to operationalize individual differences in executive control (Tabert et al., 2001). The results showed that the total number of words produced during verbal fluency tasks predicted the level of state anxiety, and it can be interpreted as support for a theoretical model of executive control capacity which may mediate emotional experience of state anxiety. Thus, an effective capacity to direct attention toward perceptual stimuli, or memory representations may be related to better retrieval or verbal coping strategies (Larsson et al., 2007). Links between executive functions and regulation of emotions are documented by neuroimaging studies. A high working memory capacity is related to an increased ability to resist putting attention on negative information. Thus, a high working capacity is characterized by a more effective attentional control (Derryberry and Reed, 2002). Personality traits such as trait anxiety may contribute to the ability to retrieve specific words. Rosen and Engle (1997) found relationships between verbal fluency and life-span working memory. There is also a study that suggests an association between personality traits and verbal fluency, i.e., Neuroticism was associated with lower scores in verbal fluency tasks (Sutin et al., 2011). Studies on verbal fluency in anxious and depressive people report that a high level of anxiety is associated with low verbal fluency scores in phonemic fluency tasks (Albus et al., 1998), both letter and semantic tasks (Beats et al., 1996), or only in semantic tasks (Fossati et al., 2003). Some cognitive impairments displayed by this group inhibit semantic strategies of retrieval and switching during verbal fluency performance (Atchley et al., 2003). Neuroimaging studies aim to show that dysfunctions of the prefrontal areas are thought to be involved in these low scores in verbal fluency tasks. Dysfunctions in activity of the prefrontal areas mirror the impairment of executive functions, and results in the use of non-effective retrieval strategies, and low switching capacities; this is reflected in low verbal fluency scores (Audenaert et al., 2002; Fossati et al., 2003). Anxiety has been found to be correlated with hypoactivation in the right prefrontal cortex in depressive patients, where verbal fluency tasks and neuroimaging techniques have been used (Liu et al., 2014).

Verbal fluency tasks may differ in their level of difficulty which may depend on the frequency of words (Ross, 2003; Ross et al., 2007). The general score in verbal fluency tasks is dependent on the frequency of the words as used in the general population; there are words of high frequency and they are generated quickly (in Polish the letter "k" is of high frequency, while "f" is of low frequency; Styczek, 1983). It means that there are less words in the Polish language starting with the letter "f," and that is why this task would be more demanding than tasks letter the letter "k." Then, tasks which include more typical words are easier than those including less typical words, the category "animals" is larger in terms of how frequently words are used, and more typical than the category "vehicles," thus, it is easier to search the words from the lexicon of "animals" than from that of "vehicles" (Strauss et al., 1998). Furthermore, non-affective tasks are easier than affective tasks. Because language comprises more words naming animals, than words naming emotions, typically people generate more non-emotional words than emotional words (Tabert et al., 2001; Rossell, 2006). We introduce all types of tasks (letter, semantic, difficult, easier, emotional, and non-emotional) to analyze the potential effect of trait anxiety on modulation upon their performance, and the putative neural substrates of this modulation. To our knowledge, this type of study is the first.

We hypothesized that trait anxiety will differentiate performance of verbal fluency, thus we expect to see differences between low-anxious and high-anxious individuals in behavioral data. Horwitz and McCaffrey (2008) stated that verbal fluency performance in anxious people depends on the task's characteristics. Hence, we additionally expect that differences in the behavioral data will be more pronounced within high-anxious group, especially for difficult and emotional tasks (specifically differences between non-emotional and negative tasks are expected because high anxiety individuals exhibit negative attention biases). And then, we expect to see differences in brain activity during verbal fluency tasks between low-anxious and high–anxious groups, in particular while performing difficult, emotional tasks. Because of this the low-anxious people are thought to use more effective strategies to search, select, and retrieve words, we expect that they will activate more prefrontal regions across verbal fluency tasks, and they will present greater activation of these brain regions which are thought to be associated with the verbal fluency tasks' performance: the superior and the inferior prefrontal gyri, the temporal middle gyrus, the fusiform gyrus, the primary and secondary occipital cortex, the precuneus, and the superior parietal areas. Likewise, for emotional tasks, activation of some parts of the limbic areas is expected, such as the amygdala, hippocampus, or/and the cingulate cortex. Because of the general integrative role of the cerebellum in language, affective, and cognitive processing, the increased activation of the cerebellum is expected in low-anxious individuals.

MATERIALS AND METHODS

Participants

The results of 35 healthy, Polish-speaking, right-handed adults aged 20–35 (18 men and 17 women) were analyzed. Participants were paid for their participation. None of the subjects had a history of neurological or psychiatric disorders (each subject completed a questionnaire during a screening phase, with relevant information on neurological, psychiatric problems, and substance abuse). The selected participants were not addicted to drugs or alcohol (screening procedure). Handedness was verified using the Edinburg Inventory (Oldfield, 1971). The experimental protocol was approved by the Local Ethics Committee of the Department of Pedagogy and Psychology of the University of Maria Curie-Sklodowska. Participants had an average level of intelligence ($M = 102$, $SD = 10$) and no memory or attention impairments. Subscales from WAIS-R (Brzezinski et al., 2004; Vocabulary and Digit Span) were used to control these variables. The State Trait Anxiety Inventory was used to measure the level of trait anxiety. Two groups were identified on the basis of the trait anxiety score: a group with a high level of anxiety ($n = 5$; five men, 5 women) and another with low anxiety ($n = 7$; 3 men, 4 women). The high and low-anxious groups were selected on the basis of the normative data for the STAI; those participants who scored above 42 were classified as high-anxious, while those who scored below 32 were classified as low-anxious (Wrześniewski et al., 2002). These two groups representing the ends of the trait anxiety continuum were chosen to better illustrate the putative differences in brain activity during the performance of verbal fluency tasks. A categorical approach is helpful in communication and has a simplifying quality. Furthermore, clinical decisions regarding treatment are generally made with respect to a binary choice, as to whether or not a patient has a disorder. Whereas the low level of anxiety represents the low end of continuum which is adaptive, a high level of anxiety represents the second end of continuum where anxiety is non-adaptive (Endler and Kocovski, 2001).

In addition, trait anxiety as a dimensional variable was used in a simple regression analysis, as a predictor for neural activity.

Procedure

Verbal fluency tasks were administered to all the subjects before the scanning procedure took place. Then, STAI, and in addition a verbal IQ estimation test, Digit Span (WAIS-R) subscale, were administrated (study outline in the **Figure 1**).

Measures

WAIS-R

The Wechsler Adult Intelligence Scale-Revised is a general test of intelligence, based on 11 subtests divided into two parts: verbal and performance. Vocabulary and Digit Span scores were used in the screening procedure to qualify and compare working memory and verbal comprehension of the participants to select only those participants without any impairments.

STAI

The State Trait Anxiety Inventory. In this analysis only the Trait Anxiety score was considered. The Polish adaptation of the STAI consisted of 20 statements describing emotional conditions. The respondent is asked to rate the applicability of each statement to him/herself according to a 4-point frequency scale: 1-rarely, 2-sometimes, 3-often, 4-usually. The reliability and validity of the STAI are very good (Wrześniewski et al., 2002).

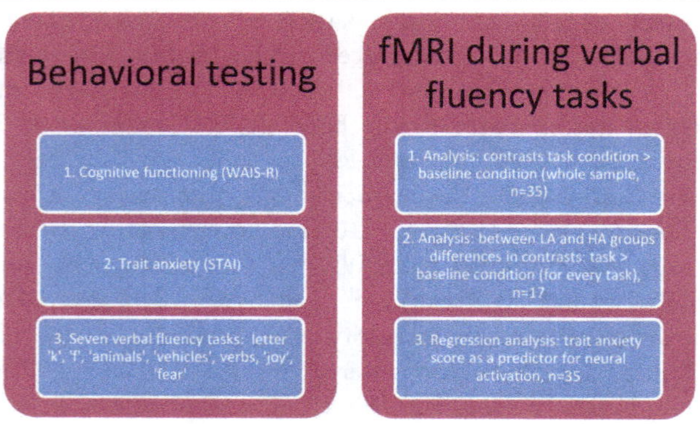

FIGURE 1 | The study outline.

Verbal fluency tasks

The subjects' fluency was tested with seven tasks in the following order: letter "k," letter "f," "animals," "vehicles," verbs, "joy," and "fear." The subjects were asked to name as many words as possible in 1 min during the stage before scanning. All generated words were recorded by the experimenter, counted for every participant and for every task. All verbal fluency tasks were performed in the same order both inside and outside of the scanner (see **Tables 1, 2**).

fMRI Procedure

Task, scanning procedure, and image acquisition

The examinations were performed in the magnetic resonance laboratory of the European Health Care Centre in Otwock (Poland). Each subject stayed in the scanner for approximately 30 min. Stimuli were presented to them in a blocked design with two alternating blocks: naming words silently (verbal fluency conditions) and to do nothing except look at a cross (baseline condition). During a sequence participants were asked to name as many items as possible related to the fluency

TABLE 2 | Descriptive statistics ($n = 17$).

Variable	Group LA* *M (SD)*	Group HA *M (SD)*	$t_{(1,15)}$
Age	27.14 (5.26)	25.40 (4.30)	−0.45ns
Education	14.70 (1.60)	14.20 (1.40)	0.15ns
Vocabulary	32.00 (13.16)	25.00 (10.09)	0.16ns
Digit span	4.57 (1.99)	3.30 (1.15)	1.71ns
Positive verbal fluency: "joy"	11.14 (5.52)	10.70 (7.02)	0.14ns
Negative verbal fluency: "fear"	10.85 (4.94)	10.40 (6.29)b	0.16ns
Number of errors	1.08 (.91)	1.10 (0.92)	0.59ns
Category "animals"	22.42 (7.13)	23.60 (6.18)	−0.36ns
Category "vehicles"	16.00 (6.75)	13.90 (4.25)	0.79ns
Verbs	18.57 (3.77)	17.70 (7.76)	0.27ns
Letter high frequency	19.71 (3.63)	17.10 (3.84)	1.41ns
Letter low frequency	16.14 (4.84)	12.09 (4.02)	1.92ns
State Anxiety	29.85 (7.31)	35.10 (5.44)	1.06ns
Trait Anxiety	30.00 (5.16)	49.10 (4.72)	7.90***

**LA, low-anxious group; HA, high-anxious group; M, mean, SD, standard deviation, ns, not significant, ***$p < 0.001$.*

TABLE 1 | The types of tasks.

Name of tasks (description)	Before the scan	During the scan (due to repetition of tasks, their equivalents were also used)
Phonemic fluency: letter high frequency k (generating word s starting with a letter "k")	X	letters: k, m, t
Phonemic fluency: letter low frequency f (generating word s starting with a letter "r")	X	letters: f, g, n
Semantic fluency category living "animals" (generating nouns naming "animals")	X	an imals, plants, birds
Semantic fluency category non-living "vehicles" (generating nouns naming "vehicles")	X	vehicles, tools, furniture
Verbs (generating verbs)	X	X
Affective fluency positive "joy" (generating words representing the category "joy")	X	joy, happiness, fun
Affective fluency negative "fear" (generating word s representing the category of "fear")	X	fear, anxiety, fright

categories which were equivalent to those used before the scanning procedure or to do nothing (baseline condition). Each sequence was preceded with instructions which were written in a textual format and shown on the screen. The LCD screen (NordicNeuroLab InroomViewingDevice) was used for visual presentation. There were seven identical functional sequences with different stimulation. Time of each sequence—3.18 min. There were repetitions of the following blocks in each sequence (each block lasted 6 vol.): 5 × (18-s display of gaze fixation point—cross, 18-s of active task) and 18-s of the cross at the end. There were seven different active tasks (see **Table 1**). The echo-planar images were acquired on a 3T Achieva Philips Medical Systems scanner using an 8-channel coil. The structural sequences (T1, T2) were assessed in order to exclude individuals with abnormal brain morphology; then high resolution T1 and SingleShot-EPI were used. The parameters of each sequence were as follows: T1 TFE high resolution sequence: TR = 7.51[ms], TE = 3.69[ms], FA = 8, FOV = 25.6 × 25.6 [cm], matrix = 256 × 256, slice thickness = 2[mm], gap = −1[mm], pixel bandwidth = 191 Hz/pix, number of slices = 181, TA = 3:18 min. A single-shot GE-EPI sequence was used for fMRI acquisition (FFE-EPI, TE = 30[ms], TR = 3000[ms], TA = 3:18 [min], slice thickness = 3[mm], gap = 0[mm], matrix = 96 × 96, FOV = 192 × 192 [mm], number of slices = 45, SENSE factor 1.8, dynamics = 66).

TABLE 3 | Brain regions which are more active for the contrasts of verbal fluency tasks > baseline condition, comparison between the LA and the HA groups ($n = 17$, two sample t- tests, $p < 0.001$, uncorr.).

Clusters			MRI coordinates			
Verbs	**Hemisphere**	**Active voxels (mm³)**	**x**	**y**	**z**	***t*-value**
Occipital Inferior gyrus	R	368	36	−82	−6	5.41
Cerebellum 8	R	328	20	−62	−56	4.74
Precuneus	R	144	4	−68	24	4.73
Inferior frontal gyrus BA 47	R	16	34	32	−20	4.08
Superior frontal gyrus	R	128	38	20	54	4.93
ANIMALS						
Fusiform gyrus	R	528	26	−66	−8	5.22
VEHICLES						
Cerebellum Crus 1	L	3240	−12	−90	−20	5.91
Temporal middle gyrus	R	344	52	−72	14	5.84
Cerebellum 6	R	936	22	−62	−16	5.75
Cerebellum Crus 1	R	808	44	−56	−38	5.65
Occipital middle gurus	R	384	34	−84	34	4.38
Fusiform gyrus	R	304	26	−62	−14	5.19
Cerebellum crus 2	L	448	−38	−68	−38	5.17
POSITIVE FLUENCY JOY						
Cerebellum 8	R	408	34	−68	−54	5.20
Cerebellum Crus1	L	560	−16	−86	−22	4.97
Occipital area BA 18	R	504	14	−94	−2	5.91
Occipital area BA 19	L	432	−30	−78	44	5.09
Superior parietal lobule	L	176	−56	−12	38	4.55
NEGATIVE FLUENCY FEAR						
Superior frontal gyrus	R	392	30	−76	−16	5.25
Cerebelum 6	R	400	34	−6	60	7.52
Fusiform gyrus	R	384	32	−76	−16	5.25
Thalamus	R	456	12	−8	12	5.59

Image preprocessing

The fMRI data after transformation from DICOM to an analysis-compatible format were analyzed using the SPM12 package (Statistical Parametric Mapping). Data preprocessing comprised five consecutive steps: (1) a quality assurance procedure—checking images for artifacts and tSNR; (2) slice time correction (each slice was acquired in 67 ms in ascending order); (3) motion correction to eliminate motion artifacts—all images were realigned to the first image in the series, trials with motion above 2 mm were rejected (2/245 series), all realignment parameters were saved and used as the regressors within a GLM (general linear model) analysis, mean motion for all sequences was 0.47 mm, there were no differences between series in motion (mean motion for all 7 sequences: 0.52, 0.42, 0.41, 0.50, 0.44, 0.52, 0.45 mm), 7/245 sequences required a scrubbing procedure; (4) normalization of the brain images (anatomical T1-weighted images coregistrated with EPI—echo planar images) to MNI template (standard space suggested by the Montreal Neurological Institute, voxel size 2 × 2 × 2 mm) to enable between-group comparisons; and (5) smoothing filters (Gaussian kernel FWHM = 6 mm) were applied to decrease morphological differences between subjects. In the analysis the Automated Anatomical Labeling Atlas was used (Tzourio-Mazoyer et al., 2002).

fMRI data analysis

Two stages of analysis were performed: a single subject analysis (SSA) at a first level and a multi subject analysis (MSA) at a second level. Each EPI series had the same epoch-based paradigm. A GLM and a standard hemodynamic response function (HRF) were fitted to the data. The time-series for each voxel were high-pass filtered (1/128 Hz cutoff) to remove low-frequency noise and signal drift. To begin with, the first-level analyses were performed on individual subjects. The aim of this analysis was to show which regions of the brain were involved in the performance of the test, in other words to show whether there was a group effect of the performed test. In the first-level analysis one contrast was calculated "fluency task vs. cross." This contrast was taken to the second-level analysis. A two sample t-test analysis, as well as a within-subject A two sample t-test was used to compare brain activation between two independent LA and HA groups (see **Table 3**), while a one sample Anova was used to compare brain activation across the whole sample (dependent variables were activations of brain regions). The main activations for contrasts tasks > baseline condition across the whole sample are presented in **Table 4**. The simple regression analyses were performed to better illustrate associations between trait anxiety and brain activation during the performance of difficult or/and easier tasks (results of regression in the text Section Results).

TABLE 4 | Brain regions which are more active for the contrasts of fluency tasks > baseline condition (one sample analysis *t*-score, *n* = 35, *t*-threshold = 4.85, *p* < 0.05, FWE correction).

Regions			MRI coordinates			
Verbs	**Hemisphere**	**Active voxels (mm^3)**	**x**	**y**	**z**	***t*-value**
Temporal superior gyrus	L	2168	−56	16	−8	14.82
Occipital inferior gyrus	L	2424	−28	−96	−8	13.01
Occipital middle gyrus	L	1720	−28	−96	−6	12.79
Cerebellum crus2	R	6376	28	−82	−48	12.25
Frontal superior gyrus	L	9688	−6	10	50	12.24
Frontal inferior gyrus	L	4744	−56	22	24	11.72
Cerebellum 8	R	3016	30	−68	−58	11.64
Occipital inferior gyrus	R	2424	38	−90	−12	10.98
Frontal superior gyrus	R	3880	2	6	64	11.12
Frontal inferior gyr. BA 47	R	2488	42	22	−6	10.20
ANIMALS						
Cerebellum crus1	R	10512	32	−68	−26	12.89
Cerebellum 6	R	3264	32	−68	−26	12.89
Cerebellum crus2	R	6720	8	−80	−28	12.37
Frontal superior gyrus	L	5512	−4	12	46	12.22
Cerebellum 8	R	2432	36	−66	−56	12.15
Anterior cingulate cortex	R	1592	−4	12	44	11.87
LETTER K						
Cerebellum 8	R	3624	34	−66	−58	14.10
Globus pallidus	L	1488	−18	6	6	13.95
Putamen	L	2384	−18	6	8	13.32
Frontal superior gyrus	L	5152	−4	10	48	12.49
Frontal inf. gyr. (pars oper.)	L	2304	−42	6	26	11.89
Precentral gyrus	L	4912	−44	6	24	11.86
Cerebellum 7b	R	1560	22	−78	−52	11.43
LETTER F						
Cerebellum 8	R	3624	28	−68	−58	12.68
Frontal superior gyrus	L	4656	−4	10	50	12.62
Frontal inf. gyr. (pars oper.)	L	2392	−42	6	26	11.85
Cerebellum 7b	R	1200	28	−74	−54	11.31
Temporal inferior gyrus	L	3248	−54	−52	−20	11.07
Putamen	L	2384	−22	8	6	10.95
Precentral gyrus	L	4888	−44	6	24	10.61
VEHICLES						
Temporal superior gyrus	L	1592	−56	16	−8	12.13
Cerebellum 6	R	2448	36	−64	−56	12.11
Precentral gyrus	L	5848	−46	6	32	11.11
Cerebellum Crus2	R	12376	38	−60	−32	11.09
Frontal inf. gyr. (pars tri.)	L	6696	−46	26	22	10.96
Frontal inf. gyr. (pars oper.)	L	3400	−40	6	28	10.53
Cerebellum Crus1	L	6912	−52	−58	−30	8.60
CerebellumCrus1	R	12376	38	−60	−32	11.09
Occipital middle area	R	496	26	−98	10	7.16

(Continued)

TABLE 4 | Continued

Regions			MRI coordinates			
Verbs	**Hemisphere**	**Active voxels (mm^3)**	**x**	**y**	**z**	***t*-value**
POSITIVE FLUENCY JOY						
Frontal superior gyrus	L	4840	−2	12	52	11.18
Occipital inferior gyrus	R	3848	38	−82	−12	11.15
Temporal superior gyrus	L	1232	−56	16	−6	11.14
Insula	L	1792	−28	20	4	10.22
Cerebellum 8	R	1920	34	−68	−54	10.08
Cerebellum Crus1	R	8000	38	−74	−26	9.95
Calcarine sulcus	R	1352	18	−96	2	9.89
Cerebellum Crus1	L	928	−30	−84	−18	7.84
Occipital lobe BA 19	L	2864	−28	−94	6	9.02
NEGATIVE FLUENCY FEAR						
Frontal superior gyrus	L	7024	−4	12	48	13.09
Temporal superior gyrus	L	1432	−54	16	−8	12.97
Cerebellum Crus1	R	10960	26	−76	−24	12.54
Occipital middle gyrus	R	1720	38	−92	4	12.12
Anterior cingulate cortex	L	1384	−4	14	44	11.30
Occipital middle gyrus	L	3624	−34	−94	4	11.06
Calcarine sulcus	R	1840	20	−102	4	11.05
Cerebellum 6	R	2136	28	−70	−26	10.85
Frontal superior gyrus	R	1848	2	10	54	9.05
Fusiform gyrus	R	192	30	−82	−6	7.38

RESULTS

Behavioral Data

There were no significant differences between the groups with low anxiety (LA) and high anxiety (HA) in terms of age, education, Vocabulary, Digit Span, number of words in positive verbal fluency, number of words in negative verbal fluency tasks, number of words in the categories of "animals," "vehicles," number of verbs, and number of words from the phonemic fluency (both low frequency and high frequency letters; see **Table 2**). The two groups differed significantly in trait anxiety, but not in state anxiety. There were also no significant sex differences in the abovementioned variables ($t = 0.94$, $p = 0.33$).

The within-group comparisons (a Wilcoxon test) for the HA group showed significant differences between scores in more difficult tasks and easier tasks (with the Bonferroni correction). Their scores were higher in easier tasks, such as: category "animals" as opposed to the harder category "vehicles" ($z = -2.80$, $p < 0.001$), letter "k" in contrast to the more difficult letter "f" ($z = 2.60$, $p < 0.01$), and verbs over category "animals" ($z = 2.31$, $p < 0.01$). These comparisons show that "vehicles," verbs, and category letter "f" are more difficult tasks for the HA, whereas "animals" and category letter "k" are easier. The most difficult category seems to be that of "vehicles." Similar comparisons for the LA group did not show significant differences between "vehicles," "animals," verbs, and letter categories (the letter "k" to the letter "f," $z = 1.40$, ns.), "animals" to verbs ($z = 1.44$, ns.), and "vehicles" to verbs ($z = -1.24$, ns). The above results show that for the LA group there are no differences between the difficult and easier tasks, whereas these differences are found for the HA group. This supports the thesis that HA individuals differ in cognitive processing between more complex and less complex tasks.

The within-group comparisons between performance on emotional ("fear," "joy") and non-emotional tasks (non-emotional means the categories of letters "k" and "f") were assessed separately within the LA and HA group. These comparisons showed that the LA group on average generated more words starting with the letter "k" than words in the category "fear" ($z = -2.37$, $p < 0.01$), and they generated more words starting with the letter "f" than in the category "fear" ($z = -2.38$, $p < 0.01$). The HA group generated more words starting with the letter "k" than in categories "joy" and "fear" ($z = -2.37$, $p < 0.01$, $z = -2.45$, $p < 0.01$, respectively). No significant differences were found for the comparisons between the number of words starting with the letter "f" and categories "joy," "fear" within the HA group. The mean number of words for the HA group is presented in **Table 2**. The above findings show a typical tendency: that people generate more non-emotional than emotional words, and that HA individuals did not generate more negative nor positive words than non-emotional. This is not in line with data suggesting negative attention biases in anxious people.

Neuroimaging Data

Interestingly, no differences were found in all behavioral data (all tasks) between the LA and the HA groups, yet differences in brain activation during the verbal fluency tasks were identified. To compare neural correlates between verbal fluency tasks between the LA and HA groups, a two sample t-test was used.

The differences in activation during the **verbs** task were found in five clusters when the following thresholds were adopted: $p = 0.001$ (uncorrected), t-threshold = 3.73, cluster size threshold = 38, alphasim $p < 0.05$. In the case of the LA group, greater activation was found in the right occipital inferior gyrus, in the right cerebellum 8, in the right precuneus, in the right superior, and in the inferior frontal gyri (see **Table 3**, **Figures 2**, **3**). A predominance of activation in the right hemispheric regions was observed in the LA group during this task, and similarly during all of the more difficult tasks. The illustration of these active regions in the right hemisphere is presented in **Figure 4**. In addition, a simple regression analysis across all participants revealed a significant weak negative correlation between trait anxiety and activation in the right occipital inferior gyrus (36, −82, −6), in the right cerebellum 8 (20, −62, −56), in the right precuneus (4, −68, 24), and in the right superior gyrus (38, 20, 54).

Another more difficult category is that of "**vehicles**," where several differences in activation between the LA and HA groups for this task were found. Activation for "vehicles" comprises the right and left cerebellum, the right temporal gyrus, the right fusiform gyrus, and the right middle occipital gyrus. A simple regression analysis with trait anxiety as predictor showed that trait anxiety is negatively and strongly correlated with the activation in the cerebellum during the performance of task "vehicles." A negative weak correlation between trait anxiety and activation in the temporal areas and activation in the occipital areas was found. It suggests that higher trait anxiety is associated with lower activation of the aforementioned brain regions.

Less demanding tasks such as that of "**animals**," the **letter "k,"** and the **letter "f"** did not elicit differences in brain activity between the LA and HA groups as it was hypothesized. Brain activation during the "animals" task was greater in the LA group only in the right fusiform gyrus. Then, the high frequency letters task elicited no differences in activation between the LA and HA groups. Similarly, low frequency letter task caused no differences in activation between LA and HA. This was surprising.

The comparisons of brain activity during the performance of the emotional tasks between the LA and HA groups showed some differences. In the case of the category "**joy**," a predominance of activation in the right hemisphere was not observed, whereas it was in category "**fear**." The performance of positive verbal fluency tasks in the LA group elicited higher activation in the right cerebellum 8, left cerebellum crus, the secondary visual cortex (the right occipital area BA 18, the left occipital area BA 19) and in the left parietal lobule. In sum, five clusters were found when the following thresholds were adopted: $p = 0.001$ (uncorrected), t-threshold = 3.73, cluster size threshold = 38,

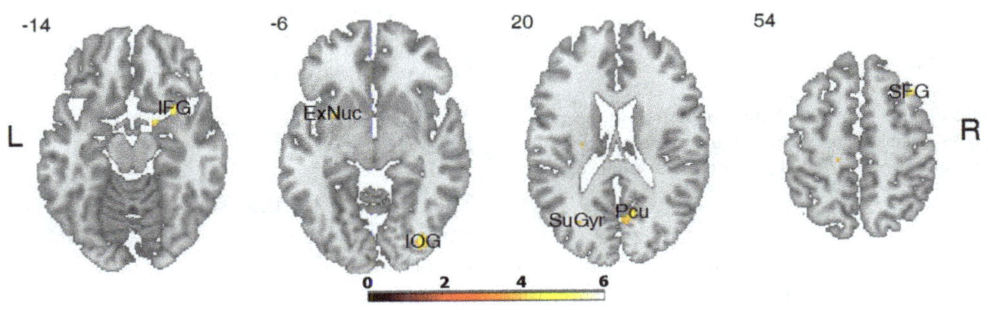

FIGURE 2 | Differences in brain activation between LA and HA groups for the contrasts verbs > baseline condition: in the right inferior frontal gyrus (IFG), right inferior occipital gyrus (IOG), right precuneus (Pcu), right superior frontal gyrus (SFG).

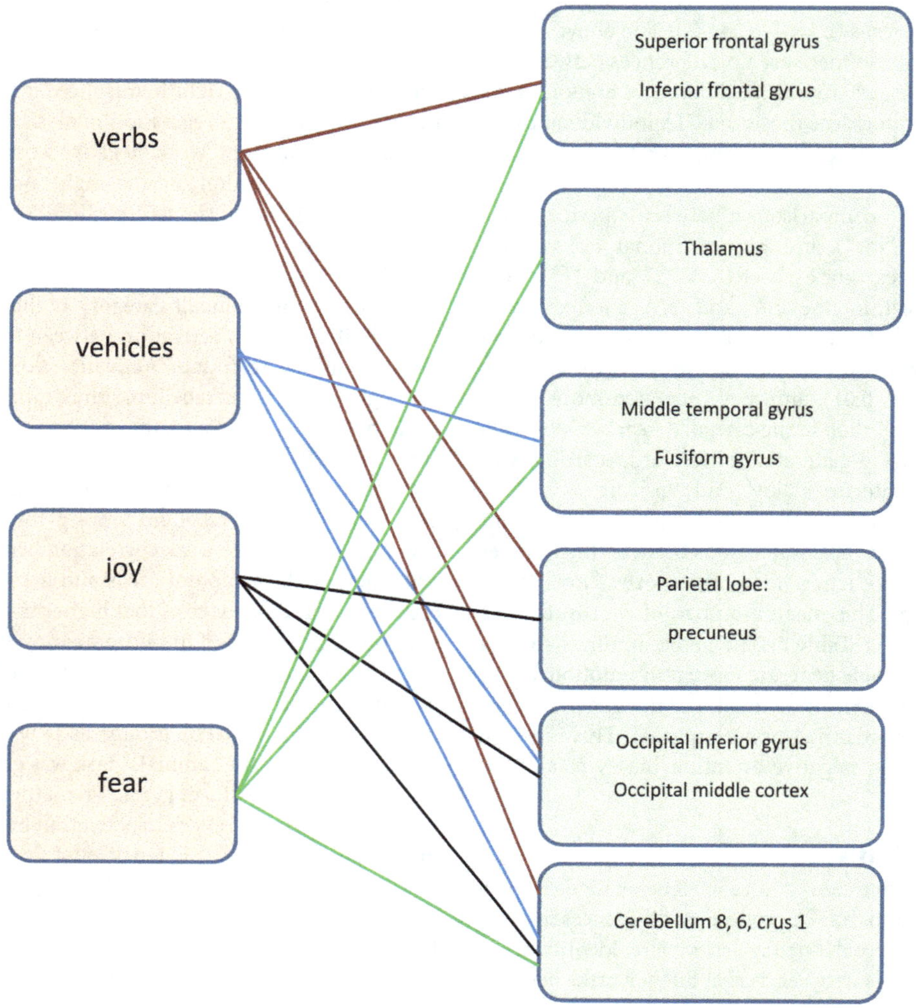

FIGURE 3 | The neural areas involved in the tasks (the right hemisphere).

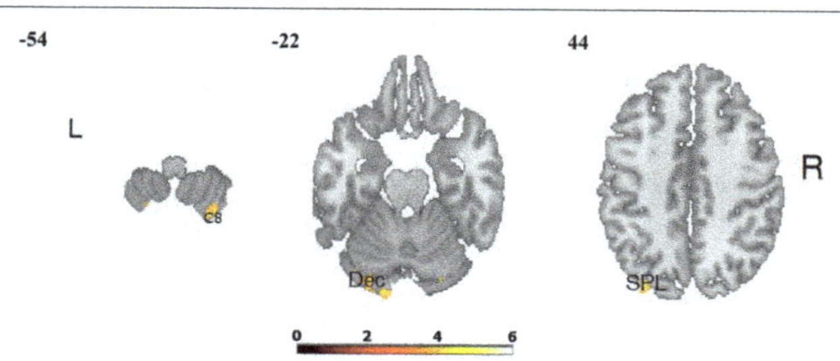

FIGURE 4 | Differences in brain activation between LA and HA groups for the contrasts "joy" > baseline condition: in the right cerebellum 8 (C 8), left cerebellum (declive—Dec), left superior parietal lobule (SPL).

see **Figure 4**. Negative verbal fluency tasks in the case of LA individuals elicited greater activation in the right frontal superior gyrus, in the right fusiform gyrus, the right cerebellum, and the right thalamus. For category "fear" four clusters were found when the following thresholds were adopted: $p = 0.001$ (uncorrected), t-threshold = 3.73, cluster size threshold = 38, alphasim $p < 0.05$ (see **Table 3**, **Figure 5**). Additionally, a simple regression analysis was conducted with trait anxiety as a predictor. It showed strong negative correlations between trait anxiety and activation in two regions: cerebellum crus1 (−16, −86, −22) and the occipital area BA 18 (14, −94, −2). Other negative correlations for emotional verbal fluency categories were weak, but they consistently show that with higher trait anxiety the activation is lower in the same brain regions as it was shown by the t-test comparisons.

DISCUSSION

The purpose of this study was to describe whether trait anxiety modulates brain activity during verbal fluency task performance. The differences in neural activation between LA and HA individuals were found, while no differences in behavioral data between these groups were identified. It suggests that different neural mechanisms may be involved in retrieval processes, yielding similar behavioral effects (Bishop, 2009).

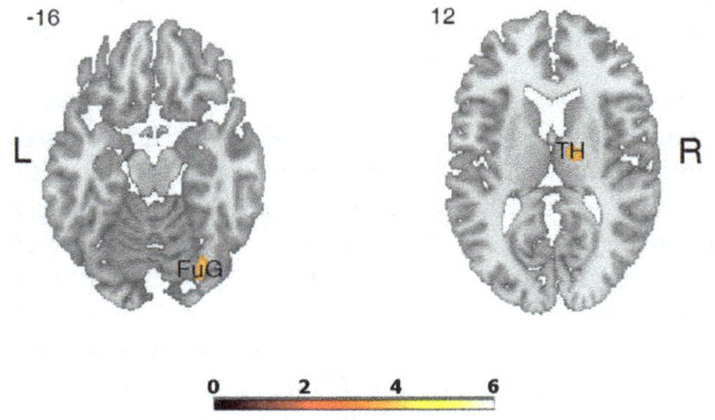

FIGURE 5 | Differences in brain activation between LA and HA groups for the contrasts "fear" > baseline condition: in the right thalamus (TH), right fusiform gyrus (FuG).

LA and HA individuals may employ other neural strategies to achieve the same results: for LA individuals it is easier to be well concentrated, while for HA people is harder to achieve the same result, activating more inappropriate brain regions, possibly HA group execute tasks with greater effort. It is in line with findings that show that trait anxiety impairs processing efficiency more than performance effectiveness (Derakshan and Eysenck, 2009). Possibly it refers also to the first general finding which was not expected: the predominance of right hemispheric activation during almost all difficult tasks in the low-anxious subjects. It may be explained in terms of data highlighting the right hemisphere's associations with explicit memory retrieval (Gabrieli et al., 1998). Possibly low-anxious individuals use more explicit and more self-relevant strategies during the performance of verbal fluency tasks. The right prefrontal cortex is associated with self-relevance during subjective evaluation, people engage more episodic retrieval during tasks of subjective evaluation (Schmitz et al., 2004). Predominance of the right hemisphere in the majority of tasks may also be interpreted as the use of novel, non-typical strategies by low-anxious people (Garoff et al., 2005). It may refer to their use of more visual strategies during verbal fluency tasks performance (Goldberg et al., 2013).

The next general finding, which was hypothesized, suggests a relationship between the task difficulty and the differences in brain activity in the LA and HA individuals: the easier the tasks the lower the differences between the LA and HA groups. This suggests that easier and more familiar tasks, such as high frequency letters and "animals" did not elicit many differences in brain activity between the groups. On the other hand, more difficult tasks coincided with more differences in brain activity between LA and HA, i.e., harder tasks such as verbs, "vehicles," "joy," and "fear" elicited more differences between the neural mechanisms of the LA and HA groups. In addition, in the HA group, significant differences between scores in the more difficult tasks and easier tasks were found. It supports the thesis that HA individuals differ in information processing between more complex and less complex tasks, and these differences are reflected in neural mechanisms. It is in line with the former findings that anxiety has a negative effect on complex or difficult tasks (Mayer, 1977), and with more recent findings (Horwitz and McCaffrey, 2008; Hartley and Phelps, 2012). It shows that trait anxiety slightly modulates brain activity associated with cognitive processes such as executive functions. For instance, the ability to selectively focus attention on a semantic category, the capacity to monitor recalled words, and/or continuously update the words that have been used. A complex tasks may elicit an uncertainty in anxious people, and this cognitive state may evoke threat-related information processing biases, and results in altered information processing (Hartley and Phelps, 2012). Studies on ambiguity, loss aversion, and risk processing in anxious individuals support the present findings that increased anxiety is associated with involvement of the different cognitive and neural mechanisms in demanding and easier tasks. Association between the difficulty of tasks and trait anxiety may be explained in terms of the cognitive noise thesis; cognitive noise may interfere with working memory (Robinson and Tamir, 2005). Authors of this thesis state that trait anxiety elicits cognitive noise which reduces cognitive flexibility in anxious people. On the contrary LA individuals do not exhibit such problems, and this was reflected in our results as lack of differences between scores in difficult and easier tasks.

We did not confirm the differences in scores for the LA and HA groups in non-emotional and emotional tasks; the within-group comparisons did not show any difference, especially in the HA group where negative verbal fluency have higher scores. However, differences in neural activity between emotional and non-emotional tasks within the LA and HA group were found. Our results present greater activation of the prefrontal regions in LA than in HA individuals, as it was hypothesized (the frontal superior gyrus in the "fear" category, and increased activity the frontal superior gyrus and frontal inferior gyrus in verbs). This seems to be linked with better attentional capacities and an unimpaired monitoring process in low-anxious individuals. Trait anxiety reduces such functions by impairing attention and task-switching capacity (Eysenck et al., 2007). Our findings correspond with data presented by low-anxious subjects as found with increased activation in the fronto-parietal networks, while highly anxious individuals showed a particular pattern of increased functioning of the cingulo-opercular and ventral attention (Sylvester et al., 2012). Attentional control theory presents the idea that anxious individuals show weaker, and insufficient or stronger (supposedly compensatory) neural activation in brain regions supporting attention (Basten et al., 2012). Greater activation of the frontal regions during verbal fluency tasks in the LA group, and lower activation of these regions in the HA group may reflect not-impaired attention, better working memory and information processing in LA individuals. Low anxiety does not involve perturbed attention allocation in appraisal (Britton et al., 2011), altering in decision, or lack of flexibility (Hartley and Phelps, 2012). Low anxiety is associated with not-impaired executive functions which refer to top-down control of cognitive processes. Increased activity of the frontal regions in group LA suggests that they engage in more effective monitoring, selection, and control of cognitive process (Shimamura, 2002). To perform verbal fluency tasks effectively the ability to selectively focus attention on a semantic category and the ability to "on-line monitor" previously recalled words and continuously update the words are all required. These abilities refer to the directed attentional system which is responsible for top-down control of attention and partly to a stimulus–driven attentional system (because instruction during study changes). These two systems are regulated by the different brain regions; top-down control of attention involves prefrontal regions of the brain, whereas a stimulus–driven attentional system engages the temporo-parietal and ventral frontal cortex (Corbetta and Shulman, 2002). These two systems interact in their functioning (Pashler et al., 2001). Effective attentional capacities require reciprocal influences of each system on the other. Anxiety may impair the balance between these two attentional systems (Corbetta and Shulman, 2002). The possibility of good balance between these systems in LA individuals in our studies is reflected in the increased activation of the frontal regions in the LA group and less differences in neural activity between difficult and easier tasks in this group.

Another noteworthy element is the fact that low-anxious individuals seem to use more adequate strategies, and they will activate brain regions which are thought to correspond with these strategies, as it was hypothesized. For example, the prefrontal cortex is thought to be involved in autobiographical memories, it modulates the amygdala-hippocampus network in the initiating, searching, and monitoring of memory (Dolcos et al., 2012). Medial and orbital prefrontal cortex activity is more associated with emotional retrieval (Markowitsch et al., 2003). These parts of the brain are connected with the thalamus to regulate memory and emotions (Barbas, 2000). These parts of the brain were more activated by the low-anxious people during the performance of verbal fluency tasks; verbs and emotional tasks. Furthermore, retrieval of words is linked to the posterior areas such as the parietal and occipital regions associated with the visual-spatial processing of information, including the processing of emotional information (Dolcos et al., 2012). And these regions were activated by the low-anxious people. Moreover, the brain areas typically involved in verbal fluency tasks, such as the middle temporal gyrus (which is thought to be responsible for semantic processing; Birn et al., 2010) and the fusiform gyrus also involved in semantic processing (Ardila et al., 2006; Noppeney, 2008; Pulvermüller, 2013; Ralph, 2014) were more active in the low-anxious individuals during verbal fluency performance. All these differences in activation between the LA and HA groups, as it was expected, support the claim that low trait anxiety enables the use of more adequate neural strategies of retrieval. The possibility that neural activation differences for LA and HA subjects could be due to differences in task-related effort inside the scanner is unlikely because the comparisons between the task condition and baseline condition (which are the indirect measure of effort) show a lot of significant differences. These comparisons show that subjects executed tasks with adequate effort, as we see in the **Table 3**, all activated brain regions are those which are typically activated during verbal fluency performance.

We did not confirm the increased activation of the limbic areas during emotional verbal fluency tasks, with one exception. Only the right thalamus was more activated during the "fear" tasks in LA individuals. The activation of the thalamus in the "fear" tasks may be interpreted in terms of Rolls' concept of the implicit-explicit emotional language. He stated that implicit emotional language is associated with activation of the thalamus, premotor, cingulate, and striatum, while explicit emotional language involves more temporal and frontal areas (Rolls, 1999). Our results show that the negative verbal fluency associated with greater activation of the thalamus, may be thought of as more implicit than the positive category. Higher activation of the amygdala and hippocampus was not found, which may be explained in the light of the recent findings. Involvement of the amygdala in emotional encoding is well-documented, however, its involvement in the retrieval of emotional memories has been difficult to demonstrate (Dolcos et al., 2012). This is because activation of the amygdala also depends on the intensity of emotional retrieval, and retrieved information such as those in our verbal fluency tasks may not be excessively charged. Higher intensity of emotional memories is associated with activation in both the amygdala and hippocampus (Botzung et al., 2010).

As it was hypothesized, our findings also show an important role of the cerebellum during retrieval in LA people. Its activation was greater especially in the difficult tasks such as "vehicles" and "joy." The cerebellum, through the connections with the prefrontal, parietal, temporal, and cingulate cortex, regulates many functions such as episodic memory, imagination, executive functions, as well as language processing (Habas et al., 2009; Stoodley et al., 2012). Our finding is in line with other evidence which shows cerebellar activation in relation to language, attention, affection, emotion, and mental imagery, and that the cerebellum is able to integrate multiple internal representations with external stimuli and self-generated responses. The cerebellar modulation permits the production of harmonious motor, cognitive, and affective behaviors. This is possible because more than half of the cerebellar cortex is interconnected with association zones of the cerebral cortex (Schmahmann and Sherman, 1998). The role of the cerebellum is well-documented, for instance, patients with cerebellar cognitive affective syndrome (which is linked to cerebellar lesions) display deficits in cognitive functioning, spatial cognition, visual-spatial memory, language, personality, and behavioral reactions, as well as affective disturbances ranging from emotional blunting and depression to disinhibition (Mariën et al., 2009). The integrative role of the cerebellum is highlighted by hypothesis of the functional cerebellar-encephalic pathways (Mariën et al., 2009). This concept holds that the cerebellum facilitates an automatic modulation of behavior, and the behavior being modulated is determined by the specificity of anatomic subcircuits within the cerebro-cerebellar system. The posterior cerebellum is involved in cognitive processes when the vermis is thought to be the limbic cerebellum. The cortico-ponto-cerebellar pathways are linked to the adjustment of emotional and cognitive process to situational context (Parvizi et al., 2001). Thus, damage to the cerebellar components of the neural circuits subserving sensorimotor, cognitive, or emotional processing disrupts the universal cerebellar transforming functions and causes the accompanying cognitive-affective deficits (Schmahmann, 2004). This shows that the cerebellum is involved in the emotional congruency, emotional regulation, cognitive flexibility, and working capacities (Annoni et al., 2003).

Greater activation of the cerebellum found in low-anxious people during the difficult verbal fluency tasks may reflect better integration of cognitive and affective capacities in low-anxious individuals, compared to the high-anxious people. In general, individuals with a high level of trait anxiety exhibit a lower level of integration of emotional and cognitive capacities (Öhman, 2008).

LIMITATIONS

The first limitation of this study was the small sample size. Second, potential factors influencing the sex differences in emotionality. We included nearly an identical number of women and men in the HA and LA groups, not find significant sex differences in cognition (by WAIS-R), and sex differences in trait/state anxiety. The results should be however interpreted with caution because of potential not-included factors influencing brain activity, such as menstrual cycle phase which was not taken into account, and might influence female brain activity (Comasco and Sundström-Poromaa, 2015).

CONCLUSION

The above findings confirm that trait anxiety slightly modulates brain activity during the performance of verbal fluency tasks. The acquired evidence shows that trait anxiety has an impact on attention, working memory, and strategies for retrieving information from memory. This impact reflects the differences in the neural mechanisms employed by low-anxious and high-anxious people, and may be observed especially during the performance of the more difficult tasks. Greater activation of the prefrontal regions, the cerebellum and the typical brain areas associated with the kind of verbal fluency task in low-anxious people reflects their better ability to selective focus attention on a semantic category, ability to perform "on-line" monitoring of recalled words, updating and switching capacities. In sum, low-anxious individuals seem to activate more adequate neural strategies of retrieval. Anxiety impairs processing efficiency more than performance effectiveness, thus anxious people may have similar behavioral results but employing information processing strategies different from non-anxious people (Derakshan and Eysenck, 2009). It may suggest that they exhibit the easier use of novel, non-typical strategies, and that they employ sensory-visual strategies more effectively, even in self-referential aspects, in comparison to highly anxious people (Northoff et al., 2006). The presented results highlight the better integration of cognitive and affective capacities in low-anxious individuals.

Our findings increase understanding trait anxiety as incorporated not only in mental organization, but also in neural representation, and as affecting cognitive functioning. They establish verbal fluency tests (with fMRI) as a useful tool in the assessment of brain mechanisms in anxious people, and/or anxiety disorders.

AUTHOR CONTRIBUTIONS

All authors listed, have made substantial, direct and intellectual contribution to the work, and approved it for publication.

ACKNOWLEDGMENTS

The authors would like to thank to dr Tomasz Wolak from Bioimaging Research Center, Institute of Physiology and Pathology of Hearing in Kajetany, and to Pawel Soluch MA from Neuro Device Group Ltd, Warsaw for cooperation and helpful comments on fMRI procedure.

REFERENCES

Albrecht, A., Bergado-Acosta, J. R., Pape, H. S., and Stork, O. (2010). Role of the neural cell adhesion molecule (NCAM) in amygdalo-hippocampal interactions and salience determination of contextual fear memory. *Int. J. Neuropsychopharmacol.* 13, 661–674. doi: 10.1017/S1461145709991106

Albus, M., Hubmann, W., Wahlheim, C., Sobizack, N., Franz, U., and Mohr, F. (1998). Contrast in neuropsychological test profile between patients with first-episode schizophrenia and first-episode affective disorders. *Acta Psychiatr. Scand.* 94, 87–93. doi: 10.1111/j.1600-0447.1996.tb09830.x

Annoni, J. M., Ptak, R., Caldara-Schnetzer, A. S., Khateb, A., and Pollerman, B. Z. (2003). Decoupling of autonomic and cognitive emotional reactions after cerebellar stroke. *Ann. Neurol.* 53, 654–658. doi: 10.1002/ana.10549

Ardila, A., Ostrosky-Solis, F., and Bernd, B. (2006). Cognitive testing toward the future: the example of semantic verbal fluency (Animals). *Int. J. Psychol.* 41, 324–332. doi: 10.1080/00207590500345542

Atchley, R. A., Ilardi, S. S., and Enole, A. (2003). Hemispheric asymmetry in the processing of emotional content in word meanings: the effect of current and past depression. *Brain Lang.* 84, 105–119. doi: 10.1016/S0093-934X(02)00523-0

Audenaert, K., Goethals, L., Van Laere, K., Lahorte, P., Brans, B., Versijpt, J., et al. (2002). SPECT neuropsychological activation procedure with the Verbal Fluency Test in attempted suicide patients. *Nucl. Med. Commun.* 23, 907–916. doi: 10.1097/00006231-200209000-00015

Barbas, H. (2000). Connections underlying the synthesis of cognition, memory, and emotion in primate prefrontal cortices. *Brain Res. Bull.* 52, 319–330. doi: 10.1016/S0361-9230(99)00245-2

Bar-Haim, Y., Lamy, D., Pergamin, L., Bakermans-Kranenburg, M. J., and van Ijzendoorn, M. H. (2007). Threat-related attentional biases in anxious and non-anxious individuals: a meta-analytic study. *Psychol. Bull.* 133, 1–24. doi: 10.1037/0033-2909.133.1.1

Barlow, D. H. (2002). *Anxiety and its Disorders: The Nature and Treatment of Anxiety and Panic.* 2nd Edn. New York, NY: Guilford Press.

Basten, U., Stelzel, C., and Fiebach, C. J. (2012). Trait anxiety and the neural efficiency of manipulation in working memory. *Cogn. Affect. Behav. Neurosci.* 12, 571–588. doi: 10.3758/s13415-012-0100-3

Beats, B. C., Sahakian, B. J., and Levy, R. (1996). Cognitive performance in tests sensitive to frontal lobe dysfunction in the elderly depressed. *Psychol. Med.* 26, 591–603. doi: 10.1017/S0033291700035662

Bertocci, M. A., Bebko, G., Olino, T., Fournier, J., Hinze, A. K., Bonar, L., et al. (2014). Behavioral and emotional dysregulation trajectories marked by prefrontal-amygdala function in symptomatic youth. *Psychol. Med.* 44, 2603–2615. doi: 10.1017/S0033291714000087

Bienvenu, O. J., Brown, C., Samuels, J. F., Liang, K. Y., Costa, P. T., Eaton, W. W., et al. (2001). Normal personality traits and comorbidity among phobic, panic, and major depressive disorders. *Psychiatry Res.* 102, 73–85. doi: 10.1016/S0165-1781(01)00228-1

Birn, R. M., Kenworthy, L., Case, L., Caravella, R., Jones, T. B., Bandettini, P. A., et al. (2010). Neural systems supporting lexical search guided by letter and semantic category cues: a self-paced overt response fMRI study of verbal fluency. *Neuroimage* 49, 1099–1107. doi: 10.1016/j.neuroimage.2009.07.036

Bishop, S. J. (2007). Neurocognitive mechanisms of anxiety: an integrative account. *Trends Cogn. Sci.* 11, 307–316. doi: 10.1016/j.tics.2007.05.008

Bishop, S. J. (2009). Trait anxiety and impoverished prefrontal control of attention. *Nat. Neurosci.* 12, 92–98. doi: 10.1038/nn.2242

Bishop, S. J., Duncan, J., and Lawrence, A. D. (2004). State anxiety modulation of the amygdala response to unattended thread-related stimuli. *J. Neurosci.* 24, 10364–10368. doi: 10.1523/JNEUROSCI.2550-04.2004

Botzung, A., Rubin, D. C., Miles, A., Cabeza, R., and Labar, K. S. (2010). Mental hoop diaries: emotional memories of a college baseketball game in rival fans. *J. Neurosci.* 30, 2130–2137. doi: 10.1523/JNEUROSCI.2481-09.2010

Bremner, J. D., Vermetten, E., Schmahl, C., Vaccarino, V., Vythilingam, M., Afzal, N., et al. (2005). Positron emission tomographic imaging of neural correlates of a fear acquisition and extinction paradigm in women with childhood sexual abuse-related post- traumatic stress disorder. *Psychol. Med.* 35, 791–806. doi: 10.1017/S0033291704003290

Britton, J. C., Lissek, S., Grillon, C., Norcross, M. A., and Pine, D. S. (2011). Development of anxiety: the role of threat appraisal and fear learning. *Depress. Anxiety* 28, 5–17. doi: 10.1002/da.20733

Brzezinski, J., Gaul, M., Hornowska, E., Jaworowska, A., Machowski, A., and Zakrzewska, M. (2004). *Skala Inteligencji D. Wechslera dla Dorosłych. Wersja Zrewidowana – Renormalizacja WAIS –R (PL). [Manual for WAIS-R], (Polished.).* Warszawa: PTP.

Butler, T., Pan, H., Tuescher, O., Engelien, A., Goldstein, M., Epstein, J., et al. (2007). Human fear-related motor circuitry. *Neuroscience* 150, 1–7. doi: 10.1016/j.neuroscience.2007.09.048

Cisler, J. M., and Kostner, E. H. W. (2010). Mechanisms of attentional biases toward threat in anxiety disorders: an integrative review. *Clin. Psychol. Rev.* 30, 203–216. doi: 10.1016/j.cpr.2009.11.003

Comasco, E., and Sundström-Poromaa, I. (2015). Neuroimaging the menstrual cycle and premenstrual dysphoric disorder. *Curr. Psychiatry Rep.* 17, 77. doi: 10.1007/s11920-015-0619-4

Corbetta, M., and Shulman, G. L. (2002). Control of goal-directed and stimulus-driven attention in the brain. *Neuroscience* 3, 201–215. doi: 10.1038/nrn755

Derakshan, N., and Eysenck, M. W. (2009). Anxiety, processing efficiency, and cognitive performance. New developments from attentional control theory. *Eur. Psychol.* 14, 168–176. doi: 10.1027/1016-9040.14.2.168

Derryberry, D., and Reed, A. M. (2002). Anxiety related attentional biases and their regulation by attentional control. *J. Abnorm. Psychol.* 111, 225–236. doi: 10.1037/0021-843X.111.2.225

Dolcos, F., Denkova, E., and Dolcos, S. (2012). Neural correlates of emotional memories: a review of evidence from brain imaging studies. *Psychologia* 55, 80–111. doi: 10.2117/psysoc.2012.80

Endler, N. S., and Kocovski, N. L. (2001). State and trait anxiety revisited. *J. Anxiety Dis.* 15, 231–245. doi: 10.1016/S0887-6185(01)00060-3

Etkin, A., Klemenhagen, K. C., Dudman, J. T., Rogan, M. T., Hen, R., Kandel, E. R., et al. (2004). Individual differences in trait anxiety predict the response of the basolateral amygdala to unconsciously processed fearful faces. *Neuron* 44, 1043–1055. doi: 10.1016/j.neuron.2004.12.006

Etkin, A., and Wager, T. D. (2007). Functional neuroimaging of anxiety: a meta-analysis of emotional processing in PTSD, social anxiety disorders, and specific phobia. *Am. J. Psychiatry* 164, 1476–1488. doi: 10.1176/appi.ajp.2007.07030504

Eysenck, M. W., Derakshan, N., Santos, R., and Calvo, M. G. (2007). Anxiety and cognitive performance: attentional control theory. *Emotion* 7, 336–353. doi: 10.1037/1528-3542.7.2.336

Fossati, P., Guillaum Le, B., Ergis, A. M., and Allilaire, J. F. (2003). Qualitative analysis of verbal fluency in depression. *Psychiatry Res.* 117, 17–24. doi: 10.1016/S0165-1781(02)00300-1

Gabrieli, J. D. E., Poldrack, R. A., and Desmond, J. E. (1998). The role of left prefrontal cortex in language and memory. *Proc. Natl. Acad. Sci. U.S.A.* 95, 906–913. doi: 10.1073/pnas.95.3.906

Garoff, R., Slotnick, S., and Schacter, D. (2005). The neural origins of specific and general memory: the role of the fusiform cortex. *Neuropsychologia* 43, 848–859. doi: 10.1016/j.neuropsychologia.2004.09.014

Goldberg, E., Roediger, D., Kucukboyaci, N. E., Carlson, C., Devinsky, O., Kuzniecky, R., et al. (2013). Hemispheric asymmetries of cortical volume of human brain. *Cortex* 49, 200–210. doi: 10.1016/j.cortex.2011.11.002

Grillon, C., Baas, J. P., Lissek, S., Smith, K., and Milstein, J. (2004). Anxious responses to predictable and unpredictable aversive events. *Behav. Neurosci.* 118, 916–924. doi: 10.1037/0735-7044.118.5.916

Haas, B. W., Omura, K., Constable, R. T., and Canli, T. (2007). Emotional conflict and neuroticism: personality dependent activation in the amygdala and subgenual anterior cingulate. *Behav. Neurosci.* 21, 249–256. doi: 10.1037/0735-7044.121.2.249

Habas, C., Komdor, N., Nguyen, D., Proter, K., Beckmann, C. F., Menon, V., et al. (2009). Distinct cerebellar contributions to intrinsic connectivity networks. *J. Neurosci.* 29, 8586–8594. doi: 10.1523/JNEUROSCI.1868-09.2009

Hartley, C. A., and Phelps, E. A. (2010). Changing fear: the neurocircuitry of emotion regulation. *Neuropsychopharmacology* 35, 136–146. doi: 10.1038/npp.2009.121

Hartley, C. A., and Phelps, E. A. (2012). Anxiety and decision making. *Biol. Psychiatry* 72, 113–118. doi: 10.1016/j.biopsych.2011.12.027

Hofmann, S. G. (2008). Cognitive processes during fear acquisition and extinction in animals and humans. *Clin. Psychol. Rev.* 28, 199–210. doi: 10.1016/j.cpr.2007.04.009

Horwitz, J. E., and McCaffrey, R. J. (2008). Effects of a third party observer and anxiety on tests of executive function. *Arch. Clinic. Neuropsychol.* 23, 409–417. doi: 10.1016/j.acn.2008.02.002

Indovina, I., Robbins, T. W., Núñez-Elizalde, A., Dunn, B., and Bishop, S. J. (2011). Fear conditioning mechanisms associated with trait vulnerability to anxiety. *Neuron* 69, 563–571. doi: 10.1016/j.neuron.2010.12.034

Kim, M. J., and Wallen, P. J. (2009). The structural integrity of an amygdala-prefrontal pathway predicts trait anxiety. *J. Neurosci.* 29, 11614–11618. doi: 10.1523/JNEUROSCI.2335-09.2009

Kindt, M. (2014). A behavioural neuroscience perspective on the aetiology and treatment of anxiety disorders. *Behav. Res. Ther.* 62, 24–36. doi: 10.1016/j.brat.2014.08.012

Knight, D. C., Waters, N. S., and Bandettini, P. A. (2009). Neural substrates of explicit and implicit fear memory. *Neuroimage* 45, 208–214. doi: 10.1016/j.neuroimage.2008.11.015

Krain, A. L., Wilson, A. M., Arbuckle, R., Castellanos, F. X., and Milham, M. P. (2006). Distinct neural mechanisms of risk and ambiguity: a meta-analysis of decision making. *Neuroimage* 32, 477–484. doi: 10.1016/j.neuroimage.2006.02.047

Larsson, M. R., Per-Olof, M., Backström, M., and Johanson, A. (2007). Baseline verbal fluency performance as predictor of state anxiety during a life hand-grenade throwing exercise – A prospective study of Swedish military conscripts. *Behav. Brain Funct.* 3:39. doi: 10.1186/1744-9081-3-39

Lemche, E., Surguladze, S. A., Brammer, M. J., Phillips, M. L., Sierra, M., David, A. S., et al. (2013). Dissociable brain correlates for depression, anxiety, dissociation, and somatization in depersonalization-derealization disorder. *CNS Spectr.* 1–8. doi: 10.1017/S1092852913000588. [Epub ahead of print].

Lissek, S., Power, A. S., McClure, E. B., Phelps, E. A., Woldehavariat, G., Grillon, C., et al. (2005). Classical fear conditioning in the anxiety disorders: a meta-analysis. *Behav. Res. Ther.* 43, 1391–1424. doi: 10.1016/j.brat.2004.10.007

Lissek, S., Rabin, S., Heller, R. E., Lukenbaugh, D., Geraci, M., Pine, D. S., et al. (2010). Overgeneralization of conditioned fear as a pathologic marker of panic disorder. *Am. J. Psychiatry* 167, 47–55. doi: 10.1176/appi.ajp.2009.09030410

Liu, X., Sun, G., Zhang, X., Xu, B., Shen, C., Shi, L., et al. (2014). Relationship between the prefrontal function and severity of the emotional symptoms during verbal fluency task in patients with major depressive disorder: a multi-channel NIRS study. *Prog. Neuropsychopharmacol. Biol. Psychiatry* 54, 114–121. doi: 10.1016/j.pnpbp.2014.05.005

Mariën, P., Baillieux, H., De Smet, H. J., Engelborghs, S., Wilssens, I., Paquier, P., et al. (2009). Cognitive, linguistic and affective disturbances following a right superior cerebellar artery infarction: a case study. *Cortex* 45, 527–536. doi: 10.1016/j.cortex.2007.12.010

Markowitsch, H. J., Vandekerckhove, M. M., Lanfermann, H., and Russ, M. (2003). Engagement of lateral and medial prefrontal areas in the ecphory of sad and happy autobiographical memories. *Cortex* 39, 643–665. doi: 10.1016/S0010-9452(08)70858-X

Mayer, R. E. (1977). Problem solving performance with task-overload: effect of self-pacing and trait anxiety. *Bull. Psychonomic Soc.* 9, 283–286. doi: 10.3758/BF03337000

Mineka, S., and Zinbarg, R. (2006). A contemporary learning theory perspective on the etiology of anxiety disorders – It's not what you thought it was. *Am. J. Psychol.* 61, 10–26. doi: 10.1037/0003-066X.61.1.10

Morgan, M. A., Romanski, L. M., and LeDoux, J. E. (1993). Extinction of emotional learning: contribution of medial prefrontal cortex. *Neurosci. Lett.* 163, 109–113. doi: 10.1016/0304-3940(93)90241-C

Most, S. B., Chun, M. M., Johnson, M. R., and Kiehl, K. A. (2006). Attentional modulation of amygdala varies with personality. *Neuroimage* 31, 934–944. doi: 10.1016/j.neuroimage.2005.12.031

Myers, K. M., and Davis, M. (2002). Behavioural and neural analysis of extinction. *Neuron* 36, 567–584. doi: 10.1016/S0896-6273(02)01064-4

Noppeney, U. (2008). The neural systems of tool and action semantics: a perspective from functional imaging. *J. Physiol. Paris* 102, 40–49. doi: 10.1016/j.jphysparis.2008.03.009

Northoff, G., Heinzel, A., de Greck, M., Bermpohl, F., Dobrowolny, H., and Panksepp, J. (2006). Self-referential processing in our brain—A meta-analysis of imaging studies on the self. *Neuroimage* 31, 440–457. doi: 10.1016/j.neuroimage.2005.12.002

Öhman, A. (2008). "Fear and anxiety: overlaps and dissociations," in *Handbook of Psychology*, eds M. Lewis, J. M. Haviland- Jones, and L. F. Barrett (New York, NY; London: The Guilford Press), 709–729.

Öhman, A., Flykt, A., and Lundqvist, D. (2000). "Unconscious emotion: evolutionary perspectives, psychophysiological data, and neuropsychological mechanisms," in *The Cognitive Neuroscience of Emotion*, eds R. Lane and L. Nadel (New York, NY: Oxford University Press), 296–327.

Oldfield, R. C. (1971). The assessment and analysis of handedness: the Edinburgh inventory. *Neuropsychologia* 9, 97–113. doi: 10.1016/0028-3932(71)90067-4

Olsson, A., Nearing, K. I., and Phelps, E. A. (2007). Learning fears by observing others: the neural system of social fear transmission. *Soc. Cogn. Affect. Neurosci.* 2, 3–11. doi: 10.1093/scan/nsm005

Parvizi, J., Anderson, S. W., Martin, C. O., Damasio, H., and Damasio, A. R. (2001). Pathological laughter and crying. A link to the cerebellum. *Brain* 124, 1708–1719. doi: 10.1093/brain/124.9.1708

Pashler, H., Johnston, J. C., and Ruthroff, E. (2001). Attention and performance. *Annu. Rev. Psychol.* 52, 629–651. doi: 10.1146/annurev.psych.52.1.629

Paulus, M. P., and Stein, M. B. (2010). Interoception in anxiety and depression. *Brain Struct. Funct.* 214, 451–463. doi: 10.1007/s00429-010-0258-9

Peters, J., Kalivas, P. W., and Quirk, G. J. (2009). Extinction circuits for fear and addiction overlap in prefrontal cortex. *Learn. Mem.* 16, 279–288. doi: 10.1101/lm.1041309

Phelps, E. A., Delgado, M. R., Nearing, K. I., and LeDoux, J. E. (2004). Extinction learning in humans: role of amygdala and vmPFC. *Neuron* 43, 897–905. doi: 10.1016/j.neuron.2004.08.042

Phelps, E. A., O'Connor, K. J., Gatenby, J. C., Gore, J. C., Grillon, C., and Davis, M. (2001). Activation of the left amygdala to a cognitive representation of fear. *Nat. Neurosci.* 4, 437–441. doi: 10.1038/86110

Pulvermüller, F. (2013). How neurons make meaning: brain mechanisms for embodied and abstract - symbolic semantics. *Trends Cogn. Sci.* 17, 458–470. doi: 10.1016/j.tics.2013.06.004

Ralph, M. (2014). Neurocognitive insights on conceptual knowledge and its breakdown. *Philos. Trans. R. Soc. B Biol. Sci.* 369, 20120392. doi: 10.1098/rstb.2012.0392

Rauch, S. L., Milad, M. R., Orr, S. P., Quinn, B. T., Fischl, B., and Pitman, R. K. (2005). Orbitofrontal thickness, retension of fear extinction, and extraversion. *Neuroreport* 16, 1909–1912. doi: 10.1097/01.wnr.0000186599.66243.50

Rende, B., Ramsberger, G., and Miyake, A. (2002). Commonalities and differences in the working memory components underlying letter and category fluency tasks: a dual-tasks investigation. *Neuropsychology* 16, 309–321. doi: 10.1037/0894-4105.16.3.309

Robinson, M. D., and Tamir, M. (2005). Neuroticism as mental noise: relation between neuroticism and reaction time standard deviations. *J. Pers. Soc. Psychol.* 89, 107–114. doi: 10.1037/0022-3514.89.1.107

Rolls, E. T. (1999). *The Brain and Emotion*. Oxford: Oxford University Press.

Rosen, M. V., and Engle, R. W. (1997). The role of working memory capacity in retrieval. *J. Exp. Psychol. Gen.* 126, 211–227. doi: 10.1037/0096-3445.126.3.211

Ross, T. (2003). The reliability cluster and switch scores for the Controlled Oral Word Association Test. *Arch. Clin. Neuropsychol.* 18, 153–164. doi: 10.1093/arclin/18.2.153

Ross, T. P., Calhoun, E., Cox, T., Wenner, C., Kono, W., and Pleasant, M. (2007). The reliability and validity of qualitative scores for the Controlled Oral Word Association Test. *Arch. Clin. Neuropsychol.* 22, 475–488. doi: 10.1016/j.acn.2007.01.026

Rossell, S. (2006). Category fluency performance in patients with schizophrenia and bipolar disorder: the influence of affective categories. *Schizophr. Res.* 82, 135–138. doi: 10.1016/j.schres.2005.10.013

Schiller, D., Levy, I., Niv, Y., LeDoux, J. E., and Phelps, E. A. (2008). From fear to safety and back: reversal of fear in the human brain. *J. Neurosci.* 28, 11517–11525. doi: 10.1523/JNEUROSCI.2265-08.2008

Schmahmann, J. D. (2004). Disorders of the cerebellum: ataxia, dysmetria of thought, and the cerebellar cognitive affective syndrome. *J. Neuropsychiatry Clin. Neurosci.* 16, 367–378. doi: 10.1176/jnp.16.3.367

Schmahmann, J. D., and Sherman, J. C. (1998). The cerebellar cognitive affective syndrome. *Brain* 121, 561–579. doi: 10.1093/brain/121.4.561

Schmidt, N. B., Mitchell, M. A., and Richey, J. A. (2008). Anxiety sensitivity as an incremental predictor of later anxiety symptoms and syndromes. *Compr. Psychiatry* 49, 407–412. doi: 10.1016/j.comppsych.2007.12.004

Schmitz, T. W., Kawahara-Baccus, T. N., and Johnson, S. C. (2004). Metacognitive evaluation, self-relevance, and the right prefrontal cortex. *Neuroimage* 22, 941–947. doi: 10.1016/j.neuroimage.2004.02.018

Sehlmeyer, C., Dannlowski, U., Schöning, S., Kugel, H., Pyka, M., Pfleiderer, B., et al. (2011). Neural correlates of trait anxiety in fear extinction. *Psychol. Med.* 41, 789–798. doi: 10.1017/S0033291710001248

Sehlmeyer, C., Schöning, S., Zwitserlood, P., Pfleiderer, B., Kircher, T., Arold, V., et al. (2009). Human fear conditioning and extinction in neuroimaging: a systematic review. *PLoS ONE* 4:e5865. doi: 10.1371/journal.pone.0005865

Shimamura, P. A. (2000). The role of prefrontal cortex in dynamic filtering. *Psychobiology* 28, 208–218. doi: 10.3758/BF03331979

Shimamura, P. A. (2002). "Memory retrieval and executive control processes," in *Principles of Frontal Lobe Function*, eds D. T. Struss and R. T. Knight (New York, NY: Oxford University Press), 210–220.

Somerville, L. H., Whalen, P. J., and Kelley, W. M. (2010). Human bed nucleus of the stria terminalis indexes hypervigilant threat monitoring. *Biol. Psychiatry* 68, 416–424. doi: 10.1016/j.biopsych.2010.04.002

Spielberger, C. D. (1979). *Understanding Stress and Anxiety*. London: Harper & Row.

Spielberger, C. D., Gorsuch, R. L., and Lushene, R. E. (1970). *Manual for the State- Trait Anxiety Inventory (STAI)*. Palo Alto, CA: Consulting Psychologists Press.

Steinfurth, E. C. K., Kanen, J. W., Raio, C. M., Clem, R. M., Huganir, R. L., and Phelps, E. A. (2014). Young and old Pavlovian fear memories can be modified with extinction training during reconsolidation in humans. *Learn. Mem.* 21, 338–341. doi: 10.1101/lm.033589.113

Stoodley, C. J., Valera, E. M., and Schmahmam, J. D. (2012). Functional topography of the cerebellum for motor and cognitive tasks: an fMRI study. *Neuroimage* 59, 1560–1570. doi: 10.1016/j.neuroimage.2011.08.065

Strauss, E., Sherman, E., and Sprenn, O. (1998). *A Compendium of Neuropsychological Tests: Administration, Norms, and Commentary*. Oxford: Oxford University Press.

Styczek, I. (1983). *Logopedia*. Warszawa: PWN.

Sutin, A. R., Terracizno, A., Kitner-Triolo, M. H., Uda, M., Schlessinger, D., and Zonderman, A. B. (2011). Personality traits prospectively predict verbal fluency in a life span sample. *Psychol. Aging* 26, 994–999. doi: 10.1037/a0024276

Sylvester, C. M., Corbetta, M., Raichle, M. E., Rodebaugh, T. L., Schlaggar, B. L., Sheline, Y. I., et al. (2012). Functional network dysfunction in anxiety and anxiety disorders. *Trends Neurosci.* 35, 527–536. doi: 10.1016/j.tins.2012.04.012

Tabert, M. H., Peery, S., Borod, J. C., Schmidt, M., Grunwald, I., and Sliwinski, M. (2001). Lexical emotional expression across the life span: quantitative and qualitative analyses of word list generation tasks. *Clin. Neuropsychol.* 15, 531–550. doi: 10.1076/clin.15.4.531.1876

Tzourio-Mazoyer, N., Landeau, B., Papathanassiou, D., Crivello, F., Etard, O., Delcroix, N., et al. (2002). Automated anatomical labeling of activation in SPM using a macroscopic anatomical parcellation of the MNI MRI single-subject brain. *Neuroimage* 15, 273–289. doi: 10.1006/nimg.2001.0978

Wrześniewski, K., Sosnowski, T., and Matusik, D. (2002). *Inwentarz Stanu i Cechy Lêku. (State and Trait Anxiety Inventory – STAI Spielberger).* Warszawa: PTP.

Conflict of Interest Statement: The authors declare that the research was conducted in the absence of any commercial or financial relationships that could be construed as a potential conflict of interest.

10

Delay Discounting without Decision-Making: Medial Prefrontal Cortex and Amygdala Activations Reflect Immediacy Processing and Correlate with Impulsivity and Anxious-depressive Traits

Vera U. Ludwig[1,2†], Corinna Nüsser[3,4†], Thomas Goschke[4], Dina Wittfoth-Schardt[5,6], Corinde E. Wiers[1,2], Susanne Erk[1], Björn H. Schott[1,7‡] and Henrik Walter[1,2‡]*

[1] Division of Mind and Brain Research, Department of Psychiatry and Psychotherapy, Charité Universitätsmedizin Berlin, Berlin, Germany, [2] Berlin School of Mind and Brain, Humboldt Universität zu Berlin, Berlin, Germany, [3] Division of Medical Psychology, University of Bonn, Bonn, Germany, [4] Department of Psychology, Technische Universität Dresden, Dresden, Germany, [5] Institute of Neuroradiology, Hannover Medical School, Hannover, Germany, [6] NICA—NeuroImaging and Clinical Applications, Hannover, Germany, [7] Leibniz-Institute for Neurobiology, Magdeburg, Germany

Edited by:
Raymond C. K. Chan,
Chinese Academy of Sciences, China

***Correspondence:**
Björn H. Schott
bjoern.schott@med.ovgu.de

†These authors have contributed equally to this work.

‡These authors share senior authorship.

Humans value rewards less when these are delivered in the future as opposed to immediately, a phenomenon referred to as delay discounting. While delay discounting has been studied during the anticipation of rewards and in the context of intertemporal decision-making, little is known about its neural correlates in the outcome phase (during reward delivery) and their relation to personality. Personality traits that have been associated with increased delay discounting include impulsivity and, potentially, anxious-depressive traits. Here we performed functional magnetic resonance imaging (fMRI) in 72 healthy participants while they carried out a monetary incentive delay (MID) task with a delay manipulation. In sixty percent of the experimental trials, participants won rewards that differed in magnitude (0.05€, 0.50€ or 1€) and delay until delivery (immediately, 10 days, or 100 days). A factor analysis on questionnaires yielded two factors reflecting Impulsivity and Anxiety/Depression, which we used to examine potential relationships between personality and delay discounting. When winning a reward, medial prefrontal cortex (mPFC) activation was higher for immediate compared to delayed rewards. Moreover, amygdala activation correlated with reward magnitude for immediate but not for delayed rewards. Amygdala activation to winning immediate rewards was higher in more impulsive participants, while mPFC activation to winning immediate rewards was higher in more anxious-depressed participants. Our results uncover neural correlates of delay discounting during reward delivery, and suggest that impulsivity and subclinical anxious-depressive traits are related to stronger neural responses for winning immediate relative to delayed rewards.

Keywords: reward, delay discounting, impulsivity, individual differences, fMRI, amygdala, prefrontal cortex

INTRODUCTION

Animals and humans typically prefer immediate over delayed rewards, even if the latter are of larger absolute value (Rachlin and Green, 1972; Mischel and Underwood, 1974; Ainslie, 1975; Mazur, 1988; Dshemuchadse et al., 2013). The phenomenon of *delay discounting* is evident in daily decisions like food choices or smoking behavior and poses a challenge to health education. To elucidate neural mechanisms of delay discounting, several studies have adapted delay discounting paradigms to functional magnetic resonance imaging (fMRI; for recent reviews, see Peters and Büchel, 2011; van den Bos and McClure, 2013). For this purpose, most previous studies worked with experimental designs that involved decisions between two rewards that differed in magnitude and delay until delivery (McClure et al., 2004, 2007; Kable and Glimcher, 2007, 2010). While this approach has yielded important insights into the neural basis of delay discounting, it has two limitations. First, decision-making is likely to engage several different cognitive processes, most prominently the valuation of rewards and action selection processes (see Rangel et al., 2008; Liu et al., 2012), and the commonly employed choice paradigms do not allow one to distinguish between these subprocesses. Second, framing effects, as proposed by cognitive delay discounting theories (Trope and Liberman, 2003; Zauberman and Lynch, 2005), may occur because valuation of one option is always affected by an available alternative (Marjorie, 1993).

Because the decision component of delay discounting may cognitively resemble other decision-making processes, the unique properties of delay discounting might actually lie in the valuation component. Valuation automatically occurs whenever humans encounter stimuli in their environment (Lebreton et al., 2009). Few studies so far have been specifically directed at the dissociation of valuation and decision-making components within delay discounting. In a two-phase paradigm employed by Liu et al. (2012), participants first evaluated two options (one immediate, one delayed; i.e., valuation phase), and made their decisions only in the second phase. In the valuation phase only, activation in ventromedial prefrontal cortex (vmPFC), ventral striatum (VS), and posterior cingulate cortex correlated with value, while the decision-making phase engaged lateral prefrontal cortices. However, given the study design participants may already have engaged in decision-making during the first phase of a trial. The safest way to exclude decision-making all together is to only present one option at a time, for example by using a monetary incentive delay (MID) task (Knutson et al., 2001a). Luo et al. (2009) adapted the MID task to study delay discounting (see also Luo et al., 2011). At the beginning of each trial, a cue predicting either an immediate reward or a delayed reward (e.g., $28 in 4 months) was presented, and participants could win the reward by responding to a target. The authors found that brain regions implicated in value processing (e.g., putamen, anterior insula) responded more strongly to immediate vs. delayed rewards, even though the immediate and the delayed rewards were preference-matched. Since only one reward was anticipated at a time, activation differences could only reflect valuation or motivational processes, but not decision-making.

Luo et al. (2009) focused on the effects of delay discounting during reward anticipation. One may argue, however, that valuation does not only occur during anticipation, but also in the outcome phase when participants have overcome the uncertainty inherent in the anticipation phase. Knutson et al. (2001b) showed that, in healthy young adults, anticipation and delivery of rewards engage largely distinct neural processes, with the VS/nucleus accumbens (NAcc) responding to cues signaling an upcoming reward, while the delivery of a previously anticipated reward is primarily associated with activation of regions in the medial prefrontal cortex (mPFC; see also Knutson et al., 2003; Schott et al., 2007). Given the role of the mPFC in coding stimulus value and personal preferences (Knutson et al., 2005; Ludwig et al., 2014; Lin et al., 2015), it seems important to consider the outcome phase when investigating the valuation component of delay discounting. In the present study, we used a variant of the MID task, but, unlike Luo et al. (2009), who only reported the neural correlates of delay discounting during reward anticipation, we focused our analyses on the outcome phase.

While high degrees of delay discounting can be observed in a number of neuropsychiatric disorders like drug addiction (Kirby and Petry, 2004; Mitchell et al., 2005), pathological gambling (Petry, 2001; Alessi and Petry, 2003), ADHD (Scheres et al., 2006, 2008), or Cluster B personality disorders (e.g., Petry, 2002), delay discounting is also subject to considerable interindividual variability within the healthy population (Odum, 2011). Despite the heterogeneity of models of personality (e.g., Costa and McCrae, 1992a; Cloninger et al., 1993), a few personality traits are widely accepted, and their corresponding constructs can be found in most established models. Among those traits, impulsivity in particular has repeatedly been associated with behavioral and neural measures of delay discounting. Impulsivity can be broadly defined as the tendency to act on arising impulses without much thinking or planning, and it is likely to be a complex, multifaceted construct (Patton et al., 1995; Evenden, 1999). A particularly strong preference for immediate compared to delayed rewards (i.e., high delay discounting) is thought to be a key feature of impulsivity. Indeed, tasks of intertemporal decision-making have consistently demonstrated a positive relationship between impulsivity and delay discounting (but see Reynolds et al., 2006; de Wit et al., 2007; Mobini et al., 2007; Koff and Lucas, 2011), in line with the increased delay discounting rates in psychiatric disorders associated with high impulsivity (e.g., Petry, 2002). At the neural level, Sripada et al. (2011) showed that more impulsive participants exhibited reduced anterior mPFC activation during decisions that involved one immediate option as compared to decisions involving only delayed options (see also Hariri et al., 2006; Luhmann et al., 2008; Jimura et al., 2013).

Another important construct widely accepted as a personality trait is the (subclinical) presence of anxious and depressive symptoms, both of which contribute to concepts like neuroticism (NEO-Five Factor Inventory [NEO-FFI]; Costa and McCrae, 1992a) or harm avoidance (Temperament and Character Inventory [TCI]; Cloninger, 1994). While impulsivity has rather consistently been linked to high delay discounting rates, a potential relationship between anxious-depressive traits and delay discounting has thus far received little attention. One study has found that individuals high on social anxiety demonstrate higher delay discounting rates than those low on social anxiety (Rounds et al., 2007). More generally, psychiatric disorders involving anxiety or depression have been associated with altered reward processing (Elman et al., 2005; Tremblay et al., 2005; Hopper et al., 2008; Sailer et al., 2008; Aupperle and Paulus, 2010). It is therefore conceivable that subclinical anxious-depressive traits may affect neural or behavioral manifestations of delay discounting, although it is not straightforward to predict the direction of the correlation: While models of approach vs. avoidance might predict, if at all, lower delay discounting in anxious or depressed individuals, the study by Rounds et al. (2007) suggests stronger delay discounting effects in more anxious-depressed individuals.

In the present study we investigate the neural underpinnings of delay discounting without decision-making in the outcome phase and further assess how individual differences in impulsivity and anxious-depressive traits relate to those neural processes. In our MID-paradigm participants could win rewards that differed in both magnitude and delay until delivery. The paradigm also included a behavioral measure: on each trial participants had to carry out a simple classification task in order to have the chance to gain a reward. Reaction times (RTs) during this task served as an indicator of participants' incentive motivation to obtain each specific reward.

Neuroanatomically, we focused on the VS, mPFC, and amygdala because these regions have been commonly associated with reward and emotional processing (Knutson et al., 2001a,b, 2003; Hommer et al., 2003; Heekeren et al., 2007; Plichta et al., 2009; Schardt et al., 2010); and activation in mPFC (Sripada et al., 2011) and in the VS (McClure et al., 2004) have specifically been linked to the processing of the immediacy of rewards (**Table 1**). We hypothesized: (i) a main effect of reward magnitude on the VS and mPFC (in line with previous findings) and (ii) a main effect of delay on the VS, the mPFC, and the amygdala in that these regions would show increased activation during winning immediate (compared to delayed) rewards ("immediacy effect"). We further hypothesized (iii) an interaction of delay and reward magnitude that was thought to reflect a stronger magnitude effect for immediate (compared to delayed) rewards.

We further aimed to assess to what extent individual differences in impulsivity and anxious-depressive traits might correlate with the differences of neural responses to immediate vs. delayed rewards. With respect to impulsivity, we hypothesized that (iv) more impulsive participants would show stronger activation in the VS or amygdala—and possibly reduced activation in the mPFC—when winning immediate (compared to delayed) rewards, as compared to less impulsive participants (e.g., Mobini et al., 2007). Regarding anxious-depressive traits, we also expected to find (v) a correlation between these traits and neural effects of immediacy during outcome although we had no specific hypotheses about the direction.

Behaviorally, we expected participants to show shorter RTs to both larger and immediate rewards compared to smaller and delayed rewards, respectively (i.e., main effects of magnitude and delay, as well as potentially an interaction of magnitude × delay). Moreover, we expected that the effect of delay would be associated with longer RTs in more impulsive individuals, while we had no directional hypothesis with respect to RTs in participants with anxious-depressive traits.

MATERIALS AND METHODS

Participants

Our study cohort consisted of seventy-two young (mean age = 23.10, range 20–29, SD = 2.23) healthy, right-handed, volunteers (35 female) recruited from the campus community of the University of Bonn, Germany. Eight additional participants were excluded from data analysis due to poor quality of the fMRI data and/or excessive movement during MRI acquisition (n = 4), incidental pathological findings in T1-weighted MR images (n = 3), and a defective anatomical image (n = 1). In all analyses involving questionnaires, we included only the 62 participants with complete data sets. In all other analyses, we included all 72 participants (62 with complete datasets + 10 with partly missing questionnaire data). All participants had normal or corrected-to-normal vision and were native speakers of German. None of the participants reported any current or past neurological, psychiatric, or medical illness (including alcohol or illegal drug abuse), or use of medication affecting cerebral blood flow or brain metabolism. Thirty-three of the participants were smokers. The study was approved by the University of Bonn Ethics Committee, and written informed consent was obtained from each participant in accordance with the Declaration of Helsinki. Participants received financial compensation for their participation.

Behavioral Paradigm and Experimental Design

Participants carried out a variant of the MID task, allowing the assessment of blood-oxygen-level dependent (BOLD) responses to reward anticipation and outcome (**Figure 1**). Each participant was first provided with both written and verbal task instructions and performed a short training version of the experiment outside the scanner to minimize learning effects during the experiment and to ensure compliance with the procedure.

At the beginning of each trial, one of nine possible rewards (3 amounts [1€, 0.50€, 0.05€] × 3 payoff times [immediately, in 10 days, in 100 days]) was presented as an abstract image cue for 1.5 s (anticipation; **Figure 1**). The reward cue was followed by a delay period during which a fixation cross was presented for 3 s. After the delay, a symbol was presented on the screen, and participants were instructed to classify it as a square or a triangle by pressing a button with their left or right index finger (counterbalanced across participants). Squares and triangles were presented in randomized order. RTs were recorded as a behavioral measure of incentive motivation. If the button press was carried out correctly and within 1.5 s after target onset,

TABLE 1 | Regions of interest (ROIs).

ROI	Type and origin of the ROI	Motivation for selecting the ROI
mPFC	ROI from the Stanford atlas of functional ROIs (Shirer et al., 2012)	- implicated in the outcome phase of MID tasks (Knutson et al., 2001b, 2003) - associated with impulsivity (e.g., Sripada et al., 2011)
VS	Combined anatomical and literature-based ROI (Zweynert et al., 2011)	- a key region for reward processing (Heekeren et al., 2007; Staudinger et al., 2011) - associated with impulsivity (e.g., Jimura et al., 2013)
Amygdala	Anatomical ROI from the AAL atlas as implemented in the WFU Pickatlas (Maldjian et al., 2003)	- a key region for reward processing and emotional processing (e.g., Hommer et al., 2003; Plichta et al., 2009; Schardt et al., 2010; Patin and Hurlemann, 2011), - associated with impulsivity (e.g., Shao et al., 2013).

An illustration of the location and extent of the ROIs can be found in Supplementary Table S1.

participants had a 60% chance of winning the anticipated reward. Participants were informed that their RTs had no influence on their chance of winning a reward, as long as the response occurred within 1.5 s. Reward delivery (win trial) or omission (omission trial) was indicated by a feedback, which was presented for another 2 s (outcome period). In win trials, the outcome screen confirmed the anticipated reward and delay in written words, while in omission trials the outcome screen stated "no win". Omission trials were included in the experimental design to prevent habituation and decreasing attention, and to minimize the correlation between the anticipation phase and the win-outcome phase. Each trial lasted 8 s. Trials were presented in a randomized order and separated by a variable inter-trial interval (range 1–6.4 s). The experiment consisted of two runs, each lasting about 23 min with a total number of 234 trials (26 of each condition).

All rewards gained in the "today" win trials were paid to the participants in cash immediately after the experiment. The gains of the "in 10 days" or "in 100 days" win trials were transferred to their bank accounts either 10 or 100 days after the experiment. The *Presentation* software package (Neurobehavioral Systems, CA, USA) was used for stimulus presentation, synchronization of the stimulus display to fMRI data acquisition, and recording of participants' behavioral responses. Stimuli were presented using video goggles (Nordic-Neuro-Lab, Norway). Behavioral responses were recorded via two fiber-optics response pads.

Questionnaire Measures

We used data from several well-established questionnaires testing anxious-depressive and/or impulsive personality traits. Specifically, we included scores from Spielberger's State-Trait Anxiety Inventory (trait score only; STAI-T; German version by Spielberger et al., 1970; Laux et al., 1981), from Beck's Depression Inventory (BDI; Beck et al., 1996; German version by Hautzinger et al., 2000), and from the NEO-FFI (Costa and McCrae, 1992b) in the German translation by

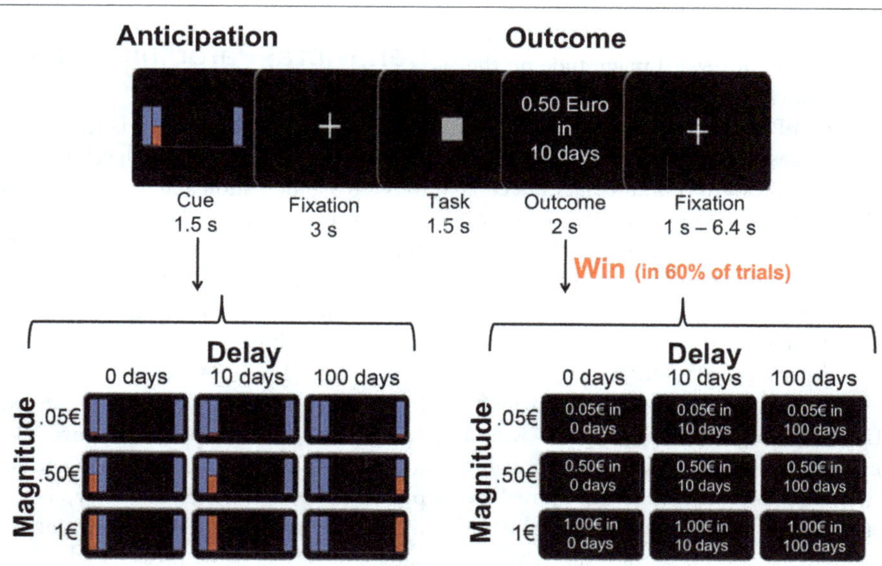

FIGURE 1 | Task and design. Participants were presented with a cue signaling the magnitude of an upcoming reward (0.05€, 0.50€ or 1€) and the delay to delivery (0, 10, or 100 days). After correctly responding to a simple task (classifying squares and triangles), participants were rewarded with the anticipated amount in 60% of trials, and they were informed about the outcome at the end of each trial.

Borkenau and Ostendorf (1993), which includes 60 items. The NEO-FFI contains the subscales neuroticism, extraversion, openness to experience, agreeableness, and conscientiousness. Furthermore, we included data from the TCI by Cloninger (1994; German version by Richter et al., 1999). This scale includes 240 items, but here we were only interested in the three subscales novelty seeking, harm avoidance, and reward dependence, corresponding to 99 items only. Finally, we used the total score of the Barratt Impulsiveness Scale (BIS-11), which consists of 30 items and assesses general impulsivity (BIS-11; Patton et al., 1995).

Factor Analysis of Questionnaire Data

The considerable overlap of the constructs assessed with currently established personality questionnaires like the NEO-FFI or the TCI has been noted by several authors (De Fruyt et al., 2000; Aluja and Blanch, 2011). Because we had no *a priori* hypothesis with respect to which questionnaire would best reflect the intermediate phenotypes of interest and in order to avoid a large number of multiple comparisons, we carried out a factor analysis on the questionnaire data to determine factors that reflected impulsive and axious-depressive traits in our variables (for similar approaches, see Whiteside and Lynam, 2003; Aluja and Blanch, 2011). We initially entered the variables BIS-11 total score, BDI, the 5 NEO-factors, STAI-T, and the 3 TCI-variables. Kaiser-Meyer-Olkin (KMO) measures of sampling adequacy (see Kaiser, 1970) for NEO openness, NEO agreeableness, and TCI reward dependence were lower than 0.50. Therefore, these variables were excluded from the factor analysis. With the remaining 8 variables included, KMO-value for the set of variables was 0.73, indicating that our data were well-suited for factor analysis. Factors were orthogonalized using direct oblimin rotation (delta = 0). Factors with eigenvalues greater than 1 were retained (Kaiser, 1960). Factor scores were calculated for each participant using the regression method. All behavioral and questionnaire data were analyzed using SPSS 19.0 (Chicago, IL, USA) software.

Analysis of the Behavior on the Visual Discrimination Task

First, participants' response accuracy was calculated to ascertain that participants were attentive and motivated during the experiment. Median instead of mean accuracy was calculated across participants because the accuracy data were not normally distributed.

Second, we calculated median RTs for all correct button presses in the visual discrimination task per condition and participant. Median instead of mean RTs were used on the single-subject level because medians are robust to outliers and non-normal distribution. At the group level, RTs did not violate assumptions of a normal distribution (Kolmogorov-Smirnov tests: all $p > 0.10$, Bonferroni-corrected). We therefore analyzed these RTs in all participants ($n = 72$) using a mixed ANOVA with the within-subject factors delay (0 days, 10 days, 100 days) and magnitude (0.05€, 0.50€, 1€). Because the within-subject factors had more than two levels, Greenhouse-Geisser correction for non-sphericity was applied to the degrees of freedom. In order to determine if the factor scores Anxiety-Depression and Impulsivity were systematically related to RTs on the task, in a second step we included these factor scores as covariates (for the 62 participants with complete datasets).

fMRI Data Acquisition and Preprocessing

Functional MRI was acquired using a 1.5T Avanto MRI system (Siemens, Erlangen, Germany). T2*-weighted MR images were acquired with a gradient-echo echoplanar imaging (EPI) sequence (TR = 2000 ms, TE = 50 ms, flip angle = 90°, ascending order). Twenty-three axial slices were collected (thickness 3.3 mm; gap 1.1 mm; field of view 210 mm) using a 4-channel head coil. Slices were oriented parallel to the anterior commissure—posterior commissure line so that they covered the mesolimbic and prefrontal regions of interest (ROI). We also collected a high-resolution T1-weighted magnetization-prepared rapid gradient echo (MP-RAGE) anatomical image (160 sagittal slices covering the whole head; thickness 1 mm; gap 0.5 mm; field of view 256 mm).

Functional MRI data were analyzed using Statistical Parametric Mapping (SPM8, Wellcome Trust Center for Neuroimaging, University College London, London, UK[1]) running on Matlab 7.11.0 (MathWorks, Natick, MA, USA). T2*-weighted EPIs were corrected for acquisition delay and spatially registered to the first acquired image (without reslicing). Each participant's high-resolution anatomical image was co-registered to the mean EPI obtained from realignment and was then segmented into gray matter, white matter, and CSF, using the segmentation algorithm provided by SPM. (*Note*: For three participants, the anatomical image was not obtained in the course of this study. In these cases, we used an anatomical image from the respective participant obtained in the course of a different study, but within 3 months of study time). The transformation parameters obtained from segmentation were used as normalization parameters for transformation of the EPIs into a standard stereotactic reference frame (Montreal Neurological Institute, MNI; voxel size = 3 × 3 × 3 mm). Normalized images were smoothed using an isotropic Gaussian kernel of 8 mm full-width half-maximum. Low frequency drifts were removed using a high pass filter with a cut-off of 128 s during the analysis. Intrinsic autocorrelations were corrected using a restricted maximum likelihood (ReML) algorithm using an autoregressive model of 1st order (AR1).

fMRI Data Analysis

Statistical analysis was performed using a two-stage mixed effects model. At the first stage, general linear model (GLM)-based analyses of brain activity patterns were performed for each participant. For each of the two runs, the GLM included nine regressors for the experimental conditions in the anticipation period (duration: 4.5 s), one regressor for the visual discrimination task (duration: 1.5 s), nine regressors for the "win" outcome periods (duration: 2 s), nine regressors for the "omission" period (duration: 2 s), and one regressor for

[1] www.fil.ion.ucl.ac.uk/spm

outcomes of missed or incorrect responses (duration: 2 s). For all regressors, stick functions at stimulus onset were convolved with the canonical hemodynamic response function (HRF) and down-sampled for each scan. Additionally, the six rigid-body transformation parameters obtained from realignment were included in the model for each session, plus a single constant representing the mean over scans. Model estimation was carried out with a ReML fit, and contrasts of interest were computed over the resulting parameter estimates.

At the second level, contrasts of parameter estimates were submitted to flexible-factorial random effects models. Specifically, we computed two separate second level ANOVA models: one for the anticipation phases, and one for the win-outcome phases. Omission-outcomes were not analyzed further. Nine first-level contrasts for anticipation (all nine conditions against baseline) or nine first-level contrasts for win-outcomes (all nine conditions against baseline) were entered as regressors into these two separate analyses. The reason for contrasting gain outcomes with baseline rather than with omission outcomes was that omissions of expected outcomes would elicit a negative prediction error (Abler et al., 2005) that would depend on the expected value (EV; the product of gain magnitude and probability; see Knutson et al., 2005) and thus on individual task performance. Because we did not include a jitter between cues and feedback stimuli, our design could not account completely for a certain degree of correlation between the anticipation phase and the win outcome phase, but we aimed to minimize this problem by keeping the average gain probability at approximately 60%, and by modeling first degree serial autocorrelations during data analysis (see below).

In these flexible factorial analyses, we specified the factors *delay* (3 levels, independence not assumed, equal variances assumed), *magnitude* (3 levels, independence not assumed, equal variances assumed), and *subject* (72 levels, accounts for task-unrelated between-subject variance, independence assumed, equal variances assumed). For both phases, the regressors in the design matrix were thus: 0.05€ in 0 days, 0.50€ in 0 days, 1€ in 0 days, 0.05€ in 10 days, 0.50€ in 10 days, 1€ in 10 days, 0.05€ in 100 days, 0.50€ in 100 days, and 1€ in 100 days, followed by one regressor per subject.

One-tailed second-level T-contrasts were then computed. In order to validate our study design, we first aimed to replicate results of previous studies by calculating effects of reward magnitude for both anticipation and win outcomes, comparing the highest with the lowest reward in both phases (1€ > 0.05, contrast: [−1 0 1 −1 0 1 -1 0 1]). Previous studies have shown that higher rewards (compared to lower rewards) elicit higher BOLD-signal in VS during anticipation and higher signal in mPFC (and sometimes VS) during win-outcomes (e.g., Knutson et al., 2001a,b; Hommer et al., 2003), and we thus expected to find the same activations if our design worked as intended. After this validation step, we tested our main hypotheses regarding immediacy and delay of rewards, using the following contrasts: effect of immediacy (0 days > 10 days and 100 days) [2 2 2 −1 −1 −1 −1 −1 −1]; effect of a short vs. a long delay (10 days > 100 days) [0 0 0 1 1 1 −1 −1 −1]; interaction of immediacy with magnitude (stronger effect for 1€ > 0.05€ for 0 days compared to 10 and 100 days): [−2 0 2 1 0 −1 1 0 −1]. Even though we were mainly interested in the outcome phase, for completeness we also calculated these contrasts for the anticipation phase.

We focused our analyses on *a priori* defined ROIs using three bilateral masks: (i) VS; (ii) mPFC; and (iii) amygdala (**Table 1**; Supplementary Figure S1). Our ROIs served to spatially constrain our analyses, and for the purpose of family-wise error (FWE)-correction for the respective ROI volumes. The voxel-wise significance level was set to $p < 0.017$, FWE-corrected for the ROI volumes (corresponding to a Bonferroni-corrected 0.05, because small-volume FWE correction was applied to each of the three ROIs separately).

Brain-Behavior Correlations

We then tested for a potential relationship between personality traits (Impulsivity, Anxiety-Depression) and BOLD responses to immediate vs. delayed rewards in the outcome phase. For this purpose, we extracted mean beta values from the regions that showed effects of immediacy at a corrected significance level (either a main effect of immediacy, or an interaction of immediacy × magnitude). To this end, we determined the group peak voxel of the second level contrasts of immediacy or immediacy × magnitude and created a spherical (r = 5 mm) ROI centered around this group peak coordinate. Mean beta values were extracted from all voxels located in this sphere for all participants using the *MarsBaR* ROI analysis toolbox.[2] We then computed the difference between the mean beta over all magnitudes for immediate rewards (0 days) minus the mean beta over all magnitudes for delayed rewards (10 days and 100 days) within these spheres as a neural marker of delay discounting. Next, correlations were computed between this neural measure of immediacy effects and the two factors Anxiety-Depression and Impulsivity (two-tailed testing). Pearson's correlations were used whenever data were normally distributed, and Spearman's correlations were used when data did not meet normal distribution.

RESULTS

Factor Analysis of the Questionnaire Data

Means and standard deviations of all questionnaires are shown in **Table 2**. In all participants, scores of the BDI and STAI-T were below clinical cut-off. Our factor analysis identified two factors in our questionnaire data that explained 70.33% of the total variance (**Table 3**). The first factor, which was termed *Anxiety-Depression* was characterized by positive contributions of NEO—Neuroticism, TCI-Harm Avoidance, STAI-T and BDI and by a negative contribution of NEO—Extraversion. The second factor, henceforth referred to as *Impulsivity*, constituted of high scores in TCI—Novelty Seeking and BIS-11 total and by low scores in NEO—Conscientiousness. To verify the reliability of the thus obtained constructs, we performed the factor analysis in an independent cohort of 125 participants who had completed a largely comparable

[2] http://marsbar.sourceforge.net/

TABLE 2 | Questionnaire data.

Questionnaire	Minimum	Maximum	Mean	*SD*
STAI-T	24	60	38.74	9.64
BDI	0	16	4.23	3.82
NEO—Neuroticism	2	37	18.11	7.73
NEO—Extraversion	14	45	31.48	7.35
NEO—Conscientiousness	12	48	30.89	8.23
TCI—Novelty seeking	1	36	22.02	7.45
TCI—Harm avoidance	0	31	11.42	6.91
BIS-11 (Total)	44	95	66.81	9.76

Descriptive statistics for all questionnaires used in the factor analysis, only for participants who had no missing values and who were therefore included in the factor analysis and in all analyses that involved factor scores (n = 62).

set of questionnaires. We essentially replicated the results of our factor analysis in that cohort (see Supplementary Table S1).

RTs During Task and their Relation to Anxiety-Depression and Impulsivity

Median accuracy for all participants on the task was 99.6% (range 92% – 100%). In the analysis of RTs to the target stimuli, we found a main effect of delay ($F_{(1.95,138.28)} = 12.97$, $p < 0.001$), and magnitude, ($F_{(1.95,138.51)} = 46.81$, $p < 0.001$), but no interaction of delay × magnitude, ($F_{(3.61,256.43)} = 1.12$, $p = 0.35$; **Figure 2**). When including the factor scores Anxiety-Depression and Impulsivity as covariates, there were no main effects of these factors and no interactions between either these factors and delay or magnitude (all $F < 1.10$, all $p > 0.30$), suggesting that neither Anxiety-Depression nor Impulsivity affected RTs. Covarying for smoking status did not change the overall pattern of results.

To follow up the main ANOVA, we carried out four *post hoc* tests to determine the nature of the significant main effects of delay and magnitude (in $n = 72$). We applied a Bonferroni-corrected significance threshold ($\alpha = 0.05/4 = 0.0125$). When testing for the main effect of delay, we found that the mean of the median RTs for immediate rewards were lower than RTs for delayed rewards (10 days, or 100 days, averaged; $T_{71} = 4.81$, $p < 0.0001$). However the mean of the median RTs for 10-days-rewards and 100-days-rewards did not differ ($T_{71} = -0.36$, $p = 0.719$). This indicates that participants

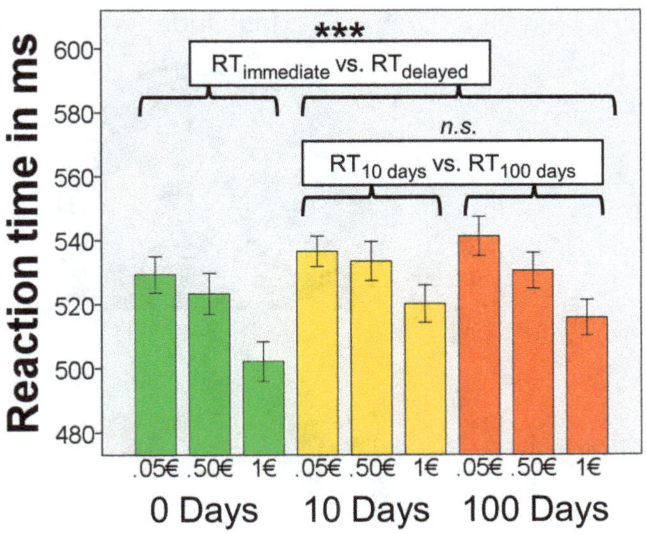

FIGURE 2 | Reaction times (RTs). Means of the median RTs per condition ($n = 72$). There were significant main effects of magnitude and delay, but there was no interaction effect of magnitude × delay. Results of the *post hoc* tests concerning effects of delay are shown in the figure. Error bars denote 95% confidence intervals (C.I.) of the mean, adjusted for within-subject designs (Loftus and Masson, 1994). ***$p < 0.001$.

responded fast for immediate rewards, and slower for delayed rewards irrespective of the period of delay. Magnitude of the reward, on the other hand, affected RTs in a value-dependent fashion, namely the mean of the median RTs for 0.05€ were longer than those for 0.50€ ($T_{71} = 2.84$, $p = 0.006$), and RTs for 0.50€ were longer than those for 1€ ($T_{71} = 6.90$, $p < 0.0001$).

TABLE 3 | Pattern matrix from the factor analysis.

Questionnaire	Component 1 Anxiety-Depression	Component 2 Impulsivity
NEO—Neuroticism	**0.84**	0.16
TCI—Harm Avoidance	**0.84**	−0.24
STAI—T	**0.82**	0.22
NEO—Extraversion	**−0.73**	0.42
BDI	**0.70**	0.23
TCI—Novelty Seeking	−0.33	**0.86**
BIS-11—Total score	0.19	**0.81**
NEO—Conscientiousness	−0.39	**−0.67**

Factor loadings higher than 0.60 are marked in bold.

fMRI Results

Validation of the Study Design: Effects of Magnitude on BOLD-Signal During Anticipation and Win-Outcome

We first aimed to validate our study design by testing for effects of reward magnitude (1€ > 0.05€) during anticipation and win-outcome. Replicating the results of previous studies, there was an effect of magnitude in the VS [peak in MNI-space [x y z] = [9 8 −2], $T = 5.38$, $p < 0.0001$, FWE-corrected for ROI volume] during anticipation. Further in line with previous studies, during the outcome phase we found effects of reward magnitude in the mPFC [peak in MNI-space [x y z] = [6 41 19], $T = 6.65$, $p < 0.00001$, FWE-corrected for ROI volume] and in the right VS/NAcc [peak in MNI-space [x y z] = [12 8 −11], $T = 4.33$, $p = 0.002$, FWE-corrected for the ROI volume; **Figure 3A**. These results indicate that our design worked as intended.

Effects of Immediacy on BOLD-Signal During the Anticipation Phase

Although the main goal of our study was to assess the neural correlates of delay discounting in the outcome phase, we also analyzed the anticipatory phase of the

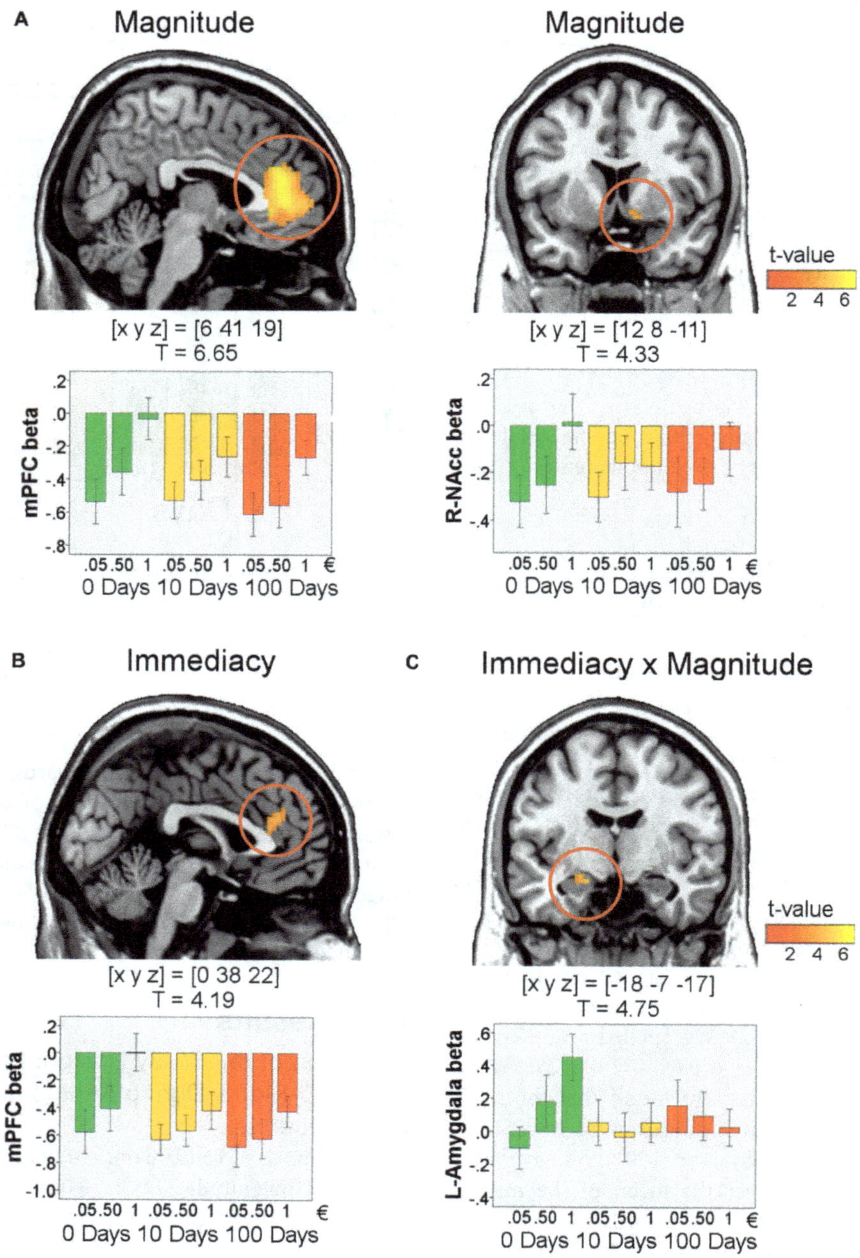

FIGURE 3 | Effects in the outcome phase for win-trials. Effects of magnitude (1€ > 0.05€, **(A)**, serves as validation of the study design), immediacy (0 days > 10 and 100 days, **(B)**), and immediacy × magnitude (1€ > 0.05€ for 0 days compared to 10 and 100 days, **(C)**; $n = 72$). For visualization, activations are shown at $p < 0.001$, uncorrected and masked by the respective ROI (medial prefrontal cortex (mPFC), amygdala, or VS). All peaks survive $p < 0.017$, FWE-correction for ROI volumes. T-values and MNI coordinates [x y z] are given for the peaks of the activations. Bar plots visualize the results by showing the mean beta values within a sphere around the peak voxel of each region (radius: 5 mm). Error bars denote 95% C.I. of the mean, adjusted for within-subject designs (Loftus and Masson, 1994).

MID task. However, we found no effects of delay (i.e., immediacy, or 10 days vs. 100 days) or of the interaction of immediacy × magnitude that were significant after correction ($p < 0.05$, FWE-corrected for the ROI volumes). Because there were no robust effects of delay during anticipation, we did not further examine influences of Anxiety-Depression or Impulsivity on brain activation during anticipation.

Effects of Immediacy on BOLD-Signal During the Win-Outcome Phase

Immediacy of reward delivery was associated with increased BOLD response within a dorsal portion of the mPFC in response to immediate as compared to delayed rewards (peak in MNI-space [x y z] = [0 38 22], $T = 4.19$, $p = 0.014$, FWE-corrected for ROI volume; **Figure 3B**). A direct comparison of the BOLD response between delay conditions (10 days vs. 100 days) yielded no reliable differences in the ROIs, even at a very liberal threshold ($p < 0.01$, $k = 5$, uncorrected).

We next tested for interactions of immediacy and reward magnitude. Specifically, we investigated which brain regions showed a more pronounced effect of magnitude (1€ vs. 0.05€) for immediate as compared to delayed rewards. Such a pattern was observed in the left amygdala (**Figure 3C**; peak in MNI-space [x y z] = [−18 −7 −17], $T = 4.75$, $k = 10$, $p = 0.00014$, FWE-corrected for ROI volume).

Correlations of Neural Delay Effects in the Win-Outcome Phase with Impulsivity and Anxiety-Depression

We then tested for a potential relationship between the BOLD response to immediate vs. delayed rewards during the outcome phase and the personality traits of interest (Impulsivity, Anxiety-Depression). To this end, we computed correlations between individual neural immediacy effects ($beta_{win\_immediate} - beta_{win\_delayed}$) in the mPFC and amygdala (betas averaged in 5 mm spheres around the peak voxel) and the Anxiety-Depression and Impulsivity scores from our factor analysis. Immediacy effects in mPFC were not normally distributed (Kolmogorov-Smirnov $p = 0.039$), while they were normally distributed in the amygdala (Kolmogorov-Smirnov $p \geq 0.20$). Therefore we used non-parametric Spearman's correlation for the mPFC analysis and parametric Pearson's correlation for the amygdala analysis.

We found that immediacy effects in the mPFC correlated positively with Anxiety-Depression ($r_s = 0.306$, $p = 0.016$, two-tailed, $n = 62$, **Figure 4A**), while immediacy effects in the left amygdala correlated positively with Impulsivity ($r = 0.407$, $p = 0.001$, two-tailed, $n = 62$, **Figure 4B**).

DISCUSSION

In the present study, we investigated the neural correlates of delay discounting during reward outcome processing in healthy participants as well as their relationship with individual differences in impulsivity and anxious-depressive traits. We found that a region within the dorsal mPFC exhibited stronger activation for delivery of immediate as opposed for delayed monetary rewards. Moreover, the left amygdala showed an interaction of immediacy and reward magnitude, in that it encoded magnitude only for immediate rewards. Personality traits that had previously been linked to altered delay discounting were found to be associated with the amygdala and mPFC responses in a trait-specific way: While the left amygdala immediacy response was more pronounced in impulsive participants, the immediacy response in the mPFC was more pronounced in participants with anxious-depressive traits.

Delay Discounting in the Outcome Phase

Effects of Immediacy on the mPFC

Previous studies have demonstrated that the mPFC responds to the delivery of predicted rewards during the outcome phase of MID tasks and that it further codes the magnitude of rewards (Knutson et al., 2001b; Hommer et al., 2003; Schott et al., 2007). The present study demonstrates that mPFC activation does not only code the mere magnitude of an outcome, but also its time of

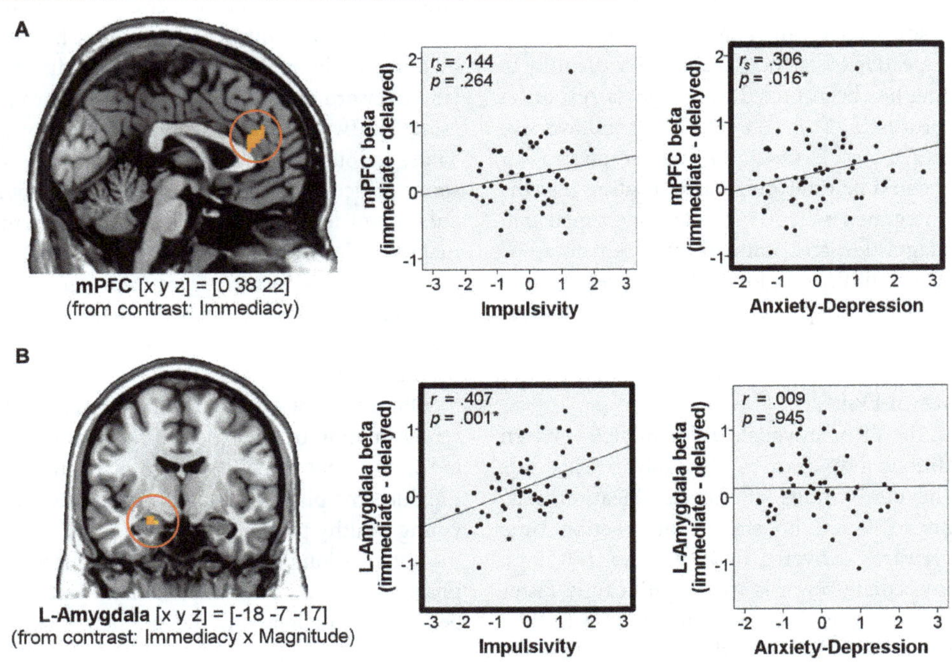

FIGURE 4 | Correlations of immediacy effects in the win-outcome phase with personality. Correlations of neural immediacy effects ($beta_{win\_immediate} - beta_{win\_delayed}$) in the mPFC **(A)** and in the left amygdala **(B)** with the factor scores Impulsivity and Anxiety-Depression ($n = 62$). On the left side of the figure, activations for these regions from the main analysis are shown at $p < 0.001$, uncorrected. Coordinates [x y z] refer to MNI-space. *Significant at $p < 0.05$ (framed in bold).

delivery: the dorsal mPFC shows a more pronounced response to immediate relative to delayed rewards. Compatibly, Sripada et al. (2011) observed that mPFC activity was higher during decisions that involved one immediate option relative to decisions between two delayed options, although in a somewhat more anterior and ventral region of the mPFC.

The most straightforward explanation of our mPFC finding is that activation in this region reflects the representation or computation of subjective value during the outcome phase. However, as subjective value was not directly measured and as the typical locus of subjective value activations in decision-making paradigms is more ventral (Rangel and Hare, 2010) alternative explanations should be considered. First, our results may relate to the role of the dorsal mPFC in triggering and mobilizing cognitive control (Botvinick et al., 2001, 2004; Ridderinkhof et al., 2004). This process might occur automatically, possibly in order to counteract the tempting nature of immediate rewards (see Fitzsimons and Bargh, 2004). Second, more pronounced mPFC responses to immediate rewards might also reflect increased self-relevance of immediate rewards, since mPFC has been related to self-referential processing (e.g., Gusnard et al., 2001) and also, more specifically, to confirmatory self-referential responses (Sajonz et al., 2010). Third, activation of the mPFC subregion might simply signal immediacy itself (see Sripada et al., 2011).

Effects of Immediacy on the Amygdala

An interaction of immediacy and magnitude was observed in the left amygdala, where magnitude was only encoded for immediate rewards. In addition to its well-known role in emotion processing, the amygdala may also, more generally, respond to stimulus salience or relevance (Liberzon et al., 2003; Ewbank et al., 2009; Mahler and Berridge, 2009; Schardt et al., 2010). In line with the notion of the amygdala as a relevance or salience detector, irrespective of valence, individual variability of dopaminergic signaling has been linked to amygdala responses during both reward processing (Schott et al., 2008) and aversive emotional stimulation (Kienast et al., 2008). With respect to our present findings, this could be interpreted as indicating that the amygdala codes an integrated salience or relevance signal that encompasses both magnitude and immediacy of an obtained reward. However, further studies employing both appetitive and aversive reinforcement will be required to systematically address this question (e.g., see Camara et al., 2009).

All-or-None Effects of Delay

Neither the mPFC nor the VS or amygdala differentiated between the two delay conditions (10 days vs. 100 days). This was mirrored by the behavioral results of the classification task, in which participants exhibited no significant reaction time differences between rewards delivered in 10 days vs. 100 days, while responses to immediate rewards were significantly faster than those to delayed rewards. This is compatible with the previous observation that the mPFC and the striatum primarily activate during choices involving immediate rewards, showing no further differentiation between rewards delivered after 2 weeks or 1 month (McClure et al., 2004). Our results expand the observation by McClure and colleagues, showing that such a pattern also applies to the valuation phase in isolation. While we cannot rule out that increasing the difference between delays even further (e.g., 5 days vs. 1 year) might ultimately lead to measurable neural differences between the delays (Kable and Glimcher, 2010), our results support the idea that immediacy *per se* is an important factor contributing to the salience of stimuli (see McClure et al., 2004, 2007). Alternatively, or additionally, because participants did not engage in decision-making, they might have—implicitly or explicitly—ignored the difference between the 10-day and 100-day delays.

Consideration on the Outcome Phase for Delayed Rewards

Finally, one might note that the outcome phase in this fMRI paradigm did not involve the receipt of an actual reward in the very same moment. It is, of course, logically impossible to receive a reward that will be delivered delayed in time (but see Prévost et al., 2010, for paradigms that involve actually waiting for the delivery of delayed rewards during neuroimaging; Jimura et al., 2013). Rather, our paradigm involved the promise to receive the amount immediately after scanning or following a certain delay after scanning, thus comparing very short to moderate and long delays.

No Delay Discounting in the Anticipation Phase

In contrast to a previous study that investigated the neural correlates of delay discounting with an MID task (Luo et al., 2009), we found no effects of delay during the anticipation of rewards. Most notably, we could not replicate the immediacy effect in the mPFC during reward anticipation, but only in the outcome phase. One reason for this might be the complexity of our paradigm that included nine different types of reward (three reward magnitudes times three delays), as compared to the (simpler) two-by-two design employed by Luo and colleagues. Thus, in our paradigm, participants might have experienced some difficulty integrating the complex symbolic anticipatory cues in order to form a mental representation of both the magnitude and the delay of the anticipated reward. Instead, they might only have formed a clear representation of the presumably most salient feature, namely the magnitude of the reward during the anticipation, which had strong effects in the VS also in the current study.

One result of our study that speaks for such an incomplete representation of the expected rewards in the anticipation phase is the fact that the VS showed a magnitude effect also during the outcome phase. Previous studies have demonstrated that, in young healthy participants, the VS is activated primarily during the anticipation phase of MID tasks, but not during the outcome phase (Knutson et al., 2001b). This pattern is, however, widely believed to depend on the predictability of rewards (Schultz et al., 2000; Berns et al., 2001; Spicer et al., 2007). In our paradigm, rewards were delivered to correct responses in only 60% of trials. Therefore, the EV of the rewards was reduced during the anticipation phase, while reward delivery during the outcome phase was likely to elicit a positive prediction error (e.g., Pagnoni et al., 2002). With respect to the mPFC, the uncertainty during reward anticipation might have led to the delayed valuation of the rewards to the outcome phase.

It must be noted, though, that during the classification task, participants exhibited shorter RTs to immediate vs. delayed rewards. It can thus not be excluded that neural activation differences during the anticipation phase might not have been picked up due to lack of statistical power, particularly when the variance explanation by the delay effects was small compared to that of the magnitude effects.

Individual Differences in the Neural Correlates of Delay Discounting in the Outcome Phase

In addition to investigating the neural correlates of the valuation component of delay discounting during the outcome phase, a second aim of our study was to investigate how delay discounting relates to interindividual variability of personality traits that are implicated in neuropsychiatric disorders. To this end, we performed a factor analysis on several well-established questionnaires, namely the NEO-FFI, the TCI, the BIS-11, the STAI-T, and the BDI. Two factors were reliably identified, and considering the contributing variables, they were labeled Anxiety-Depression and Impulsivity (**Table 3**). With previous studies demonstrating that impulsivity is associated with increased delay discounting (e.g., de Wit et al., 2007; Mobini et al., 2007), and some evidence for a correlation of delay discounting with anxiety-related traits (Rounds et al., 2007), we aimed to correlate the brain activation patterns observed as a function of immediacy with these two traits.

Correlation of Impulsivity with Immediacy Effects in the Amygdala

Previous studies investigating the relationship between impulsivity and the neural correlates of reward processing have mostly focused on the response of the striatum. Those studies have yielded partly conflicting results, as both positive (e.g., Forbes et al., 2007) and negative (Beck et al., 2009) correlations between ventral striatal reward responses and impulsivity have been reported. A recent meta-analysis suggests that the relationship between impulsivity-related personality traits and the striatal reward response might depend on the population investigated, with healthy participants showing positive correlations of impulsivity and striatal reward responses, while patient populations with clinically relevant levels of impulsivity may show the opposite pattern (Plichta and Scheres, 2014).

With the focus of the present study being the investigation of delay effects, we did not compute correlations of individual differences with the striatal reward response, as striatal activity was not modulated by delay. Rather we tested for correlations in the amygdala and the mPFC, which both showed effects of immediacy in the outcome phase. We found that the factor *Impulsivity* correlated positively with the response of the left amygdala to immediate vs. delayed rewards in the outcome phase. As discussed above, the amygdala, apart from its well-characterized function in emotion processing, is also believed to convey the signaling of stimulus salience or relevance (Liberzon et al., 2003; Ewbank et al., 2009; Mahler and Berridge, 2009; Schardt et al., 2010). Studies of the neural mechanisms of impulsivity have previously identified the amygdala as an important anatomical structure mediating impulsivity. Volumetric investigations point to a role of the amygdala in motor impulsivity (Gopal et al., 2013), and impulsivity correlates positively with the amygdala response to winning monetary rewards in a slot-machine game (Shao et al., 2013). Our results are in line with the latter finding and extend it by showing that high impulsivity is not only associated with a more pronounced amygdala response to winning rewards in general, but rather, that impulsive individuals are also specifically more responsive to winning *immediate* as compared to delayed rewards. This is in line with most definitions of impulsivity that center around the idea that impulsive individuals are focused on the present and on short-term gratification (e.g., see Evenden, 1999). It also complies with a recent connectionist model of intertemporal choice in which impulsivity was modeled as a reduced response threshold, leading to faster choices and an attenuated influence of the value of delayed rewards (Scherbaum et al., 2012). In summary, our results strengthen the notion that, in addition to the well-known role of the striatum in impulsivity, the preference for immediate rewards in impulsive individuals may at least in part be mediated by the amygdala.

From a clinical point of view, the positive direction of the correlation between immediacy-related amygdala responses and impulsivity is noteworthy, as amygdala hyperactivity has been repeatedly observed in Borderline personality disorder (BPD; Krause-Utz et al., 2014), a psychiatric condition characterized by dysfunctional levels of impulsivity that often lead to self-harming behaviors in the affected patients. Delay discounting is very pronounced in BPD patients (Barker et al., 2015), and future studies should investigate a potential role of amygdala hyperactivity in delay discounting in this patient group.

Correlation of Anxiety-Depression with Immediacy Effects in the mPFC

While the positive relationship between Impulsivity and immediacy-related amygdala activity was well in line with our hypotheses, the observation that Anxiety-Depression correlated positively with the mPFC immediacy response was not predicted. As the immediacy effect in the mPFC itself has no satisfying single explanation, as discussed above, the interpretation of correlations within the mPFC remains largely speculative. We will constrain our discussion to two possibilities.

The first explanation relates to the possible role of the mPFC in coding subjective value (Hare et al., 2009; Kahnt et al., 2011; Park et al., 2011). The correlation of mPFC activation with Anxiety-Depression would then suggest that (subclinical) anxious-depressive individuals overvalue immediate and/or undervalue delayed rewards. This is compatible with a cardinal feature of clinical depression, the so-called Beck's triad (Beck, 1987), which is a pessimistic view of the self, the world and, relevant to this interpretation, the future. It is also in line with findings by Rounds et al. (2007) who reported increased delay discounting in individuals with social anxiety.

A second possibility is that the correlative findings relate to a role of the mPFC in triggering or mobilizing cognitive control in the outcome phase of immediate rewards (Botvinick et al., 2004; Ridderinkhof et al., 2004). In this case the described would mean that anxious-depressive participants trigger or mobilize more cognitive control for immediate rewards, for example because they might ruminate and worry more about receiving—or not receiving—rewards. However, these interpretations are highly tentative at this point and will have to be tested in future, specifically designed experiments.

Future research should expand this approach to populations with clinically relevant levels of anxious-depressive traits, like patients with affective disorders, anxiety or personality disorders like Borderline or avoidant personality disorder. One previous study has suggested reduced delay discounting in patients with social anxiety disorder (Rounds et al., 2007), and several authors have pointed out the role of medial prefrontal and rostral anterior cingulate dysfunction—and possibly hyperfunction—in these disorders (Lemogne et al., 2012; Holtmann et al., 2013; Adhikari, 2014). The observation that anxious-depressive traits correlate positively with the neural immediacy effect in healthy participants points to the possibility that mPFC dysfunction in patients with clinical levels of depression or anxiety might also result in increased delay discounting.

Subjective Value as an Alternative Explanation

One potential limitation of the present study design is that the effects of immediacy and magnitude might also be, at least in part, attributable to subjective value, as an immediate reward of a certain magnitude has a higher overall subjective value than a delayed reward of the same magnitude. Luo et al. (2009) aimed to circumvent this problem by creating preference-matched stimuli for each participant and could still observe delay discounting effects. In the present study, however, we decided against this approach, because we were interested in individual differences of the valuation process in relation to impulsive and anxious-depressive personality traits. We argued that the correlation of delay discounting effects with decreased overall subjective value is inherent to the phenomenon, since delay discounting is a process of devaluation. Nevertheless, this might constitute a potential limitation of the current study. That is, we can, as of now, not exclude the possibility that, even though we focused on brain structures that responded to immediacy or immediacy-magnitude interactions rather than reward magnitude *per se*, the observed brain-behavior correlations also relate to overall subjective value of the rewards.

CONCLUSION

Taken together, our study demonstrates that immediate vs. delayed delivery of rewards engages activity of mPFC and the amygdala during the processing of reward outcome. This pattern of activation is further associated with individual differences in both impulsivity and anxious-depressive traits, with impulsivity correlating positively with immediacy-related amygdala activity, while anxious-depressive traits correlate with immediacy-related mPFC activity.

AUTHOR CONTRIBUTIONS

HW and CN designed the study. CN and DW-S carried out the research. VUL and BHS analyzed the data based on and extending earlier analyses by CN, supervised by HW and SE. In collaboration with the other authors, VUL, BHS, and HW interpreted the results of these analyses. VUL, BHS and HW wrote the article, partly based on the doctoral dissertation by CN, and aided by CEW and TG. All authors revised the manuscript critically for important intellectual content.

ACKNOWLEDGMENTS

BHS and TG received support from the Deutsche Forschungsgemeinschaft (SFB 779, TP A8 and SFB 940/1 respectively). CN and DWS received support from the Volkswagen (VW) Foundation (grants II/80777, II/8077). VUL and CEW were funded by the Berlin School of Mind and Brain, and VUL was additionally funded by the German National Academic Foundation. We thank Ilja Veer for helpful comments on the manuscript.

REFERENCES

Abler, B., Walter, H., and Erk, S. (2005). Neural correlates of frustration. *Neuroreport* 16, 669–672. doi: 10.1097/00001756-200505120-00003

Adhikari, A. (2014). Distributed circuits underlying anxiety. *Front. Behav. Neurosci.* 8:112. doi: 10.3389/fnbeh.2014.00112

Ainslie, G. (1975). Specious reward: a behavioral theory of impulsiveness and impulse control. *Psychol. Bull.* 82, 463–496. doi: 10.1037/h0076860

Alessi, S. M., and Petry, N. M. (2003). Pathological gambling severity is associated with impulsivity in a delay discounting procedure. *Behav. Processes* 64, 345–354. doi: 10.1016/s0376-6357(03)00150-5

Aluja, A., and Blanch, A. (2011). The five and seven factors personality models: differences and similitude between the TCI-R, NEO-FFI-R and ZKPQ-50-CC. *Span. J. Psychol.* 14, 659–666. doi: 10.5209/rev_sjop.2011.v14.n2.14

Aupperle, R. L., and Paulus, M. P. (2010). Neural systems underlying approach and avoidance in anxiety disorders. *Dialogues Clin. Neurosci.* 12, 517–531.

Barker, V., Romaniuk, L., Cardinal, R. N., Pope, M., Nicol, K., and Hall, J. (2015). Impulsivity in borderline personality disorder. *Psychol. Med.* 45, 1955–1964. doi: 10.1017/S0033291714003079

Beck, A., Schlagenhauf, F., Wüstenberg, T., Hein, J., Kienast, T., Kahnt, T., et al. (2009). Ventral striatal activation during reward anticipation correlates with impulsivity in alcoholics. *Biol. Psychiatry* 66, 734–742. doi: 10.1016/j.biopsych.2009.04.035

Beck, A. T. (1987). Cognitive models of depression. *J. Cogn. Psychother.* 1, 5–37.

Beck, A. T., Steer, R. A., Ball, R., and Ranieri, W. (1996). Comparison of beck depression inventories -IA and -II in psychiatric outpatients. *J. Pers. Assess.* 67, 588–597. doi: 10.1207/s15327752jpa6703_13

Berns, G. S., McClure, S. M., Pagnoni, G., and Montague, P. R. (2001). Predictability modulates human brain response to reward. *J. Neurosci.* 21, 2793–2798.

Borkenau, P., and Ostendorf, E. (1993). *NEO-Fünf-Faktoren-Inventar (NEO-FFI) nach Costa und McCrae.* Göttingen: Hogrefe.

Botvinick, M. M., Braver, T. S., Barch, D. M., Carter, C. S., and Cohen, J. D. (2001). Conflict monitoring and cognitive control. *Psychol. Rev.* 108, 624–652. doi: 10.1037/0033-295X.108.3.624

Botvinick, M. M., Cohen, J. D., and Carter, C. S. (2004). Conflict monitoring and anterior cingulate cortex: an update. *Trends Cogn. Sci.* 8, 539–546. doi: 10.1016/j.tics.2004.10.003

Camara, E., Rodriguez-Fornells, A., and Münte, T. F. (2009). Functional connectivity of reward processing in the brain. *Front. Hum. Neurosci.* 2:19. doi: 10.3389/neuro.09.019.2008

Cloninger, C. R. (1994). *The Temperament and Character Inventory (TCI): A Guide to its Development and Use.* St. Louis, MO: Center for Psychobiology of Personality, Washington University.

Cloninger, C. R., Svrakic, D. M., and Przybeck, T. R. (1993). A psychobiological model of temperament and character. *Arch. Gen. Psychiatry* 50, 975–990. doi: 10.1001/archpsyc.1993.01820240059008

Costa, P. T. Jr., and McCrae, R. R. (1992a). Four ways five factors are basic. *Pers. Individ. Dif.* 13, 653–665. doi: 10.1016/0191-8869(92)90236-i

Costa, P. T., and McCrae, R. R. (1992b). *Revised NEO Personality Inventory (NEO PI-R) and NEO Five Factor Inventory. Professional Manual.* Odessa, FL: Psychological Assessment Resources.

De Fruyt, F., Van De Wiele, L., and Van Heeringen, C. (2000). Cloninger's psychobiological model of temperament and character and the five-factor model of personality. *Pers. Individ. Dif.* 29, 441–452. doi: 10.1016/s0191-8869(99)00204-4

de Wit, H., Flory, J. D., Acheson, A., Mccloskey, M., and Manuck, S. B. (2007). IQ and nonplanning impulsivity are independently associated with delay discounting in middle-aged adults. *Pers. Individ. Dif.* 42, 111–121. doi: 10.1016/j.paid.2006.06.026

Dshemuchadse, M., Scherbaum, S., and Goschke, T. (2013). How decisions emerge: action dynamics in intertemporal decision making. *J. Exp. Psychol. Gen.* 142, 93–100. doi: 10.1037/a0028499

Elman, I., Ariely, D., Mazar, N., Aharon, I., Lasko, N. B., Macklin, M. L., et al. (2005). Probing reward function in post-traumatic stress disorder with beautiful facial images. *Psychiatry Res.* 135, 179–183. doi: 10.1016/j.psychres.2005.04.002

Evenden, J. L. (1999). Varieties of impulsivity. *Psychopharmacology (Berl)* 146, 348–361. doi: 10.1007/pl00005481

Ewbank, M. P., Barnard, P. J., Croucher, C. J., Ramponi, C., and Calder, A. J. (2009). The amygdala response to images with impact. *Soc. Cogn. Affect. Neurosci.* 4, 127–133. doi: 10.1093/scan/nsn048

Fitzsimons, G. M., and Bargh, J. A. (2004). "Automatic self-regulation," in *Handbook of Self-Regulation*, eds. R. F. Baumeister and K. D. Vohs (New York: Guilford Press), 151–170.

Forbes, E. E., Brown, S. M., Kimak, M., Ferrell, R. E., Manuck, S. B., and Hariri, A. R. (2007). Genetic variation in components of dopamine neurotransmission impacts ventral striatal reactivity associated with impulsivity. *Mol. Psychiatry* 14, 60–70. doi: 10.1038/sj.mp.4002086

Gopal, A., Clark, E., Allgair, A., D'Amato, C., Furman, M., Gansler, D. A., et al. (2013). Dorsal/ventral parcellation of the amygdala: relevance to impulsivity and aggression. *Psychiatry Res.* 211, 24–30. doi: 10.1016/j.pscychresns.2012.10.010

Gusnard, D. A., Akbudak, E., Shulman, G. L., and Raichle, M. E. (2001). Medial prefrontal cortex and self-referential mental activity: relation to a default mode of brain function. *Proc. Natl. Acad. Sci. U S A* 98, 4259–4264. doi: 10.1073/pnas.071043098

Hare, T. A., Camerer, C. F., and Rangel, A. (2009). Self-control in decision-making involves modulation of the vmPFC valuation system. *Science* 324, 646–648. doi: 10.1126/science.1168450

Hariri, A. R., Brown, S. M., Williamson, D. E., Flory, J. D., de Wit, H., and Manuck, S. B. (2006). Preference for immediate over delayed rewards is associated with magnitude of ventral striatal activity. *J. Neurosci.* 26, 13213–13217. doi: 10.1523/jneurosci.3446-06.2006

Hautzinger, M., Bailer, M., Worall, H., and Keller, F. (2000). *Beck-Depressions-Inventar (BDI). Testhandbuch.* Bern: Huber.

Heekeren, H. R., Wartenburger, I., Marschner, A., Mell, T., Villringer, A., and Reischies, F. M. (2007). Role of ventral striatum in reward-based decision making. *Neuroreport* 18, 951–955. doi: 10.1097/wnr.0b013e3281532bd7

Holtmann, J., Herbort, M. C., Wustenberg, T., Soch, J., Richter, S., Walter, H., et al. (2013). Trait anxiety modulates fronto-limbic processing of emotional interference in borderline personality disorder. *Front. Hum. Neurosci.* 7:54. doi: 10.3389/fnhum.2013.00054

Hommer, D. W., Knutson, B., Fong, G. W., Bennett, S., Adams, C. M., and Varnera, J. L. (2003). Amygdalar recruitment during anticipation of monetary rewards: an event-related fMRI study. *Ann. N. Y. Acad. Sci.* 985, 476–478. doi: 10.1111/j.1749-6632.2003.tb07103.x

Hopper, J. W., Pitman, R. K., Su, Z., Heyman, G. M., Lasko, N. B., Macklin, M. L., et al. (2008). Probing reward function in posttraumatic stress disorder: expectancy and satisfaction with monetary gains and losses. *J. Psychiatr. Res.* 42, 802–807. doi: 10.1016/j.jpsychires.2007.10.008

Jimura, K., Chushak, M. S., and Braver, T. S. (2013). Impulsivity and self-control during intertemporal decision making linked to the neural dynamics of reward value representation. *J. Neurosci.* 33, 344–357. doi: 10.1523/JNEUROSCI.0919-12.2013

Kable, J. W., and Glimcher, P. W. (2007). The neural correlates of subjective value during intertemporal choice. *Nat. Neurosci.* 10, 1625–1633. doi: 10.1038/nn2007

Kable, J. W., and Glimcher, P. W. (2010). An "as soon as possible" effect in human intertemporal decision making: behavioral evidence and neural mechanisms. *J. Neurophysiol.* 103, 2513–2531. doi: 10.1152/jn.00177.2009

Kahnt, T., Heinzle, J., Park, S. Q., and Haynes, J.-D. (2011). Decoding different roles for vmPFC and dlPFC in multi-attribute decision making. *Neuroimage* 56, 709–715. doi: 10.1016/j.neuroimage.2010.05.058

Kaiser, H. F. (1960). The application of electronic computers for factor analysis. *Educ. Psychol. Meas.* 20, 141–151. doi: 10.1177/001316446002000116

Kaiser, H. F. (1970). A second generation little jiffy. *Psychometrika* 35, 401–415. doi: 10.1007/BF02291817

Kienast, T., Hariri, A. R., Schlagenhauf, F., Wrase, J., Sterzer, P., Buchholz, H. G., et al. (2008). Dopamine in amygdala gates limbic processing of aversive stimuli in humans. *Nat. Neurosci.* 11, 1381–1382. doi: 10.1038/nn.2222

Kirby, K. N., and Petry, N. M. (2004). Heroin and cocaine abusers have higher discount rates for delayed rewards than alcoholics or non-drug-using controls. *Addiction* 99, 461–471. doi: 10.1111/j.1360-0443.2003.00669.x

Knutson, B., Adams, C. M., Fong, G. W., and Hommer, D. (2001a). Anticipation of increasing monetary reward selectively recruits nucleus accumbens. *J. Neurosci.* 21:RC159.

Knutson, B., Fong, G. W., Adams, C. M., Varner, J. L., and Hommer, D. (2001b). Dissociation of reward anticipation and outcome with event-related fMRI. *Neuroreport* 12, 3683–3687. doi: 10.1097/00001756-200112040-00016

Knutson, B., Fong, G. W., Bennett, S. M., Adams, C. M., and Hommer, D. (2003). A region of mesial prefrontal cortex tracks monetarily rewarding outcomes: characterization with rapid event-related fMRI. *Neuroimage* 18, 263–272. doi: 10.1016/s1053-8119(02)00057-5

Knutson, B., Taylor, J., Kaufman, M., Peterson, R., and Glover, G. (2005). Distributed neural representation of expected value. *J. Neurosci.* 25, 4806–4812. doi: 10.1523/jneurosci.0642-05.2005

Koff, E., and Lucas, M. (2011). Mood moderates the relationship between impulsiveness and delay discounting. *Pers. Individ. Dif.* 50, 1018–1022. doi: 10.1016/j.paid.2011.01.016

Krause-Utz, A., Winter, D., Niedtfeld, I., and Schmahl, C. (2014). The latest neuroimaging findings in borderline personality disorder. *Curr. Psychiatry Rep.* 16, 014–0438. doi: 10.1007/s11920-014-0438-z

Laux, L., Glanzmann, P., Schaffner, P., and Spielberger, C. D. (1981). *Das State-Trait-Angstinventar (Testmappe mit Handanweisung, Fragebogen STAI-G Form X 1 und Fragebogen STAI-G Form X 2).* Weinheim: Beltz.

Lebreton, M., Jorge, S., Michel, V., Thirion, B., and Pessiglione, M. (2009). An automatic valuation system in the human brain: evidence from functional neuroimaging. *Neuron* 64, 431–439. doi: 10.1016/j.neuron.2009.09.040

Lemogne, C., Delaveau, P., Freton, M., Guionnet, S., and Fossati, P. (2012). Medial prefrontal cortex and the self in major depression. *J. Affect. Disord.* 136, e1–e11. doi: 10.1016/j.jad.2010.11.034

Liberzon, I., Phan, K. L., Decker, L. R., and Taylor, S. F. (2003). Extended amygdala and emotional salience: a PET activation study of positive and negative affect. *Neuropsychopharmacology* 28, 726–733. doi: 10.1038/sj.npp.1300113

Liu, L., Feng, T., Wang, J., and Li, H. (2012). The neural dissociation of subjective valuation from choice processes in intertemporal choice. *Behav. Brain Res.* 231, 40–47. doi: 10.1016/j.bbr.2012.02.045

Lin, W. J., Horner, A. J., Bisby, J. A., and Burgess, N. (2015). Medial prefrontal cortex: adding value to imagined scenarios. *J. Cogn. Neurosci.* 27, 1957–1967. doi: 10.1162/jocn_a_00836

Loftus, G. R., and Masson, M. E. J. (1994). Using confidence intervals in within-subject designs. *Psychon. Bull. Rev.* 1, 476–490. doi: 10.3758/bf03210951

Ludwig, V. U., Stelzel, C., Krutiak, H., Magrabi, A., Steimke, R., Paschke, L. M., et al. (2014). The suggestible brain: posthypnotic effects on value-based decision-making. *Soc. Cogn. Affect. Neurosci.* 9, 1281–1288. doi: 10.1093/scan/nst110

Luhmann, C. C., Chun, M. M., Yi, D.-J., Lee, D., and Wang, X.-J. (2008). Neural dissociation of delay and uncertainty in intertemporal choice. *J. Neurosci.* 28, 14459–14466. doi: 10.1523/JNEUROSCI.5058-08.2008

Luo, S., Ainslie, G., Giragosian, L., and Monterosso, J. R. (2009). Behavioral and neural evidence of incentive bias for immediate rewards relative to preference-matched delayed rewards. *J. Neurosci.* 29, 14820–14827. doi: 10.1523/JNEUROSCI.4261-09.2009

Luo, S., Ainslie, G., Giragosian, L., and Monterosso, J. R. (2011). Striatal hyposensitivity to delayed rewards among cigarette smokers. *Drug. Alcohol Depend.* 116, 18–23. doi: 10.1016/j.drugalcdep.2010.11.012

Mahler, S. V., and Berridge, K. C. (2009). Which cue to "want?" central amygdala opioid activation enhances and focuses incentive salience on a prepotent reward cue. *J. Neurosci.* 29, 6500–6513. doi: 10.1523/JNEUROSCI.3875-08.2009

Maldjian, J. A., Laurienti, P. J., Kraft, R. A., and Burdette, J. H. (2003). An automated method for neuroanatomic and cytoarchitectonic atlas-based interrogation of fMRI data sets. *Neuroimage* 19, 1233–1239. doi: 10.1016/S1053-8119(03)00169-1

Marjorie, K. S. (1993). Outcome signs, question frames and discount rates. *Manage. Sci.* 39, 806–815. doi: 10.1287/mnsc.39.7.806

Mazur, J. E. (1988). Estimation of indifference points with an adjusting-delay procedure. *J. Exp. Anal. Behav.* 49, 37–47. doi: 10.1901/jeab.1988.49-37

McClure, S. M., Ericson, K. M., Laibson, D. I., Loewenstein, G., and Cohen, J. D. (2007). Time discounting for primary rewards. *J. Neurosci.* 27, 5796–5804. doi: 10.1523/jneurosci.4246-06.2007

McClure, S. M., Laibson, D. I., Loewenstein, G., and Cohen, J. D. (2004). Separate neural systems value immediate and delayed monetary rewards. *Science* 306, 503–507. doi: 10.1126/science.1100907

Mischel, W., and Underwood, B. (1974). Instrumental ideation in delay of gratification. *Child Dev.* 45, 1083–1088. doi: 10.2307/1128098

Mitchell, J. M., Fields, H. L., D'Esposito, M., and Boettiger, C. A. (2005). Impulsive responding in alcoholics. *Alcohol. Clin. Exp. Res.* 29, 2158–2169. doi: 10.1097/01.alc.0000191755.63639.4a

Mobini, S., Grant, A., Kass, A. E., and Yeomans, M. R. (2007). Relationships between functional and dysfunctional impulsivity, delay discounting and cognitive distortions. *Pers. Individ. Dif.* 43, 1517–1528. doi: 10.1016/j.paid.2007.04.009

Odum, A. L. (2011). Delay discounting: trait variable? *Behav. Processes* 87, 1–9. doi: 10.1016/j.beproc.2011.02.007

Pagnoni, G., Zink, C. F., Montague, P. R., and Berns, G. S. (2002). Activity in human ventral striatum locked to errors of reward prediction. *Nat. Neurosci.* 5, 97–98. doi: 10.1038/nn802

Park, S. Q., Kahnt, T., Rieskamp, J., and Heekeren, H. R. (2011). Neurobiology of value integration: when value impacts valuation. *J. Neurosci.* 31, 9307–9314. doi: 10.1523/JNEUROSCI.4973-10.2011

Patin, A., and Hurlemann, R. (2011). Modulating amygdala responses to emotion: evidence from pharmacological fMRI. *Neuropsychologia* 49, 706–717. doi: 10.1016/j.neuropsychologia.2010.10.004

Patton, J. H., Stanford, M. S., and Barratt, E. S. (1995). Factor structure of the barratt impulsiveness scale. *J. Clin. Psychol.* 51, 768–774. doi: 10.1002/1097-4679(199511)51:6<768::aid-jclp2270510607>3.0.co;2-1

Petry, N. (2002). Discounting of delayed rewards in substance abusers: relationship to antisocial personality disorder. *Psychopharmacology (Berl)* 162, 425–432. doi: 10.1007/s00213-002-1115-1

Peters, J., and Büchel, C. (2011). The neural mechanisms of inter-temporal decision-making: understanding variability. *Trends Cogn. Sci.* 15, 227–239. doi: 10.1016/j.tics.2011.03.002

Petry, N. M. (2001). Pathological gamblers, with and without substance use disorders, discount delayed rewards at high rates. *J. Abnorm. Psychol.* 110, 482–487. doi: 10.1037//0021-843x.110.3.482

Plichta, M. M., and Scheres, A. (2014). Ventral-striatal responsiveness during reward anticipation in ADHD and its relation to trait impulsivity in the healthy population: a meta-analytic review of the fMRI literature. *Neurosci. Biobehav. Rev.* 38, 125–134. doi: 10.1016/j.neubiorev.2013.07.012

Plichta, M. M., Vasic, N., Wolf, R. C., Lesch, K.-P., Brummer, D., Jacob, C., et al. (2009). Neural hyporesponsiveness and hyperresponsiveness during immediate and delayed reward processing in adult attention-deficit/hyperactivity disorder. *Biol. Psychiatry* 65, 7–14. doi: 10.1016/j.biopsych.2008.07.008

Prévost, C., Pessiglione, M., Météreau, E., Cléry-Melin, M.-L., and Dreher, J.-C. (2010). Separate valuation subsystems for delay and effort decision costs. *J. Neurosci.* 30, 14080–14090. doi: 10.1523/JNEUROSCI.2752-10.2010

Rachlin, H., and Green, L. (1972). Commitment, choice and self-control. *J. Exp. Anal. Behav.* 17, 15–22. doi: 10.1901/jeab.1972.17-15

Rangel, A., Camerer, C., and Montague, P. R. (2008). A framework for studying the neurobiology of value-based decision making. *Nat. Rev. Neurosci.* 9, 545–556. doi: 10.1038/nrn2357

Rangel, A., and Hare, T. (2010). Neural computations associated with goal-directed choice. *Curr. Opin. Neurobiol.* 20, 262–270. doi: 10.1016/j.conb.2010.03.001

Reynolds, B., Ortengren, A., Richards, J. B., and de Wit, H. (2006). Dimensions of impulsive behavior: personality and behavioral measures. *Pers. Individ. Dif.* 40, 305–315. doi: 10.1016/j.paid.2005.03.024

Richter, J., Eisemann, M., Richter, G., and Cloninger, C. (1999). *Das Temperament und Charakter Inventar (TCI): ein Leitfaden über seine Entwicklung und Anwendung.* Göttingen: Swets Test Services mbH.

Ridderinkhof, K. R., Ullsperger, M., Crone, E. A., and Nieuwenhuis, S. (2004). The role of the medial frontal cortex in cognitive control. *Science* 306, 443–447. doi: 10.1126/science.1100301

Rounds, J. S., Beck, J. G., and Grant, D. M. (2007). Is the delay discounting paradigm useful in understanding social anxiety? *Behav. Res. Ther.* 45, 729–735. doi: 10.1016/j.brat.2006.06.007

Sailer, U., Robinson, S., Fischmeister, F. P., König, D., Oppenauer, C., Lueger-Schuster, B., et al. (2008). Altered reward processing in the nucleus accumbens and mesial prefrontal cortex of patients with posttraumatic stress disorder. *Neuropsychologia* 46, 2836–2844. doi: 10.1016/j.neuropsychologia.2008.05.022

Sajonz, B., Kahnt, T., Margulies, D. S., Park, S. Q., Wittmann, A., Stoy, M., et al. (2010). Delineating self-referential processing from episodic memory retrieval: common and dissociable networks. *Neuroimage* 50, 1606–1617. doi: 10.1016/j.neuroimage.2010.01.087

Schardt, D. M., Erk, S., Nüsser, C., Nöthen, M. M., Cichon, S., Rietschel, M., et al. (2010). Volition diminishes genetically mediated amygdala hyperreactivity. *Neuroimage* 53, 943–951. doi: 10.1016/j.neuroimage.2009.11.078

Scherbaum, S., Dshemuchadse, M., and Goschke, T. (2012). Building a bridge into the future: dynamic connectionist modeling as an integrative tool for research on intertemporal choice. *Front. Psychol.* 3:514. doi: 10.3389/fpsyg.2012.00514

Scheres, A., Dijkstra, M., Ainslie, E., Balkan, J., Reynolds, B., Sonuga-Barke, E., et al. (2006). Temporal and probabilistic discounting of rewards in children and adolescents: effects of age and ADHD symptoms. *Neuropsychologia* 44, 2092–2103. doi: 10.1016/j.neuropsychologia.2005.10.012

Scheres, A., Lee, A., and Sumiya, M. (2008). Temporal reward discounting and ADHD: task and symptom specific effects. *J. Neural Transm.* 115, 221–226. doi: 10.1007/s00702-007-0813-6

Schott, B. H., Minuzzi, L., Krebs, R. M., Elmenhorst, D., Lang, M., Winz, O. H., et al. (2008). Mesolimbic functional magnetic resonance imaging activations during reward anticipation correlate with reward-related ventral striatal dopamine release. *J. Neurosci.* 28, 14311–14319. doi: 10.1523/JNEUROSCI.2058-08.2008

Schott, B. H., Niehaus, L., Wittmann, B. C., Schütze, H., Seidenbecher, C. I., Heinze, H.-J., et al. (2007). Ageing and early-stage parkinson's disease affect separable neural mechanisms of mesolimbic reward processing. *Brain* 130, 2412–2424. doi: 10.1093/brain/awm147

Schultz, W., Tremblay, L., and Hollerman, J. R. (2000). Reward processing in primate orbitofrontal cortex and basal ganglia. *Cereb. Cortex* 10, 272–284. doi: 10.1093/cercor/10.3.272

Shao, R., Read, J., Behrens, T. E. J., and Rogers, R. D. (2013). Shifts in reinforcement signalling while playing slot-machines as a function of prior experience and impulsivity. *Transl. Psychiatry* 3:e213. doi: 10.1038/tp.2012.134

Shirer, W. R., Ryali, S., Rykhlevskaia, E., Menon, V., and Greicius, M. D. (2012). Decoding subject-driven cognitive states with whole-brain connectivity patterns. *Cereb. Cortex* 22, 158–165. doi: 10.1093/cercor/bhr099

Spicer, J., Galvan, A., Hare, T. A., Voss, H., Glover, G., and Casey, B. J. (2007). Sensitivity of the nucleus accumbens to violations in expectation of reward. *Neuroimage* 34, 455–461. doi: 10.1016/j.neuroimage.2006.09.012

Spielberger, C. D., Gorsuch, R. L., and Lushene, R. (1970). *Test Manual for the State-Trait Anxiety Inventory.* Palo Alto, Califorina: Consulting Psychologists Press.

Tremblay, L. K., Naranjo, C. A., Graham, S. J., Herrmann, N., Mayberg, H. S., Hevenor, S., et al. (2005). Functional neuroanatomical substrates of altered reward processing in major depressive disorder revealed by a dopaminergic probe. *Arch. Gen. Psychiatry* 62, 1228–1236. doi: 10.1001/archpsyc.62.11.1228

Trope, Y., and Liberman, N. (2003). Temporal construal. *Psychol. Rev.* 110, 403–421. doi: 10.1037/0033-295X.110.3.403

van den Bos, W., and McClure, S. M. (2013). Towards a general model of temporal discounting. *J. Exp. Anal. Behav.* 99, 58–73. doi: 10.1002/jeab.6

Whiteside, S. P., and Lynam, D. R. (2003). Understanding the role of impulsivity and externalizing psychopathology in alcohol abuse: application of the UPPS impulsive behavior scale. *Exp. Clin. Psychopharmacol.* 11, 210–217. doi: 10.1037/1064-1297.11.3.210

Zauberman, G., and Lynch, J. G. Jr. (2005). Resource slack and propensity to discount delayed investments of time versus money. *J. Exp. Psychol. Gen.* 134, 23–37. doi: 10.1037/0096-3445.134.1.23

Zweynert, S., Pade, J. P., Wüstenberg, T., Sterzer, P., Walter, H., Seidenbecher, C. I., et al. (2012). Motivational salience modulates hippocampal repetition suppression and functional connectivity in humans. *Front. Hum. Neurosci.* 5:144. doi: 10.3389/fnhum.201100144

Conflict of Interest Statement: The authors declare that the research was conducted in the absence of any commercial or financial relationships that could be construed as a potential conflict of interest.

11

Increased Prevalence of Intermittent Rhythmic Delta or Theta Activity (IRDA/IRTA) in the Electroencephalograms (EEGs) of Patients with Borderline Personality Disorder

Edited by:
Raymond C. K. Chan,
Chinese Academy of Sciences, China

***Correspondence:**
Ludger Tebartz van Elst
tebartzvanelst@uniklinik-freiburg.de

Ludger Tebartz van Elst[1], Max Fleck[1], Susanne Bartels[1], Dirk-Matthias Altenmüller[2], Andreas Riedel[1], Emanuel Bubl[3], Swantje Matthies[1], Bernd Feige[1], Evgeniy Perlov[1] and Dominique Endres[1]*

[1] Section for Experimental Neuropsychiatry, Department for Psychiatry and Psychotherapy, University Medical Center Freiburg, Freiburg, Germany, [2] Department of Neurosurgery, Freiburg Epilepsy Center, University Medical Center Freiburg, Freiburg, Germany, [3] Department for Psychiatry and Psychotherapy, Saarland University Medical Center, Homburg, Germany

Introduction: An increased prevalence of pathological electroencephalography (EEG) signals has been reported in patients with borderline personality disorder (BPD). In an elaborative case description of such a patient with intermittent rhythmic delta and theta activity (IRDA/IRTA), the BPD symptoms where linked to the frequency of the IRDAs/IRTAs and vanished with the IRDAs/IRTAs following anticonvulsive therapy. This observation raised a question regarding the prevalence of such EEG abnormalities in BPD patients. The aim of this retrospective study was to identify the frequency of EEG abnormalities in a carefully analyzed psychiatric collective. Following earlier reports, we hypothesized an increased prevalence of EEG abnormalities in BPD patients.

Participants and Methods: We recruited 96 consecutive patients with BPD from the archive of a university clinic for psychiatry and psychotherapy, and compared the prevalence of EEG abnormalities to those of 76 healthy controls subjects. The EEGs were rated by three different blinded clinicians, including a consultant specializing in epilepsy from the local epilepsy center.

Results: We found a significant increase in the prevalence of IRDAs and IRTAs in BPD patients (14.6%) compared to the control subjects (3.9%; $p = 0.020$).

Discussion: In this blinded retrospective case-control study, we were able to confirm an increased prevalence of pathological EEG findings (IRDAs/IRTAs only) in BPD patients. The major limitation of this study is that the control group was not matched on age and gender. Therefore, the results should be regarded as preliminary findings of an open uncontrolled, retrospective study. Future research performing prospective, controlled studies is needed to verify our findings and answer the question of whether such EEG findings might predict a positive response to anticonvulsive pharmacological treatment.

Keywords: IRDA, IRTA, local area network inhibition, EEG, borderline personality disorder

INTRODUCTION

Electroencephalography (EEG) represents a method by which the functional integrity of the brain can be investigated with high temporal, but poor spatial, resolution. The discovery of this method by Hans Berger (Berger, 1969; Shipton, 1975) marks the advent of modern biological psychiatry. This paper focuses on EEG abnormalities in patients with Borderline Personality Disorder (BPD).

The concept of BPD was developed in the 1970s and was introduced as a specific diagnostic category in DSM-III in 1980 (Goldstein, 1983). It is characterized by the core features of emotional instability, impulsivity, and instability of self-image and interpersonal relationships (Lieb et al., 2004). Since, episodic dissociative phenomena that are often related to very aversive states of inner tension also belong to the features of BPD and because this is reminiscent of complex partial epileptic seizures, a pathophysiological link to epilepsy has been discussed in the past (Harris et al., 2002; Williams et al., 2006; Tebartz van Elst et al., 2011). Further, there has been discussion as to whether patients with specific epilepsy syndromes such as juvenile myoclonic epilepsy might develop BPD features more often than people with other forms of epilepsy or healthy controls (de Araujo Filho and Yacubian, 2013).

Early EEG studies found an increased prevalence of generally diffuse EEG pathology in BPD patients (De La Fuente et al., 1998; Reeves et al., 2003). In a meta-analysis by Shelley et al. (2008), the respective prevalence rates were estimated to be between 5.8 and 46%. However, most of the summarized studies were hampered by methodological problems, the samples sizes were rather small or the EEG ratings had not been done in a blinded way.

In this context, we recently published the case of a patient with BPD and the EEG pathology of intermittent rhythmic delta and theta activity (IRDA and IRTA) with very severe dissociative states of inner tension and autoaggressive behavior. Anticonvulsive treatment with valproate led to remission of clinical symptoms and a significant reduction in the frequency of IRTAs. Based on these observations, we have put forward the hypothesis of "local area network inhibition" (LANI hypothesis), which holds that non-ictal, paroxysmal neuronal activity (like sharp waves, polyspikes, spike-wave complexes [SWCs], IRDAs, IRTAs) induces inhibitory adaptation processes in local networks in an attempt by the brain to maintain the excitatory-inhibitory homeostasis of the affected networks. Rare and distributed trigger activity may induce sub-threshold inhibition, which can fade away without producing neuropsychiatric symptoms, while frequent and focal trigger activity could eventually induce supra-threshold LANI, which then results in neuropsychiatric symptoms depending on the affected cerebral site or circuit (Tebartz van Elst et al., 2011).

IRDAs were originally described by Cobb in 1945 (Cobb, 1945). According to the local distribution, IRDAs can be categorized as frontal IRDAs (FIRDAs), temporal IRDAs (TIRDAs), and occipital IRDAs (OIRDAs). Without any local specification, it is appropriate to simply refer to IRDAs. They are regarded as a pathological EEG pattern of unknown pathophysiological significance (Brigo, 2011). Within the framework of the LANI model, we hypothesized that IRDAs may have the pathophysiological potential to induce adaptive homeostatic processes, potentially leading to functional alternations of the affected neuronal networks. This assumption is, for example, supported by observations that such EEG phenomena are linked to complex neuropsychiatric symptoms in the context of limbic encephalitis (van Vliet et al., 2012) or to symptoms of migraine (Kakisaka et al., 2014).

The LANI model could explain the pathophysiology of some symptoms in a subgroup of patients with BPD (i.e., those who present with EEG abnormalities like IRDAs or IRTAs). One might put forward the hypothesis, that—as in the case mentioned above (Tebartz van Elst et al., 2011)—such patients could well respond to therapy with anticonvulsants. Following this line of thought, it is remarkable that the therapeutic efficacy of anticonvulsants in cases of BPD has been described for a number of different substances (Bellino et al., 2005; Loew et al., 2006; Stoffers et al., 2010; Vita et al., 2011; Ripoll, 2012). Given these considerations, it is noteworthy that in clinical practice many patients with BPD do not receive a diagnostic work-up that includes a thorough EEG investigation. However, before calling for such laborious procedures, it is important to clarify how often such EEG phenomena can be expected in unselected patients with BPD.

Rationale for our Study

In our clinic, we have a ward that specializes in providing in-patient treatment for BPD patients through employing dialectic behavioral therapy (Lynch et al., 2007). Even though the focus of this ward is psychotherapy, we traditionally perform EEG analyses for all hospitalized patients of our clinic. The current clinical study takes advantage of this fact in that it enables us to retrospectively analyze the frequency of relevant EEG pathologies in these patients. Thus, the aim of this retrospective study was to clarify the frequency of EEG abnormalities (i.e., SWCs, IRDAs, and IRTAs) in BPD patients. Based on the findings of earlier studies (Shelley et al., 2008), we hypothesized an increased prevalence of EEG abnormalities in BPD patients.

PARTICIPANTS AND METHODS

The study received approval from the Ethics Committee of the University of Freiburg (EK-Fr 233/14).

Composition of the Patient Group

We included patients suffering from BPD who had been admitted to our hospital for in-patient treatment between 2001 and 2011. Since visual, high-quality EEG analysis is very time consuming, we were not able to include all datasets. In the absence of reliable and expectable prevalence rates from earlier controlled studies, we decided to adopt a pragmatic approach and included the first 100 consecutive patients who fulfilled all inclusion and exclusion criteria. Due to *post-hoc* information, we had to exclude four BPD patients, which led to 96 BPD patients being included.

The BPD patients were diagnosed according to the standards of our specialized unit, i.e., the Borderline diagnosis was established by senior consultant psychiatrists based on a detailed structured psychiatric interview (Structured Clinical Interview for DSM-IV, SCID I and II; First et al., 1996, 1997) that integrated common psychiatric and somatic differential diagnoses as well as the patients' medical histories. We included more female patients (93 out of 96) because our in-patient treatment is especially designed for female BPD patients.

Patients with known comorbid organic psychiatric disorders, psychotic disorders, or other personality disorders were excluded from the study. We also excluded patients with any neurological disorder, a history of birth complications, febrile convulsions or encephalitic disease in the past. A family history of epilepsy also led to exclusion from our study. Antiepileptic medication can reduce epileptic EEG patterns (Duncan, 1987) and so might lead to the underestimation of EEG abnormalities, while clozapine is known to be the most proconvulsive medication and can lead to an overestimation of EEG abnormalities (Welch et al., 1994; Meyer, 2004; Alper et al., 2007). Therefore, we also excluded patients taking anticonvulsant medication or the proconvulsant drug clozapine. For patients who received more than one EEG, we selected the initial one for this study.

Composition of the Control Group

In our daily clinical practice, we do not analyze the EEGs of healthy controls. Therefore, we included controls from an earlier, large EEG study conducted in-house. Again, any psychiatric or neurological diagnoses lead to exclusion. Nicotine consumption was not an exclusion criterion. We were able to include all 76 datasets for which electronic records were available (Feige et al., 2008). In addition, we compared the findings of our BPD sample to figures from the literature. Based on published data, EEG abnormalities in healthy controls who received neurological as well as psychiatric assessments were found in about 0.5% of cases (study of 13,658 trainee pilots; Gregory et al., 1993). For the statistical analysis, we conservatively assumed EEG abnormalities in 1% of the general population (Shelley et al., 2008).

EEG Reading and Classification

All EEGs were recorded using the international 10/20 system for 20 min, including a hyperventilation phase of more than 3 min, which was used as a provocation method. Sintered Ag-AgCl bridge electrode impedances were kept below 5 kOhm. Signals were acquired using a Schwarzer 25-channel USB amplifier, filtered between 0.07 and 100 Hz, sampled with a rate of 256 Hz and continuously stored on disc for later analysis. Neurofile® software was used for visual EEG analysis following typical clinical standards. Longitudinal rows were used as standard montage. In cases of pathological findings in the bipolar longitudinal rows, we correlated abnormalities with bipolar transverse rows and reference electrodes. All EEGs were analyzed by the same blinded trained expert rater (MF), who identified all normal EEGs in a first step. The abnormal and all nebulous EEG findings were reevaluated in a second step by a board certified neurologist (SB). All EEGs that were deemed abnormal following this second step were rated by a board certified consultant epileptologist from the local university epilepsy center (DMA). All raters were blinded throughout the diagnostic process. Final diagnosis was established as a consensus diagnosis of all raters. All abnormalities were documented (i.e., each IRDA, IRTA, and SWC). **Figure 1** shows an exemplary EEG with IRTA. To define clear outcome criteria and to avoid the overestimation of pathological EEGs based on diffuse slowing due to drowsiness or hyperventilation, we took care to exclude such phenomena of physiological slowing and did not rate any unclear EEG slowing as a pathological phenomenon.

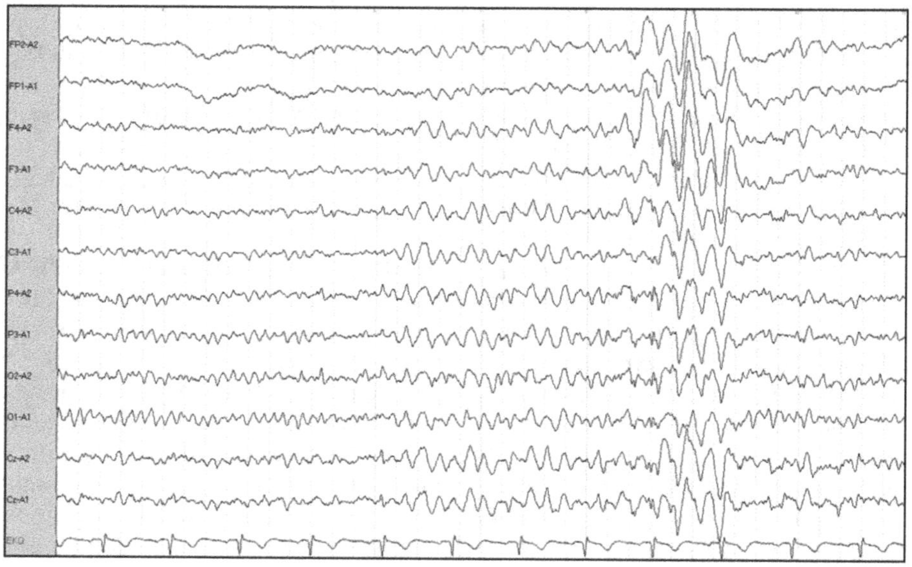

FIGURE 1 | Example of a clinical electroencephalogram (EEG) of a patient with borderline personality disorder. The X-axis illustrates intermittent rhythmic theta activity (IRTA), and Y-axis shows a referential montage to the ears. FP, frontoparietal; A, ear; F, frontal; C, central; P, parietal; O, occipital; Cz, central zero; EKG, electrocardiography.

TABLE 1 | Demographic and clinical characteristics of borderline personality disorder and control group.

	Borderline personality disorder (n = 96)	Control group (n = 76)	Statistics
Age	27.0 ± 6.9	37.8 ± 10.8	$t = -7.7$, $df = 121.1$, $p \leq 0.001$
Gender	93 F:3 M	38 F:38 M	$X^2 = 51.3$, $df = 1$, $p \leq 0.001$
SCHOOL EDUCATION			
No degree	4 (4.2%)	Not available	
Low degree	27 (28.1%)	Not available	
Medium degree	35 (36.5%)	Not available	
High degree	28 (29.2%)	Not available	
Unknown	2 (2.1%)	Not available	
PROFESSIONAL DEGREE			
None/semiskilled	53 (55.2%)	Not available	
Vocational training	31 (32.3%)	Not available	
University degree	10 (10.4%)	Not available	
Unknown	2 (2.1%)	Not available	
MEDICATION			
Medication on discharge	55 (57.3%)	Unmedicated	
No medication	41 (42.7%)	Unmedicated	
ABNORMAL PSYCHOPATHOLOGICAL FINDINGS*			
Attention and memory	50 (52.1%)	Not inquired	
Formal thought disorder	18 (18.8%)	Not inquired	
Fear and compulsion	26 (27.1%)	Not inquired	
Affectivity	86 (89.6%)	Not inquired	
Energy and psychomotor domain	51 (53.1%)	Not inquired	
Circadian rhythm	32 (33.3%)	Not inquired	
Suicidal tendency	17 (17.7%)	Not inquired	
PSYCHIATRIC COMORBIDITY			
Psychiatric overall comorbidity	60 (62.5%)	Excluded	
ADHD	29 (30.2%)	Excluded	
Major Depression	Current: 25 (26%) Remitted: 5 (5.2%)	Excluded	
Eating disorder	11 (11.5%)	Excluded	
Adaptation disorder	4 (4.2%)	Excluded	
Others**	12 (12.5%)	Excluded	

*Documented on discharge; **Phobia (in 3 patients), alcohol abuse (3), obsessive compulsive disorder (2), dysthymia (1), bipolar disorder (1), tic disorder (1), somatoform disorder (1). F, female; M, male; ADHD, attention deficit hyperactivity disorder.*

Demographic and Psychometric Data

All demographic and psychometric information was assessed using our clinic's electronic documentation system. This data comprised demographic data, psychopathological symptoms following the standardized AMDP system (Arbeitsgemeinschaft für Methodik und Dokumentation in der Psychiatrie, www.amdp.de), medical and psychiatric history, medication, and social information. Only patients with complete documentation were included.

Data Handling and Statistical Analysis

All EEG, demographic, and psychometric information was carefully evaluated and entered into a data bank using the Statistical Package for the Social Sciences (SPSS 20). Age was compared using two-sided independent-sample t-tests, while gender was analyzed using Pearson's two-sided X^2-test. The prevalence of EEG abnormalities between groups was compared using Pearson's two-sided X^2-test. We compared the prevalence rates of the BPD patients with both our own and a historical control group. Moreover, we compared age matched groups, after the exclusion of the oldest control subjects. In addition, we compared only female patients and female controls. To exclude any effects of medication, we compared the unmedicated BPD patients with the control group. A $p < 0.05$ served as the criterion of significance.

RESULTS

Demographic Data

Table 1 summarizes the clinical and demographic data of our patients and the control group. The BPD patients turned out to be significantly younger than the members of the control group. Also, since the control group was not specifically generated to be matched with this study, it consisted of a significantly higher number of male subjects.

Prevalence of EEG Abnormalities

Only IRDAs and IRTAs were found in the patient and control groups. No patient showed clear-cut epileptiform potentials such as sharp waves, polyspikes, or spike-wave complexes. Still, the BPD patients demonstrated significantly higher rates of EEG abnormalities ($X^2 = 5.4, df = 1, p = 0.020$). When comparing the rate of EEG abnormalities to the 1% estimated from figures in the literature, this difference became even more significant ($X^2 = 12.8, df = 1, p \leq 0.001$).

When comparing only unmedicated BPD patients ($n = 41$) to all controls, we also found increased percentages of EEG abnormalities ($X^2 = 4.3, df = 1, p = 0.038$; **Table 2**). Comparing only female BPD patients ($n = 93$, age: 27.1 ± 6.9) and female controls ($n = 38$; age: 40.1 ± 11.7; $p_{age} \leq 0.001$), we find higher rates of EEG pathologies in the female patients (15.1 vs. 5.3% in the controls), showing a non-significant trend in the X^2-test ($X^2 = 2.4$, $df = 1$, $p = 0.120$). Due to the small sample size of male patients ($n = 3$), we have not compared the male groups. After excluding the oldest controls, we analyzed the age matched groups (96 BPD patients vs. 41 controls). Again, the EEG pathologies were higher in the BPD group (14.6 vs. 7.3% in the controls), which was not significant ($X^2 = 1.4$, $df = 1$, $p = 0.237$).

Clinical Characteristics of BPD Patients with IRDAs/IRTAs

Table 3 summarizes the clinical characteristics of the 14 BPD patients with EEG abnormalities. All patients were female and suffered mostly from mental tension, self-injuries and dissociative symptoms. Five patients had attempted suicide.

TABLE 2 | EEG abnormalities in borderline personality disorder.

	Borderline personality disorder ($n = 96$)	Control group ($n = 76$)	Statistics (Pearson-X^2-test)
IRDAs/ IRTAs	14 (14.6%)	3 (3.9%)	$X^2 = 5.4$; $df = 1$; **$p = 0.020$**
	Unmedicated borderline personality disorder group ($n = 41$)	**Control group ($n = 76$)**	
IRDAs/ IRTAs	6 (14.6%)	3 (3.9%)	$X^2 = 4.3$; $df = 1$; **$p = 0.038$**
	Borderline personality disorder ($n = 96$)	**Historical control group** (Gregory et al., 1993; Shelley et al., 2008)	
IRDAs/ IRTAs	14 (14.6%)	1%	$X^2 = 12.8$; $df = 1$; **$p \leq 0.001$**

IRDAs, intermittent rhythmic delta activity; IRTAs, intermittent rhythmic theta activity.

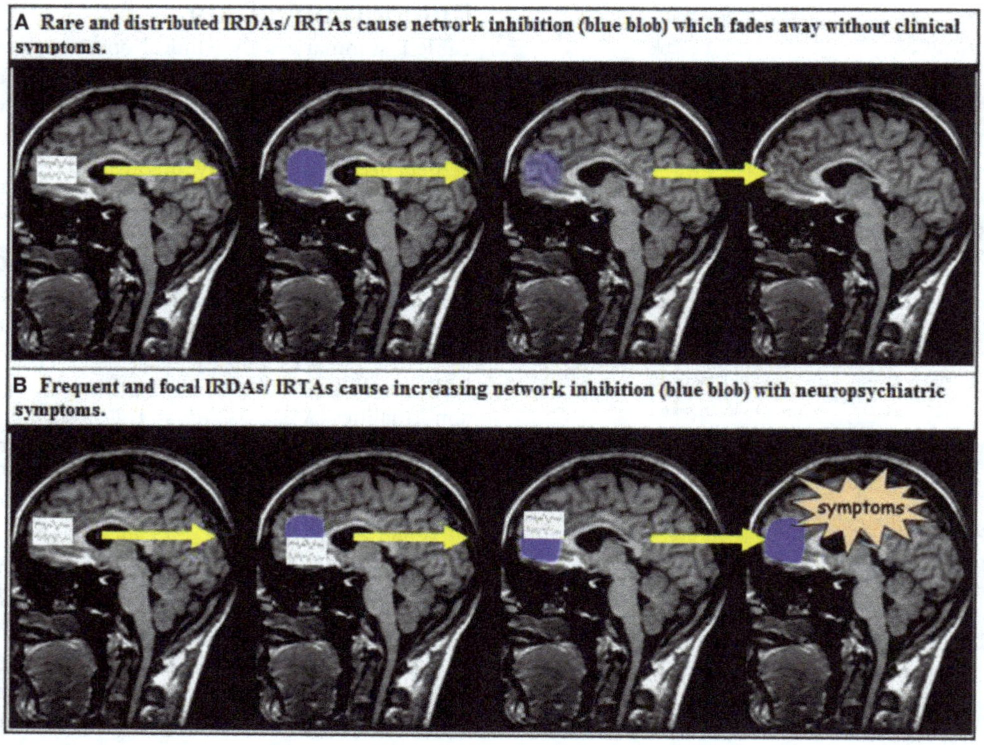

FIGURE 2 | The local area network inhibition (LANI) model as a potential paraepileptic pathomechanism (Tebartz van Elst et al., 2011; Tebartz van Elst and Perlov, 2013). IRDA, intermittent rhythmic delta activity; IRTA, intermittent rhythmic theta activity.

Six out of 14 patients were unmedicated, while eight patients were taking antidepressants. Depression was the most frequent comorbidity in patients with IRDAs/IRTAs. Three patients had a comorbid eating disorder.

DISCUSSION

The main result of our study is that, among the BPD patients, there was a significant subgroup of 14.6% who displayed clear-cut EEG abnormalities in terms of IRDAs and IRTAs. In contrast to other studies, no epileptic patterns could be detected. However, due to the not exactly matched control group, our results should be regarded as only preliminary findings.

Comparison with Previous Studies

Our finding is well within the range of EEG abnormalities in BPD patients reported in the review by Shelley and colleagues (5.8–46%; Shelley et al., 2008; **Table 4**). In our study, only IRDAs and IRTAs were found, as in some previous studies involving BPD patients (Snyder and Pitts, 1984; De La Fuente et al., 1998). Snyder and Pitts (1984) found significantly more abnormalities

TABLE 3 | Characterization of patients with IRDAs/IRTAs.

Nr.	Patient characteristics	Paroxysmal symptoms	Comorbidity	Medication	EEG-abnormalities
1	21 years, female, trainee nurse	Dissociative symptoms, self injuries, suicidal tendency, several suicidal attempts	Depression, PTSD	None	IRDAs with frontal maximum
2	26 years, female, industrial clerk	Mental tension, difficulties controlling anger, self injuries, several suicidal attempts	Atypical bulimia nervosa	None	IRDAs with frontal maximum
3	28 years, female, commercial clerk	Affective instability, self injuries	Depression (currently remitted)	Citalopram	FIRTAs
4	22 years, female, media worker	Mental tension, self injuries, affective instability	None	None	IRTAs
5	19 years, female, no professional training	Mental tension, self injuries, dissociative symptoms, suicidal tendency, one suicidal attempt	Past alcohol abuse	None	IRTAs with fronto-central maximum
6	19 years, female, school for domestic science	Dissociative seizures, mental tension, self injuries	None	None	IRTAs
7	22 years, female, no professional training	Mental tension, self injuries	Mild depression, past substance abuse, two suicidal attempts	Venlafaxine	IRDAs with frontal maximum
8	25 years, female, no professional training	Dissociative states, mental tension, self injuries, three suicidal attempts	Anorexia nervosa, depression	Quetiapine, fluoxetine, benperidol	IRTAs with parieto-temporal maximum
9	22 years, female, trainee office clerk	Mental tension, self injuries, suicidal tendency, several suicidal attempts	Depression (currently remitted)	Venlafaxine, prothipendyl, chlorprothixene	FIRTAs
10	19 years, female, trainee hotel clerk	Mental tension, self injuries	None	None	FIRTAs
11	26 years, female, insurance clerk	Dissociative states, mental tension, suicidal tendency	Depression, ADHD, PTSD	Methylphenidate, fluspirilene	FIRTAs
12	25 years, female, insurance clerk	Mental tension, self injuries, dissociative states with depersonalization and derealization, suicidal tendency	Atypical bulimia nervosa, depression (currently remitted)	Citalopram, perazine	FIRTAs
13	34 years, female, profession unclear	Mental tension, self injuries, derealization, hallucinations	None	Risperidone, zopiclone, chlorprothixene, fluoxetine, tetrazepam	FIRTAs
14	27 years, female, office clerk	Dissociative symptoms, mental tension, self injuries, suicidal tendency	ADHD, abuse of alcohol	Venlafaxine, zopiclone	FIRTAs

EEG, electroencephalogram; PTSD, Post-Traumatic Stress Disorder; ADHD, attention deficit hyperactivity disorder; IRDA, intermittent rhythmic delta activity; IRTA, intermittent rhythmic theta activity; FIRTA, frontal intermittent rhythmic theta activity.

in 37 male BPD patients, mostly slow wave activity. De La Fuente et al. (1998) described diffuse slow activity in 40% of the mostly female patients in a collective of 20 patients. In a study by Archer et al. (1988), dysrhythmia was found in 31.3%, while in a study by Cornelius et al. (1986) it was detected in 18.8% of the BPD patients. Ogiso et al. (1993) depicted an association between positive spikes and high impulsivity. Our low overall prevalence rates might be explained by our strict inclusion and exclusion criteria, which excluded all patients with any evidence of organic comorbidities and relevant medication effects. Also, due to our desire to avoid an overestimation of pathological EEG and in contrast to many other studies in the literature, we did not rate unclear EEG slowing as pathological phenomena. Moreover, differences in the reference electrodes in earlier studies might have influenced the analysis process and findings.

Pathological EEG findings in Healthy Subjects

In order to judge whether or not such findings are relevant, it is important to clarify how often similar pathological EEG findings are obtained in the general population without BPD. Depending on the inclusion and exclusion criteria, EEG abnormalities were identified in 0.3–18.6%, showing a broad range of "normality" (Gregory et al., 1993; Boutros et al., 2005; Shelley et al., 2008). However, after the exclusion of possible contaminating factors, epileptiform dysrhythmia in healthy control groups can be

TABLE 4 | Previous EEG findings in borderline personality disorder (following Boutros et al., 2003; Shelley et al., 2008).

Study	N (PBD/ controls)	Gender patients (F/M)	Medication	Comorbidity	EEG-abnormalities	Characteristics
Tebartz van Elst et al., 2011	1/0	1/0	None	None	Epileptiform discharges	Remission with valporate
De La Fuente et al., 1998	20/0	15/5	None	None current	Diffuse slow activity in 40%	More frequent in medicated patients
Ogiso et al., 1993	18/21	18/0	Anxiolytics, antipsychotics, antidepressants	Depression, substance abuse	Positive spikes in patients with high impulsivity; Wave and spike phantoms in patients with interpersonal relationship dysfunction	
Drake et al., 1992	6/0	Not reported	Not reported	Not reported	Normal findings in patients with pseudo-seizures	
Schmid et al., 1989	1/0	1/0	Antidepressant, antipsychotic	Depression	Normal	
Cowdry et al., 1985	39/20 (unipolar depressed patients)	36/3	Not reported	No current Axis I disorder, Axis II not reported	More frequent epileptiform discharges in BPD; mostly paroxysmal posterior sharp waves	
Messner, 1986	1/0	0/1	None	None	Focal temporal lobe slow-wave activity	
Archer et al., 1988	16/83 (10 with non-BPD personality disorders, 39 with dysthymic disorders, 34 with other mixed diagnosis)	Not reported	None	None	Dysrhytmics in 31.3%; 6.3% had spike and wave discharges	No significant differences compared with control groups; wake and sleep EEG
Cornelius et al., 1986	69/22 (non-BPD personality disorders)	52/17	None	None current	Dysrhythmias in 18.8% of BPD patients; severe abnormalities in 5.8%	No significant differences compared with non-BPD personality disorder group
Snyder and Pitts, 1984	37/31 (dysthymic disorder)	0/37	None	None	Significantly more abnormalities, mostly slow-wave activity	Only male patients

BPD, borderline personality disorder; F, female; M, male; EEG, electroencephalogram.

assumed to account for less than 1% of cases (Shelley et al., 2008). Therefore, the authors of review articles regarding EEG abnormalities in control groups and in psychiatric collectives argue for stricter inclusion and exclusion criteria, such as those enforced in our study (Boutros et al., 2005; Shelley et al., 2008).

Limitations

The major limitation of this study is that it is a retrospective analysis without adequate control group. Therefore, the results should basically be regarded as preliminary findings of an open uncontrolled study and statistical calculations should be regarded as only exploratory in nature. We cannot be sure about what is driving the difference in occurrence of EEG abnormalities in this sample. In any retrospective analysis of EEG patient collectives, it is difficult to generate suitable control groups because controls are not routinely investigated. Therefore, further and prospective studies are needed to confirm the findings raised in this paper.

For this study, we were able to use a control group of healthy participants who took part in an earlier project involving sleep research (Feige et al., 2008). However, this control group was smaller than our patient group and was not well matched with respect to gender and age. The BPD patients were younger than the controls and females were more common than in the control group. The control subjects did not receive a thorough neurological or psychiatric assessment. Earlier evidence from basic clinical EEG research illustrates that the less strictly the EEG control samples were defined in terms of neurological and psychiatric evaluations, the higher the resulting prevalence of EEG pathologies turned out to be (Tebartz van Elst and Perlov, 2013). In large cohorts of well investigated pilots who had received not only neurological but also internistic and psychiatric evaluations, pathological EEGs proved to be very rare, with a prevalence of between 0.3 and 0.6% (Thorner, 1942; Bennett, 1967; Gregory et al., 1993). In contrast, less well defined control samples produced prevalence figures for pathological EEG findings in 5–8% of cases (Iida et al., 1985; Okubo et al., 1993). In that sense, our control sample is comparable to the clinical samples published by Iida et al. (1985) and Okubo et al. (1993), with pathological findings in 3.9% of cases. Therefore, we would have detected false positive EEG pathologies in our control group.

Moreover, the effect of medication could not be completely eliminated since we were unable to include only unmedicated patients. We excluded patients who were currently taking the most proconvulsive (clozapine; Duncan, 1987; Meyer, 2004; Alper et al., 2007) and typical anticonvulsive medications (antiepileptics). However, other neuroleptics or antidepressants might have influenced our results. Neuroleptics (e.g., olanzapine) could reduce the seizure threshold to a lesser extent compared with clozapine; some antidepressants—mainly selective serotonin reuptake inhibitors—might have the opposite effect and actually increase the seizure threshold (Alper et al., 2007; Tebartz van Elst and Perlov, 2013).

However, six of the 14 BPD patients with pathological EEGs were unmedicated and nine were medicated. A total of 41 out of the 96 BPD patients were unmedicated. When restricting the analysis to these 41 unmedicated patients and comparing EEG abnormalities with our control group, the prevalence of pathological EEG findings was the same (14.6%). This means that our overall prevalence rates cannot be explained by a medication effect.

Following clinical practice, the data analysis was performed based on clinical expert ratings and was thus investigator-dependent. Therefore, this kind of clinical data analysis is prone to rater bias. For that reason, all clinical raters were blinded with respect to the identity of the EEGs of interest. For this reason, we can reject the suggestion that a rating bias might have increased the prevalence of pathological EEG findings in our BPD group.

Further, all EEGs deemed to be pathological were ultimately assessed by a team of three experts, including one board certified consultant neurologist (SB) and another very experienced board certified consultant neurologist and epileptologist from the local university epilepsy center (DMA). Therefore, we think that the quality of the clinical rating of the EEGs corresponds to the highest clinical standards. However, since the first line trained rater (MF) is not an experienced epileptologist, we cannot rule out the fact that false negative EEG ratings might have lowered the prevalence of pathological EEG findings. In further studies, an automatic and quantitative means of detecting IRDAs and IRTAs should be performed to verify our results.

The sample size could have been larger than the 96 patients we decided to include in this project. However, since visual EEG analysis in general and the algorithm of analysis we chose in this study in particular is extremely time consuming, for practical reasons we were not able to create a larger sample. Also, the size of our sample compares well to publications in the literature, as can be deduced from **Table 4**.

The way we defined our sample does have an impact on the generalizability of our findings. In order to avoid an overestimation of the rate of EEG pathologies, we excluded patients with any kind of neurological comorbidity as well as those with a history of birth complications, febrile seizures, a history of meningitis, or encephalitis, and a family history of epilepsy. All of these factors could have contributed to pathological EEG findings and were therefore excluded. We were not able to exclude a medication effect in the overall sample but, as mentioned above, the rate of EEG pathologies in the unmedicated BPD patients was the same as that in the mixed group. Since in the general medical settings quite a few BPD patients do fulfill at least one of the exclusion criteria mentioned above, we cannot generalize our findings to this clinical sample.

Also, in order to simulate the classical clinical diagnostic setting, we assessed only routine EEG studies of 20 min length. Repeated and prospective EEG studies, including sleep and sleep deprivation recordings, would most likely have produced higher prevalence rates of pathological findings, possibly including classical epileptiform activity. Therefore, our detection rate of EEG abnormalities has to be regarded as a minimum detection rate and it is very likely that the prevalence of pathological EEG findings will be even higher if such exclusion criteria are not applied or repeated and more elaborate assessment methods are applied.

Despite these limitations, we here present the largest study to date into possible EEG pathologies in BPD patients and produce evidence that a considerable subgroup of 14.6% of BPD patients do display EEG pathologies in terms of IRDAs or IRTAs. Thus, a question arises as to what this might mean from a pathophysiological point of view and with respect to treatment.

Clinical Relevance of IRDAs/IRTAs in BPD

The clinical relevance of intermittent rhythmic delta or theta EEG activity is poorly understood. As discussed in the introduction, both IRDAs and IRTAs are clearly regarded as pathological EEG patterns (Brigo, 2011). However, it is unclear precisely what their presence means in terms of disturbed neuronal information processing. Clearly, none of our patients do suffer from epilepsy. The LANI hypothesis outlined in the introduction is a pathophysiological model that can explain why patients exhibiting IRDAs or IRTAs may develop clinical neuropsychiatric symptoms at one time (i.e., when IRDAs are focal and frequent enough to stimulate above threshold reactive neuronal network inhibition) but not at another time (i.e., when IRDAs are distributed or rare so that reactive neuromodulation remains subthreshold and can fade away before another IRDA event occurs) (Tebartz van Elst et al., 2011). If true, the IRDA/IRTA model would be a model of a paraepileptic pathomechanism, i.e., a pathophysiology in which non-ictal, but paroxysmal EEG activity results in neuropsychiatric symptoms via reactive network modulation (**Figure 2**). It is important to stress that this assumed mechanism cannot be regarded as epilepsy (Tebartz van Elst et al., 2011). Another well-established example of such a paraepileptic pathomechanism is that of Todd's paresis (Fisher and Schachter, 2000), where epileptic seizure activity also induces neuromodulatory processes that result in long-term functional alterations of the neurophysiology and affected neuronal networks (Fisher and Schachter, 2000; Schulze-Bonhage and Tebartz van Elst, 2010; Tebartz van Elst et al., 2011).

However, in Todd's paresis the diagnosis is necessarily linked to classical seizures whereas the LANI hypothesis is based on non-ictal paroxysmal activity acting as the trigger mechanism, which means that a diagnosis of epilepsy cannot be made (Tebartz van Elst et al., 2011).

The idea that non-ictal epileptiform activity in the brain causes secondary modulation of the neurophysiology of neuronal networks, which in turn causes psychiatric symptoms, is not new to neuropsychiatry (Stevens, 1988, 1995, 1999; Bruton et al., 1994; Heimer, 2000, 2003; Tatlidil, 2000; Läppchen et al., 2008, 2011). Such models are difficult to prove and the present study was a first step in that direction as it validated the prevalence of the EEG phenomenon of IRDAs or IRTAs in a fairly typical sample of BPD patients in the tertiary referral setting of a specialized center offering specific therapy.

At the end of the day, the question of the precise pathophysiology and meaning of IRDAs and IRTAs is a rather academic matter and it will take a while until we are able to clarify it. However, from a clinical point of view, another more important therapeutic question arises, i.e., whether or not the observation of such EEG pathologies in BPD patients might have therapeutic implications. We recently described a patient with IRTAs and severe dissociative and auto-aggressive symptoms who responded very well to therapy with valproate as well as topiramate later in the course (Tebartz van Elst et al., 2011). Based on this observation, one might speculate that the presence of IRDAs or IRTAs in BPD patients might be a biological predictor of a positive response to anticonvulsive treatment options. To our knowledge, there are no studies published in the literature focusing on this question. However, the answer to this question might be very important for the therapy of a subgroup of BPD patients. Clearly, further research is needed to resolve this important clinical issue.

SUMMARY

To our knowledge, this uncontrolled study is the largest survey to date on the prevalence of EEG pathology in a carefully selected, retrospectively defined sample of BPD patients where all possible risk factors for pathological EEG findings led to exclusion. The EEG readings followed high standards and were conducted by blinded highly qualified raters. We found a prevalence of IRDAs or IRTAs in 14.6% of BPD patients. Further research is needed to clarify whether or not such pathological EEG findings might predict the response to anticonvulsive pharmacotherapy in these patients.

AUTHOR CONTRIBUTIONS

All authors listed, have made substantial, direct and intellectual contribution to the work, and approved it for publication.

ACKNOWLEDGMENTS

The study was funded by the Clinic for Psychiatry and Psychotherapy at the University Medical Center Freiburg.

REFERENCES

Alper, K., Schwartz, K. A., Kolts, R. L., and Khan, A. (2007). Seizure incidence in psychopharmacological clinical trials: an analysis of Food and Drug Administration (FDA) summary basis of approval reports. *Biol. Psychiatry* 62, 345–354. doi: 10.1016/j.biopsych.2006.09.023

Archer, R. P., Struve, F. A., Ball, J. D., and Gordon, R. A. (1988). EEG in borderline personality disorder. *Biol. Psychiatry* 24, 731–732. doi: 10.1016/0006-3223(88)90156-4

Bellino, S., Paradiso, E., and Bogetto, F. (2005). Oxcarbazepine in the treatment of borderline personality disorder: a pilot study. *J. Clin. Psychiatry* 66, 1111–1115. doi: 10.4088/JCP.v66n0904

Bennett, D. R. (1967). Spike-wave complexes in "normal" flying personnel. *Aerosp. Med.* 38, 1276–1282.

Berger, H. (1969). On the electroencephalogram of man. *Electroencephalogr. Clin. Neurophysiol.* Suppl. 28, 37–73.

Boutros, N., Mirolo, H. A., and Struve, F. (2005). Normative data for the unquantified EEG: examination of adequacy for neuropsychiatric research. *J. Neuropsychiatry Clin. Neurosci.* 17, 84–90. doi: 10.1176/jnp.17.1.84

Boutros, N. N., Torello, M., and McGlashan, T. H. (2003). Electrophysiological aberrations in borderline personality disorder: state of the evidence. *J. Neuropsychiatry Clin. Neurosci.* 15, 145–154. doi: 10.1176/jnp.15.2.145

Brigo, F. (2011). Intermittent rhythmic delta activity patterns. *Epilepsy Behav.* 20, 254–256. doi: 10.1016/j.yebeh.2010.11.009

Bruton, C. J., Stevens, J. R., and Frith, C. D. (1994). Epilepsy, psychosis, and schizophrenia: clinical and neuropathologic correlations. *Neurology* 44, 34–42. doi: 10.1212/WNL.44.1.34

Cobb, W. A. (1945). Rhythmic slow discharges in the electroencephalogram. *J. Neurol. Neurosurg. Psychiatry* 8, 65–78. doi: 10.1136/jnnp.8.3-4.65

Cornelius, J. R., Brenner, R. P., Soloff, P. H., Schulz, S. C., and Tumuluru, R. V. (1986). EEG abnormalities in borderline personality disorder: specific or nonspecific. *Biol. Psychiatry* 21, 977–980. doi: 10.1016/0006-3223(86)90275-1

Cowdry, R. W., Pickar, D., and Davies, R. (1985). Symptoms and EEG findings in the borderline syndrome. *Int. J. Psychiatry Med.* 15, 201–211. doi: 10.2190/3Y0C-HAUK-04JX-GBPN

de Araujo Filho, G. M., and Yacubian, E. M. T. (2013). Juvenile myoclonic epilepsy: psychiatric comorbidity and impact on outcome. *Epilepsy Behav.* 28(Suppl. 1), 74–80. doi: 10.1016/j.yebeh.2013.03.026

De La Fuente, J. M., Tugendhaft, P., and Mavroudakis, N. (1998). Electroencephalographic abnormalities in borderline personality disorder. *Psychiatry Res.* 77, 131–138. doi: 10.1016/S0165-1781(97)00149-2

Drake, M. E., Pakalnis, A., and Phillips, B. B. (1992). Neuropsychological and psychiatric correlates of intractable pseudoseizures. *Seizure* 1, 11–13. doi: 10.1016/1059-1311(92)90048-6

Duncan, J. S. (1987). Antiepileptic drugs and the electroencephalogram. *Epilepsia* 28, 259–266. doi: 10.1111/j.1528-1157.1987.tb04216.x

Feige, B., Al-Shajlawi, A., Nissen, C., Voderholzer, U., Hornyak, M., Spiegelhalder, K., et al. (2008). Does REM sleep contribute to subjective wake time in primary insomnia? A comparison of polysomnographic and subjective sleep in 100 patients. *J. Sleep Res.* 17, 180–190. doi: 10.1111/j.1365-2869.2008.00651.x

First, M. B., Gibbon, M., Spitzer, R. L., Williams, J. B. W., and Benjamin, L. S. (1997). *Structured Clinical Interview for DSM-IV Axis II Personality Disorders, (SCID-II).* Washington, D.C: American Psychiatric Press.

First, M. B., Spitzer, R. L., Gibbon, M., and Williams, J. B. W. (1996). *Structured Clinical Interview for DSM-IV Axis I Disorders, Clinician Version (SCID-CV).* Washington, DC: American Psychiatric Press.

Fisher, R. S., and Schachter, S. C. (2000). The postictal state: a neglected entity in the management of epilepsy. *Epilepsy Behav.* 1, 52–59. doi: 10.1006/ebeh.2000.0023

Goldstein, W. N. (1983). DSM-III and the diagnosis of borderline. *Am. J. Psychother.* 37, 312–327.

Gregory, R. P., Oates, T., and Merry, R. T. (1993). Electroencephalogram epileptiform abnormalities in candidates for aircrew training. *Electroencephalogr. Clin. Neurophysiol.* 86, 75–77. doi: 10.1016/0013-4694(93)90069-8

Harris, C. L., Dinn, W. M., and Marcinkiewicz, J. A. (2002). Partial seizure-like symptoms in borderline personality disorder. *Epilepsy Behav.* 3, 433–438. doi: 10.1016/S1525-5050(02)00521-8

Heimer, L. (2000). Basal forebrain in the context of schizophrenia. *Brain Res. Brain Res. Rev.* 31, 205–235. doi: 10.1016/S0165-0173(99)00039-9

Heimer, L. (2003). A new anatomical framework for neuropsychiatric disorders and drug abuse. *Am. J. Psychiatry* 160, 1726–1739. doi: 10.1176/appi.ajp.160.10.1726

Iida, N., Okada, S., and Tsuboi, T. (1985). EEG abnormalities in nonepileptic patients. *Folia Psychiatr. Neurol. Jpn.* 39, 43–58. doi: 10.1111/j.1440-1819.1985.tb01943.x

Kakisaka, Y., Jin, K., Kato, K., Iwasaki, M., and Nakasato, N. (2014). Temporal intermittent rhythmic delta activity and abdominal migraine. *Neurol. Sci.* 35, 627–628. doi: 10.1007/s10072-013-1625-0

Läppchen, C. H., Feil, B., Fauser, S., Glocker, F. X., and Schulze-Bonhage, A. (2011). Changes in interhemispheric inhibition following successful epilepsy surgery: a TMS study. *J. Neurol.* 258, 68–73. doi: 10.1007/s00415-010-5683-4

Läppchen, C. H., Feil, B., Fauser, S., Wuwer, Y., Glocker, F. X., and Schulze-Bonhage, A. (2008). Changes in intracortical excitability after successful epilepsy surgery. *Epilepsy Res.* 79, 55–62. doi: 10.1016/j.eplepsyres.2007.12.010

Lieb, K., Zanarini, M. C., Schmahl, C., Linehan, M. M., and Bohus, M. (2004). Borderline personality disorder. *Lancet* 364, 453–461. doi: 10.1016/S0140-6736(04)16770-6

Loew, T. H., Nickel, M. K., Muehlbacher, M., Kaplan, P., Nickel, C., Kettler, C., et al. (2006). Topiramate treatment for women with borderline personality disorder: a double-blind, placebo-controlled study. *J. Clin. Psychopharmacol.* 26, 61–66. doi: 10.1097/01.jcp.0000195113.61291.48

Lynch, T. R., Trost, W. T., Salsman, N., and Linehan, M. M. (2007). Dialectical behavior therapy for borderline personality disorder. *Annu. Rev. Clin. Psychol.* 3, 181–205. doi: 10.1146/annurev.clinpsy.2.022305.095229

Messner, E. (1986). Covert complex partial seizures in psychotherapy. *Am. J. Orthopsychiatry* 56, 323–326. doi: 10.1111/j.1939-0025.1986.tb02735.x

Meyer, A. (2004). Anfallssteigernde Wirkung von Medikamenten. *Nervenheilkunde* 23, 186–240.

Ogiso, Y., Moriya, N., Ikuta, N., Maher-Nishizono, A., Takase, M., Miyake, Y., et al. (1993). Relationship between clinical symptoms and EEG findings in borderline personality disorder. *Jpn. J. Psychiatry Neurol.* 47, 37–46. doi: 10.1111/j.1440-1819.1993.tb02027.x

Okubo, Y., Matsuura, M., Asai, T., Kato, M., Kojima, T., and Toru, M. (1993). A follow-up study of healthy children with epileptiform EEG discharges. *J. Epilepsy* 6, 250–256.

Reeves, R. R., Struve, F. A., and Patrick, G. (2003). EEG does not predict response to valproate treatment of aggression in patients with borderline and antisocial personality disorders. *Clin. Electroencephalogr.* 34, 84–86. doi: 10.1177/155005940303400207

Ripoll, L. H. (2012). Clinical psychopharmacology of borderline personality disorder: an update on the available evidence in light of the Diagnostic and Statistical Manual of Mental Disorders - 5. *Curr. Opin. Psychiatry* 25, 52–58. doi: 10.1097/YCO.0b013e32834c3f19

Schmid, E. M., Handleman, M. J., and Bidder, T. G. (1989). Seizure disorder misdiagnosed as borderline syndrome. *Am. J. Psychiatry* 146, 400–401.

Schulze-Bonhage, A., and Tebartz van Elst, L. (2010). Postictal psychosis: evidence for extrafocal functional precursors. *Epilepsy Behav.* 18, 308–312. doi: 10.1016/j.yebeh.2010.02.009

Shelley, B. P., Trimble, M. R., and Boutros, N. N. (2008). Electroencephalographic cerebral dysrhythmic abnormalities in the trinity of nonepileptic general population, neuropsychiatric, and neurobehavioral disorders. *J. Neuropsychiatry Clin. Neurosci.* 20, 7–22. doi: 10.1176/jnp.2008.20.1.7

Shipton, H. W. (1975). EGG analysis: a history and a prospectus. *Annu. Rev. Biophys. Bioeng.* 4, 1–13.

Snyder, S., and Pitts, W. M. (1984). Electroencephalography of DSM-III borderline personality disorder. *Acta Psychiatr. Scand.* 69, 129–134. doi: 10.1111/j.1600-0447.1984.tb02476.x

Stevens, J. R. (1988). Epilepsy, psychosis and schizophrenia. *Schizophr. Res.* 1, 79–89. doi: 10.1016/0920-9964(88)90044-8

Stevens, J. R. (1995). Clozapine: the Yin and Yang of seizures and psychosis. *Biol. Psychiatry* 37, 425–426. doi: 10.1016/0006-3223(95)00151-6

Stevens, J. R. (1999). Epilepsy, schizophrenia, and the extended amygdala. *Ann. N. Y. Acad. Sci.* 877, 548–561. doi: 10.1111/j.1749-6632.1999.tb09288.x

Stoffers, J., Völlm, B. A., Rücker, G., Timmer, A., Huband, N., and Lieb, K. (2010). Pharmacological interventions for borderline personality disorder. *Cochrane Database Syst. Rev.* 16:CD005653 doi: 10.1002/14651858.CD005653.pub2

Tatlidil, R. (2000). Persistent postictal hyperperfusion demonstrated with PET. *Epilepsy Res.* 42, 83–88. doi: 10.1016/S0920-1211(00)00135-2

Tebartz van Elst, L., Krishnamoorthy, E. S., Schulze-Bonhage, A., Altenmüller, D.-M., Richter, H., Ebert, D., et al. (2011). Local area network inhibition: a model of a potentially important paraepileptic pathomechanism in neuropsychiatric disorders. *Epilepsy Behav.* 22, 231–239. doi: 10.1016/j.yebeh.2011.06.016

Tebartz van Elst, L., and Perlov, E. (2013). *Epilepsie und Psyche: Psychische Störungen bei Epilepsie - epileptische Phänomene in der Psychiatrie, 1st edn.* Stuttgart: Kohlhammer.

Thorner, M. W. (1942). *Procurement of Electroencephalograph Tracings in 1000 Flying Cadets for Evaluating the Gibbs Technique in Relation to Flying Ability.* USAD School of Aviation Medical Research Report, 7–1.

van Vliet, J., Mulleners, W., and Meulstee, J. (2012). EEG leading to the diagnosis of limbic encephalitis. *Clin. EEG Neurosci.* 43, 161–164. doi: 10.1177/1550059411433612

Vita, A., Peri, L., de, and Sacchetti, E. (2011). Antipsychotics, antidepressants, anticonvulsants, and placebo on the symptom dimensions of borderline personality disorder: a meta-analysis of randomized controlled and open-label trials. *J. Clin. Psychopharmacol.* 31, 613–624. doi: 10.1097/JCP.0b013e31822c1636

Welch, J., Manschreck, T., and Redmond, D. (1994). Clozapine-induced seizures and EEG changes. *J. Neuropsychiatry Clin. Neurosci.* 6, 250–256.

Williams, L. M., Sidis, A., Gordon, E., and Meares, R. A. (2006). "Missing links" in borderline personality disorder: loss of neural synchrony relates to lack of emotion regulation and impulse control. *J. Psychiatry Neurosci.* 31, 181–188.

Conflict of Interest Statement: The authors declare that the research was conducted in the absence of any commercial or financial relationships that could be construed as a potential conflict of interest.

12

The Alteration of Gray Matter Volume and Cognitive Control in Adolescents with Internet Gaming Disorder

Edited by:
Raymond C. K. Chan, Institute of Psychology, Chinese Academy of Sciences, China

***Correspondence:**
*Kai Yuan, School of Life Science and Technology, Xidian University, Xi'an, Shaanxi Province, 710071, China
kyuan@xidian.edu.cn;
Ming Zhang, Department of Medical Imaging, The First Affiliated Hospital of Medical College, Xi'an Jiaotong University, Xi'an, Shaanxi Province, 710061, China
zhangming01@mail.xjtu.edu.cn*

Hongmei Wang[1], Chenwang Jin[1], Kai Yuan[2,3], Tahir Mehmood Shakir[1], Cuiping Mao[1], Xuan Niu[1], Chen Niu[1], Liping Guo[1] and Ming Zhang[1]**

[1] Department of Medical Imaging, The First Affiliated Hospital of Medical College, Xi'an Jiaotong University, Xi'an, China, [2] School of Life Science and Technology, Xidian University, Xi'an, China, [3] Engineering Research Center of Molecular and Neuro Imaging Ministry of Education, Xi'an, China

Objective: Internet gaming disorder (IGD) has been investigated by many behavioral and neuroimaging studies, for it has became one of the main behavior disorders among adolescents. However, few studies focused on the relationship between alteration of gray matter volume (GMV) and cognitive control feature in IGD adolescents.

Methods: Twenty-eight participants with IAD and twenty-eight healthy age and gender matched controls participated in the study. Brain morphology of adolescents with IGD and healthy controls was investigated using an optimized voxel-based morphometry (VBM) technique. Cognitive control performances were measured by Stroop task, and correlation analysis was performed between brain structural change and behavioral performance in IGD group.

Results: The results showed that GMV of the bilateral anterior cingulate cortex (ACC), precuneus, supplementary motor area (SMA), superior parietal cortex, left dorsal lateral prefrontal cortex (DLPFC), left insula, and bilateral cerebellum decreased in the IGD participants compared with healthy controls. Moreover, GMV of the ACC was negatively correlated with the incongruent response errors of Stroop task in IGD group.

Conclusion: Our results suggest that the alteration of GMV is associated with the performance change of cognitive control in adolescents with IGD, which indicating substantial brain image effects induced by IGD.

Keywords: internet addiction disorder, gray matter, cognitive control, anterior cingulate cortex, color-word stroop

Adolescence is a particular developmental period with rapid alterations in physical, psychological, and social development (Casey et al., 2008). As a big challenge in social adjustment and feelings of vulnerability associated with the relatively immature cognitive control performance, it may elicit a higher incidence of affective disorders and addiction among adolescents (Steinberg, 2005). Internet addiction (IA), as a new disorder, has been a public issue with fast developing of internet in recent years. Data from the China Youth Internet Association (announced on February 2, 2010) showed that the incidence of IA for Chinese urban youths is about 14% with the total number of 24 million (Yuan et al., 2011). IA consists of three subtypes: Internet gaming disorder (IGD), sexual preoccupations, and email/text messaging (Block, 2007). In China, the most important subtype of IA is IGD, and appendix of Diagnostic and Statistical Manual of Mental Disorders (5th Ed., DSM-5) also includes IGD, which emphasized that more research is needed to explore its clinical relevance and underlying neural mechanisms (Brand et al., 2014). The problem of IA drew much focus from education experts, psychologists and psychiatrists, so a lot of researches were performed on IA to investigate its brain mechanism and behavioral intervention (Ko et al., 2009, 2013a; Ding et al., 2013). However, currently the mechanism of IA is not clear and there is no standardized treatment for IGD available.

Adolescents with IGD spend ever-increasing amounts of time for online activities, leading to social withdrawal, self-neglect, poor diet and family problems (Murali and George, 2007; Young, 2007; Kim and Haridakis, 2009). It has been regarded as a behavioral disorder like pathological gambling (King et al., 2012), sexual activity (Holden, 2001), for they shared similar clinical symptoms including excessive use, withdrawal, tolerance, and negative repercussions (Beard and Wolf, 2001). A research showed that cognitive control has been altered in participants with heavy gamblers relative to controls (Toneatto et al., 1997), which suggested that addiction may compromise the cognitive control function. Cao et al. reported a specific relationship between cognitive control and IA by using questionnaires, and the IGD subjects exhibited more impulsivity than control group (Cao et al., 2007).

Cognitive control refers to the ability to control one's own actions, behavior, and even thoughts (Cools and D'Esposito, 2011), as well as the capacity to flexibly adapt thoughts and behavior to current goals by selecting and integrating relevant information from the environment (Blasi et al., 2006). Studies have revealed that the anterior cingulate cortex (ACC) was involved in value assessment for cues pictures, emotional responses induced by craving, and the dorsal lateral prefrontal cortex (DLPFC) participated in cognitive processing for expecting reward and response after received reward (Sun et al., 2012; Brand et al., 2014; Ding et al., 2014). Several studies found cognitive control ability of IGD subjects was altered, for they showed more response errors and longer reaction time (RT) in Stroop task and Go-Nogo tasks in comparison with controls. For Stroop task, the response time, and response errors or mean error rates during the incongruent condition has been key indicators to assessing cognitive control function in IGD studies (Dong et al., 2013a, 2014; Yuan et al., 2013a). In details, Yuan et al. observed that both groups showed significant Stroop effect, where the RT was longer during the incongruent than the congruent condition. The IGD group committed more errors than the control group during the incongruent condition (Yuan et al., 2013a,b; Xing et al., 2014). Dong et al. consistently reported that the IGD group showed reduced efficiency of response-inhibition processes relative to healthy controls, for they demonstrated a non-significant trend for longer RTs (Dong et al., 2012, 2013a,b, 2014). On the other side, Go-Nogo and/or Go-stop tasks have been used to study behavioral characteristics of IGD. One study found that the scores of participants with IGD were significantly correlated with the number of failed no-go trials, suggesting that the low gaming-related inhibition or high impulsivity in IGD group (van Holst et al., 2012). Li et al. reported that the percentage of successfully inhibited responses was significantly lower in IA group than controls in a Go-stop task, which further supported that response inhibition in IA adolescents was impaired (Li et al., 2014).

Furthermore, many studies with neuroimaging and electrophysiological techniques investigated brain changes and cognitive control function in IGD. Dong et al. found that greater activity in the anterior (and also posterior) cingulate cortex for the interference condition of Stroop paradigm in participants with IGD compared with control subjects (Dong et al., 2012). Increased brain activities in the inferior frontal cortex and ACC may be implicated in altered cognitive control ability (Dong et al., 2013a). Yuan et al. also found that cortical thickness and amplitude of low frequency fluctuation (ALFF) values of prefrontal cortex correlated with the Stroop effect, providing brain image evidence for dysfunction in cognitive control performance of IGD. An Event-related potential (ERP) study also found that IGD group demonstrated lower NoGo-N2 amplitude, higher NoGo-P3 amplitude, and longer NoGo-P3 peak latency, indicating that they engaged in more cognitive endeavors, less efficiency in information processing, and lower impulse control than their normal peers (Dong et al., 2010). Another ERP study reported that people with IGD showed reduced medial frontal negativity (MFN) deflection in incongruent conditions than controls, which implied impaired cognitive control in IGD (Dong et al., 2011). However, few researches focused on the relationship between alteration of gray matter volume (GMV) and cognitive control ability in IGD.

The main purposes of the present study were: (1) to investigate cognitive control function with color-word Stroop task; (2) to explore stops aaddiction alteration of brain GMV using voxel-based morphometry (VBM) method; (3) to investigate the correlation between neuroimaging measures and behavioral performances in IGD. Based on the published literature on IGD, we hypothesized that IGD participants will show compromised performance for Stroop task and reduced GMV of the prefrontal cortex. Moreover, the prefrontal cortex GMV will be negatively correlated with the Stroop task performance in IGD individuals.

Materials and Methods

All research procedures were approved by the First Affiliated Hospital of Medical College in Xi'an Jiaotong University Subcommittee on Human Studies and were conducted in accordance with the Declaration of Helsinki.

Subjects

Twenty-eight college students with IGD were recruited in our study based on the criteria of the modified Young Diagnostic Questionnaire for Internet addiction (YDQ) by Beard and Wolf (Young, 1998; Beard and Wolf, 2001). Young suggested that respondents who answered five or more "yes" for the eight questions were considered to be an internet dependent user (Young, 1998). Beard and Wolf modified the YDQ criteria (Beard and Wolf, 2001), proposed that respondents who answered "yes" to questions 1 to 5 and at least to any one of the remaining three questions were classified as suffering from IA, which was used for screening subjects for the present study. We asked the subjects to recall their life-style when they were initially addicted to the internet, which was a retrospective measure for the addiction is a gradual process and we planned to explore linear changes of the brain structure. We retested them with the YDQ criteria modified by Beard and Wolf (Brand et al., 2014) to verify that they qualified for IA diagnosis. By communicating with their parents via telephone we confirmed the reliability of the self-reports from the IGD subjects. We also confirmed this information from their roommates and classmates that if they often played internet game till late night so that disturbing others' life. Twenty-eight age and gender matched ($p > 0.05$) healthy controls without personal or family history of psychiatric disorders were also recruited in our study. In order to ensure that the healthy controls were not suffering from IGD, they were administered by modified YDQ for Internet addiction of Beard and Wolf. All recruited participants were native Chinese speakers, right-handed. Urine test was performed for all subjects to exclude substance abuse before magnetic resonance imaging (MRI) scanning. Exclusion criteria for both groups were (1) neurological disorders or physical illness, including brain tumor, hepatitis, or epilepsy assessed by clinical evaluations and medical records; (2) alcohol, nicotine or drug abuse; and (3) pregnancy or menstrual period in women; Written consent forms were obtained by all the patients and controls. More detailed demographic information was given in **Table 1**.

TABLE 1 | Demographics of internet gaming disorder and control groups.

Items	IGD	Control	*p* value
Age (years)	18.8±1.33	19.3±2.56	>0.05
Gender	M18,F10	M20,F8	>0.05
Education (years)	12.18±0.48	12.2±0.56	>0.05
Hours of internet use(/day)	7.9±1.35	2.6±0.96	*
Days of internet use(/week)	5.35±1.31	2±0.71	*
Internet addiction test(IAT)	65.3±11.31	30.4±5.85	*
Duration of online gaming (years)	5.25±2.15	2.81±1.38	*

$^*p < 0.005$.

MRI Data Acquisition

Brain imaging scan was performed on a 3T GE scanner at imaging center of Xi'an Jiontong university first affiliated hospital. A standard birdcage head coil and restraining foam pads were used to minimize head motion and protect hearing. The axial 3D T1-weighted images were obtained with a spoiled gradient recall sequence and the following parameters: repetition time (TR) = 8.5 ms; echo time (TE) = 3.4 ms; flip angle (FA) = 12°; field of view (FOV) = 240×240 mm^2; data matrix = 240×240; slices = 140; voxel size = $1 \times 1 \times 1$ mm.

MRI Data Analysis

MRI structure data was analyzed with FSL-VBM (Douaud et al., 2007),[1] an optimized VBM protocol (Good et al., 2001) of FSL (Smith et al., 2004). First, structural images were brain-extracted and segmented gray matter was registered to the MNI 152 standard space using non-linear registration (Andersson et al., 2007). The resulting images were averaged and flipped along *x*-axis to create a left-right symmetric, study-specific gray matter template. Second, all native gray matter images were non-linearly registered to this study-specific template and "modulated" to correct for local expansion (or contraction) due to the non-linear component of the spatial transformation. The modulated gray matter images were then smoothed with an isotropic Gaussian kernel with a sigma of 3 mm. Finally, voxel wise GLM was applied by correcting for multiple comparisons across space. Regional structure in gray matter were assessed by permutation-based non-parametric testing (5000 times) (Nichols and Holmes, 2002).

Behavioral Data Collection

Color-word Stroop task was implemented by E-prime 2.0 software. This task included a block design with three conditions, i.e., congruent, incongruent and rest. Red, Blue, and Green, three words were displayed in three colors (red, blue and green) as the congruent and incongruent stimuli. During rest, the subjects just focused their eyes on the cross displayed at the center of the screen. We designed two runs with different sequences of congruent and incongruent blocks (Xing et al., 2014). We tested participants individually in a quiet room and the participants kept a calm state of mind. Each of them was instructed to respond to the displayed color as fast as possible by pressing a button on a Serial Response Box TM with the right hand. The index, middle, and ring finger of right hand corresponding to red, blue, and green were used to press button respectively. The behavior data was collected two or three days before MRI scanning after practice.

The Process of Correlation Analysis

Analysis of covariance (ANCOVA) was employed with age, gender effects and total intracranial volume as covariates. We used a *post hoc* correlation analysis to investigate relationship between GMV and behavioral performances in IGD group, and response errors and response time for incongruent condition of color-word Stroop task were employed to be the factors of correlation respectively of IGD group.

Results

Our results showed that the average ages of IGD and control group were 18.8 ± 1.33 and 19.3 ± 2.56 years old, and there is no statistical difference between them ($p > 0.05$). According to their self-report of Internet use, the time spending by IGD adolescents per day and per week were more than the control group ($p < 0.005$).The IGD individuals spent longer duration of time on online gaming ($p < 0.005$) (**Table 1**).

Behavioral Results

A significant Stroop effect were observed in both group, where the RT was longer for the incongruent relative to the

[1]http://fsl.fmrib.ox.ac.uk/fsl/fslwiki/FSLVBM

congruent condition (IGD group: 628.24 ± 59.20 vs. 549.38 ± 44.17 and control group: 707.52 ± 66.43 vs. 581.97 ± 39.35; $p < 0.005$). The IGD group committed more errors than the control group during the incongruent condition (IGD group: 8.67 ± 5.41 vs. control group: 6.64 ± 3.65; $p < 0.05$), and the response delay (RD) measured by RT during the incongruent condition minus congruent conditions was significantly different between these two groups (IGD group: 78.87 ± 45.38 vs. control group :125.56 ± 49.20; $p < 0.05$) (**Table 2**).

Brain Imaging Results

VBM comparison indicated decreased GMV in several brain areas, i.e., the bilateral ACC, precuneus, supplementary motor area (SMA), superior parietal cortex, left DLPFC, left insula and bilateral cerebellum in the IGD group compared with the control group (**Figure 1**).

Correlation Analysis Results

Correlation analysis showed that the GMV of the ACC negatively correlated with Stroop task response errors for incongruent condition in the IGD group (**Figure 1**), but there was no statistical correlation between the GMV and RT for incongruent condition in the IGD group.

Discussion

Adolescence is a period with significant changes in both the social landscape and brain development, which is also a time with higher incidence of affective and addiction problems (Casey et al., 2008). Many scientist in Asia have reported that IGD became a public health problems in teenagers and youth (Ko et al., 2007; Park et al., 2008). It is difficult to have a valid therapy based on the unclear mechanism of IA. The brain structure changes and cognitive control deficits were observed in IGD adolescents. However, investigating relationship between brain structure and cognitive control in IGD is critical for developing possible intervention for this disorder. In the present study, reduced cognitive control ability and abnormal brain GMV in the IGD adolescents were observed compared with the control group, and more importantly, there was a negative correlation between the GMV of ACC and response errors for incongruent condition in the color-word Stroop task in IGD group.

TABLE 2 | Behavioral results for internet gaming disorder and control groups.

Items	IGD		Control	
	Congruent	Incongruent	Congruent	Incongruent
RT (ms)	549.38±44.17	628.24±59.20	581.97±39.35	707.52±66.43
Errors	3.21±2.38	8.67±5.41	3±2.04	6.64±3.65
RD (ms)	78.87±45.38		125.56±49.20	

Form: Mean ± standard deviation.

The Alteration of Behavior Changes and Gray Matter Volume in IGD Group

In order to verify impaired cognitive control ability in adolescents with IGD, a color-word Stroop task was used in the current study. Consistent with previous findings (Dong et al., 2011, 2013a; Yuan et al., 2013a,b), the IGD group committed more errors than the control group during the incongruent condition, which demonstrated that adolescents with IGD showed impaired cognitive control ability, as measured by the color-word Stroop test. The result that the RT during incongruent condition and RD of IGD group were shorter than control group may be imply that IGD subjects showed a different reaction pattern relative to controls, and they responded fast but taking the risk of making more errors, which was clearly a change in the response strategy. The study also found that the GMV of the ACC, DLPFC, precuneus, SMA, superior parietal cortex, insula, and cerebellum in the IGD group changed, which is in line with published IGD studies. Zhou and Weng et al. reported GMV reduction or abnormal activation in some brain areas in IGD subjects (Yuan et al., 2011; Zhou et al., 2011; Sun et al., 2012; Ko et al., 2013b; Weng et al., 2013). Although no study reported GMV of the precuneus decreased, fMRI study reported that the precuneus showed abnormal activation during cue-induced task in IGD subject (Ko et al., 2013a,b). The superior parietal cortex was found to be related with cognitive control (Durston et al., 2002, 2003; Ko et al., 2013a).

The Relationship between Gray Matter Volume of ACC and Performance of Color-Word Stroop Task

The correlation between the GMV of ACC and response errors showed that less GMV of ACC in IGD group was associated with more response errors during the incongruent condition in color-word Stroop task, which is a promising finding for the present study. The role of the ACC in cognitive control was well established and has been reported in a number of fMRI studies on Stroop interference paradigm in normal participants. Botvinick et al. reported the ACC was involved with conflict-monitoring function, for the ACC was more active under conditions of high conflict (Botvinick et al., 1999). Another research of Angus W. MacDonald III discovered that the activity of ACC was dissociable from top–down control, and it played a consistent role in monitoring conflict during response period (MacDonald et al., 2000). The study of Kerns revealed that the conflict-related activity of ACC predicted both greater prefrontal cortex activity and adjustments in behavior, supporting a role of ACC in conflict monitoring and cognitive control (Kerns et al., 2004). Furthermore, Matsumoto demonstrated that the cognitive control recruited by the ACC may be "consequential" based on conflicts between evoked plans and concrete actions (Matsumoto and Tanaka, 2004). A large body of experimental evidence on numerous diseases has accrued to support the important function of ACC in cognitive control. Akio Soeda et al. studied traumatic brain injury (TBI) patients

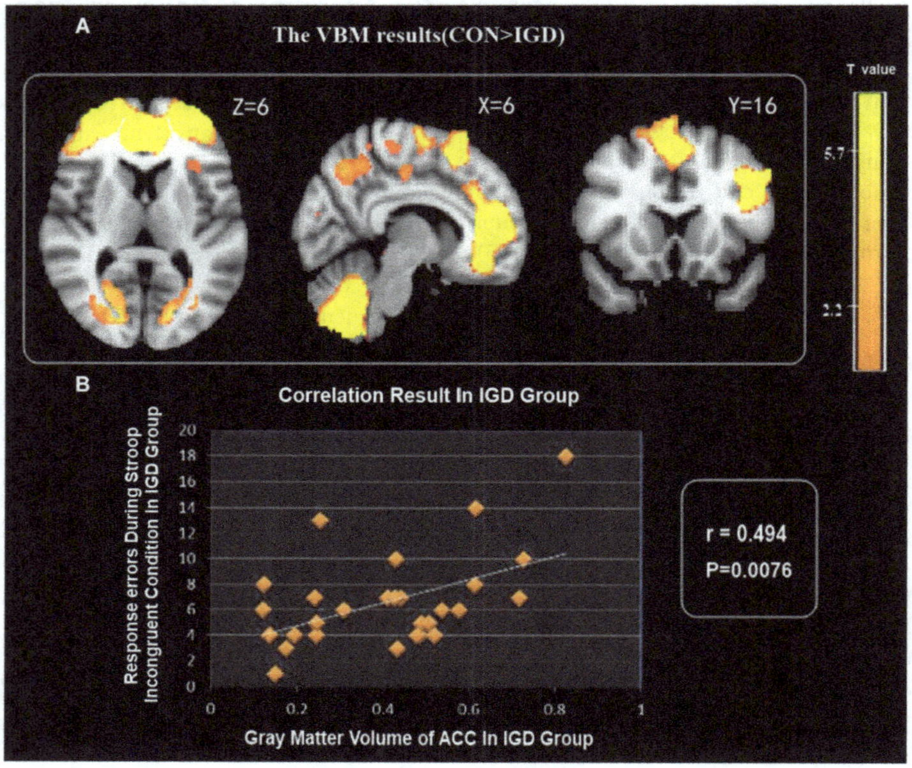

FIGURE 1 | (A) IGD group showed reduced gray matter volume (GMV) in the bilateral ACC, precuneus, SMA, superior parietal cortex, cerebellum, left DLPFC and left insula. **(B)** Correlation between GMV of ACC and Stroop task response errors during incongruent condition in IGD group.

and found out that the decreased activation in the ACC may be associated with alteration in functional cerebral activity, which may reflect either cortical disinhibition attributable to disconnection or compensation for an inefficient cognitive process (Soeda et al., 2005). Abnormal activity of ACC has been found in many mental problems, including obsessive--compulsive disorder (OCD), attention deficit-hyperactivity disorder (ADHD), and major depressive disorder (MDD; Ursu et al., 2003; Liotti et al., 2005; Murali and George, 2007). Recent neuroimaging studies also found altered activation of the ACC in heroin- and opioid-dependent individuals in GO/NOGO paradigm (Forman et al., 2004), suggesting the ACC is a key area in response inhibition (Fu et al., 2008). The research on cocaine users confirmed activity of ACC in inhibitory control (Kaufman et al., 2003; Goldstein et al., 2007, 2009). A Magnetic Resonance Spectroscopy (MRS) study on nicotine dependence showed that glutamate + glutamine (Glx) levels reduced in ACC, indicating the ACC was involved in cognitive control by modulating behavior (Wheelock et al., 2014). In a word, the ACC is important for cognitive control ability. The ACC's structural abnormalities and dysfunction in IGD have been reported in previous studies. The VBM results of Zhou et al. showed that the GMV of ACC decreased in IGD compared with controls (Yuan et al., 2011; Zhou et al., 2011). Many researches on IGD indicated that the ACC participated in the cognitive control, such as inhibitory control, error monitoring, and decision making (Dong et al., 2012, 2013a,b).

Conclusion

In the present study we found GMVs reduced in the ACC and other brain regions, as well as behavior pattern altered in cognitive control processing, which is consistent with published brain image studies on IGD and other addiction, suggesting IGD compromised both behavioral activity and neural structure in adolescents with IGD. Furthermore, we also found that ACC volume negatively correlated with incongruent response errors for Stroop paradigm, indicating a totally different response pattern in IGD individuals and its negative impacts on brain structure in adolescents.

Acknowledgments

ZM and KY were responsible for the study concept and design. HW, CJ, XN, GL and CN contributed to the acquisition of MRI data. HW, CM and KY performed the data analysis and interpretation of findings. HW and KY drafted the manuscript. STM corrected mistakes in grammar. All authors critically reviewed content and approved final version for publication. This research was supported by National Science Foundation of China (81371530, 81271546, 81101036).

References

Andersson, J., Jenkinson, M., and Smith, S. (2007). *Non-Linear Registration, Aka Spatial Normalisation.* FMRIB Analysis Group Technical Reports: TR07JA02. Available online at: www.fmrib.ox.ac.uk/analysis/techrep

Beard, K. W., and Wolf, E. M. (2001). Modification in the proposed diagnostic criteria for internet addiction. *Cyberpsychol. Behav.* 4, 377–383. doi: 10.1089/109493101300210286

Blasi, G., Goldberg, T. E., Weickert, T., Das, S., Kohn, P., Zoltick, B., et al. (2006). Brain regions underlying response inhibition and interference monitoring and suppression. *Eur. J. Neurosci.* 23, 1658–1664. doi: 10.1111/j.1460-9568.2006.04680.x

Block, J. J. (2007). Prevalence underestimated in problematic internet use study. *CNS Spectr.* 12, 14–15.

Botvinick, M., Nystrom, L. E., Fissell, K., Carter, C. S., and Cohen, J. D. (1999). Conflict monitoring versus selection-for-action in anterior cingulate cortex. *Nature* 402, 179–181. doi: 10.1038/46035

Brand, M., Young, K. S., and Laier, C. (2014). Prefrontal control and internet addiction: a theoretical model and review of neuropsychological and neuroimaging findings. *Front. Hum. Neurosci.* 8:375. doi: 10.3389/fnhum.2014.00375

Cao, F., Su, L., Liu, T., and Gao, X. (2007). The relationship between impulsivity and internet addiction in a sample of Chinese adolescents. *Eur. Psychiatry* 22, 466–471. doi: 10.1016/j.eurpsy.2007.05.004

Casey, B. J., Jones, R. M., and Hare, T. A. (2008). The adolescent brain. *Ann. N Y Acad. Sci.* 1124, 111–126. doi: 10.1196/annals.1440.010

Cools, R., and D'Esposito, M. (2011). Inverted-U-Shaped dopamine actions on human working memory and cognitive control. *Biol. Psychiatry* 69, e113–e125. doi: 10.1016/j.biopsych.2011.03.028

Ding, W. N., Sun, J. H., Sun, Y. W., Chen, X., Zhou, Y., Zhuang, Z. G., et al. (2014). Trait impulsivity and impaired prefrontal impulse inhibition function in adolescents with internet gaming addiction revealed by a Go/No-Go fMRI study. *Behav. Brain Funct.* 10:20. doi: 10.1186/1744-9081-10-20

Ding, W. N., Sun, J. H., Sun, Y. W., Zhou, Y., Li, L., Xu, J. R., et al. (2013). Altered default network resting-state functional connectivity in adolescents with internet gaming addiction. *PLoS One* 8:e59902. doi: 10.1371/journal.pone.0059902

Dong, G., Devito, E. E., Du, X., and Cui, Z. (2012). Impaired inhibitory control in 'internet addiction disorder': a functional magnetic resonance imaging study. *Psychiatry Res.* 203, 153–158. doi: 10.1016/j.pscychresns.2012.02.001

Dong, G., Hu, Y., Lin, X., and Lu, Q. (2013a). What makes internet addicts continue playing online even when faced by severe negative consequences? Possible explanations from an fMRI study. *Biol. Psychol.* 94, 282–289. doi: 10.1016/j.biopsycho.2013.07.009

Dong, G., Lin, X., Zhou, H., and Lu, Q. (2014). Cognitive flexibility in internet addicts: fMRI evidence from difficult-to-easy and easy-to-difficult switching situations. *Addict. Behav.* 39, 677–683. doi: 10.1016/j.addbeh.2013.11.028

Dong, G., Shen, Y., Huang, J., and Du, X. (2013b). Impaired error-monitoring function in people with internet addiction disorder: an event-related fMRI study. *Eur. Addict. Res.* 19, 269–275. doi: 10.1159/000346783

Dong, G., Zhou, H., and Zhao, X. (2010). Impulse inhibition in people with internet addiction disorder: electrophysiological evidence from a Go/NoGo study. *Neurosci. Lett.* 485, 138–142. doi: 10.1016/j.neulet.2010.09.002

Dong, G., Zhou, H., and Zhao, X. (2011). Male internet addicts show impaired executive control ability: evidence from a color-word stroop task. *Neurosci. Lett.* 499, 114–118. doi: 10.1016/j.neulet.2011.05.047

Douaud, G., Smith, S., Jenkinson, M., Behrens, T., Johansen-Berg, H., Vickers, J., et al. (2007). Anatomically related grey and white matter abnormalities in adolescent-onset schizophrenia. *Brain* 130, 2375–2386. doi: 10.1093/brain/awm184

Durston, S., Davidson, M. C., Thomas, K. M., Worden, M. S., Tottenham, N., Martinez, A., et al. (2003). Parametric manipulation of conflict and response competition using rapid mixed-trial event-related fMRI. *Neuroimage* 20, 2135–2141. doi: 10.1016/j.neuroimage.2003.08.004

Durston, S., Thomas, K. M., Worden, M. S., Yang, Y., and Casey, B. J. (2002). The effect of preceding context on inhibition: an event-related fMRI study. *Neuroimage* 16, 449–453. doi: 10.1006/nimg.2002.1074

Forman, S. D., Dougherty, G. G., Casey, B. J., Siegle, G. J., Braver, T. S., Barch, D. M., et al. (2004). Opiate addicts lack error-dependent activation of rostral anterior cingulate. *Biol. Psychiatry* 55, 531–537. doi: 10.1016/j.biopsych.2003.09.011

Fu, L. P., Bi, G. H., Zou, Z. T., Wang, Y., Ye, E. M., Ma, L., et al. (2008). Impaired response inhibition function in abstinent heroin dependents: an fMRI study. *Neurosci. Lett.* 438, 322–326. doi: 10.1016/j.neulet.2008.04.033

Goldstein, R. Z., Alia-Klein, N., Tomasi, D., Carrillo, J. H., Maloney, T., Woicik, P. A., et al. (2009). Anterior cingulate cortex hypoactivations to an emotionally salient task in cocaine addiction. *Proc. Natl. Acad. Sci. U S A* 106, 9453–9458. doi: 10.1073/pnas.0900491106

Goldstein, R. Z., Tomasi, D., Rajaram, S., Cottone, L. A., Zhang, L., Maloney, T., et al. (2007). Role of the anterior cingulate and medial orbitofrontal cortex in processing drug cues in cocaine addiction. *Neuroscience* 144, 1153–1159. doi: 10.1016/j.neuroscience.2006.11.024

Good, C. D., Johnsrude, I. S., Ashburner, J., Henson, R. N., Friston, K. J., and Frackowiak, R. S. (2001). A voxel-based morphometric study of ageing in 465 normal adult human brains. *Neuroimage* 14, 21–36. doi: 10.1006/nimg.2001.0786

Holden, C. (2001). 'Behavioral' addictions: do they exist? *Science* 294, 980–982. doi: 10.1126/science.294.5544.980

Kaufman, J. N., Ross, T. J., Stein, E. A., and Garavan, H. (2003). Cingulate hypoactivity in cocaine users during a GO-NOGO task as revealed by event-related functional magnetic resonance imaging. *J. Neurosci.* 23, 7839–7843.

Kerns, J. G., Cohen, J. D., MacDonald, A. W. 3rd, Cho, R. Y., Stenger, V. A., and Carter, C. S. (2004). Anterior cingulate conflict monitoring and adjustments in control. *Science* 303, 1023–1026. doi: 10.1126/science.1089910

Kim, J., and Haridakis, P. M. (2009). The role of internet user characteristics and motives in explaining three dimensions of internet addiction. *J. Comput. Mediat. Commun.* 14, 988–1015. doi: 10.1111/j.1083-6101.2009.01478.x

King, D. L., Delfabbro, P. H., Griffiths, M. D., and Gradisar, M. (2012). Cognitive-behavioral approaches to outpatient treatment of internet addiction in children and adolescents. *J. Clin. Psychol.* 68, 1185–1195. doi: 10.1002/jclp.21918

Ko, C. H., Liu, G. C., Hsiao, S., Yen, J. Y., Yang, M. J., Lin, W. C., et al. (2009). Brain activities associated with gaming urge of online gaming addiction. *J. Psychiatr. Res.* 43, 739–747. doi: 10.1016/j.jpsychires.2008.09.012

Ko, C. H., Liu, G. C., Yen, J. Y., Chen, C. Y., Yen, C. F., and Chen, C. S. (2013a). Brain correlates of craving for online gaming under cue exposure in subjects with internet gaming addiction and in remitted subjects. *Addict. Biol.* 18, 559–569. doi: 10.1111/j.1369-1600.2011.00405.x

Ko, C. H., Liu, G. C., Yen, J. Y., Yen, C. F., Chen, C. S., and Lin, W. C. (2013b). The brain activations for both cue-induced gaming urge and smoking craving among subjects comorbid with internet gaming addiction and nicotine dependence. *J. Psychiatr. Res.* 47, 486–493. doi: 10.1016/j.jpsychires.2012.11.008

Ko, C.-H., Yen, J.-Y., Yen, C.-F., Lin, H.-C., and Yang, M.-J. (2007). Factors predictive for incidence and remission of internet addiction in young adolescents: a prospective study. *Cyberpsychol. Behav.* 10, 545–551. doi: 10.1089/cpb.2007.9992

Li, B., Friston, K. J., Liu, J., Liu, Y., Zhang, G., Cao, F., et al. (2014). Impaired frontal-basal ganglia connectivity in adolescents with internet addiction. *Sci. Rep.* 4:5027. doi: 10.1038/srep05027

Liotti, M., Pliszka, S. R., Perez, R., Kothmann, D., and Woldorff, M. G. (2005). Abnormal brain activity related to performance monitoring and error detection in children with ADHD. *Cortex* 41, 377–388. doi: 10.1016/s0010-9452(08)70274-0

MacDonald, A. W. 3rd, Cohen, J. D., Stenger, V. A., and Carter, C. S. (2000). Dissociating the role of the dorsolateral prefrontal and anterior cingulate cortex in cognitive control. *Science* 288, 1835–1838. doi: 10.1126/science.288.5472.1835

Matsumoto, K., and Tanaka, K. (2004). Neuroscience. Conflict and cognitive control. *Science* 303, 969–970. doi: 10.1126/science.1094733

Murali, V., and George, S. (2007). Lost online: an overview of internet addiction. *Adv. Psychiatr. Treat.* 13, 24–30. doi: 10.1192/apt.bp.106.002907

Nichols, T. E., and Holmes, A. P. (2002). Nonparametric permutation tests for functional neuroimaging: a primer with examples. *Hum. Brain Mapp.* 15, 1–25. doi: 10.1002/hbm.1058

Park, S. K., Kim, J. Y., and Cho, C. B. (2008). Prevalence of internet addiction and correlations with family factors among South Korean adolescents. *Adolescence* 43, 895–909.

Smith, S. M., Jenkinson, M., Woolrich, M. W., Beckmann, C. F., Behrens, T. E. J., Johansen-Berg, H., et al. (2004). Advances in functional and structural MR image analysis and implementation as FSL. *Neuroimage* 23, S208–S219. doi: 10.1016/j.neuroimage.2004.07.051

Soeda, A., Nakashima, T., Okumura, A., Kuwata, K., Shinoda, J., and Iwama, T. (2005). Cognitive impairment after traumatic brain injury: a functional magnetic resonance imaging study using the stroop task. *Neuroradiology* 47, 501–506. doi: 10.1007/s00234-005-1372-x

Steinberg, L. (2005). Cognitive and affective development in adolescence. *Trends Cogn. Sci.* 9, 69–74. doi: 10.1016/j.tics.2004.12.005

Sun, Y., Ying, H., Seetohul, R. M., Xuemei, W., Ya, Z., Qian, L., et al. (2012). Brain fMRI study of crave induced by cue pictures in online game addicts (male adolescents). *Behav. Brain Res.* 233, 563–576. doi: 10.1016/j.bbr.2012.05.005

Toneatto, T., Blitz-Miller, T., Calderwood, K., Dragonetti, R., and Tsanos, A. (1997). Cognitive distortions in heavy gambling. *J. Gambl. Stud.* 13, 253–266. doi: 10.1023/A:1024983300428

Ursu, S., Stenger, V. A., Shear, M. K., Jones, M. R., and Carter, C. S. (2003). Overactive action monitoring in obsessive-compulsive disorder: evidence from functional magnetic resonance imaging. *Psychol. Sci.* 14, 347–353. doi: 10.1111/1467-9280.24411

van Holst, R. J., Lemmens, J. S., Valkenburg, P. M., Peter, J., Veltman, D. J., and Goudriaan, A. E. (2012). Attentional bias and disinhibition toward gaming cues are related to problem gaming in male adolescents. *J. Adolesc. Health* 50, 541–546. doi: 10.1016/j.jadohealth.2011.07.006

Weng, C. B., Qian, R. B., Fu, X. M., Lin, B., Han, X. P., Niu, C. S., et al. (2013). Gray matter and white matter abnormalities in online game addiction. *Eur. J. Radiol.* 82, 1308–1312. doi: 10.1016/j.ejrad.2013.01.031

Wheelock, M. D., Reid, M. A., To, H., White, D. M., Cropsey, K. L., and Lahti, A. C. (2014). Open label smoking cessation with varenicline is associated with decreased glutamate levels and functional changes in anterior cingulate cortex: preliminary findings. *Front. Pharmacol.* 5:158. doi: 10.3389/fphar.2014.00158

Xing, L., Yuan, K., Bi, Y., Yin, J., Cai, C., Feng, D., et al. (2014). Reduced fiber integrity and cognitive control in adolescents with internet gaming disorder. *Brain Res.* 1586, 109–117. doi: 10.1016/j.brainres.2014.08.044

Young, K. S. (1998). Internet addiction: the emergence of a new clinical disorder. *Cyberpsychol. Behav.* 1, 237–244. doi: 10.1089/cpb.1998.1.237

Young, K. S. (2007). Cognitive behavior therapy with internet addicts: treatment outcomes and implications. *Cyberpsychol. Behav.* 10, 671–679. doi: 10.1089/cpb.2007.9971

Yuan, K., Cheng, P., Dong, T., Bi, Y., Xing, L., Yu, D., et al. (2013a). Cortical thickness abnormalities in late adolescence with online gaming addiction. *PLoS One* 8:e53055. doi: 10.1371/journal.pone.0053055

Yuan, K., Jin, C., Cheng, P., Yang, X., Dong, T., Bi, Y., et al. (2013b). Amplitude of low frequency fluctuation abnormalities in adolescents with online gaming addiction. *PLoS One* 8:e78708. doi: 10.1371/journal.pone.0078708

Yuan, K., Qin, W., Wang, G., Zeng, F., Zhao, L., Yang, X., et al. (2011). Microstructure abnormalities in adolescents with internet addiction disorder. *PLoS One* 6:e20708. doi: 10.1371/journal.pone.0020708

Zhou, Y., Lin, F. C., Du, Y. S., Qin, L. D., Zhao, Z. M., Xu, J. R., et al. (2011). Gray matter abnormalities in internet addiction: a voxel-based morphometry study. *Eur. J. Radiol.* 79, 92–95. doi: 10.1016/j.ejrad.2009.10.025

Conflict of Interest Statement: The authors declare that the research was conducted in the absence of any commercial or financial relationships that could be construed as a potential conflict of interest.

13

Dorsal Anterior Cingulate Cortex Responses to Repeated Social Evaluative Feedback in Young Women with and without a History of Depression

Edited by:
Raymond C. K. Chan,
Chinese Academy of Sciences, China

***Correspondence:**
Katarina Dedovic
katarina.dedovic@mail.mcgill.ca

Katarina Dedovic[1,2], George M. Slavich[3], Keely A. Muscatell[4,5], Michael R. Irwin[3] and Naomi I. Eisenberger[1]*

[1] Social and Affective Neuroscience Laboratory, University of California, Los Angeles, Los Angeles, CA, USA, [2] Addiction Research Studies and Laboratory, Douglas Hospital Research Centre, McGill University, Montreal, QC, Canada, [3] Cousins Center for Psychoneuroimmunology and Department of Psychiatry and Biobehavioral Sciences, University of California, Los Angeles, Los Angeles, CA, USA, [4] The Robert Wood Johnson Foundation Health and Society Scholars Program, University of California, San Francisco/University of California, Berkeley, San Francisco, CA, USA, [5] Department of Psychology, University of California, Berkeley, Berkeley, CA, USA

The dorsal anterior cingulate cortex (dACC) is recruited when a person is socially rejected or negatively evaluated. However, it remains to be fully understood how this region responds to repeated exposure to personally-relevant social evaluation, in both healthy populations and those vulnerable to Major Depressive Disorder (MDD), as well as how responding in these regions is associated with subsequent clinical functioning. To address this gap in the literature, we recruited 17 young women with past history of MDD (previously depressed) and 31 healthy controls and exposed them to a social evaluative session in a neuroimaging environment. In two bouts, participants received an equal amount of positive, negative, and neutral feedback from a confederate. All participants reported increases in feelings of social evaluation in response to the evaluative task. However, compared to healthy controls, previously depressed participants tended to show greater increases in depressed mood following the task. At the neural level, in response to negative (vs. positive) feedback, no main effect of group or evaluation periods was observed. However, a significant interaction between group and evaluation periods was found. Specifically, over the two bouts of evaluation, activity in the dACC decreased among healthy participants while it increased among previously depressed individuals. Interestingly and unexpectedly, in the previously depressed group specifically, this increased activity in dACC over time was associated with lower levels of depressive symptoms at baseline and at 6-months following the evaluation session (controlling for baseline levels). Thus, the subset of previously depressed participants who showed increases in the recruitment of the dACC over time in response to the negative evaluation seemed to fair better emotionally. These findings suggest that examining how the dACC responds *to repeated bouts* of negative evaluation reveals a new dimension to the role of the dACC in processing exclusion and contributing to mental health outcomes in a population vulnerable to MDD. Further, investigation of the dynamics of the dACC response to negative social evaluation is warranted.

Keywords: social evaluation, social rejection, dorsal anterior cingulate cortex, major depressive disorder, vulnerability, resilience

INTRODUCTION

Major Depressive Disorder (MDD) is a severe, debilitating disorder, affecting approximately twice as many women compared to men (Marcus et al., 2012; Ferrari et al., 2013). It is characterized by the presence of depressed mood and/or loss of interest for at least 2 weeks, along with a combination of several psychophysiological symptoms such as sleep disturbances, fatigue, poor concentration, and feelings of guilt/worthlessness, which all contribute to impaired social and occupational functioning (American Psychiatric Association, 2000).

Experiences of psychological stress, particularly social stressors such as social evaluation or social rejection, are intricately linked with the development of depression. Specifically, individuals experiencing social rejection are 22 times more likely to develop depression (Kendler et al., 2003), and do so more quickly (Slavich et al., 2009), than persons not experiencing such stress. It has been suggested that maladaptive responses to social rejection at the neural, psychological, and physiological levels interact with each other as well as with other vulnerability factors, such as past history of depression, levels of early life stress, and genetic factors, to increase a person's vulnerability to depression (Slavich et al., 2010). Notably, being able to adaptively respond to *repeated* experiences of psychological stress is an important aspect of one's vulnerability or resilience to MDD (Southwick et al., 2005). However, the neural mechanisms subserving this dynamic process remain unclear. Here, we addressed this question by exposing female participants with and without prior history of MDD to two bouts of social evaluation in a neuroimaging environment.

Past history of MDD is an important moderator of the association between experiences of social evaluation and vulnerability to depression. Indeed, while the onset of the first lifetime depressive episode is tightly linked with highly stressful life experiences, it has been shown that once the first depressive episode has been experienced, subsequent episodes can be triggered by much milder stressors (Stroud et al., 2011), especially interpersonal stressors (Slavich et al., 2011). Moreover, with each new depressive episode experienced, the risk for subsequent episodes increases (Burcusa and Iacono, 2007; Koppers et al., 2011). Therefore, prior history of depression is an important context in which to examine mechanisms underlying the link between repeated experiences of social evaluation and rejection and subsequent risk for depression.

Previous studies in healthy samples have shown that when a person experiences social rejection or negative evaluation compared to social acceptance or positive evaluation, there is heightened activity in the dorsal anterior cingulate cortex (dACC; Eisenberger et al., 2003, 2011; Kross et al., 2011; Rotge et al., 2015); c.f., (Somerville et al., 2006). The dACC has been proposed to be part of the "neural alarm system" (Eisenberger and Lieberman, 2004; Spunt et al., 2012) and as such is involved in both detection and appraisal of social exclusion (Kawamoto et al., 2015), which are dynamic processes.

Along these lines, it has recently been suggested that dACC activity changes over the course of an episode of social rejection or exclusion (Kawamoto et al., 2015; Rotge et al., 2015). Specifically, several studies focusing primarily on event-related potentials have reported that, in healthy individuals, activity in dACC decreases over repeated exposure to social rejection (Crowley et al., 2009; Moor et al., 2012; Kawamoto et al., 2013; Themanson et al., 2013). For example, it was observed that in healthy young adults, across two sets of 20 exclusion trials each, N2 (reflecting ACC—based neural alarm activation) and P3b components (reflecting conscious cognitive control and attentional processes), were larger during the first 20 complete-exclusion event trials compared to the second 20 in a computerized game of social exclusion called Cyberball (Themanson et al., 2013). Similarly, Kawomoto and colleagues investigated the P3b component in healthy adults and observed a decrease in amplitude in the second half compared to first half of exclusion period of Cyberball (Kawamoto et al., 2013). Furthermore, an fMRI study with healthy adolescents and young adults observed that dACC activity was higher during the first block of exclusion compared to the middle or last block of exclusion in Cyberball (Moor et al., 2012). Overall, these findings suggest that, in healthy individuals, dACC activity decreases over periods of negative social experiences.

With depressed individuals, however, the overall response of the dACC is more mixed. Specifically, a meta-analysis found a hyperactive dACC response to processing negative information in MDD individuals (Hamilton et al., 2011; Graham et al., 2013), while other studies using more cognitive tasks showed decreased dACC activity in MDD (e.g., Crocker et al., 2013; Ubl et al., 2015). Another meta-analysis revealed that patients with MDD compared to controls show overall heightened levels of dACC activity across many study paradigms (Graham et al., 2013). With respect to the temporal dynamics of the dACC response, one study investigated activity in medial prefrontal cortex including dACC in response to a social evaluative threat task in depressed individuals with and without co-morbid anxiety compared to controls and individuals with anxiety (Waugh et al., 2012). In this study, participants were first asked to relax for 2 min, then to prepare to give a speech for another 2 min, and finally to simply relax since in the end they would not need to give a speech. The authors observed that while all depressed individuals exhibited a resurgence of medial frontal cortex including dACC activation during the late speech preparation period, participants without depression (controls and those with non-comorbid anxiety) exhibited a return to baseline during this period (Waugh et al., 2012). Thus, depressed individuals may show an increase in dACC activity over the course of a stressful task.

In healthy individuals, overall increased activity in dACC tracks with key psychological factors associated with vulnerability to depression, such as interpersonal sensitivity and low self-esteem such that the higher the levels of the vulnerability factor, the greater the overall dACC activity in response to rejection over acceptance (e.g., Eisenberger et al., 2003, 2011; Kong et al., 2015; Rotge et al., 2015). With respect to dynamic change in dACC activity, one study revealed that it is also associated with psychological variables. Specifically, Themanson and colleagues have observed that the increase in P3b amplitude from inclusion to the initial exclusion phase of Cyberball was associated with less positive affect and less feelings of control (Themanson et al., 2013). In MDD, the associations between the dynamic dACC response and psychological measures have not been explored (Waugh et al., 2012).

While all these studies offer insight into the link between vulnerability to MDD and nature of dACC activity in response to processing various types of negative information, there is an absence of empirical research examining whether past experience of depression is associated with a differential activity in the dACC particularly in response to repeated personally-relevant social evaluation, an important aspect of vulnerability to MDD. In addition, it remains unclear how, in this population, does the change of activity over repeated bouts of social evaluation in dACC track with psychological responses to social evaluation, as well as current and future clinical functioning?

To address some of the gaps in the current literature with respect to the association between repeated experiences of social evaluation and subsequent vulnerability to depression, the current study exposed young women with a past history of depression (previously depressed) and healthy controls to two bouts of social evaluation in a Magnetic Resonance Imaging (MRI) scanner. We focused on female participants due to the fact that: (a) approximately twice as many women compared to men suffer from depression (Marcus et al., 2012; Ferrari et al., 2013) and (b) women are particularly sensitive to interpersonal stressors (Stroud et al., 2002). We expected that, compared to the controls, previously depressed participants would show overall greater activity in dACC in response to negative (vs. positive) social-evaluative feedback. In addition, we hypothesized that whereas previously depressed participants would show an increase in activity in the dACC over the two exposures to social evaluation, controls would show a decrease. Furthermore, we also explored how changes in activity in the dACC in response to repeated bouts of social evaluation related to psychological responses to social evaluation, current clinical functioning, as well as vulnerability to depression at 6 and 12 months following the evaluation. We expected that the increase in dACC activity over the course of the social evaluative session in previously depressed sample would be related to poorer psychological and clinical outcomes.

METHODS AND MATERIALS

Subject Selection

General eligibility criteria for participation in this study were: (a) being female; (b) aged between 18 and 25 years; (c) being right handed; (d) meeting safety criteria to participate in functional MRI (fMRI) research; (e) not having present or past history of autoimmune, liver or other severe chronic diseases; (f) not using hormonal contraception; and (g) no substance/alcohol abuse in the past 6 months. Additionally, participants in the control group needed to meet the following eligibility criteria: (a) no current or past history of any Axis I disorder, including MDD, and (b) no current or past history of taking psychiatric medication. Specific eligibility criteria for the previously depressed group were: (a) having had one or two lifetime major depressive episodes; (b) no Major Depressive Episode or major Axis I disorder in the past month; (c) no history of chronic, unremitting depression; (d) no psychiatric medication in past month; and (e) no past history of Post-traumatic Stress Disorder, mania, psychosis, delusions, or bipolar disorder. Consistent with other related studies (e.g., LeMoult et al., 2009; Harkness et al., 2010), potential previously depressed participants were not excluded if they had a history of general anxiety disorder, social anxiety disorder, or dysthymia in addition to depression.

Procedure

Through university online classifieds and campus posters, we recruited 17 previously depressed and 31 control females to participate in a study that examined "the link between how the brain and body respond to first impressions and vulnerability to depression." Initial eligibility was established during a telephone-screening interview and was verified on a separate day, in an in-person session, via a Structured Clinical Interview for DSM Diagnosis (SCID; First et al., 1995). During this time, participants also completed a screener for safety criteria for participation in fMRI research. Eligible participants then completed a personally relevant interview—the "impressions interview"—that was videotaped (to be used later for the social evaluative session). Within 1–3 days following the impressions interview, subjects completed the fMRI safety screening again and then participated in an fMRI scanning session. The fMRI testing session always occurred within 2 weeks of the SCID. Furthermore, participants completed follow-up questionnaires online at ~6 and 12 months following the fMRI session to assess their depressive symptoms during the year following the baseline study visits. The Institutional Review Board of the University of California, Los Angeles approved the study, and all participants provided written informed consent.

Impressions Interview

Participants were told that, in order to examine how the brain and body respond to first impressions, all participants first needed to complete an "impressions interview." The interview consisted of answering personally relevant questions while being videotaped, for approximately 10 min. Some of the questions included "What are you most proud of that you have done in your life so far?" or "What are some of your shortcomings?." They were also informed that, on the scan day, they would be paired with another participant, and at that time, the experimenters would choose one of them to form an impression of the other based on the video of the interview. Meanwhile, the other person would be scanned while they saw the impression being formed of them. Unbeknownst to the participant, the "other participant" was always a confederate and thus, the subject was always scanned (and thus the one being evaluated).

Scan Day

On the scan day, all participants arrived at the scanning facility at 12:30 p.m.; they were met by two experimenters and were introduced to the other "participant," actually a confederate. The participant and confederate interacted for 2 min to establish a rapport, after which point they were placed in separate testing rooms, where they stayed for the first hour. During this time, participants acclimatized to the testing environment and completed socio-demographic and psychological trait questionnaires, including the Beck Depression Inventory—II (Beck et al., 1996), State Trait Anxiety Inventory (STAI) (Spielberger, 1983), Rosenberg Self-Esteem Scale (Rosenberg, 1965), Fear of Evaluation Scale (Leary, 1983), and Mehrabian Sensitivity to Rejection Scale (Mehrabian, 1976). Twenty-five minutes prior to the scan, participants completed an in-house state questionnaire which asked them to provide their impression of the other participant including their feelings of social evaluation ("I feel evaluated by the other participant;" "I feel judged by the other participant") on a scale ranging from 1 (*not at all*) to 7 (*very much*). They also completed an abridged version of the depressed mood subscale of the Profile of Mood States questionnaire (McNair et al., 1992), which assessed their current feelings of depression, from 0 (*not at all*) to 4 (*extremely*), for the following feelings: unhappy, blue, miserable, sad, discouraged, hopeless, worthless, helpless.

After completing the pre-scan state questionnaires, the participant was reunited with the confederate. At this point, the participant was informed that she was chosen to complete the fMRI scan and have her video interview evaluated by the confederate. While addressing both the participant and the confederate, the experimenter explained the details of the social evaluative task, as well as the full scanning procedure. Specifically, it was explained that the confederate would be outside of the scanner in the control room where she would be watching the participant's video on one screen and providing feedback on how the participant was coming across by using an impressions user interface on another screen (see below for technical details). The participant, on the other hand, was told that she would not be able to see her full video; rather, she would only be shown a couple of clips to remind her of what the confederate was seeing and the rest of the time she would be viewing the impressions user interface with the confederate's feedback. The participant was also asked to report, by pressing buttons on a button box, how she felt in response to receiving the feedback. In addition, the participant was informed that before and after the social evaluative task, she would view evaluations of nature scenes and that she would also undergo a structural imaging scan.

Social Evaluative Task

The social evaluative scan task (Eisenberger et al., 2011; Muscatell et al., 2014) started with a short 5 s clip of the start of the participant's own interview, which was then followed by a display of the "impressions user interface"—a 4 × 6 word grid where positive, neutral, and negative adjectives were displayed. Adjectives were selected based on pilot testing with an independent sample of UCLA undergraduates ($N = 74$). The participant saw a mouse moving over the adjectives (believed to be controlled by the evaluator) and, every 10 s, she saw a mouse click over an adjective button indicating the evaluator's rating of the participant's performance in the impressions interview video (**Figure 1**). Notably, the user interface was in fact a pre-made evaluation video, and all participants saw exactly the same video. During the first part of the evaluation, which lasted 4 min and 28 s, participants saw 6 negative, 9 neutral, and 7 positive adjectives being selected. Then, participants were again shown a short 5 s clip, this time corresponding to the middle of their own interview. This was again followed up by the evaluation video lasting 4 min and 24 s containing 9 negative, 6 neutral, and 8 positive adjectives being selected. Importantly, adjectives in both parts of the evaluation were presented in a pseudorandom order such that no more than two adjectives of the same valence could be presented consecutively. A fixation crosshair (10 s), presented pre- and post-social evaluative task formed the implicit baseline. Participants were instructed that every time they received an evaluation, they were to respond using a button box with four buttons about how they felt at that moment using a 1–4 scale (1 = *really bad*, 4 = *really good*; reverse-coded for manipulation check analyses, so higher numbers indicate feeling worse). Participants were told that the evaluator would have no knowledge of these personal responses.

After the completion of the scanning session, participants returned to the behavioral testing room where they completed the post-scan state questionnaires. Throughout the session, participants also provided biological samples; however, these data are not the subject of the present manuscript.

Follow-Up Sessions

At approximately 6 and 12 months following the scanning session, participants who agreed to be contacted for the online follow-up assessments were sent instructions on how to complete several questionnaires, including the BDI-II. Due to subject attrition, the sample sizes for analyses related to the 6-month and 12-month assessments were as follows: in controls, at 6 months, $N = 26$, and at 12 months, $N = 19$; in the previously depressed group, at 6 months, $N = 13$, and at 12 months, $N = 12$.

Statistical Analyses of Sociodemographic and Psychological Trait and State Measures

If participants were missing an answer to one item for a given questionnaire, the value for that missing value was replaced either by the mean score of that questionnaire or, if the questionnaire contained subscales, by the mean score of the subscale that the

A

B

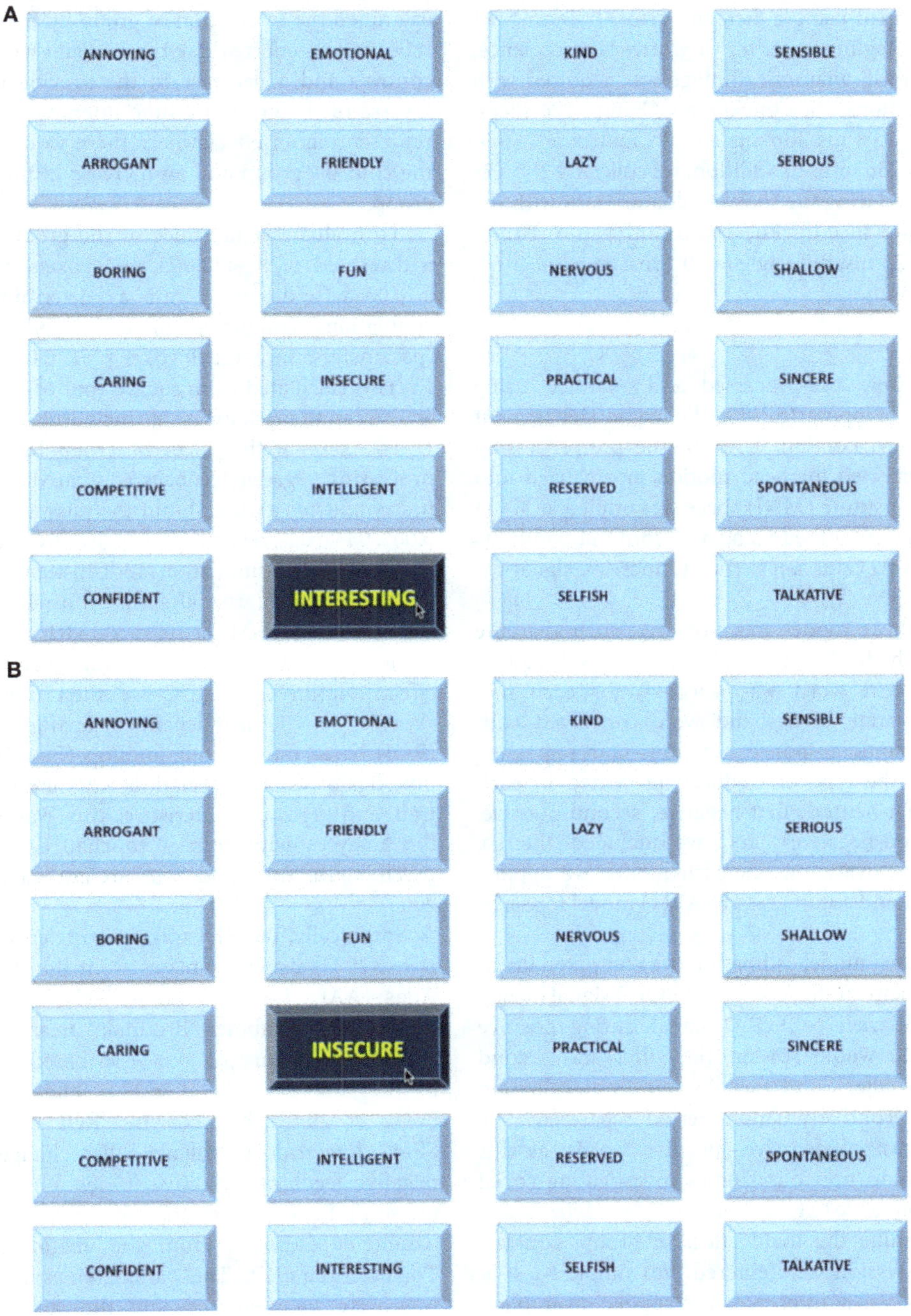

FIGURE 1 | The "impressions user interface" used in the social evaluative session. Every 10 s, a participant saw a mouse click over an adjective button indicating the evaluator's rating of the participant's performance in the impressions interview video. The rating could be **(A)** positive, **(B)** negative, or neutral (not shown).

missing item belonged to, for that subject (Osborne, 2013). In the present sample, one HC participant was missing one item on the BDI-II completed on the day of the scan. Furthermore, two participants from the HC group had a missing item each on the Sensitivity to Rejection Scale; one other HC participant had a missing item on the STAI.

For continuous socio-demographic and psychological trait data, an independent t-test examined group differences. When data were not normally distributed, group differences were examined using the non-parametric Mann-Whitney U statistic. Group differences on categorical data were assessed using tests of independence (i.e., χ^2 statistic or Fisher's exact test). A two-way mixed design ANOVA was conducted to examine group differences with respect to changes in psychological state and trait measures over time. Significant interactions were decomposed using simple main effects analyses.

fMRI Image Acquisition

Participants were scanned using a Siemens Trio 3.0 Tesla MRI scanner at the UCLA Staglin Center for Cognitive Neuroscience. A T1-weighted MPRAGE anatomical image was acquired with the following specifications: slice thickness = 1 mm, 176 slices, $TR = 2300$ ms, $TE = 2.98$ ms, flip angle = 9°, matrix = 256 × 256, Field-Of-View = 256 mm. In addition, we collected 288 T2-weighted EPI volumes during the social evaluation task with the following specifications: slice thickness = 3 mm, gap = 1 mm, $TR = 2000$ ms, $TE = 25$ ms, flip angle = 90°, matrix = 64 × 64, Field-Of-View = 200 mm.

fMRI Analyses

Neuroimaging data were pre-processed and analyzed using Statistical Parametric Mapping (SPM8; Wellcome Department of Cognitive Neurology, London, UK). In the pre-processing step, images were corrected for head motion, normalized into Montreal Neurologic Institute (MNI) space (resampled at 3 × 3 × 3 mm), and spatially smoothed using an 8 mm full-width-at-half-maximum (FWHM) Gaussian kernel, to increase signal-to-noise ratio.

Next, a general linear model was prepared such that the presentations of each feedback word and the subsequent 11–12 s (until the next word was selected) for each half were modeled as separate blocks and were convolved with a canonical hemodynamic response function. Our regressor-of-interest coded for the type of feedback presented in each half (first-positive, first-neutral, first-negative, second-positive, second-neutral, second-negative), and we included the six motion parameters as covariates. For each model, we applied 128 Hz high-pass filter and autoregressive AR(1) model for serial correlations.

Following the classical model estimation, we computed linear contrasts for each participant that compared BOLD signal during the negative feedback trials to BOLD signal during positive feedback, first for the whole session (i.e., first and second evaluation periods together), and then for the first evaluation period and for the second evaluation period separately. We focused on the contrast of negative—positive words, as this is the most analogous to previous studies investigating social rejection vs. social acceptance (e.g., Eisenberger et al., 2003; Rotge et al., 2015). To examine the main effect of group, contrast images for the whole session were entered into simple t-test at the group level for statistical inference. We applied an implicit mask, as well as an explicit whole brain gray matter mask. Note that the main group effect had to be explored within the simple t-test framework, as specifying the group contrast within the mixed design flexible factorial framework is not possible. To examine the main effect of evaluation periods, as well as group × evaluation periods interaction contrast images for each period of the evaluation for each participant were entered into flexible factorial analyses at the group level for statistical inference. The following factors were included in the flexible factorial: subject, group (controls vs. previously depressed) and evaluation period (first vs. second bout). Again, we applied an implicit mask, as well as an explicit whole brain gray matter mask. Following the classical model estimation, we examined the contrast for the main effect of time. We also examined the interaction of group by time (0 0 0 0 −1 1 1 −1) reflecting an effect where there would be an increase within the controls and a decrease in the previously depressed, and the inverse of the group by time interaction (0 0 0 0 1 −1 −1 1) representing an effect where there would be a decrease within the controls group and an increase in the previously depressed group.

To evaluate significance of the group main effect, we used a threshold of $p < 0.005$, 104 voxels, which corresponds to a 0.05 false-discovery rate as determined by Monte Carlo simulations conducted in the AFNI program 3dClustSim (parameters: individual voxel $p = 0.005$; 10,000 simulations; FWHM calculated from square root of ResMS at 11.78 × 14.95 × 12.27 mm; mask image file including 43,755 voxels).

To examine the effect of group by evaluation period on processing negative feedback compared to positive feedback, we first conducted a whole-brain analysis and used a threshold of $p <$ 0.005, 94 voxels, reflecting 0.05 false-discovery rate as determined by Monte Carlo simulations (3dClustSim parameters: individual voxel $p = 0.005$; 10,000 simulations; FWHM calculated from square root of ResMS at 10.84 × 14.02 × 12.51 mm; mask image file including 43,755 voxels). If this analysis revealed significant effects within the dACC we then used previously defined (Way et al., 2009), independent anatomical regions-of-interest (ROI) based on previous findings (Eisenberger et al., 2011) to investigate dACC association with measures of psychological trait and state characteristics; this was done to ensure that the analyses with respect to change in neural activity and psychological traits and states are not biased (Kriegeskorte et al., 2009).

Specifically, the ROI was constructed in PickAtlas (Maldjian et al., 2003) using templates from the Automated Anatomical Atlas (AAL; Tzourio-Mazoyer et al., 2002). Specifically, the dACC ROI combined Brodman areas 32 and 24, and used a rostral boundary of $y = +36$ based on criteria established by Vogt et al. (2003), and a caudal boundary of $y = 0$ (Way et al., 2009). For the ROI analyses, we first used SPM's *imagecalc* to calculate the change in activity for the negative feedback—positive feedback from the first period to the second period of evaluation (i.e., t2–t1). Then, we extracted parameter estimates from the anatomical ROI using SPM Toolbox MarsBaR. The parameter estimates obtained in this way were then entered into the custom model within the univariate ANCOVA framework to model the group effect, the effect of the covariate (i.e., change in activity in the structural dACC ROI) and the interaction effect between the group factor and the covariate on the dependent variable of interest (e.g., psychological responses to social evaluation, depression symptoms at baseline, 6 and 12 months). A significant interaction effect would reveal that the regression slope between the change in activity in the dACC ROI and the psychological variable of interest differs between the previously depressed and controls. For the psychological state measures, the model was set up to examine the impact of the interaction on the measure taken post the evaluative session while controlling for the pre-scan levels.

RESULTS

We evaluated BDI-II scores for all participants on the scan day and found that one previously depressed participant scored at clinical levels (BDI-II = 21) and one healthy participant at near-clinical levels (BDI-II = 19). These participants were excluded from subsequent analyses, leaving the total number of subjects per group at 30 for the controls and 16 for the previously depressed group.

Self-Report Data

Sociodemographic Data

The previously depressed participants were older compared to the controls ($M = 20.1$ years vs. $M = 18.9$ years, $U = 137$, $p = 0.013$). Groups did not differ based on their racial or ethnic background ($ps = 0.67$).

Psychological Traits

At the time of the social evaluative session, previously depressed participants had average BDI-II score within the normal range ($M = 6.13$, $SD = 5.35$); yet, these levels were nevertheless higher compared to controls ($M = 2.97$, $SD = 3.61$, $U = 148$, $p = 0.031$) (**Table 1**). The previously depressed group also showed higher scores on the Fear of Evaluation scale [$t_{(44)} = -2.18$, $p = 0.034$], higher trait anxiety scores on STAI [$t_{(21.8)} = -2.9$, $p = 0.008$], and lower scores on trait levels of self-esteem [$t_{(44)} = 2.71$, $p = 0.009$]; the groups did not differ with respect to Sensitivity to Rejection [$t_{(44)} = 1.53$, $p = 0.13$] (**Table 1**).

A Group (previously depressed, controls) by Time (baseline, 6, 12 months) ANOVA, revealed a significant Group effect [$F_{(1, 29)} = 6.17$, $p = 0.019$, Partial $\eta^2 = 0.18$], such that the previously depressed participants had overall higher BDI-II scores compared to control participants (**Table 1**). No other effects (Time, or Time by Group interaction) were significant ($ps > 0.25$).

Moment-to-Moment Responses to the Social Evaluative Task

To ensure that the evaluative task was having the intended effect, we examined whether participants' feelings in response to the evaluative feedback varied depending upon whether they were seeing negative, positive, or neutral adjectives in the scanner. A three-way mixed ANOVA [Group (previously depressed vs. controls) by Feedback Type (positive, negative, neutral) by Evaluation period (first bout vs. second bout of evaluation)] yielded a significant main effect of Evaluation period, revealing that all participants felt worse over time [$F_{(1, 44)} = 12.21$, $p = 0.001$, Partial $\eta^2 = 0.22$]. We also observed a main effect of Feedback Type [$F_{(1.39, 61.14)} = 150.34$, $p < 0.001$, Partial $\eta^2 = 0.77$], confirming that all participants felt worse in response to negative compared to neutral feedback [$t_{(45)} = 14.97$, $p < 0.001$] and worse in response to neutral compared to positive feedback [$t_{(45)} = 8.21$, $p < 0.001$]. Finally, we observed a significant Feedback Type by Group interaction [$F_{(1.39, 61.14)} = 6.05$, $p = 0.009$, Partial $\eta^2 = 0.12$]. Decomposing the interaction revealed that in response to positive feedback, the previously depressed participants endorsed greater levels of negative feelings ($M = 1.90$; $SD = 0.65$) compared to the controls ($M = 1.40$; $SD = 0.42$) [$F_{(1, 44)} = 11.45$, $p = 0.002$], but there were no differences for negative [$F_{(1, 44)} = 0.13$, $p = 0.72$] or neutral feedback [$F_{(1, 44)} = 0.55$, $p = 0.46$]. No other effects (i.e., main effect of Group, Group × Evaluation period, Evaluation period × Feedback Type, Group × Feedback × Evaluation period interaction) were significant.

Changes in Psychological States from Pre- to Post-evaluation

Feelings of social evaluation

To examine whether the task was successful in increasing feelings of social evaluation, we conducted a two-factor mixed-design ANOVA (Group by Time pre- vs. post-scan). The analysis showed only a significant effect of Time reflecting increased

TABLE 1 | Sociodemographic data and psychological profile of study participants.

	Controls $N = 30$ Mean ± Standard Deviation	Previously depressed $N = 16$ Mean ± Standard Deviation
Age	18.9 ± 1.06	20.13 ± 1.78*
BDI-II at the evaluative testing session	2.97 ± 3.61	6.13 ± 5.35*
BDI-II at 6 months post-testing session	4.23 ± 4.88 ($N =$ **26**)	9.00 ± 8.80 ($N =$ **13**)
BDI-II at 12 months post-testing session	5.47 ± 5.84 ($N =$ **19**)	7.42 ± 6.14 ($N =$ **12**)
Mehrabian sensitivity to rejection	−4.80 ± 19.46	−13.06 ± 12.75
Fear of evaluation scale	33.03 ± 7.01	37.62 ± 6.37*
State-trait anxiety inventory	33.80 ± 6.53	41.94 ± 10.16*
Rosenberg self-esteem	57.6 ± 8.2	49.9 ± 10.68*
RACIAL/ETHNIC BACKGROUND		
White	6	5
Asian/Filipino/Polynesian	7	4
Latino	7	2
Middle Eastern/East Indian	2	0
Other/mixed	8	5

*BDI-II, Beck Depression Inventory-II; *p < 0.05 compared to controls. Note the reduction in sample size, written in bold, for analyses involving BDI-II at 6 and 12 months.*

feelings of social evaluation post-task ($M = 5.09$; $SD = 1.50$) compared to pre-task ($M = 3.09$; $SD = 1.44$) in all participants [$F_{(1, 44)} = 84.47$, $p < 0.001$, Partial $\eta^2 = 0.66$; **Figure 2A**]. No other effects (Group, Group × Time interaction) were significant ($ps > 0.12$).

Depressed mood

A Group by Time (pre- vs. post-scan) ANOVA for depressed mood revealed a significant main effect of Group [$F_{(1, 44)} = 5.87$, $p = 0.02$, Partial $\eta^2 = 0.12$], showing overall greater levels of depressed mood in previously depressed participants compared to controls. We also observed a main effect of Time [$F_{(1, 44)} = 4.17$, $p = 0.047$, Partial $\eta^2 = 0.09$] reflecting an increase in depressed mood over time. Importantly, the Time effect was primarily driven by a bigger increase in depressed mood over time in the previously depressed group as suggested by the tendency for Group by Time interaction [$F_{(1, 44)} = 3.29$, $p = 0.077$, Partial $\eta^2 = 0.07$; **Figure 2B**].

Neuroimaging Data

Whole Brain Analysis

The whole brain Group effect revealed no significant activations in the dACC or in any other neural regions. Furthermore, there was no significant effect of the Evaluation period (first vs. second bout of evaluation). However, there was a significant Group by Evaluation period interaction effect only in the dACC (cluster = 127, corrected $p < 0.05$, MNI coordinates $x = 12$, $y = 20$, $z = 31$; **Figures 3A,B**; **Table 2**), such that there was a decrease over the two bouts of evaluation in dACC activity within the control group and an increase in the previously depressed group. Lowering the voxel threshold to $p < 0.005$, and the cluster extent to 40, revealed additional regions including anterior insula (MNI coordinates, $x = -27$, $y = 17$, $z = 1$; see Table S1).

In order to decompose the whole brain interaction effect for dACC, we extracted parameter estimates directly from the significant dACC cluster and entered these into SPSS. These analyses revealed that the activity within dACC was reduced over the two evaluation bouts among the controls [$F_{(1, 44)} = 6.49$, $p = 0.014$] but increased among the previously depressed participants [$F_{(1, 44)} = 7.65$, $p = 0.008$]. In addition, the groups did not differ with respect to activity in dACC during the first

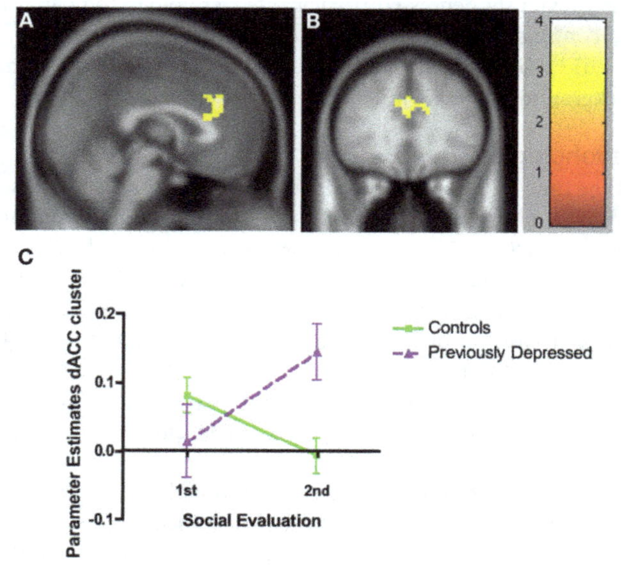

FIGURE 3 | Whole brain analyses of group × time interaction reflecting effect where neural activity increases over time in the previously depressed women but decreases in controls. (A) Sagittal view revealing a significant cluster in dorsal anterior cingulate cortex (dACC). **(B)** Coronal view of the same dACC cluster. **(C)** Parameter estimates extracted from the dACC cluster showing that within the control group activity within the dACC decreases, while in the previously depressed group, it increases. Note that extracted parameter estimates from this dACC cluster are taken from non-independent voxels and thus are used here simply to illustrate the observed effect at the whole brain level.

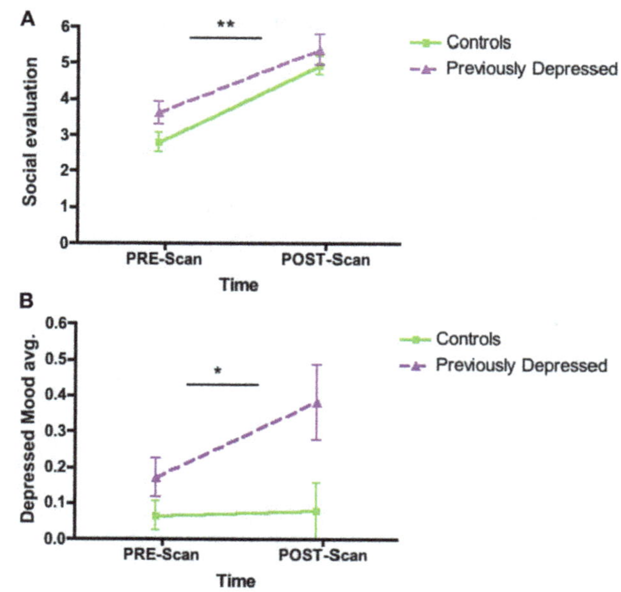

FIGURE 2 | Change in Psychological States from Pre- to Post-scan during the Social Evaluative Session. (A) Feelings of social evaluation. **(B)** Depressed mood. Main effect of Time shown. **$p < 0.001$; *$p < 0.05$.

TABLE 2 | Whole brain analyses of group × time interaction reflecting effect where neural activity increases over time in the previously depressed women but decreases in controls.

	Anatomical region	Brodmann Area	*x*	*y*	*z*	*t*	*k*
GROUP × TIME							
↑Previously Depressed							
↓Controls							
Whole Brain							
	dACC	24	12	20	31	4.04	127
		32	*−12*	*26*	*28*	*3.86*	
		32	*0*	*32*	*31*	*3.63*	

Effects are significant at p < 0.05 corrected. Montreal Neurological Institute coordinates; coordinate in italics connote peaks within a same cluster; dACC, dorsal anterior cingulate cortex.

bout of the evaluation [$F_{(1, 44)} = 1.65, p = 0.21$], but previously depressed (vs. healthy controls) had higher levels of activity during the second bout of the evaluation [$F_{(1, 44)} = 10.30, p = 0.002$] (**Figure 3C**). It is important to note that extracted parameter estimates from this dACC cluster are taken from non-independent voxels, which can lead to biases in additional statistical analyses. Thus, the extracted parameter estimates and these additional analyses are used simply to illustrate which effect in which group is driving the observed effect at the whole brain level.

To examine group differences with respect to how change in dACC activity was associated with changes in psychological responses to the task as well as depressive symptoms at baseline, 6 and 12 months, we extracted parameter estimates from an independent anatomical dACC ROI and conducted the statistical analyses using SPSS (see Methods and Materials for details). We used the independent anatomical dACC ROI in order to ensure that these correlational analyses were independent of the whole brain group × evaluation period interaction analyses (Kriegeskorte et al., 2009).

Correlations between Changes in dACC ROI Activity Over Evaluation Periods and Self-Reported Psychological Responses to the Task

There were no group differences in how changes in dACC activity correlated with changes in either feelings of social evaluation or depressed mood.

Correlations between Changes in dACC ROI Activity Over Evaluation Periods and Depressive Symptoms at Baseline, 6 Months, and 12 Months Post-task

Baseline depressive symptoms

We observed a significant interaction effect between Group and Change in activity in the dACC ROI (**Figure 4A**) on baseline depressive symptoms (evaluated via the BDI-II), [$F_{(1, 42)} = 7.56, p = 0.009$, Partial $\eta^2 = 0.15$]. Thus, among the previously depressed, the greater the increase in activity in dACC over the two bouts of the evaluation, the *lower* the depressive symptoms on the day of the evaluation ($B = -21.25, t = -3.01, p = 0.009$), but no relationship was found among the controls ($B = -0.015, t = -0.004, p = 0.99$; **Figure 4B**).

Depressive symptoms at 6 and 12 months post-task

Finally, we also investigated whether there was a Group difference with respect to regression slopes between the Change in the dACC ROI and the BDI-II scores assessed at 6 and 12 months. We found a significant interaction effect for 6 months [$F_{(1, 35)} = 4.56, p = 0.04$, Partial $\eta^2 = 0.12$; **Figure 4C**], but not 12 months [$F_{(1, 27)} = 1.98, p = 0.17$, Partial $\eta^2 = 0.07$]. The significant interaction for the BDI-II levels at 6 months revealed that, only among the previously depressed, the greater increase in activity in the dACC over the two bouts of evaluation, the *lower* the BDI-II score at 6 months post-social evaluative session (previously depressed group: $B = -33.87, t = -2.92, p = 0.014$; controls group: $B = -10.23, t = -1.93, p = 0.07$; **Figure 3C**).

To examine whether the relationship between changes in dACC activity and depressive symptoms at 6 months

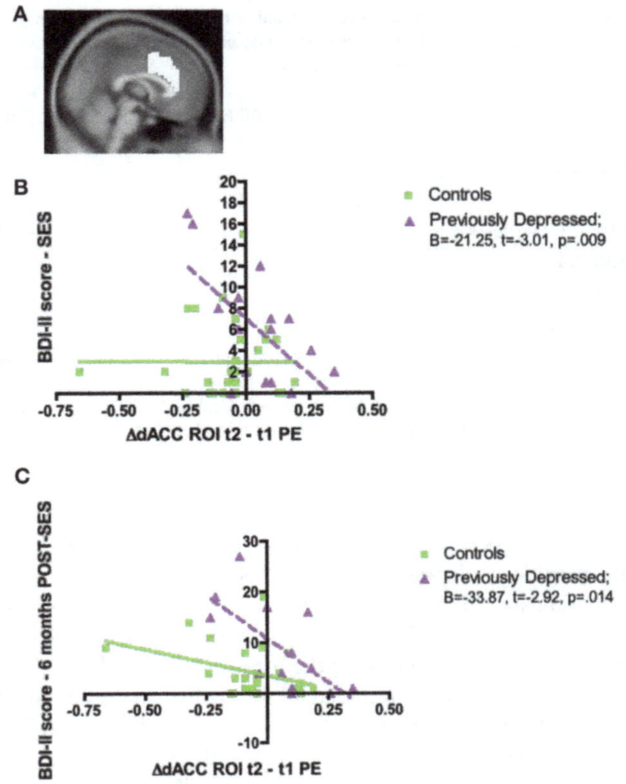

FIGURE 4 | Significant associations between the increase in activity over time in dorsal anterior cingulate cortex (dACC) independent, structural region of interest (ROI), and psychological measures in the previously depressed women compared to controls. (A) Sagittal view of the independent, structural dACC region of interest used to extract parameter estimates for subsequent analyses; **(B)** Beck Depression Inventory-II (BDI-II) score at the social evaluative session (SES); **(C)** BDI-II score at 6 months following the social evaluative session (SES).

in the previously depressed participants was independent of participants' depressive symptoms at the time of the social evaluative session, we conducted a hierarchical regression. We first entered the BDI-II scores at the time of the social evaluative session and, in the next step, entered the parameter estimates from the dACC ROI. There was a significant change in the fitness of the model upon the introduction of the dACC ROI (F change $= 5.02, p = 0.049$), with only the second model that included both BDI-II scores and dACC ROI being significant [$F_{(2, 10)} = 4.14, p = 0.049$]. Specifically, the second model revealed that change in activity in dACC ROI significantly contributed to the BDI-II at 6 months, $t = -2.24, p = 0.049$, controlling for baseline BDI-II levels (**Table 3**).

DISCUSSION

The present study aimed to investigate neural mechanisms underlying the association between repeated exposure to social evaluation and depressive symptoms in psychiatrically healthy and previously depressed young women. Although, both groups reported increases in feelings of social evaluation in response

TABLE 3 | Hierarchical regression reveals significant and unique contribution of increase in activity in dorsal anterior cingulate cortex (dACC) to depression levels at 6 months following the social evaluative session in the previously depressed women.

	b	SE *B*	β	*p*
MODEL 1				
Constant	4.22	3.861		0.298
BDI-II at testing session	0.683	0.442	0.422	0.151
MODEL 2				
Constant	13.659	5.352		0.029
BDI-II at testing session	−0.324	0.587	−0.201	0.593
ΔdACC t2-t1	−41.74	18.624	−0.814	0.049

Adjusted R^2 for Model 2 = 0.344; F change between Model 2 vs. Model 1, $p = 0.049$; Δ, change in activity in dACC from first bout (t1) to second bout (t2) of social evaluation; BDI-II, Beck Depression Inventory-II.

to a brief socially evaluative stressor, we found evidence that previously depressed participants experienced this social evaluation in a unique way. Namely, the previously depressed (compared to controls) tended to show increased levels of depressed mood in response to the social evaluation. In addition, previously depressed compared to the controls showed more negative feelings in response to positive feedback, which is consistent with the role of anhedonia in depression (e.g., Eshel and Roiser, 2010; Beevers et al., 2013). Overall, these findings are in line with the idea that the previously depressed represent a population vulnerable to developing depression.

With regard to neural activity, we did not observe an overall group effect or time effect. However, as expected, the previously depressed participants did show increased activity over repeated bouts of social evaluation within the dACC in response to negative compared to positive feedback, while controls showed a decline in this contrast. Interestingly, and surprisingly, this increase within the dACC in the previously depressed was linked with lower levels of depressive symptoms at baseline, and most notably, with lower levels of depressive symptoms 6 months after the social evaluative session—an effect that held even after controlling for baseline depression levels. Thus, those previously depressed women who showed increases over time in dACC responses to negative compared to positive feedback seemed to show traces of resilience with respect to their current psychological state and well as their depression symptoms 6 months later.

It has been suggested that the dACC plays an important role in responding to social exclusion (Kawamoto et al., 2012), with experiences of negative social evaluation or rejection consistently being associated with overall heightened activity in the dACC in healthy samples (Eisenberger et al., 2003, 2011; Kross et al., 2011; Rotge et al., 2015). Further, in healthy samples, this engagement of dACC was found to wane over the course of playing a computerized game of social exclusion (Crowley et al., 2009; Moor et al., 2012; Kawamoto et al., 2013; Themanson et al., 2013). Therefore, the decrease over time in dACC activity in response to negative compared to positive feedback in the healthy sample observed here could represent an adaptive response to negative social evaluation. Indeed, this pattern of response is consistent with the idea that if one mounts a physiological response to a personally-relevant stressful situation, that response should be followed by a successful recovery, if it is to be adaptive (Fredrickson et al., 2003; Tugade and Fredrickson, 2004).

The previously depressed group did not show difference in the overall activity in dACC, which suggests that abnormalities in overall dACC activity previously observed in MDD patients (Hamilton et al., 2011; Crocker et al., 2013; Graham et al., 2013; Ubl et al., 2015) could be a characteristic of being in a depressive state (Hamilton et al., 2011). The increase in dACC activity over the course of the social evaluation task, however, is similar to what was previously observed in MDD patients (Waugh et al., 2012). Still, it is not yet clear what function the dACC is serving during the task. Waugh and colleagues proposed that the resurgence of medial frontal cortex activity including dACC over the course of their stress paradigm in MDD patients may represent either rumination about negative aspects of the stress task or, alternatively, generation of arousal necessary for anticipated effort in performing the task (Waugh et al., 2012). Future work will be needed to more fully examine these alternatives.

Surprisingly, in the current study, increased dACC activity over the two social evaluation periods was associated with *lower* depressive symptoms at baseline as well as at 6 months following the social evaluative session. Although, running contrary to what one would expect from the previous findings of heightened dACC activity during a given experience of social evaluation, these findings are in line with previous studies showing that heightened risk for developing depression could be linked with a blunted neural response to emotional contexts (McCabe et al., 2012; Kujawa et al., 2014; Chester et al., 2015), a phenomenon that has also been observed in persons experiencing a depressive episode (e.g., Miller et al., 2015; Ubl et al., 2015). Specifically, a blunted neural response in the dACC to both negative and positive stimuli (e.g., food or monetary) has been observed in children and young adults at heightened vulnerability to develop depression due to family history (McCabe et al., 2012; Kujawa et al., 2014). In addition, another study in young adults with heightened subclinical levels of alexythimia, a condition with strong links to depression (Honkalampi et al., 2000), revealed that participants who tended to have difficulty identifying their feelings felt more rejected on a daily basis in part because of diminished dACC activity during social rejection experiences (Chester et al., 2015). It was proposed that the blunted dACC response resulted in a failure of these individuals to adjust their behavioral tendencies to achieve social inclusion in the future (Chester et al., 2015). Therefore, it is possible that increased dACC activity over time may represent a form of emotional context sensitivity, which is considered an adaptive emotional response even among those remitted from depression (Rottenberg et al., 2005; Waugh and Koster, 2014), and therefore may constitute a sign of resilience. As we did not include a third bout of evaluation, we could not evaluate whether these individuals were also able to show the appropriate adaptive recovery of this increased response; this should be evaluated in future studies. Future work is needed to better understand why increasing neural sensitivity over time in previously depressed participants was related to better subsequent outcomes.

Although, the current study reveals important details with respect to the role of the dACC during the processing of *repeated* social evaluation and vulnerability/resilience to depression, it does have some notable limitations. First, the study has uneven sample sizes per study groups with small sample size affecting the previously depressed group; this is due to difficulty in recruiting previously depressed participants who at the time of testing had a healthy psychological profile. Nevertheless, the sample size within the previously depressed group is adequate and within the guidelines for the employed statistical tests (Field, 2005). Second, due to careful selection of the previously depressed sample in order to limit sources of variability and the fact that we investigated a university student sample, it is possible that the current results are not generalizable to all participants with a past history of depression. Study results should be replicated in a larger, community-based sample. Furthermore, the social evaluative task had only two repetitions of social evaluations, which provides only limited insight into the nature of temporal dynamics of dACC activity; future studies should include multiple repetitions of social evaluative sessions.

Overall, the study revealed that while young women with a past history of MDD tend to be particularly sensitive to repeated bouts of social evaluation in terms of its effects on depressed mood, those who showed increases in dACC activity over the course of the social evaluative session to negative compared to positive feedback showed lower depressive symptoms at baseline and 6 months later. Changes in dACC activity over repeated bouts of social evaluation may be an important mechanism underlying the association between experiences of repeated social evaluation and individual differences in continued resilience and vulnerability to depression. Given that the change in dACC activity *over time* in response to negative evaluation reveals a new dimension to the role of the dACC in processing exclusion and its association with mental health outcomes in a sample with distinct vulnerability to depression, further investigation of the dynamics of dACC response to negative social evaluation is warranted.

AUTHOR CONTRIBUTIONS

KD: study design, study execution, analyses, manuscript writing and editing. GS: study design, study execution, manuscript editing. KM: study design, study execution, manuscript editing. MI: study design, manuscript editing. NE: study design, manuscript writing and editing.

FUNDING

This work was supported by a National Alliance for Research on Schizophrenia and Depression (NARSAD) Young Investigator Award (NE), a UCLA Cousins Center for Psychoneuroimmunology Seed Grant (NE), a UCLA Clinical & Translational Science Institute (CTSI) Seed Grant (NE), the NIH/National Center for Advancing Translational Science (NCATS) UCLA CTSI Grant Number UL1TR000124, the UCLA Older Americans Independence Center Inflammatory Biology Core (funded by NIA/NIH Grant Number AG028748), the National Science Foundation Graduate Research Fellowship Program (KM), NIH Pre-Doctoral Institutional Training Grant T32 MH015750 (KM), and the Canadian Institutes of Health Research Postdoctoral Fellowship program (KD).

ACKNOWLEDGMENTS

The authors wish to thank the Staglin IMHRO Center for Cognitive Neuroscience at UCLA, the UCLA Clinical and Translational Research Center, and the Cousins Center for Psychoneuroimmunology Inflammatory Biology Core Laboratory for supporting this research. We also acknowledge the contributions of Brittany Branscomb, Stephanie Chan, Christie Fung, Joyce Gorman, Ashley Guzman, Adrienne Healey, Evelyn Ho, Patil Kodchian, Becky Phan, and Shizue Reid for serving as confederates and research assistants.

SUPPLEMENTARY MATERIAL

The Supplementary Material for this article can be found online at: http://journal.frontiersin.org/article/10.3389/fnbeh.2016.00064

REFERENCES

American Psychiatric Association (2000). *Diagnostic and Statistical Manual of Mental Disorders (DSM-IV-TR)*. Washington DC: American Psychiatric Association.

Beck, A. T., Steer, R. A., and Brown, G. K. (1996). *Manual for the Beck Depression Inventory-II*. San Antonio, TX: Psychological Corporation.

Beevers, C. G., Worthy, D. A., Gorlick, M. A., Nix, B., Chotibut, T., and Todd Maddox, W. (2013). Influence of depression symptoms on history-independent reward and punishment processing. *Psychiatry Res.* 207, 53–60. doi: 10.1016/j.psychres.2012.09.054

Burcusa, S. L., and Iacono, W. G. (2007). Risk for recurrence in depression. *Clin. Psychol. Rev.* 27, 959–985. doi: 10.1016/j.cpr.2007.02.005

Chester, D. S., Pond, R. S. Jr., and DeWall, C. N. (2015). Alexithymia is associated with blunted anterior cingulate response to social rejection: implications for daily rejection. *Soc. Cogn. Affect. Neurosci.* 10, 517–522. doi: 10.1093/scan/nsu082

Crocker, L. D., Heller, W., Warren, S. L., O'Hare, A. J., Infantolino, Z. P., and Miller, G. A. (2013). Relationships among cognition, emotion, and motivation: implications for intervention and neuroplasticity in psychopathology. *Front. Hum. Neurosci.* 7:261. doi: 10.3389/fnhum.2013.00261

Crowley, M. J., Wu, J., McCarty, E. R., David, D. H., Bailey, C. A., and Mayes, L. C. (2009). Exclusion and micro-rejection: event-related potential response predicts mitigated distress. *Neuroreport* 20, 1518–1522. doi: 10.1097/WNR.0b013e328330377a

Eisenberger, N. I., Inagaki, T. K., Muscatell, K. A., Byrne Haltom, K. E., and Leary, M. R. (2011). The neural sociometer: brain mechanisms underlying state self-esteem. *J. Cogn. Neurosci.* 23, 3448–3455. doi: 10.1162/jocn_a_00027

Eisenberger, N. I., and Lieberman, M. D. (2004). Why rejection hurts: a common neural alarm system for physical and social pain. *Trends Cogn. Sci. (Regul. Ed).* 8, 294–300. doi: 10.1016/j.tics.2004.05.010

Eisenberger, N. I., Lieberman, M. D., and Williams, K. D. (2003). Does rejection hurt? *An FMRI study of social exclusion. Science* 302, 290–292. doi: 10.1126/science.1089134

Eshel, N., and Roiser, J. P. (2010). Reward and punishment processing in depression. *Biol. Psychiatry* 68, 118–124. doi: 10.1016/j.biopsych.2010.01.027

Ferrari, A. J., Charlson, F. J., Norman, R. E., Patten, S. B., Freedman, G., Murray, C. J., et al. (2013). Burden of depressive disorders by country, sex, age, and year: findings from the global burden of disease study 2010. *PLoS Med.* 10:e1001547. doi: 10.1371/journal.pmed.1001547

Field, A. (2005). *Discovering Statistics using SPSS.* London: Sage Publications.

First, M. B., Gibbon, M., Spitzer, R. L., and Williams, J. B. (1995). *User's Guide for the Structured Clinical Interview for DSM-IV Axis I Disorders (SCID-I, version 2.0, Final Version).* New York, NY: New York State Psychiatric Institute.

Fredrickson, B. L., Tugade, M. M., Waugh, C. E., and Larkin, G. R. (2003). What good are positive emotions in crises? A prospective study of resilience and emotions following the terrorist attacks on the United States on September 11th, 2011. *J. Pers. Soc. Psychol.* 84, 365–376. doi: 10.1037/0022-3514.84.2.365

Graham, J., Salimi-Khorshidi, G., Hagan, C., Walsh, N., Goodyer, I., Lennox, B., et al. (2013). Meta-analytic evidence for neuroimaging models of depression: state or trait? *J. Affect. Disord.* 151, 423–431. doi: 10.1016/j.jad.2013.07.002

Hamilton, J. P., Glover, G. H., Hsu, J. J., Johnson, R. F., and Gotlib, I. H. (2011). Modulation of subgenual anterior cingulate cortex activity with real-time neurofeedback. *Hum. Brain Mapp.* 32, 22–31. doi: 10.1002/hbm.20997

Harkness, K. L., Jacobson, J. A., Duong, D., and Sabbagh, M. A. (2010). Mental state decoding in past major depression: effect of sad versus happy bood induction. *Cogn. Emot.* 24, 3. doi: 10.1080/02699930902750249

Honkalampi, K., Hintikka, J., Tanskanen, A., Lehtonen, J., and Viinamäki, H. (2000). Depression is strongly associated with alexithymia in the general population. *J. Psychosom. Res.* 48, 99–104. doi: 10.1016/S0022-3999(99)00083-5

Kawamoto, T., Nittono, H., and Ura, M. (2013). Cognitive, affective, and motivational changes during ostracism: an ERP, EMG, and EEG study using a computerized cyberball task. *Neurosci J.* 2013:304674. doi: 10.1155/2013/304674

Kawamoto, T., Onoda, K., Nakashima, K., Nittono, H., Yamaguchi, S., and Ura, M. (2012). Is dorsal anterior cingulate cortex activation in response to social exclusion due to expectancy violation? *An fMRI study. Front. Evol. Neurosci.* 4:11. doi: 10.3389/fnevo.2012.00011

Kawamoto, T., Ura, M., and Nittono, H. (2015). Intrapersonal and interpersonal processes of social exclusion. *Front. Neurosci.* 9:62. doi: 10.3389/fnins.2015.00062

Kendler, K. S., Hettema, J. M., Butera, F., Gardner, C. O., and Prescott, C. A. (2003). Life event dimensions of loss, humiliation, entrapment, and danger in the prediction of onsets of major depression and generalized anxiety. *Arch. Gen. Psychiatry* 60, 789–796. doi: 10.1001/archpsyc.60.8.789

Kong, F., Wang, X., Hu, S., and Liu, J. (2015). Neural correlates of psychological resilience and their relation to life satisfaction in a sample of healthy young adults. *Neuroimage* 123, 165–172. doi: 10.1016/j.neuroimage.2015.08.020

Koppers, D., Peen, J., Niekerken, S., Van, R., and Dekker, J. (2011). Prevalence and risk factors for recurrence of depression five years after short term psychodynamic therapy. *J. Affect. Disord.* 134, 468–472. doi: 10.1016/j.jad.2011.05.027

Kriegeskorte, N., Simmons, W. K., Bellgowan, P. S. F., and Baker, C. I. (2009). Circular analysis in systems neuroscience: the dangers of double dipping. *Nat. Neurosci.* 12, 535–540. doi: 10.1038/nn.2303

Kross, E., Berman, M. G., Mischel, W., Smith, E. E., and Wager, T. D. (2011). Social rejection shares somatosensory representations with physical pain. *Proc. Natl. Acad. Sci. U.S.A.* 108, 6270–6275. doi: 10.1073/pnas.1102693108

Kujawa, A., Proudfit, G. H., and Klein, D. N. (2014). Neural reactivity to rewards and losses in offspring of mothers and fathers with histories of depressive and anxiety disorders. *J. Abnorm. Psychol.* 123, 287–297. doi: 10.1037/a0036285

Leary, M. R. (1983). A brief version of the Fear of Negative Evaluation Scale. *Pers. Soc. Psychol. Bull.* 9, 371–376. doi: 10.1177/0146167283093007

LeMoult, J., Joormann, J., Sherdell, L., Wright, Y., and Gotlib, I. H. (2009). Identification of emotional facial expressions following recovery from depression. *J. Abnorm. Psychol.* 118, 828–833. doi: 10.1037/a0016944

Maldjian, J. A., Laurienti, P. J., Kraft, R. A., and Burdette, J. H. (2003). An automated method for neuroanatomic and cytoarchitectonic atlas-based interrogation of fMRI data sets. *Neuroimage* 19, 1233–1239. doi: 10.1016/S1053-8119(03)00169-1

Marcus, M., Yasamy, T. M., van Ommeren, M., Chisholm, D., and Saxena, S. (2012). *Depression: A Global Public Health Concern.* Geneva: WHO Department of Mental Health and Substance Abuse.

McCabe, C., Woffindale, C., Harmer, C. J., and Cowen, P. J. (2012). Neural processing of reward and punishment in young people at increased familial risk of depression. *Biol. Psychiatry* 72, 588–594. doi: 10.1016/j.biopsych.2012.04.034

McNair, D. M., Lorr, M., and Droppleman, L. P. (1992). *EdITS Manual for the Profile of Mood States.* San Diego, CA: Educational and Industrial Testing Service.

Mehrabian, A. (1976). Questionnaire measures of affiliative tendency and sensitivity to rejection. *Psychol. Rep.* 38, 199–209. doi: 10.2466/pr0.1976.38.1.199

Miller, C. H., Hamilton, J. P., Sacchet, M. D., and Gotlib, I. H. (2015). Meta-analysis of functional neuroimaging of major depressive disorder in youth. *JAMA Psychiatry* 72, 1045–1053. doi: 10.1001/jamapsychiatry.2015.1376

Moor, B. G., Güroğlu, B., Op de Macks, Z. A., Rombouts, S. A. R. B., Van der Molen, M. W., and Crone, E. A. (2012). Social exclusion and punishment of excluders: neural correlates and developmental trajectories. *Neuroimage* 59, 708–717. doi: 10.1016/j.neuroimage.2011.07.028

Muscatell, K. A., Dedovic, K., Slavich, G. M., Jarcho, M. R., Breen, E. C., Bower, J. E., et al. (2014). Greater amygdala activity and dorsomedial prefrontal-amygdala coupling are associated with enhanced inflammatory responses to stress. *Brain Behav. Immun.* 43, 46–53. doi: 10.1016/j.bbi.2014.06.201

Osborne, J. W. (2013). *Best Practices in Data Cleaning.* Los Angeles, CA: SAGE Publication Inc.

Rosenberg, M. (1965). *Society and the Adolescent Self-Image.* Princeton, NJ: Princeton University Press.

Rotge, J. Y., Lemogne, C., Hinfray, S., Huguet, P., Grynszpan, O., Tartour, E., et al. (2015). A meta-analysis of the anterior cingulate contribution to social pain. *Soc. Cogn. Affect. Neurosci.* 10, 19–27. doi: 10.1093/scan/nsu110

Rottenberg, J., Gross, J. J., and Gotlib, I. H. (2005). Emotion context insensitivity in major depressive disorder. *J. Abnorm. Psychol.* 114, 627–639. doi: 10.1037/0021-843X.114.4.627

Slavich, G. M., Monroe, S. M., and Gotlib, I. H. (2011). Early parental loss and depression history: associations with recent life stress in major depressive disorder. *J. Psychiatr. Res.* 45, 1146–1152. doi: 10.1016/j.jpsychires.2011.03.004

Slavich, G. M., O'Donovan, A., Epel, E. S., and Kemeny, M. E. (2010). Black sheep get the blues: a psychobiological model of social rejection and depression. *Neurosci. Biobehav. Rev.* 35, 39–45. doi: 10.1016/j.neubiorev.2010.01.003

Slavich, G. M., Thornton, T., Torres, L. D., Monroe, S. M., and Gotlib, I. H. (2009). Targeted rejection predicts hastened onset of major depression. *J. Soc. Clin. Psychol.* 28, 223–243. doi: 10.1521/jscp.2009.28.2.223

Somerville, L. H., Heatherton, T. F., and Kelley, W. M. (2006). Anterior cingulate cortex responds differentially to expectancy violation and social rejection. *Nat. Neurosci.* 9, 1007–1008. doi: 10.1038/nn1728

Southwick, S. M., Vythilingam, M., and Charney, D. S. (2005). The psychobiology of depression and resilience to stress: implications for prevention and treatment. *Annu. Rev. Clin. Psychol.* 1, 255–291. doi: 10.1146/annurev.clinpsy.1.102803.143948

Spielberger, C. D. (1983). *Manual for the State-Trait Anxiety Inventory.* Palo Alto, CA: Consulting Psychologicsts Press.

Spunt, R. P., Lieberman, M. D., Cohen, J. R., and Eisenberger, N. I. (2012). The phenomenology of error processing: the dorsal ACC response to stop-signal errors tracks reports of negative affect. *J. Cogn. Neurosci.* 24, 1753–1765. doi: 10.1162/jocn_a_00242

Stroud, C. B., Davila, J., Hammen, C., and Vrshek-Schallhorn, S. (2011). Severe and nonsevere events in first onsets versus recurrences of depression: evidence for stress sensitization. *J. Abnorm. Psychol.* 120, 142–154. doi: 10.1037/a0021659

Stroud, L. R., Salovey, P., and Epel, E. S. (2002). Sex differences in stress responses: social rejection versus achievement stress. *Biol. Psychiatry* 52, 318–327. doi: 10.1016/S0006-3223(02)01333-1

Themanson, J. R., Khatcherian, S. M., Ball, A. B., and Rosen, P. J. (2013). An event-related examination of neural activity during social interactions. *Soc. Cogn. Affect. Neurosci.* 8, 727–733. doi: 10.1093/scan/nss058

Tugade, M. M., and Fredrickson, B. L. (2004). Resilience individuals use positive emotions to bounce back from negative emotional experiences. *J. Pers. Soc. Psychol.* 86, 320–333. doi: 10.1037/0022-3514.86.2.320

Tzourio-Mazoyer, N., Landeau, B., Papathanassiou, D., Crivello, F., Etard, O., Delcroix, N., et al. (2002). Automated anatomical labeling of activations in SPM using a macroscopic anatomical parcellation of the MNI MRI single-subject brain. *Neuroimage* 15, 273–289. doi: 10.1006/nimg.2001.0978

Ubl, B., Kuehner, C., Kirsch, P., Ruttorf, M., Diener, C., and Flor, H. (2015). Altered neural reward and loss processing and prediction error signalling in depression. *Soc. Cogn. Affect. Neurosci.* 10, 1102–1112. doi: 10.1093/scan/nsu158

Vogt, B. A., Berger, G. R., and Derbyshire, S. W. (2003). Structural and functional dichotomy of human midcingulate cortex. *Eur. J. Neurosci.* 18, 3134–3144. doi: 10.1111/j.1460-9568.2003.03034.x

Waugh, C. E., Hamilton, J. P., Chen, M. C., Joormann, J., and Gotlib, I. H. (2012). Neural temporal dynamics of stress in comorbid major depressive disorder and social anxiety disorder. *Biol. Mood Anxiety Disord.* 2, 1–15. doi: 10.1186/2045-5380-2-11

Waugh, C. E., and Koster, E. H. W. (2014). A resilience framework for promoting stable remission from depression. *Clin. Psychol. Rev.* 41, 49–60. doi: 10.1016/j.cpr.2014.05.004

Way, B. M., Taylor, S. E., and Eisenberger, N. I. (2009). Variation in the mu-opioid receptor gene (OPRM1) is associated with dispositional and neural sensitivity to social rejection. *Proc. Natl. Acad. Sci. U.S.A.* 106, 15079–15084. doi: 10.1073/pnas.0812612106

Conflict of Interest Statement: The authors declare that the research was conducted in the absence of any commercial or financial relationships that could

14

Interaction Effect between Handedness and CNTNAP2 Polymorphism (rs7794745 Genotype) on Voice-specific Frontotemporal Activity in Healthy Individuals: An fMRI Study

Edited by:
Morten L. Kringelbach,
University of Aarhus, Denmark;
University of Oxford, UK

***Correspondence:**
Michihiko Koeda,
Department of Neuropsychiatry,
Graduate School of Medicine, Nippon Medical School, 1-1-5, Sendagi,
Bunkyo-Ku, Tokyo 113-8603, Japan
mkoeda@nms.ac.jp

Michihiko Koeda[1], Atsushi Watanabe[2,3], Kumiko Tsuda[4], Miwako Matsumoto[4], Yumiko Ikeda[5], Woochan Kim[1], Amane Tateno[1], Banyar Than Naing[2,3], Hiroyuki Karibe[5], Takashi Shimada[3], Hidenori Suzuki[6], Masato Matsuura[4] and Yoshiro Okubo[1]*

[1] Department of Neuropsychiatry, Graduate School of Medicine, Nippon Medical School, Tokyo, Japan, [2] Division of Personalized Genetic Medicine, Nippon Medical School Hospital, Tokyo, Japan, [3] Department of Biochemistry and Molecular Biology, Graduate School of Medicine, Nippon Medical School, Tokyo, Japan, [4] Department of Biofunctional Informatics, Tokyo Medical and Dental University, Tokyo, Japan, [5] Department of Pediatric Dentistry, Nippon Dental University, Tokyo, Japan, [6] Department of Pharmacology, Graduate School of Medicine, Nippon Medical School, Tokyo, Japan

Recent neuroimaging studies have demonstrated that Contactin-associated protein-like2 (*CNTNAP2*) polymorphisms affect left-hemispheric function of language processing in healthy individuals, but no study has investigated the influence of these polymorphisms on right-hemispheric function involved in human voice perception. Further, although recent reports suggest that determination of handedness is influenced by genetic effect, the interaction effect between handedness and *CNTNAP2* polymorphisms for brain activity in human voice perception and language processing has not been revealed. We aimed to investigate the interaction effect of handedness and *CNTNAP2* polymorphisms in respect to brain function for human voice perception and language processing in healthy individuals. Brain function of 108 healthy volunteers (74 right-handed and 34 non-right-handed) was examined while they were passively listening to reverse sentences (rSEN), identifiable non-vocal sounds (SND), and sentences (SEN). Full factorial design analysis was calculated by using three factors: (1) rs7794745 (A/A or A/T), (2) rs2710102 [G/G or A carrier (A/G and A/A)], and (3) voice-specific response (rSEN or SND). The main effect of rs7794745 (A/A or A/T) was significantly revealed at the right middle frontal gyrus (MFG) and bilateral superior temporal gyrus (STG). This result suggests that rs7794745 genotype affects voice-specific brain function. Furthermore, interaction effect was significantly observed among MFG-STG activations by human voice perception, rs7794745 (A/A or A/T), and handedness. These results suggest that *CNTNAP2* polymorphisms could be one of the important factors in the neural development related to vocal communication and language processing in both right-handed and non-right-handed healthy individuals.

Keywords: *CNTNAP2*, fMRI, voice, handedness, SNPs, autism, schizophrenia

Introduction

It is believed that most people process language predominantly in the left hemisphere, but the biological and molecular mechanisms are unclear. In respect to brain function, previous neuroimaging studies of language processing in healthy subjects have demonstrated cerebral activation at the left hemispheric frontotempo-parietal cortices by using functional magnetic resonance imaging (fMRI) (Frost et al., 1999; Springer et al., 1999; Price, 2000; Koeda et al., 2006a, 2007). On the other hand, recent genetic neuroimaging studies have verified the influence of single nucleotide polymorphisms (SNPs) in relation to brain structure and brain function (Camara et al., 2010; Frielingsdorf et al., 2010; Cuenco et al., 2011; Chen et al., 2012; Forbes et al., 2012; Hajek et al., 2012; Blasi et al., 2013; Clemm Von Hohenberg et al., 2013).

The contactin-associated protein-like 2 (*CNTNAP2*) gene is known as a transcriptional factor regulated by forkhead box P2 (*FOXP2*) gene related to language processing (Grigorenko, 2009; Newbury and Monaco, 2010; Catani et al., 2011; Penagarikano and Geschwind, 2012; Graham and Fisher, 2013; Rodenas-Cuadrado et al., 2014). Recent studies have reported that *CNTNAP2* is associated with human brain development as cell adhesion molecules (Ip et al., 2011; Huang et al., 2013; Muntané et al., 2014). Two studies have shown that genotypes of *CNTNAP2* affect brain function in healthy subjects (Whalley et al., 2011; Kos et al., 2012). One study has demonstrated that the group with A/T genotype in rs7794745, one of the SNPs in *CNTNAP2*, shows significantly greater activation in the right inferior frontal gyrus (IFG) and right temporal lobe compared with the group with A/A genotype during verbal fluency task (Whalley et al., 2011). Another study of event-related potential (ERP) has demonstrated that the waveform in P600 changes in the A/T genotype group in rs7794745 compared with the A/A genotype group (Kos et al., 2012).

Recent reports have indicated that *CNTNAP2* polymorphisms affect brain function for language processing in neurodevelopmental disorders as well as in healthy subjects. *CNTNAP2* has been reported to be an important genetic factor for differentiating the pathogenesis of language impairment in autism spectrum disorder (ASD) or attention-deficit hyperactivity disorder (ADHD) (Sizoo et al., 2010). A study has shown that A/T in rs7794745 of *CNTNAP2* is a risk genotype of autism compared with A/A (Li et al., 2010). The risk allele of *CNTNAP2* is closely associated with reduced white matter volume in ASD, and with a reduction of fractal anisotropy in the cerebellum and frontotemporal cortex (Tan et al., 2010). Further, previous studies have reported that rs2710102 of *CNTNAP2* is associated with language acquisition in early language development (Whitehouse et al., 2011), or language development disorder (Alarcon et al., 2008; Vernes et al., 2008).

Language is processed predominantly in the left hemisphere in most people. According to previous reports, about 95% of right-handed (RH) subjects are left hemispheric dominant (Binder et al., 1997; Springer et al., 1999). In contrast, about 75% of non-right-handed (non-RH) subjects are left hemispheric dominant (Pujol et al., 1999; Szaflarski et al., 2002). This rate of language being processed in the left hemisphere is significantly less in non-RH subjects than in RH subjects. Further, in non-RH subjects, the rate of predominant left hemispheric language dominance with a family history of non-RH subjects is significantly less than that without such a family history (Szaflarski et al., 2002; Liu et al., 2009). These results suggest that genetic effect may affect acquisition of handedness in the stage of language development.

Recent research has reported that SNPs on several genes related to language development affect brain volumes or brain function (Geschwind et al., 2002; Medland et al., 2006; Sun and Walsh, 2006). Especially, there is evidence of SNPs on *CNTNAP2* associated with brain function for language comprehension (Whalley et al., 2011). However, to our knowledge, no study has investigated the interaction effect between handedness and SNPs on *CNTNAP2* for brain activity in language processing. Further, it is unclear whether *CNTNAP2* affects brain function in human voice perception as well as in language processing. Recent neuroimaging studies demonstrated predominantly right hemispheric activation at the bilateral superior temporal gyrus (STG) during passive listening to human voice (Belin et al., 2000; Fecteau et al., 2004; Koeda et al., 2006a; Charest et al., 2013). In addition, studies of patients with autism and schizophrenia have revealed impairment of brain function at the right STG during human voice perception (Ocklenburg et al., 2013). Based on these findings, it seems important to verify the genetic influence on brain function during listening to human voice as well as language, although, to our knowledge, no such study has been documented. Additionally, recent neuroimaging studies have demonstrated that language dominance in non-RH healthy people is different from RH subjects (Szaflarski et al., 2002; Greve et al., 2013; Perlaki et al., 2013), but the genetic influence on handedness and brain function during auditory processing such as language, human voice, and environmental sounds remains unclear.

We aimed to (1) investigate the phenotypic influence of the genotype of *CNTNAP2* in order to verify the cerebral response to human voice perception and lexical-semantic processing in language processing by using fMRI, and (2) clarify whether brain function of language dominance and human voice perception is affected by genetic factor(s) and handedness.

In this study, to clarify the specific polymorphism(s) related to language processing and human voice perception, 2 SNPs (rs7794745 and rs2710102) in *CNTNAP2* were selected. These SNPs are known as biological high-risk markers for ASD, epilepsy, mental retardation, schizophrenia, and cognitive impairment (Friedman et al., 2008; Li et al., 2010; Stein et al., 2011; Clemm Von Hohenberg et al., 2013; Ji et al., 2013; Sampath et al., 2013). We investigated whether these 2 SNPs affect brain function in healthy individuals.

Materials and Methods

Subjects of fMRI Study

One hundred and eight healthy subjects (53 males and 55 females, mean age 26.3 years, $SD = 6.9$) participated in the present study. All 108 volunteers were native speakers of Japanese. None of the control subjects was taking alcohol or medication at the time, nor did they have a history of psychiatric disorder, significant physical illness, head injury, neurological disorder, or alcohol or drug dependence based on the contents of the Japanese version of Diagnostic Interview for Genetic Studies (DIGS). After complete explanation of the study, written informed consent was obtained from all subjects. The study protocol was approved by the Gene Institutional Review Board of Nippon Medical School. The mean period of education (mean ± SD) was 15.7 ± 0.7 years (male: 15.9 ± 0.7 years; female: 15.6 ± 0.7 years). According to data from the UNESCO Institute for Statistics (http://hdr.undp.org/en/data), the expected years of schooling in 2011 in Japan were as follows: male: 15.4; female: 15.1, respectively. The results of one-sample t-test for these expected years of schooling were as follows: male [$t_{(52)} = 5.08, p < 0.001$]; female [$t_{(54)} = 5.21, p < 0.001$], respectively. Based on the Edinburgh Handedness Inventory (EHI) (Oldfield, 1971) and according to the definition of previous studies (Oldfield, 1971; Springer et al., 1999; Szaflarski et al., 2002; Koeda et al., 2013), handedness of RH subjects was defined as equal to or more than 50 in the score of EHI, whereas that of non-RH subjects was defined as less than 50. Accordingly, handedness was 74 RH and 34 non-RH according to EHI (Oldfield, 1971). Mean (±SD) EHI in the 74 RH subjects was 88.5 ± 11.1, and that of the 34 non-RH subjects was −39.6 ± 38.3.

Sample Collection, Preparation, and Genotyping

Genomic DNA samples were extracted from peripheral blood using standard procedures. Genotype screening for each SNP was performed by small amplicon genotyping (SAG) method based on high-resolution melting curve analysis (Watanabe et al., 2011). *Two* SNPs, rs7794745 located at intron2 and rs2710102 located at intron13 in *CNTNAP2*, were examined. PCR primers were designed to flank the one base pair just adjacent to the target SNP: 5′-GCAGGACCTGGAAAGGCCTAA-3′ (forward), 5′-GGCCTTTGACACTTAGTCTTATCA-3′ (reverse) in rs7794745 and 5′-GGGCCTTTGTTTTTCCTTCTTTCTC-3′ (forward), 5′-GCGGTTAACATTTACTCTGAGACC-3′ (reverse) in rs2710102. We added external GC at the 5′ end of each primer to adjust the GC percentage (shown with underlines). All primers were designed with the LightScanner Primer Design software program (Idaho Technology, UT, USA). DNA amplification was performed with a 96-well plate at a 10-μl final volume containing 4 μl of 2.5× high-sensitivity genotyping master mix (Idaho Technology), 1 μM of each primer, and 20 ng of genomic DNA. The thermocycling conditions were: 2 min at 95°C, followed by 45 cycles of 30 s at 94°C and 30 s at 67°C in a CFX96 Real-Time PCR detection system (Bio-Rad Laboratories, CA, USA). After PCR, high-resolution melting was performed with a 96-well plate LightScanner (Idaho Technology), which collected data from 55°C to 98°C at a ramp rate of 0.10°C/s. The genotyping of all subjects was determined in comparison with control DNA confirmed by sequencing in the SNP pattern. Genotype of rs7794745 is A/A, A/T, and T/T; that of rs2710102 is G/G, G/A, A/A. In our study, the dominant DNA sequence was presumed to be T in rs7794745 and G in rs2710102 according to the Japanese Hapmap ratio (**Table 1**). The genotypes were classified into A/A and A/T in rs7794745, and G/G and A carriers (G/A and A/A) in rs2710102, respectively. In rs2710102, the genotypes of C/C, C/T, and T/T were used in some studies (Whalley et al., 2011; Whitehouse et al., 2011; Zhou et al., 2012; Clemm Von Hohenberg et al., 2013; Sampath et al., 2013), and the genotypes of G/G, G/A, and A/A in an opposite strand were used in other studies (Stein et al., 2011; Ji et al., 2013). In this study, we used the genotypes of G/G, G/A, and A/A in rs2710102.

Experiment Design of fMRI

Based on a previously published fMRI protocol (Koeda et al., 2006a,b, 2007), passive listening fMRI experiments were performed (**Figure 1**). The subjects listened to three types of stimuli: forward-played sentences (SEN); the same sentences, but played in reverse (rSEN); and identifiable nonvocal sounds (SND). The duration of each stimulus (SEN, rSEN, and SND) was 20 s. The subjects listened to these 3 stimuli, each followed by a silence of 20 s, alternately. In our fMRI study, a set of the experiment, silence-stimulus-silence-stimulus-silence-stimulus, was repeated six times. These three stimuli (rSEN, SND, SEN) were played pseudo-randomly in each set of the experiment (**Figure 1**). Contents of SEN stimuli used are shown in Appendix 1. Total scanning time was 720 s (120 s × 6). After the subjects were scanned by fMRI, they answered a questionnaire in order to confirm the performance based on previous studies (Koeda et al., 2006a,b, 2007). Regarding rSEN, the subjects were asked about the type of sounds (i.e., human or non-human), gender of sounds, and whether these sounds included intonation or meaning (See Appendix 2). Questions of Appendix 2 were asked after the subject listened to rSEN stimuli. As for SND, the subjects were asked what kind of sounds they listened to. Concerning SEN, the subjects were asked several questions regarding the contents of each story in multiple choice format.

Instruments Used For Presentation of Stimuli

Stimuli were presented by the use of Media Studio Pro (version 6.0 Ulead Systems, Inc., Taiwan) running under Windows XP. Subjects listened to the sound stimuli through headphones attached to an air conductance sound delivery system. The average sound pressure of stimulus amplitude was kept at 80 dB.

fMRI Acquisition

Images were acquired with a Phillips 3.0 Tesla scanner. Functional images of 395 volumes were acquired with T2*-weighted gradient echo planar imaging sequences sensitive to blood oxygenation level-dependent (BOLD) contrast. Each volume consisted of 35 transaxial contiguous slices, slice thickness 4 mm, to cover almost the whole brain (flip angle, 72.5°; time to echo [TE], 23 ms; repetition time [TR], 1.6 s; matrix, 52 × 30 × 64; field of view, 208 × 120 × 256).

Image Processing

Data analysis was performed with statistical parametric mapping software SPM8 (Wellcome Department of Cognitive Neurology, London, United Kingdom) running with MATLAB (Mathworks, Natick, MA). All volumes of functional EPI images were realigned to the first volume of each session to correct for subject motion. These images were spatially normalized to the standard space defined by Montreal Neurological Institute (MNI)

TABLE 1 | Baseline characteristics of subjects.

Total subject number	105
M/F	52/53
Handedness (non-RH/RH)	34/71
EHI	RH: 88.5 ± 11.1
	non-RH: −39.6 ± 38.3
LFH (Y/N)	39/66

rs7794745	**A/A**	**A/T**		***p*-value**
n	57	48		–
M/F	27/30	25/23	$X^2 = 0.23$	n.s.
Age	26.2 ± 6.8	26.2 ± 7.0	$t_{(103)} = 0.03$	n.s.
Handedness (non-RH/RH)	19/38	15/33	$X^2 = 0.05$	n.s.
EHI	RH: 87.5 ± 12.5	RH: 90.2 ± 9.4	$t_{(69)} = -1.04$	n.s.
	non-RH: −35.2 ± 39.1	non-RH: −45.1 ± 37.9	$t_{(32)} = 0.74$	n.s.
LFH (Y/N)	19/38	20/28	$X^2 = 0.78$	n.s.
Education (years)	15.7 ± 0.7	15.7 ± 0.6	$t_{(103)} = 0.24$	n.s.
Hapmap (ss44810024) [ratio (%)]/our current study [ratio (%)]	43/54.3	57/45.7	$X^2 = 2.42$	n.s.

rs2710102	**G/G**	**A carriers (G/A and A/A)**		***p*-value**
n	54	51		–
M/F	29/25	23/28	$X^2 = 0.78$	n.s.
Age	25.9 ± 6.5	26.6 ± 7.3	$t_{(103)} = -0.55$	n.s.
Handedness (non-RH/RH)	20/34	14/37	$X^2 = 1.10$	n.s.
EHI	RH: 89.3 ± 11.0	RH: 88.3 ± 11.5	$t_{(69)} = 0.37$	n.s.
	non-RH: −43.3 ± 39.0	non-RH: −34.3 ± 38.1	$t_{(32)} = -0.66$	n.s.
LFH (Y/N)	23/31	16/35		n.s.
Education (years)	15.7 ± 0.6	15.7 ± 0.7	$t_{(103)} = -0.31$	n.s.
Hapmap (ss44810024) [ratio (%)]/our current study [ratio (%)]	55.3/51.4	44.7/48.6	$X^2 = 0.32$	n.s.

Characteristics of two SNPs (rs7794745 and rs2710102) of CNTNAP2. Bottom line: comparison of allele frequency between international HapMap Project (http://www.ncbi.nlm.nih.gov/projects/SNP/) and our current study. Abbreviations: n, number of subjects; M/F, males/females; RH, right-handed subjects; non-RH, non-right-handed subjects; EHI, Edinburgh Handedness Inventory; LFH, left-handed family history (LFH).

template. After normalization, all scans had a final resolution of $2 \times 2 \times 2\,\text{mm}^3$. Functional images were spatially smoothed with a 3-D isotropic Gaussian kernel (full width at half maximum of 8 mm). Low-frequency noise was removed by applying a high-pass filter temporal smoothing function to the fMRI time series to enhance the temporal signal-to-noise ratio. The significance of hemodynamic changes in each condition was examined using the general linear model with boxcar functions convoluted with a hemodynamic response function. Statistical parametric maps for each contrast of the t-statistics were calculated on a voxel-by-voxel basis. The *t*-values were then transformed to unit normal distribution, resulting in z-scores. Data were excluded if the motion artifact was more than 2 mm on the head location (x, y, z translation; pitch, roll, and yaw) at the stage of realignment based on a previous study (Christodoulou et al., 2013).

The models of 3 contrasts (rSEN, SND, and SEN) were created by blocked design during the fMRI experiments (**Figure 1**). At first, investigating the SNP effect on cerebral activation in auditory processing, cerebral activation under the 3 contrasts was analyzed.

Next, based on our previous studies (Koeda et al., 2006a,b, 2007), to clarify cerebral activation in human voice perception, cerebral activation under rSEN minus SND was examined. Further, cerebral activation under SEN minus rSEN was examined to verify the effect of cerebral activation on language processing (**Figure 1**).

Statistical Analysis

Group analysis (2nd-level analysis in SPM8) was performed on the data of the 108 control subjects using a random effect model on a voxel-by-voxel basis. First, in order to examine the effects of SNPs on cerebral activation in general auditory processing, fMRI data were analyzed based on the $2 \times 2 \times 3$ full factorial model with the factors of A carriers (A/A or A/T) in rs2710102, [G/G, or A carriers (G/A and A/A)] in rs2710102, and task (rSEN or SND or SEN) [voxel level: $p < 0.001$, cluster level $p < 0.05$ corrected for multiple comparisons, Monte-Carlo simulation ($n = 1000$)]. This statistical threshold was determined based on a previous fMRI study (Slotnick et al., 2003). Second, in order to investigate the effects of SNPs on the cerebral activation of human voice perception, fMRI data were analyzed based on the $2 \times 2 \times 2$ full

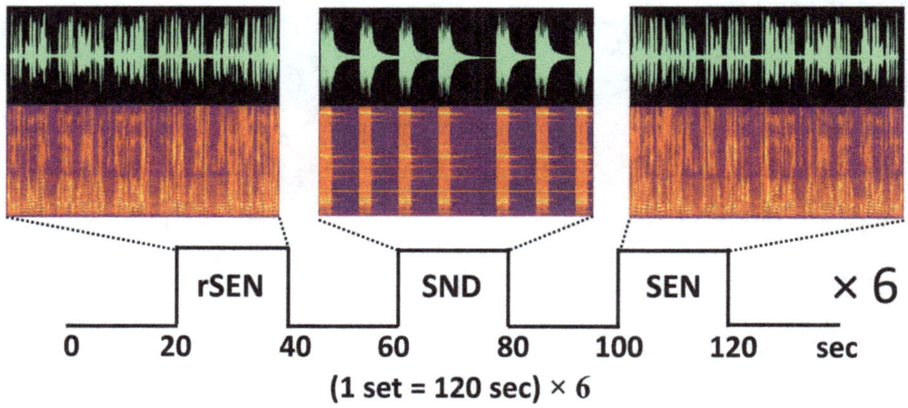

FIGURE 1 | Protocol of fMRI experiment. The subjects passively listened to reverse sentences (rSEN), identifiable non-vocal sounds (SND), and sentences (SEN) during MRI scanning. The top row shows the time-domain waveforms, the horizontal axis shows the tone domain, and the vertical axis shows the power of the sound. The middle row shows the sound spectrograms under the three sound conditions. The horizontal axis shows the time domain, and the vertical axis shows the frequency (about 0–4000 Hz) of the tone domain.

factorial model with the factors of task (rSEN or SND), rs7794745 (A/A or A/T) and rs2710102 [G/G, or A carriers (G/A and A/A)], [voxel level: $p < 0.005$, cluster level $p < 0.05$ corrected for multiple comparisons, Monte-Carlo simulation ($n = 1000$)]. Third, to investigate the effects of SNPs in *CNTNAP2* on cerebral activation of language processing, fMRI data were analyzed based on the $2 \times 2 \times 2$ full factorial model with the factors of task (rSEN or SEN), A carriers (A/A or A/T) in rs7794745 and G/G, or A carriers (G/A and A/A) in rs2710102 [voxel level: $p < 0.005$, cluster level $p < 0.05$ corrected for multiple comparisons, Monte-Carlo simulation ($n = 1000$)]. By using rfxplot (Glascher, 2009), cerebral activation at the regions of interests (ROIs) was investigated. In the main effect of task, ROIs were focused on sphere voxels of 10 mm radius from the coordinates of the peak voxel of activation.

Results

Baseline Characteristics of Subjects

The fMRI data of 3 subjects were excluded due to motion artifacts, and thus the data of 105 subjects were analyzed in this study. **Table 1** shows the baseline characteristics of the subjects. Among the 105 subjects, 57 subjects possessed A/A genotype in rs7794745, and 48 possessed A/T genotype, whereas in rs2710102, 54 possessed G/G genotype, 41 G/A genotype, and 10 A/A genotype. Finally, in the current study, since A/A genotype in rs2710102 was seen in only a few subjects, two phenotypes were compared: (1) G/G in rs2710102, and (2) A carrier (G/A and A/A) in rs2710102.

For each genotype of both rs7794745 and rs2710102, the rates of gender (M/F), age, handedness, EHI, LFH, and education are summarized in **Table 1**. No significant differences were observed in these factors between rs7794745 genotypes (A/A or A/T), and between rs2710102 genotypes [G/G or A carrier (G/A, and A/A)] (**Table 1**). Further, the genotype frequency of the known rate of Japanese, based on the database of the international HapMap Project (http://hapmap.ncbi.nlm.nih.gov/), was compared with the subjects' rates in the current study (**Table 1**). The Hapmap Japanese rate was examined by using the following websites: rs7794745: http://www.ncbi.nlm.nih.gov/projects/SNP/snp_ref.cgi?rs=7794745; rs2710102: http://www.ncbi.nlm.nih.gov/projects/SNP/snp_ref.cgi?rs=2710102. NCBI Assay IDs in this project were rs7794745: ss44810024; rs2710102: ss11865581, respectively. No significant difference was observed between the HapMap Japanese rate and our subjects (rs7794745: $\chi^2 = 2.42, p > 0.05$; rs2710102: $\chi^2 = 0.32, p > 0.05$).

Behavioral Data (Accuracy)

In the fMRI experiment, the mean percentages (±SD) of accuracy of rs7794745 for rSEN, SND, and SEN were as follows: [rs7794745 A/A] rSEN: 95.1 ± 1.3, SND: 95.2 ± 1.5, SEN 93.0 ± 1.4, [rs7794745 A/T] rSEN: 96.3 ± 1.3, SND: 91.2 ± 2.0, SEN: 93.8 ± 1.4, [rs2710102 G/G] rSEN: 96.3 ± 1.2, SND: 93.5 ± 1.6, SEN: 93.3 ± 1.3, [rs2710102 A carriers (G/A and A/A)] rSEN: 94.9 ± 1.4, SND 93.1 ± 1.9, SEN 93.4 ± 1.5. The 2×3 mixed ANOVA was not significantly different from the main effect of rs7794745 [$F_{(1, 103)} = 0.36, p > 0.05$; effect size (Partial Eta Squared) < 0.01], main effect of task [$F_{(2, 206)} = 1.70, p > 0.05$; effect size (Partial Eta Squared) = 0.02], and interaction effect [$F_{(2, 206)} = 1.83, p > 0.05$; effect size (Partial Eta Squared) = 0.02] (**Figure 2**; **Table 2**; Supplemental Table 1). Similarly, the 2×3 mixed ANOVA was not significantly different from the main effect of rs2710102 [$F_{(1, 103)} = 0.23, p > 0.05$; effect size (Partial Eta Squared) < 0.01], main effect of task [$F_{(1, 103)} = 2.92, p > 0.05$; effect size (Partial Eta Squared) = 0.03], and interaction effect [$F_{(2, 206)} = 0.13, p > 0.05$; effect size (Partial Eta Squared) < 0.01] (**Figure 2**; **Table 2**; Supplemental Table 1), respectively.

fMRI Data

Full Factorial Design Analysis

In order to investigate genetic effects on cerebral activation in general auditory processing, fMRI data was analyzed based on

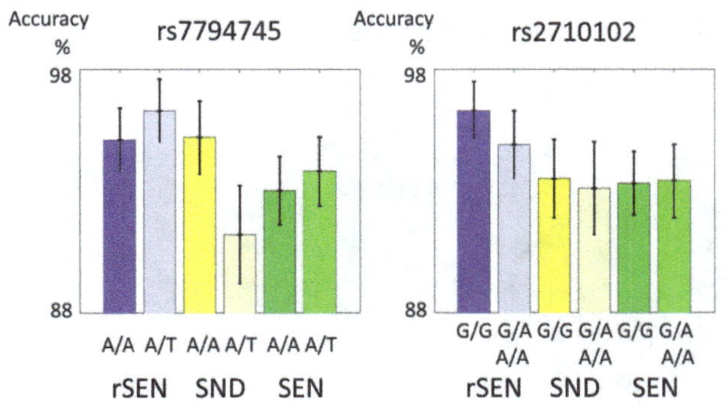

FIGURE 2 | Performance during fMRI experiments. These two figures show the distribution of fMRI performance in rs7794745 (left side) and rs2710102 (right side) of *CNTNAP2* gene. In both SNPs, there were no significant differences in the performance of rSEN, SND, and SEN ($p > 0.05$). (1) rSEN: rs7794745 A/A: blue bar, rs7794745 A/T: light blue bar, (2) SND: rs7794745 A/A: yellow bar, rs7794745 A/T: light yellow bar, (3) SEN: rs7794745 A/A: green bar, rs7794745 A/T: light green bar, (4) rSEN: rs2710102 G/G: blue bar, rs2710102 G/A and A/A: light blue bar, (5) SND: rs2710102 G/G: yellow bar, rs2710102 G/A and A/A: light yellow bar, (6) SEN: rs2710102 G/G: green bar, rs2710102 G/A and A/A: light green bar.

TABLE 2 | Performance ratio (%).

		rSEN	SND	SEN
rs7794745	A/A	95.1 ± 1.3	95.2 ± 1.5	93.0 ± 1.4
	AT	96.3 ± 1.3	91.2 ± 2.0	93.8 ± 1.4
rs2710102	G/G	96.3 ± 1.2	93.5 ± 1.6	93.3 ± 1.3
	G/A and A/A	94.9 ± 1.4	93.1 ± 1.9	93.4 ± 1.5

Mean (±SE) of performance in each allele of rs7794745 (upper part) and rs2710102 (lower part) during fMRI experiments.

TABLE 3 | (A) *CNTNAP2* (rs7794745) effect of cerebral activation of general auditory processing. (B) *CNTNAP2* (rs7794745) effect of cerebral response to human voice perception. (C) *CNTNAP2* (rs7794745) effect of cerebral response to language processing.

Brain Regions	BA	Coordinate			$F_{(1, 303)}$	z-value	P (cluster-level, corrected)
		x	y	z			
A							
A/A < A/T							
R MFG	11	42	46	−10	21.85	4.44	<0.001 (<0.05/4)
A/A > A/T							
L STG	22	−54	−30	8	17.33	3.94	0.001 (<0.05/4)
R STG	22	56	−24	4	16.78	3.87	0.002 (<0.05/4)
R Precuneus	31	8	−72	22	16.12	3.79	0.002 (<0.05/4)
B							
A/A < A/T							
R MFG	11	46	48	0	14.18	3.52	0.005 (<0.05/3)
A/A > A/T							
R STG	22	56	−24	4	12.58	3.30	0.010 (<0.05/3)
L STG	22	−54	−30	6	11.89	3.20	0.013 (<0.05/3)
C							
A/A > A/T							
R MFG	11	42	46	−8	11.35	3.12	0.019 (<0.05)

Note for Table A: Peak coordinates (x, y, z) and their z-values of cerebral activation of general auditory processing with main effect of rs7794745 (A/A or A/T) by full factorial design analysis. Abbreviations: L, left hemisphere; R, right hemisphere; BA, Broadmann's area; MFG, middle frontal gyrus; STG, superior temporal gyrus.

Note for Table B: Peak coordinates (x, y, z) and their z-values of cerebral activation of human voice perception with main effect of rs7794745 in full factorial design analysis. Abbreviations: L, left hemisphere; R, right hemisphere; BA, Brodmann's area; MFG, middle frontal gyrus, STG, superior temporal gyrus.

Note for Table A: Peak coordinates (x, y, z) and their z-values of cerebral activation of language processing with main effect of rs7794745 in full factorial design analysis. R, right hemisphere; BA, Brodmann's area.

the 2 × 2 × 3 full factorial design with three factors: rs7794745 (A/A or A/T), rs2710102 [G/G or A carriers (G/A and A/A)], and task (rSEN or SND or SEN) [voxel level: $p < 0.001$, cluster level $p < 0.05$ corrected for multiple comparisons, Monte-Carlo simulation ($n = 1000$)]. Main effect of rs7794745 (A/A or A/T) was significantly observed in the bilateral STG, R precuneus, and R MFG (voxel level: $p < 0.001$, cluster level $p < 0.05$ corrected, R: right) (**Figure 3** and **Table 3A**), whereas main effect of rs2710102 [G/G, or A carriers (G/A, and A/A)] was not significantly different. From the results of main effect of rs7794745 on cerebral response to general auditory processing, ROIs were set on 4 regions: L STG [−54, −30, 8], R Precuneus [8, −72, 22], R STG [56, −24, 4], and R MFG [42, 46, −10] (L: left).

In order to examine the genetic effects on cerebral response to human voice perception, fMRI data were analyzed based on the 2 × 2 × 2 full factorial design with the three factors: rs7794745 (A/A or A/T), rs2710102 [G/G, or A carriers (G/A and A/A)], and task (rSEN or SND) [voxel level: $p < 0.001$, cluster level $p < 0.05$ corrected for multiple comparisons, Monte-Carlo simulation ($n = 1000$)]. Main effect of rs7794745 (A/A or A/T) was significantly observed in bilateral STG and R MFG (voxel level: $p < 0.005$, cluster level $p < 0.05$ corrected) (**Figure 4** and **Table 3B**), whereas main effect of rs2710102 [G/G, or A carriers (G/A and A/A)] was not significantly different. From the results of main effect of rs7794745, ROIs were set on 3 regions: L STG [−54, −30, 6], R STG [56, −24, 4], and R MFG [46, 48, 0]. In these ROIs, beta values under rSEN or SND conditions were calculated by using rfxplot (Glascher, 2009). In **Figure 4**, cerebral activations between rSEN and SND were compared by Wilcoxon Signed Rank Test. In rs7794745 A/A, the beta values of rSEN were significantly greater than those of SND [L STG: $Z = -3.01, p = 0.002$ ($p < 0.05/3$); R STG: $Z = -4.38$, $p < 0.001$ ($p < 0.05/3$); R MFG: $-3.33, p = 0.001$, ($p < 0.05/3$)], whereas in rs7794745 A/T, the beta values were not significantly different between rSEN and SND (L STG: $Z = -0.39, p > 0.05/3$; R STG: $Z = -1.90, p > 0.05/3$; R MFG: $Z = -0.17, p > 0.05/3$).

In order to investigate the genetic effects on cerebral activation in language processing, fMRI data were analyzed based on the 2 × 2 × 2 full factorial design with the three factors: rs7794745 (A/A or A/T), rs2710102 [G/G or A carriers (G/A and A/A)], and task (rSEN or SEN) [voxel level: $p < 0.001$, cluster level

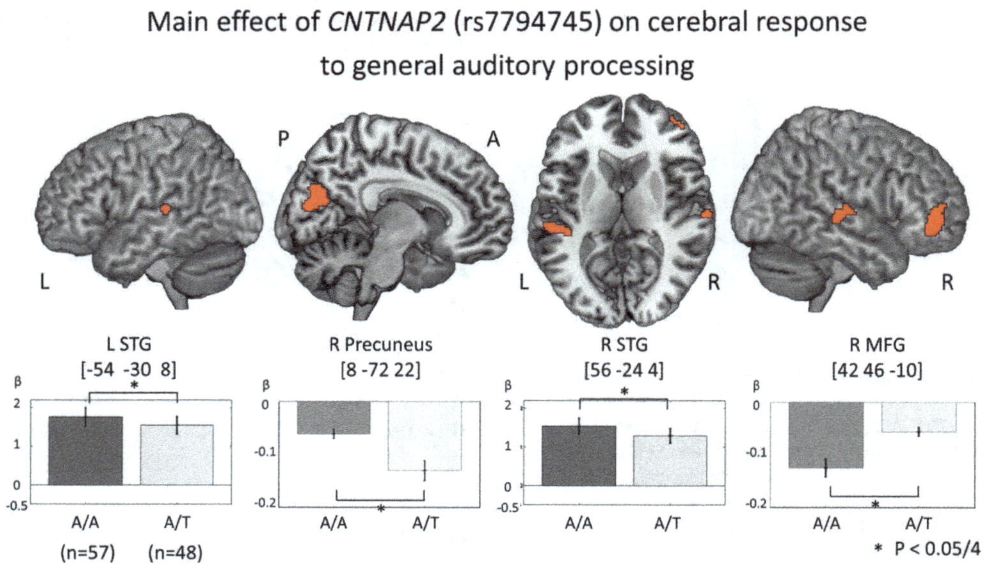

FIGURE 3 | Main effect of *CNTNAP2* (rs7794745) on cerebral response to general auditory processing. The results of the main effect of rs7794745 (A/A or A/T) in the analysis of full factorial design are shown (voxel level: $p < 0.001$, cluster level: $p < 0.05/4$, Monte–Carlo simulation). The bars show the distribution of beta values of brain function in general auditory processing at the MNI coordinates of peak activation (A/A: gray, rs7794745 A/T: light gray). Asterisk (*) shows a significant rs7794745 effect (A/A and A/T) with Bonferroni correction in 4 ROIs ($p < 0.05/4$). Abbreviations: L, left; R, right; A, anterior; P, posterior.

$p < 0.05$ corrected for multiple comparisons, Monte-Carlo simulation ($n = 1000$)]. Main effect of rs7794745 (A/A or A/T) was significantly observed in R MFG (voxel level: $p < 0.005$, cluster level $p < 0.05$ corrected) (**Figure 5** and **Table 3C**), whereas main effect of rs2710102 [G/G, or A carriers (G/A and A/A)] was not significantly different.

In **Figure 5**, cerebral activations between rSEN and SEN were compared by Wilcoxon Signed Rank Test. In rs7794745 A/A, the beta value of rSEN was significantly greater than that of SEN [R MFG: $Z = -4.53, p < 0.001$ ($p < 0.05/3$)], whereas in rs7794745 A/T, the beta value was not significantly different between rSEN and SEN (R MFG: $Z = -1.57, p > 0.05/3$).

Figure 6 shows the distribution of cerebral response to human voice perception (cerebral activation under rSEN-SND contrast) in the 3 ROIs (L STG, R STG, and R MFG) in RH and non-RH subjects. In mixed ANOVA [3 ROIs × rs7794745 (A/A or A/T) × LFH × handedness], main effect was not significantly revealed in 3 ROIs, rs7794745 (A/A or A/T), LFH, and handedness (**Table 4**). Remarkably, interaction effect among the 3 ROIs, rs7794745 (A/A or A/T), and handedness was significantly observed [$F_{(1,\,97)} = 9.94$, $p = 0.002$ ($p < 0.05/3$); **Table 4**], whereas other interaction effects were not significantly observed (**Table 4**).

TABLE 4 | *CNTNAP2* (rs7794745) effect of cerebral response to human voice perception between RH and non-RH subjects.

Mixed ANOVA: 3 ROIs × rs7794745 (A/A or A/T) × LFH × Handedness		
Main effect	***F*-value**	***p***
3 ROIs	$F_{(1.9,\,182.4)} = 1.19$	n.s.
rs7794745 (A/A, A/T)	$F_{(1,\,97)} = 0.01$	n.s.
LFH	$F_{(1,\,97)} = 1.21$	n.s.
Handedness	$F_{(1,\,97)} = 0.97$	n.s.
INTERACTION EFFECT		
3 ROIs × rs7794745 (A/A, A/T)	$F_{(1,\,97)} = 2.97$	n.s.
3 ROIs × LFH	$F_{(1,\,97)} = 1.02$	n.s.
3 ROIs × Handedness	$F_{(1,\,97)} = 1.14$	n.s.
3 ROIs × rs7794745 (A/A, A/T) × LFH	$F_{(1,\,97)} = 0.33$	n.s.
3 ROIs × rs7794745 × Handedness	$F_{(1,\,97)} = 9.94$	0.002*
3 ROIs × LFH × Handedness	$F_{(1,\,97)} = 0.86$	n.s.
3 ROIs × rs7794745 × LFH × Handedness	$F_{(1,\,97)} = 0.67$	n.s.

Mixed ANOVA (3 ROIs × rs7794745 × LFH × handedness) was calculated for cerebral activation in human voice perception. Interaction effects among the 3 ROIs, rs7794745 and handedness (EHI < 50, or EHI = 50) were significantly observed. Asterisk (*) shows p < 0.05/3.

Discussion

We aimed to investigate the interaction effect between *CNTNAP2* polymorphism and handedness on linguistic and voice-specific brain activity in healthy individuals. In the current study, the effect of rs7794745 genotype (A/A or A/T) was observed at the bilateral STG, R precuneus, and R MFG on cerebral activation in general auditory processing. Further, the effect of rs7794745 genotype was observed at the bilateral STG and R MFG on cerebral activation in human voice perception, and the effect of rs7794745 genotype was observed at the R MFG on cerebral activation in language processing. Notably, among handedness, rs7794745, and MFG-STG activations by human

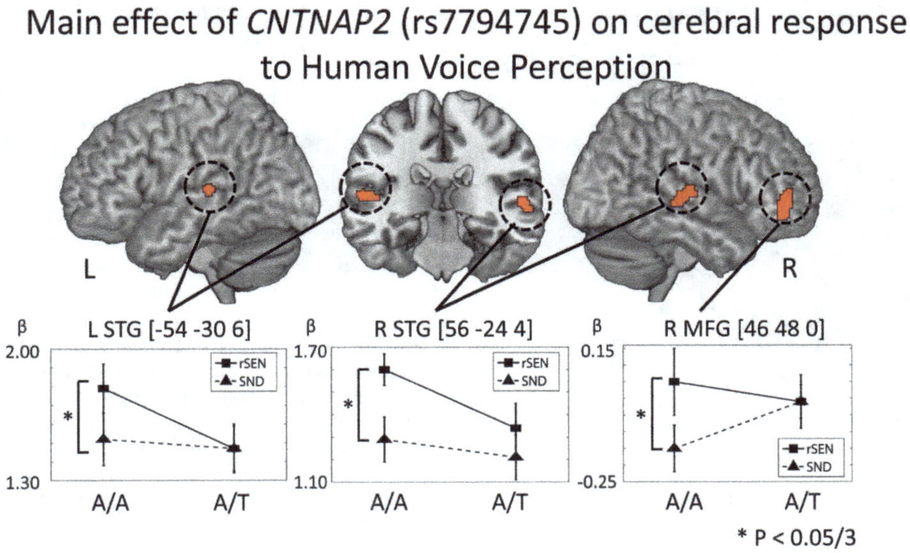

FIGURE 4 | *CNTNAP2* (rs7794745) effect on cerebral response to human voice perception. The results of the main effect of rs7794745 in the analysis of full factorial design are shown (voxel level: $p < 0.001$, cluster level: $p < 0.05/3$, Monte–Carlo simulation). The error bar shows the distribution of beta values in cerebral activation under rSEN minus baseline (mean: black squares, line) and under SND minus baseline (mean: black triangles, dashed line) at the peak coordinates with the main effect of rs7794745. Asterisks (*) show significant differences with Bonferroni correction in the 3 ROIs ($p < 0.05/3$). Abbreviations: L, left hemisphere; R, right hemisphere; MFG, middle frontal gyrus; STG, superior temporal gyrus.

voice perception, interaction effect was significantly observed. These results suggest that the difference of the specific allele in *CNTNAP2* gene has an influence on brain activity of human voice perception between RH and non-RH subjects.

The Effect of *CNTNAP2* Polymorphisms on Cerebral Response to Auditory Processing in Healthy Individuals

In our present results, although the means of the performance ratio were not significantly different between A/A and A/T in rs7794745 (**Figure 2** and **Table 2**), the effect of rs7794745 genotype was significantly observed at the R MFG, bilateral STG, and R precuneus on brain activity to general auditory processing with SEN, rSEN, and SND (**Figure 3** and **Table 3A**). These findings suggest that A/T in rs7794745 of *CNTNAP2* has an influence on the reduction of brain activity in general auditory processing. Further, on brain activity in human voice perception, the effect of rs7794745 genotype was significantly revealed at the bilateral STG and R MFG (**Figure 4** and **Table 3B**). These results indicate that A/T in rs7794745 of *CNTNAP2* affects the decrease in voice-specific brain activity. Recent studies have shown that several SNPs of *CNTNAP2* are biological high-risk markers in ASD, epilepsy, mental retardation, schizophrenia, and cognitive impairment (Friedman et al., 2008; Stein et al., 2011; Li and Bartlett, 2012; Clemm Von Hohenberg et al., 2013; Ji et al., 2013; Sampath et al., 2013). Especially, A/T in rs7794745 was reported to be one of the risks in ASD in the Chinese Han population (Li et al., 2010). In addition, recent neuroimaging studies in healthy subjects demonstrated cerebral activation at the bilateral STG predominantly in the right hemisphere while listening to human voice (Belin et al., 2000; Fecteau et al., 2004; Koeda et al., 2006a; Charest et al., 2013). In contrast, neuroimaging studies in patients with autism showed hypo-activation in R STG (Ocklenburg et al., 2013). However, to our knowledge, no study has investigated the influence of *CNTNAP2* genotype in relation to cerebral response to human voice perception. Our current findings indicate that A/T in rs7794745 of *CNTNAP2*, which is related to neuropsychiatric disorders, affects brain activity of human voice perception in healthy subjects. Voice-specific brain activity is significantly different by the difference of rs7794745 genotype (**Figure 4**). Voice-specific response was clearly observed in genotype A/A, but it was not revealed in genotype A/T. These findings indicate that A/T in rs7794745 more severely affects the reduction of cerebral response to human voice perception.

CNTNAP2 and Language Processing in the Brain

Our results demonstrated the main effect by the difference of rs7794745 genotype at R MFG in lexical-semantic processing of language processing (**Figure 5** and **Table 3C**). A recent neuroimaging study demonstrated increasing brain activity at the right frontotemporal region in language processing by T/T in rs7794745 compared with A carriers (A/A and A/T) (Whalley et al., 2011). On the other hand, our results showed a reduction in right frontal activity of language processing in healthy subjects by rs7794745 A/T compared with A/A. These opposing findings in right frontal activity could be due to differences in the fMRI experiments. The previous fMRI study used a sentence completion paradigm with sentences with the last words missing, asking to silently think of an appropriate word to complete the sentences and press a button when they had done so (Whalley et al., 2011), whereas we investigated brain activity when the subjects were passively listening to contents of the story.

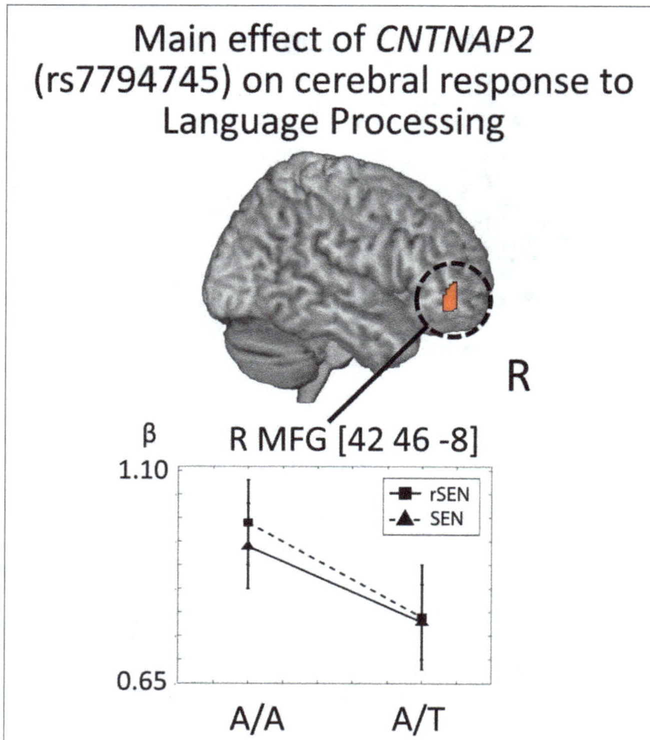

FIGURE 5 | *CNTNAP2* (rs7794745) effect on cerebral response to language processing. The results of the main effect of rs7794745 (A/A or A/T) in the analysis of full factorial design are shown. The error bar shows the distribution of beta values of cerebral activation under rSEN minus baseline (mean: black squares; dashed line) and under SEN minus baseline (mean: black triangles; line) at the peak coordinates with the main effect of rs7794745 (A/A or A/T). Significant difference was observed in right MFG. Abbreviations: R, right hemisphere; MFG, middle frontal gyrus.

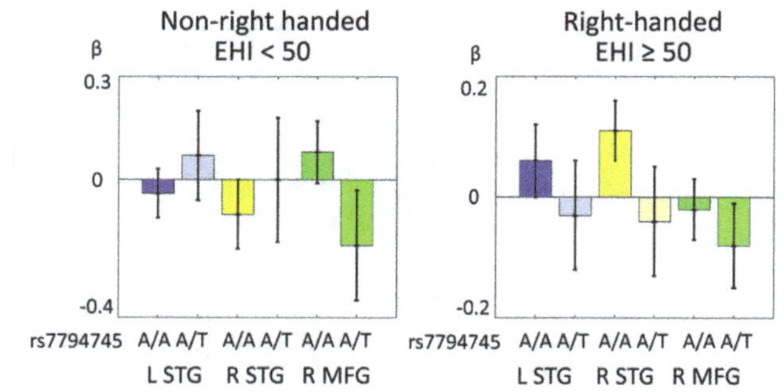

FIGURE 6 | Comparison of *CNTNAP2* (rs7794745) effect of cerebral response to human voice perception between right-handed (RH) and non-right-handed (non-RH) subjects. Distributions of BOLD signals of 3 ROIs in human voice perception in non-RH subjects (rs7795745 A/A: $n = 38$; A/T: $n = 33$, left side) and RH subjects (rs7794745 A/A: $n = 19$; A/T: $n = 14$, right side). LTG (A/A: blue, A/T: light blue), STG (A/A: yellow, A/T: light yellow), MFG (A/A: green, A/T: light green), L, left; R, right; EHI, Edinburgh Handedness Inventory.

However, taking these findings into account, these results suggest that rs7794745 A/T genotype at least affects right hemispheric activity in language processing. In our present study, the effect of rs7794745 genotype was revealed in the right frontal region in language processing despite the lack of significant difference in the performance ratio. In contrast, the effect of rs2710102 genotype was not observed in brain activity of language processing. A recent neuroimaging study reported that, in healthy individuals, rs2710102 is associated with right frontal activity, whereas rs7794745 is related to right temporal activity in language processing (Whalley et al., 2011). In our current study, although rs7794745 genotype of *CNTNAP2* does not influence right temporal activity but rather right frontal activity in language processing, these results do suggest that the genotype of *CNTNAP2* is closely associated with right hemispheric activity in language processing. Recent neuroimaging studies of ASD have shown increasing right frontal activity in language processing (Harris et al., 2006; Knaus et al., 2008; Tesink et al., 2011; Eigsti et al., 2012; Pina-Camacho et al., 2012; Shen et al., 2012). In our current study, the effect of rs7794745 genotype could influence right frontal activity in language processing in healthy subjects. Some neuroimaging studies demonstrated that frontal brain activity in language processing was changed by *FOXP2* gene, which is related to language impairment (Jamadar et al., 2011; Ocklenburg et al., 2013). Taking the previous reports and our current results into consideration, some SNPs of *CNTNAP2* and *FOXP2*, related to language impairment, may directly affect brain activity of language processing as an endophenotype in healthy subjects.

Influence of *CNTNAP2* on Voice-Specific Brain Activity and Handedness

We investigated the interaction effect between *CNTNAP2* polymorphism and handedness regarding cerebral response to human voice perception. In mixed ANOVA, interaction effect was revealed between *CNTNAP2* polymorphism [rs7794745 (A/A and A/T)] and handedness regarding the MFG-STG activations to human voice perception (**Table 4**). **Figure 6** shows the distribution of these interaction effects. In our results, the activation in bilateral STG at A/A in rs7794745 was observed as a negative value in non-RH subjects (**Figure 6**), whereas it was observed as a positive value in RH subjects (**Figure 6**). In addition, frontal activation at A/A in rs7794745 in non-RH subjects was positive (**Figure 6**), but that in RH subjects was negative (**Figure 6**). These results indicate that the activity of MFG-STG by human voice perception shows a differential pattern according to the subject's handedness and type of A/A or A/T in rs7794745 of *CNTNAP2*. On the other hand, the frontal activation in rs7794745 (A/T) showed negative beta values in both RH and non-RH subjects (**Figure 6**). Further, the left temporal activation at A/T in rs7794745 demonstrated negative beta values in RH subjects (**Figure 6**), while positive beta values were shown in non-RH subjects (**Figure 6**). These findings suggest that the effect of rs7794745 genotype on voice-specific brain activity is opposite by the difference of handedness. A previous study has demonstrated that two SNPs in FOXP2 gene, which has been shown to be related to speech development, affect cognitive performance during dichotic listening task (Ocklenburg et al., 2013). Further, a recent neuroimaging study has demonstrated that some SNPs in *FOXP2* gene are associated with the determination of language dominance in the frontotemporal cortices during reading task (Pinel et al., 2012). However, to our knowledge, no study has as yet investigated the genetic effects on handedness and brain activity in auditory processing. Our results demonstrated an interaction effect among *CNTNAP2*, handedness, and cerebral response to human voice perception, although they showed no significant difference between handedness and brain activity in language processing. These findings suggest that the allele of rs7794745 affects cerebral response and laterality to human voice perception in MFG-STG in healthy individuals. A recent research has shown that the allele of rs7794745 affects patients with ASD (Li et al., 2010). Further, studies of patients with autism and schizophrenia have demonstrated impairment of voice-specific brain activity at the right STG (Ocklenburg et al., 2013). Taking this into account, in the evaluation of voice-specific response, this suggests that the difference of rs7794745 allele would be an important factor, as well as handedness.

Previous neuroimaging studies have shown that language dominance is affected by the difference of handedness (Pujol et al., 1999; Szaflarski et al., 2002). Especially, since language dominance is impacted by a family history of non-RH subjects (Szaflarski et al., 2002; Liu et al., 2009), genetic factor language-related gene, such as *CNTNAP2*, could associate with reduced language dominance or reversed language dominance. In our study, interaction effect between *CNTNAP2* genotype and handedness was not significantly observed in brain activity of language processing. These results suggest that rs7794745 and rs2710102 genotypes do not influence brain activity of language processing. On the other hand, our current findings, rs7794745 genotype affects voice-specific brain activity by the difference of handedness, suggest that cerebral response to human voice perception is genetically more susceptible than cerebral response to language processing. Regarding as voice-specific response in RH subjects, the group of genotype A/A in rs7794745 was observed at bilateral STG, whereas no bilateral STG activation was observed in the group of genotype A/T. In addition, concerning voice specific response in non-RH subjects, genotype A/A in rs7794745 was not shown at bilateral STG. These results may reflect that the group of rs7794745 genotype A/A can more easily respond to cerebral response to human voice perception than the rs7794745 genotype A/T group.

There are some limitations to the present study. First, although the allele effect on *CNTNAP2* was demonstrated in brain activity by passive listening task in our study, it is unclear whether the same genetic effect can be observed in any language processing. By each language processing task, the influence of *CNTNAP2* allele on brain activity could be different. Second, in our present study, behavior performance was not significantly different. Since behavior performance in every subject was extremely high, by the ceiling effect, it may be difficult to conclude whether the allele of *CNTNAP2* affecting brain activity is associated with any differences in language abilities. In behavioral performance, it was a very small effect size. These results may also be related to the ceiling effect due to the high performance of most subjects. Third, in our current study, we collected healthy volunteers without any psychiatric diseases, history of head injury, neurological disorder, alcohol, or drug dependence on the basis of interviews. However, a family history of these risks was not considered. Further, the subjects did not undergo verbal IQ and personality trait tests. Although educational levels of all subjects were more than 12 years, we should have considered the possibility that some of the subjects included a language impairment despite their high educational attainment.

Conclusion

We investigated the influence of *CNTNAP2* on voice-specific brain activity, language-related brain activity, and handedness. Our results indicated that rs7794745 A/T in *CNTNAP2* is associated with a decrease in cerebral activation at R MFG and bilateral STG in human voice perception. This finding suggests that *CNTNAP2* polymorphisms could have a direct impact on right hemispheric activity for vocal communication as an endophenotype in healthy individuals. In addition, A/T in rs7794745 influences the activation of R MFG in language processing. This genotype may be related to a change in frontal activity in language processing of healthy subjects. Finally, our results demonstrated that rs7794745 has some influence on the difference in voice-specific brain activity between RH and non-RH subjects. These results suggest that *CNTNAP2* could be an important factor in the neural development related to vocal communication in both RH and non-RH subjects.

Acknowledgments

We gratefully acknowledge the staff of Yaesu Clinic, Nippon Medical School Hospital; Section of Biofunctional Informatics, Tokyo Medical and Dental University; and Voice Neurocognition Laboratory, University of Glasgow. This work was supported by a Health and Labor Sciences Research Grant for Research on Psychiatric and Neurological Diseases and Mental Health (H23-seishin-ippan-002) from the Japanese Ministry of Health, Labor and Welfare.

Supplementary Material

The Supplementary Material for this article can be found online at: http://www.frontiersin.org/journal/10.3389/fnbeh.2015.00087/abstract

References

Alarcon, M., Abrahams, B. S., Stone, J. L., Duvall, J. A., Perederiy, J. V., Bomar, J. M., et al. (2008). Linkage, association, and gene-expression analyses identify CNTNAP2 as an autism-susceptibility gene. *Am. J. Hum. Genet.* 82, 150–159. doi: 10.1016/j.ajhg.2007.09.005

Belin, P., Zatorre, R. J., Lafaille, P., Ahad, P., and Pike, B. (2000). Voice-selective areas in human auditory cortex. *Nature* 403, 309–312. doi: 10.1038/35002078

Binder, J. R., Frost, J. A., Hammeke, T. A., Cox, R. W., Rao, S. M., and Prieto, T. (1997). Human brain language areas identified by functional magnetic resonance imaging. *J. Neurosci.* 17, 353–362.

Blasi, G., De Virgilio, C., Papazacharias, A., Taurisano, P., Gelao, B., Fazio, L., et al. (2013). Converging evidence for the association of functional genetic variation in the serotonin receptor 2a gene with prefrontal function and olanzapine treatment. *JAMA Psychiatry* 70, 921–930. doi: 10.1001/jamapsychiatry.2013.1378

Camara, E., Kramer, U. M., Cunillera, T., Marco-Pallares, J., Cucurell, D., Nager, W., et al. (2010). The effects of COMT (Val108/158Met) and DRD4 (SNP -521) dopamine genotypes on brain activations related to valence and magnitude of rewards. *Cereb. Cortex* 20, 1985–1996. doi: 10.1093/cercor/bhp263

Catani, M., Craig, M. C., Forkel, S. J., Kanaan, R., Picchioni, M., Toulopoulou, T., et al. (2011). Altered integrity of perisylvian language pathways in schizophrenia: relationship to auditory hallucinations. *Biol. Psychiatry* 70, 1143–1150. doi: 10.1016/j.biopsych.2011.06.013

Charest, I., Pernet, C., Latinus, M., Crabbe, F., and Belin, P. (2013). Cerebral processing of voice gender studied using a continuous carryover FMRI design. *Cereb. Cortex* 23, 958–966. doi: 10.1093/cercor/bhs090

Chen, J., Calhoun, V. D., Pearlson, G. D., Ehrlich, S., Turner, J. A., Ho, B. C., et al. (2012). Multifaceted genomic risk for brain function in schizophrenia. *Neuroimage* 61, 866–875. doi: 10.1016/j.neuroimage.2012.03.022

Christodoulou, A. G., Bauer, T. E., Kiehl, K. A., Feldstein Ewing, S. W., Bryan, A. D., and Calhoun, V. D. (2013). A quality control method for detecting and suppressing uncorrected residual motion in fMRI studies. *Magn. Reson. Imaging* 31, 707–717. doi: 10.1016/j.mri.2012.11.007

Clemm Von Hohenberg, C., Wigand, M. C., Kubicki, M., Leicht, G., Giegling, I., Karch, S., et al. (2013). CNTNAP2 polymorphisms and structural brain connectivity: a diffusion-tensor imaging study. *J. Psychiatr. Res.* 47, 1349–1356. doi: 10.1016/j.jpsychires.2013.07.002

Cuenco, K. T., Friedland, R., Baldwin, C. T., Guo, J., Vardarajan, B., Lunetta, K. L., et al. (2011). Association of TTR polymorphisms with hippocampal atrophy in Alzheimer disease families. *Neurobiol. Aging* 32, 249–256. doi: 10.1016/j.neurobiolaging.2009.02.014

Eigsti, I. M., Schuh, J., Mencl, E., Schultz, R. T., and Paul, R. (2012). The neural underpinnings of prosody in autism. *Child Neuropsychol.* 18, 600–617. doi: 10.1080/09297049.2011.639757

Fecteau, S., Armony, J. L., Joanette, Y., and Belin, P. (2004). Is voice processing species-specific in human auditory cortex? An fMRI study. *Neuroimage* 23, 840–848. doi: 10.1016/j.neuroimage.2004.09.019

Forbes, C. E., Poore, J. C., Barbey, A. K., Krueger, F., Solomon, J., Lipsky, R. H., et al. (2012). BDNF polymorphism-dependent OFC and DLPFC plasticity differentially moderates implicit and explicit bias. *Cereb. Cortex* 22, 2602–2609. doi: 10.1093/cercor/bhr337

Friedman, J. I., Vrijenhoek, T., Markx, S., Janssen, I. M., Van Der Vliet, W. A., Faas, B. H., et al. (2008). CNTNAP2 gene dosage variation is associated with schizophrenia and epilepsy. *Mol. Psychiatry* 13, 261–266. doi: 10.1038/sj.mp.4002049

Frielingsdorf, H., Bath, K. G., Soliman, F., Difede, J., Casey, B. J., and Lee, F. S. (2010). Variant brain-derived neurotrophic factor Val66Met endophenotypes: implications for posttraumatic stress disorder. *Ann. N.Y. Acad. Sci.* 1208, 150–157. doi: 10.1111/j.1749-6632.2010.05722.x

Frost, J. A., Binder, J. R., Springer, J. A., Hammeke, T. A., Bellgowan, P. S., Rao, S. M., et al. (1999). Language processing is strongly left lateralized in both sexes. Evidence from functional MRI. *Brain 122 (Pt 2)*, 199–208.

Geschwind, D. H., Miller, B. L., Decarli, C., and Carmelli, D. (2002). Heritability of lobar brain volumes in twins supports genetic models of cerebral laterality and handedness. *Proc. Natl. Acad. Sci. U.S.A.* 99, 3176–3181. doi: 10.1073/pnas.052494999

Glascher, J. (2009). Visualization of group inference data in functional neuroimaging. *Neuroinformatics* 7, 73–82. doi: 10.1007/s12021-008-9042-x

Graham, S. A., and Fisher, S. E. (2013). Decoding the genetics of speech and language. *Curr. Opin. Neurobiol.* 23, 43–51. doi: 10.1016/j.conb.2012.11.006

Greve, D. N., Van Der Haegen, L., Cai, Q., Stufflebeam, S., Sabuncu, M. R., Fischl, B., et al. (2013). A surface-based analysis of language lateralization and cortical asymmetry. *J. Cogn. Neurosci.* 25, 1477–1492. doi: 10.1162/jocn_a_00405

Grigorenko, E. L. (2009). Speaking genes or genes for speaking? Deciphering the genetics of speech and language. *J. Child Psychol. Psychiatry* 50, 116–125. doi: 10.1111/j.1469-7610.2008.02006.x

Hajek, T., Kopecek, M., and Hoschl, C. (2012). Reduced hippocampal volumes in healthy carriers of brain-derived neurotrophic factor Val66Met polymorphism: meta-analysis. *World J. Biol. Psychiatry* 13, 178–187. doi: 10.3109/15622975.2011.580005

Harris, G. J., Chabris, C. F., Clark, J., Urban, T., Aharon, I., Steele, S., et al. (2006). Brain activation during semantic processing in autism spectrum disorders via functional magnetic resonance imaging. *Brain Cogn.* 61, 54–68. doi: 10.1016/j.bandc.2005.12.015

Huang, H., Jeon, T., Sedmak, G., Pletikos, M., Vasung, L., Xu, X., et al. (2013). Coupling diffusion imaging with histological and gene expression analysis to examine the dynamics of cortical areas across the fetal period of human brain development. *Cereb. Cortex* 23, 2620–2631. doi: 10.1093/cercor/bhs241

Ip, B. K., Bayatti, N., Howard, N. J., Lindsay, S., and Clowry, G. J. (2011). The corticofugal neuron-associated genes ROBO1, SRGAP1, and CTIP2 exhibit an anterior to posterior gradient of expression in early fetal human neocortex development. *Cereb. Cortex* 21, 1395–1407. doi: 10.1093/cercor/bhq219

Jamadar, S., Powers, N. R., Meda, S. A., Gelernter, J., Gruen, J. R., and Pearlson, G. D. (2011). Genetic influences of cortical gray matter in language-related regions in healthy controls and schizophrenia. *Schizophr. Res.* 129, 141–148. doi: 10.1016/j.schres.2011.03.027

Ji, W., Li, T., Pan, Y., Tao, H., Ju, K., Wen, Z., et al. (2013). CNTNAP2 is significantly associated with schizophrenia and major depression in the Han Chinese population. *Psychiatry Res.* 207, 225–228. doi: 10.1016/j.psychres.2012.09.024

Knaus, T. A., Silver, A. M., Lindgren, K. A., Hadjikhani, N., and Tager-Flusberg, H. (2008). fMRI activation during a language task in adolescents with ASD. *J. Int. Neuropsychol. Soc.* 14, 967–979. doi: 10.1017/S1355617708081216

Koeda, M., Takahashi, H., Matsuura, M., Asai, K., and Okubo, Y. (2013). Cerebral responses to vocal attractiveness and auditory hallucinations in schizophrenia: a functional MRI study. *Front. Hum. Neurosci.* 7:221. doi: 10.3389/fnhum.2013.00221

Koeda, M., Takahashi, H., Yahata, N., Asai, K., Okubo, Y., and Tanaka, H. (2006a). A functional MRI study: cerebral laterality for lexical-semantic processing and human voice perception. *Am. J. Neuroradiol.* 27, 1472–1479. Available online at: http://www.ajnr.org/content/27/7/1472.long

Koeda, M., Takahashi, H., Yahata, N., Matsuura, M., Asai, K., Okubo, Y., et al. (2006b). Language processing and human voice perception in schizophrenia: a functional magnetic resonance imaging study. *Biol. Psychiatry* 59, 948–957. doi: 10.1016/j.biopsych.2006.01.013

Koeda, M., Takahashi, H., Yahata, N., Matsuura, M., Asai, K., Okubo, Y., et al. (2007). Neural responses to human voice and hemisphere dominance for lexical-semantic processing–an fMRI study. *Methods Inf. Med.* 46, 247–250. Available online at: http://methods.schattauer.de/en/contents/archivestandard/issue/671/manuscript/7962.html

Kos, M., Van Den Brink, D., Snijders, T. M., Rijpkema, M., Franke, B., Fernandez, G., et al. (2012). CNTNAP2 and language processing in healthy individuals as measured with ERPs. *PLoS ONE* 7:e46995. doi: 10.1371/journal.pone.0046995

Li, N., and Bartlett, C. W. (2012). Defining the genetic architecture of human developmental language impairment. *Life Sci.* 90, 469–475. doi: 10.1016/j.lfs.2012.01.016

Li, X., Hu, Z., He, Y., Xiong, Z., Long, Z., Peng, Y., et al. (2010). Association analysis of CNTNAP2 polymorphisms with autism in the Chinese Han population. *Psychiatr. Genet.* 20, 113–117. doi: 10.1097/YPG.0b013e32833a216f

Liu, H., Stufflebeam, S. M., Sepulcre, J., Hedden, T., and Buckner, R. L. (2009). Evidence from intrinsic activity that asymmetry of the human brain is controlled by multiple factors. *Proc. Natl. Acad. Sci. U.S.A.* 106, 20499–20503. doi: 10.1073/pnas.0908073106

Medland, S. E., Duffy, D. L., Wright, M. J., Geffen, G. M., and Martin, N. G. (2006). Handedness in twins: joint analysis of data from 35 samples. *Twin Res. Hum. Genet.* 9, 46–53. doi: 10.1375/twin.9.1.46

Muntané, G., Horvath, J. E., Hof, P. R., Ely, J. J., Hopkins, W. D., Raghanti, M. A., et al. (2014). Analysis of synaptic gene expression in the neocortex of primates reveals evolutionary changes in glutamatergic neurotransmission. *Cereb. Cortex.* doi: 10.1093/cercor/bht354. [Epub ahead of print].

Newbury, D. F., and Monaco, A. P. (2010). Genetic advances in the study of speech and language disorders. *Neuron* 68, 309–320. doi: 10.1016/j.neuron.2010.10.001

Ocklenburg, S., Arning, L., Gerding, W. M., Epplen, J. T., Gunturkun, O., and Beste, C. (2013). FOXP2 variation modulates functional hemispheric

asymmetries for speech perception. *Brain Lang.* 126, 279–284. doi: 10.1016/j.bandl.2013.07.001
Oldfield, R. C. (1971). The assessment and analysis of handedness: the Edinburgh inventory. *Neuropsychologia* 9, 97–113. doi: 10.1016/0028-3932(71)90067-4
Penagarikano, O., and Geschwind, D. H. (2012). What does CNTNAP2 reveal about autism spectrum disorder? *Trends Mol. Med.* 18, 156–163. doi: 10.1016/j.molmed.2012.01.003
Perlaki, G., Horvath, R., Orsi, G., Aradi, M., Auer, T., Varga, E., et al. (2013). White-matter microstructure and language lateralization in left-handers: a whole-brain MRI analysis. *Brain Cogn.* 82, 319–328. doi: 10.1016/j.bandc.2013.05.005
Pina-Camacho, L., Villero, S., Fraguas, D., Boada, L., Janssen, J., Navas-Sanchez, F. J., et al. (2012). Autism spectrum disorder: does neuroimaging support the DSM-5 proposal for a symptom dyad? A systematic review of functional magnetic resonance imaging and diffusion tensor imaging studies. *J. Autism Dev. Disord.* 42, 1326–1341. doi: 10.1007/s10803-011-1360-4
Pinel, P., Fauchereau, F., Moreno, A., Barbot, A., Lathrop, M., Zelenika, D., et al. (2012). Genetic variants of FOXP2 and KIAA0319/TTRAP/THEM2 locus are associated with altered brain activation in distinct language-related regions. *J. Neurosci.* 32, 817–825. doi: 10.1523/JNEUROSCI.5996-10.2012
Price, C. J. (2000). The anatomy of language: contributions from functional neuroimaging. *J. Anat.* 197(Pt 3), 335–359. doi: 10.1046/j.1469-7580.2000.19730335.x
Pujol, J., Deus, J., Losilla, J. M., and Capdevila, A. (1999). Cerebral lateralization of language in normal left-handed people studied by functional MRI. *Neurology* 52, 1038–1043. doi: 10.1212/WNL.52.5.1038
Rodenas-Cuadrado, P., Ho, J., and Vernes, S. C. (2014). Shining a light on CNTNAP2: complex functions to complex disorders. *Eur. J. Hum. Genet.* 22, 171–178. doi: 10.1038/ejhg.2013.100
Sampath, S., Bhat, S., Gupta, S., O'connor, A., West, A. B., Arking, D. E., et al. (2013). Defining the contribution of CNTNAP2 to autism susceptibility. *PLoS ONE* 8:e77906. doi: 10.1371/journal.pone.0077906
Shen, M. D., Shih, P., Ottl, B., Keehn, B., Leyden, K. M., Gaffrey, M. S., et al. (2012). Atypical lexicosemantic function of extrastriate cortex in autism spectrum disorder: evidence from functional and effective connectivity. *Neuroimage* 62, 1780–1791. doi: 10.1016/j.neuroimage.2012.06.008
Sun, T., and Walsh, C. A. (2006). Molecular approaches to brain asymmetry and handedness. *Nat. Rev. Neurosci.* 7, 655–662. doi: 10.1038/nrn1930
Szaflarski, J. P., Binder, J. R., Possing, E. T., Mckiernan, K. A., Ward, B. D., and Hammeke, T. A. (2002). Language lateralization in left-handed and ambidextrous people: fMRI data. *Neurology* 59, 238–244. doi: 10.1212/WNL.59.2.238
Tan, G. C., Doke, T. F., Ashburner, J., Wood, N. W., and Frackowiak, R. S. (2010). Normal variation in fronto-occipital circuitry and cerebellar structure with an autism-associated polymorphism of CNTNAP2. *Neuroimage* 53, 1030–1042. doi: 10.1016/j.neuroimage.2010.02.018
Tesink, C. M., Buitelaar, J. K., Petersson, K. M., Van Der Gaag, R. J., Teunisse, J. P., and Hagoort, P. (2011). Neural correlates of language comprehension in autism spectrum disorders: when language conflicts with world knowledge. *Neuropsychologia* 49, 1095–1104. doi: 10.1016/j.neuropsychologia.2011.01.018
Vernes, S. C., Newbury, D. F., Abrahams, B. S., Winchester, L., Nicod, J., Groszer, M., et al. (2008). A functional genetic link between distinct developmental language disorders. *N. Engl. J. Med.* 359, 2337–2345. doi: 10.1056/NEJMoa0802828
Watanabe, A., Karasugi, T., Sawai, H., Naing, B. T., Ikegawa, S., Orimo, H., et al. (2011). Prevalence of c.1559delT in ALPL, a common mutation resulting in the perinatal (lethal) form of hypophosphatasia in Japanese and effects of the mutation on heterozygous carriers. *J. Hum. Genet.* 56, 166–168. doi: 10.1038/jhg.2010.161
Whalley, H. C., O'connell, G., Sussmann, J. E., Peel, A., Stanfield, A. C., Hayiou-Thomas, M. E., et al. (2011). Genetic variation in CNTNAP2 alters brain function during linguistic processing in healthy individuals. *Am. J. Med. Genet. B Neuropsychiatr. Genet.* 156B, 941–948. doi: 10.1002/ajmg.b.31241
Whitehouse, A. J., Bishop, D. V., Ang, Q. W., Pennell, C. E., and Fisher, S. E. (2011). CNTNAP2 variants affect early language development in the general population. *Genes Brain Behav.* 10, 451–456. doi: 10.1111/j.1601-183X.2011.00684.x
Zhou, S., Zhu, Z., Qiu, X., Wu, W., Wang, W., Liu, Z., et al. (2012). Association study of IL-17RC, CHL1, DSCAM and CNTNAP2 genes polymorphisms with adolescent idiopathic scoliosis susceptibility in a Chinese Han population. *Stud. Health Technol. Inform.* 176, 47–51. doi: 10.3233/978-1-61499-067-3-47

Conflict of Interest Statement: The authors declare that the research was conducted in the absence of any commercial or financial relationships that could be construed as a potential conflict of interest.

Appendix 1: Contents of the Sentences

We used the following sentences in the task.

1. Ms. Keiko Ueda, who lives in Kitakyushu city and works as a licensed cook at a company cafeteria, notified the police near the station that 56,000 yen was stolen when she was mugged at Odouri last night.
2. Last night, when Mr. Ichiro Sato was driving a 10-ton truck full of eggs along the road to Yokohama, near the mouth of the Tama River the axle of the truck broke, and the truck slipped off the road and was buried in a ditch.
3. These days, "Casual Day," during which businessmen work in plain clothes with no tie, have been established, but the apparel business has developed and is marketing a "Dressed-Up Monday Campaign" that advertises "Let's be smartly dressed in a suit every Monday."
4. Today, the designs of Northern Europe have become increasingly popular, and a cultural event showing a collection of Swedish designs, music and images, etc., called "Swedish style 2001," will be held at various locations in Tokyo.

Appendix 2: Contents of the Questions in the Pilot Study

Appendix Questionnaire

Please answer the following question after listening to 2 sounds.

As what did you recognize these sounds? Please circle the appropriate one.

1. Human voice
2. Animal sound
3. Machine sound
4. Environmental sound

If you circled no. 1, please answer these questions.

As what did you recognize the first sound?

1. Male voice
2. Female voice

As what did you recognize the second sound?

1. Male voice
2. Female voice

Did you recognize these sounds as having intonation?

Yes No

Did you recognize a message from these sounds?

Yes No

15

Dimensional Schizotypy and Social Cognition: Sn fMRI Imaging Study

Edited by:
John D. Salamone, University of Connecticut, USA

***Correspondence:**
*Raymond C. K. Chan, Institute of Psychology, Chinese Academy of Sciences, 16 Lincui Road, Beijing 10101, China
rckchan@psych.ac.cn*

***Yi Wang** [1], **Wen-hua Liu** [2], **Zhi Li** [1,3], **Xin-hua Wei** [4], **Xin-qing Jiang** [4], **David L. Neumann** [5], **David H. K. Shum** [5], **Eric F. C. Cheung** [6] **and Raymond C. K. Chan** [1]**

[1] Neuropsychology and Applied Cognitive Neuroscience Laboratory, Key Laboratory of Mental Health, Institute of Psychology, Chinese Academy of Sciences, Beijing, China, [2] School of Health Management, Guangzhou Medical University, Guangzhou, China, [3] University of Chinese Academy of Sciences, Beijing, China, [4] Department of Radiology, Guangzhou First People's Hospital, Guangzhou, China, [5] Menzies Health Institute Queensland and School of Applied Psychology, Griffith University, Gold Coast, QLD, Australia, [6] Castle Peak Hospital, Hong Kong, China

Impairment in empathy has been demonstrated in patients with schizophrenia and individuals with psychosis proneness. In the present study, we examined the neural correlates underlying theory of mind (ToM) and empathy and the relationships between these two social cognitive abilities with schizotypy. Fifty-six first-year college students (31 males, 25 females) between 17 and 21 years of age (M = 19.3, SD = 0.9) from a medical university in China participated. All participants undertook a comic strips functional imaging task that specifically examined both empathy and ToM. In addition, they completed two self-report scales: the Chapman Psychosis Proneness scale and the Interpersonal Responsivity Index (IRI). Results showed that both empathy and ToM conditions of the task were associated with brain activity in the middle temporal gyrus, the temporo-parietal junction (TPJ), the precuneus and the posterior cingulate gyrus. In addition, we found positive correlations between negative schizotypy and brain activity in regions involved in social cognition, namely, the middle temporal gyrus, the TPJ, as well as the medial prefrontal gyrus. These findings highlight that different dimensions of schizotypy may show different associations with brain regions involved in social cognitive abilities. More importantly, the positive correlation between brain activity and anhedonia suggests the presence of compensatory mechanisms in high-risk populations.

Keywords: schizotypy, theory of mind, empathy, fMRI, anhedonia

Introduction

Theory of mind (ToM) refers to the ability to understand others' mental state and infer their aims, intentions, and beliefs (Premack and Woodruff, 1978). It is an important ability that influences social functioning in humans. Deficits in ToM performance in patients with schizophrenia have been well-established (Sprong et al., 2007; Bora et al., 2009). ToM impairment has also been observed in first onset schizophrenia patients, unaffected relatives of schizophrenia patients, ultra-high risk individuals (Bora and Pantelis, 2013), as well as individuals with psychometrically-defined schizotypy (Morrison et al., 2013). However, the mechanism underlying ToM deficit in schizophrenia spectrum disorders and its association with clinical symptoms are not fully understood. Studies that measure dimensions and extent of schizotypy has the advantage of avoiding the confounding effects of medication and illness duration in patients with schizophrenia. Recent studies suggest that schizotypy has multiple dimensions, such as positive schizotypy (e.g., magical ideation and perceptual aberration, similar to positive symptoms in schizophrenia), negative schizotypy (e.g., anhedonia, similar to negative symptoms in schizophrenia) and that these different dimensions may have unique behavioral, cognitive, and brain correlates (Nelson et al., 2013; Ettinger et al., 2014).While some studies found no significant association between schizotypal traits and ToM performance (Jahshan and Sergi, 2007; Fernyhough et al., 2008; McCleery et al., 2012), other studies showed that ToM deficits are related to positive schizotypy (Pickup, 2006; Barragan et al., 2011; Gooding and Pflum, 2011; Pflum et al., 2013) and negative schizotypy (Aldebot Sacks et al., 2012). The multidimensional nature of schizotypy may be an important confounding factor contributing to the inconsistent findings in research on schizotypy.

Concerning the neural correlates of ToM, it has been shown that the medial prefrontal region and the superior temporal sulcus (STS) are involved in ToM processing (Frith and Frith, 2005), and these areas are considered key areas for mentalizing (Blakemore, 2008). In schizophrenia patients, reduction of gray matter volume in the ventral medial prefrontal cortex (Hooker et al., 2011) and the STS (Koelkebeck et al., 2013) are positively correlated with impaired ToM performance. Abnormal activation in the medial prefrontal cortex (MPFC), the STS and the temporo-parietal junction (TPJ) in response to ToM tasks in patients with schizophrenia have also been observed (Brunet-Gouet and Decety, 2006; Bosia et al., 2012). On the other hand, previous studies have found increased brain activation in individuals at-risk of developing schizophrenia (Brune et al., 2011) as well as individuals with psychosis proneness as measured by the positive subscale of the Community Assessment of Psychic Experiences questionnaire (Modinos et al., 2010) to controls. Although preliminary, these results suggest that high risk individuals already show changes in neural activity when performing ToM tasks in the absence of significant behavioral changes.

ToM is now conceptualized as having two components, namely, cognitive, and affective ToM (Shamay-Tsoory et al., 2007): the former refers to making inference about others' beliefs and intentions and the latter refers to making inference about others' emotions. Shamay-Tsoory et al. (2007) suggested that performance on cognitive and affective ToM are dissociated in patients with schizophrenia, and negative symptoms may have unique associations with affective ToM. Empathy is a construct related to ToM and refers to the ability to infer and share others' emotional state, which is an important requirement in social cognition (Green et al., 2008). Empathy has also been considered to have both cognitive and affective components. In terms of psychological processing, affective ToM is similar to the cognitive component of empathy, as both require inferring the emotions of others (Sebastian et al., 2012). In contrast to findings in ToM, empirical findings have shown that negative schizotypy (such as the anhedonia score measured by the Chapman Psychosis Proneness Scale (Chapman et al., 1995) or the "no close friends" subscale score of the Schizotypal Personality Questionnaire (SPQ, Raine, 1991) is associated with empathy (Henry et al., 2008; Wang et al., 2013a).

Vollm et al. (2006) used a functional imaging task that included both ToM and empathy conditions and examined the neural correlates of each condition and their differences in 13 healthy participants (Vollm et al., 2006). The results showed that brain regions like the MPFC, the TPJ and the temporal poles were commonly activated in both conditions, while affective empathy triggered the activation of brain regions involved in emotional processing, such as the cingulate and the amygdala. Adopting a similar paradigm, Benedetti and his colleagues observed abnormal activations in the superior temporal gyrus, the TPJ as well as the prefrontal cortex for both cognitive and affective ToM conditions in chronic schizophrenia patients (Benedetti et al., 2009).

The purpose of the present study was to examine the associations between the various dimensions of schizotypal traits as measured by the Chapman Psychosis Proneness Scale and brain activity during a functional imaging task consisting of both ToM and empathy conditions. We hypothesized that brain areas, including the STS/TPJ and the MPFC, would be activated in both the ToM and empathy conditions of the imaging task. We further hypothesized that positive and negative schizotypy would be associated with different patterns of brain activation under ToM and empathy conditions. Since positive schizotypy have been found to be associated with deficits in ToM performance, and negative schizotypy have been found to be related to mentalization of emotions, we hypothesized that between schizotypal traits and The Interpersonal Reactivity Index (IRI) scores, the association between higher negative schizotypy (anhedonia) and poorer empathic ability would be found. Furthermore, while positive schizotypy may be associated with brain activity changes in the TPJ/STS in the ToM conditions, negative schizotypy may be associated with abnormal brain activity changes in the temporal and parietal lobes in empathy conditions.

Materials and Methods

Participants

Fifty-six first-year college students (31 males and 25 females) aged between 17 and 21 years ($M = 19.3$ years, $SD = 0.9$) from the Guangzhou Medical University participated in this study. All were right-handed as assessed by the Annett Handedness Scale (Annett, 1970). None had a history of psychiatric disorder, drug abuse or neurological disorders. Participants who scored higher than 13 on the Beck Depression Inventory (Beck et al., 1961) were excluded (four participants). IQ of the participants were estimated using the information, arithmetic, similarity and digit span subtests of the Chinese Version Wechsler Adult Intelligence Scale-Revised (WAIS-R) (Gong and Dai, 1984). The estimated IQ of participants ranged from 88 to 139, with a mean of 118.32 ($SD = 9.84$). The present study was approved by the Ethics Committee of the Institute of Psychology, the Chinese Academy of Sciences. Written informed consent was obtained from each participant.

Measures

Imaging Task

A visual ToM functional MRI task consisting of a series of comic strips was used in the present study. It was adapted into Chinese from a task used by Vollm et al. (2006). The task was presented in a block design with eight blocks in total. There were four kinds of stories: ToM, empathy (Emp), physical causality with one character and physical causality with two characters. The ToM and Emp conditions had one or two characters in them. Each kind of story was presented twice and all blocks were presented in a random order. In each block, five trials consisting of comic strips belonging to the same kind of stories were presented. In each trial, three pictures depicting a short story were displayed in the upper half of the screen for 6 s. Next, two pictures appeared in the lower half of the screen for another 6 s. During the second 6-s period, participants were asked to choose one of the two pictures from the lower half of the screen as the appropriate ending to the story by pressing the corresponding button. One trial lasted for 12 s; and each block consisted of an initial instruction slide and five trials and lasted for 66 s in total. The duration of the whole task was 8 min and 48 s. For a more detailed description of this task, please refer to Vollm et al. (2006) and Neumann et al. (2014). Before entering the scanner, all participants were given time to practice to make sure that they understood the task.

Self-report Scales

All participants were also asked to complete self-report scales that measure schizotypal traits and empathy. *The Chinese version of the Chapman Psychosis-Proneness Scales* (Chapman et al., 1995), including the Revised Social Anhedonia Scale (40 items), the Physical Anhedonia scale (61 items), the Magical Ideation Scale (40 items), and the Perceptual Aberration Scale (35 items) were used to determine the positive and negative dimensions of schizotypy (Wang et al., 2012). The former two Chapman scales were used to capture negative schizotypal traits (anhedonia) and the latter two scales were used to capture positive schizotypal traits (psychotic-like positive symptoms). The higher the participants scored, the higher was their level of schizotypy. The Cronbach's coefficients alpha of the four scales ranged from 0.75 to 0.89 in the present study.

The Interpersonal Reactivity Index (IRI) is a 28-item self-report scale that measures empathy and it consists of four subscales: perspective taking, fantasy, personal distress, and empathic concern (Davis, 1983). The first two subscales were designed to capture cognitive empathy and the last two scales captured affective empathy. In the Chinese version of the IRI, six items were deleted and the remaining 22 items have been shown to have good reliability and validity in both normal and schizophrenia populations (Chan, 1986). The Cronbach's alpha coefficients were 0.82 for the personal distress, 0.77 for the perspective taking, 0.73 for the fantasy and 0.63 for the empathic concern subscale.

Images Acquisition and Preprocessing

All MRI scans were acquired using a 3T SIEMENS Verio MR scanner at the Guangzhou First People's Hospital, Guangzhou, China. Functional imaging data were acquired using a T2-weighted echo planar imaging (EPI) sequence; 264 whole-brain volumes were collected with slice thickness = 4 mm, echo time (TE) = 28 ms, repetition time (TR) = 2000 ms, flip angle = 90°, matrix size = 64 × 64, 32 slices in coronal plane, field of view (FOV) = 210 × 210 mm, voxel size = 3 × 3 × 4 mm, bandwidth = 2232 Hz/Px. Scans were screened by a radiologist to exclude any incidental clinical abnormalities before further analyses. Preprocessing was performed using the Statistical Parametric Mapping software (SPM8, Wellcome Department of Imaging Neuroscience, Institute of Neurology and the National Hospital for Neurology and Neurosurgery; London, England). The first eight volumes were removed. Time delay in image acquisition and head motion were corrected. The fMRI images were further spatially normalized to the Montreal Neurological Institute (MNI) EPI template and re-sliced to 3 mm cubic voxels and then smoothed using a 10 mm full width at half maximum (FWHM) Gaussian kernel. Using the general linear model, contrast images, and beta images were generated for each participant, including "ToM minus physical causality with one character," and "Empathy minus physical causality with two characters." The head motion parameters in six directions were taken as covariates.

Statistical Analysis

For the behavioral data, we calculated the descriptive statistics of the scores on the self-report scales, including the IRI and the Chapman scales, as well as performance on the imaging task. Since gender has been identified as a confounding variable in previous empathy studies (e.g., Wang et al., 2013a), we also examined gender differences for the behavioral variables. To examine the associations between schizotypy and ToM/empathy, we calculated correlations between dimensional schizotypal traits measured by self-report scales and the IRI scores.

For the functional imaging data, all participants' contrast images, including contrast images for the ToM condition modeled as "ToM minus physical causality with one character" and the empathy condition modeled as "Empathy minus physical causality with two characters" were taken into the second level analysis. We first conducted one-sample t-tests using the contrast images for ToM and empathy conditions to examine brain activation in both conditions. In addition, we also conducted conjunction analysis to confirm the common areas for both conditions. The clusters were reported with a threshold of $p < 0.001$ and a cluster size of >50 voxels (corresponding to a cluster-level AlphaSim corrected $p < 0.01$ for multiple comparisons). After identifying the brain regions involved in the ToM and/or empathy conditions, we extracted the percentage signal change of those regions during the ToM and empathy blocks and calculated the correlations between the percentage signal change and schizotypy scores on the Chapman scales. Regions of interest were defined according to the results of the one sample t-tests and conjunction analysis. The percentage signal changes of all ROIs for each participant were extracted using the Marsbar v0.43 (Matthew et al., 2002) toolbox.

Results

Self-reported Scores and Behavioral Performance

Table 1 shows age, estimated IQ, IRI scores and the Chapman Psychosis Proneness scores for the whole sample. Results of independent sample t-tests showed that female participants

TABLE 1 | Descriptive analyses and gender effect on behavioral results.

	Whole sample ($n = 56$)		Male ($n = 31$)		Female ($n = 25$)		Gender effect	
	Mean	SD	Mean	SD	Mean	SD	t	p
Age	19.25	0.88	19.35	0.95	19.12	0.78	1.02	0.315
IQ estimates	118.32	9.84	117.42	9.56	119.44	10.26	−0.76	0.450
IRI SCALE								
PD	2.65	0.72	2.33	0.61	3.04	0.65	**−4.20**	**0.000**
PT	3.78	0.51	3.81	0.58	3.74	0.42	0.56	0.582
FA	3.56	0.67	3.42	0.70	3.73	0.60	−1.79	0.079
EC	3.71	0.54	3.63	0.51	3.81	0.57	−1.28	0.208
SCHIZOTYPY								
CSAS	7.80	5.58	8.16	6.26	7.36	4.68	0.53	0.598
CPAS	12.36	10.35	12.87	10.95	11.72	9.75	0.41	0.683
PAS	6.87	7.54	7.32	9.02	6.32	5.28	0.49	0.625
MIS	10.73	5.75	9.68	5.02	12.04	6.41	−1.55	0.128
IMAGING TASK (ACCURACY)								
ToM	0.80	0.16	0.83	0.14	0.76	0.18	1.62	0.112
Empathy	0.94	0.08	0.96	0.07	0.91	0.09	**2.61**	**0.012**
Physical causality with one character	0.90	0.11	0.92	0.10	0.88	0.12	1.23	0.223
Physical causality with two characters	0.83	0.15	0.86	0.15	0.80	0.15	1.36	0.180

Two sample t-tests were conducted to explore the gender effect, two-tailed. IRI, The Interpersonal Reactivity Index; PD, personal distress; PT, perspective taking; FA, fantasy; EC, empathic concern; CSAS, Chinese version of social anhedonia scale; CPAS, Chinese version of physical anhedonia scale; PAS, Chinese version of perceptual aberration scale; MIS, Chinese version of magical ideation scale; ToM, Theory of Mind. Values in bold indicate that they are statistical significant.

reported higher scores on the IRI personal distress subscale ($t = 4.20$, $p < 0.001$). Concerning the behavioral performance in the imaging task, the mean accuracy across all trials were higher than 0.80, and there was no significant gender effect except that males had higher accuracy in the empathy condition ($t = 2.61$, $p < 0.05$).

Functional Imaging Results

We conducted a series of one sample t-tests to examine the brain activation associated with the ToM and empathy conditions. Compared to the physical causality condition, we found increased activity in the bilateral cuneus, the bilateral middle temporal gyrus, the left precuneus, the left superior frontal cortex and the right TPJ during the ToM condition. For the empathy condition relative to the physical causality condition, we found a similar increase in brain activations in the bilateral cuneus, the left precuneus and the right middle temporal gyrus. The results are shown in **Table 2** and **Figure 1**. Using conjunction analysis, we further confirmed the common areas activated by both the ToM and the empathy conditions, namely the bilateral cuneus, the middle temporal gyrus and the TPJ (**Table 2**). Further comparisons showed that the left TPJ and the lingual gyrus were activated more strongly during the ToM condition than the empathy condition.

Associations between Schizotypy and Brain Activity

We then extracted the percentage signal changes of significant clusters related to the ToM or the empathy conditions in our imaging task. We calculated the correlations between schizotypy and IRI scores, as well as the percentage signal changes of ROIs, with and without gender as covariates.

We found significant negative correlations between social anhedonia and IRI empathic concern subscale scores ($r = -0.24$, $p < 0.05$), between physical anhedonia and IRI fantasy subscale scores ($r = -0.30$, $p < 0.05$) and IRI empathic concern subscale scores ($r = -0.35$, $p < 0.01$). We also found positive correlations between magical ideation subscale scores and IRI personal distress subscale scores ($r = 0.30$, $p < 0.05$) and fantasy subscale scores ($r = 0.30$, $p < 0.05$). Using gender as covariate, we also found significant positive correlations between both physical and social anhedonia and IRI personal distress subscale scores (see **Table 3** for details).

Concerning the correlations with percentage signal changes, in the ToM condition, positive correlations were found between social anhedonia and brain activity in the right cuneus, the bilateral middle temporal gyrus, the medial frontal gyrus, and the right TPJ. We also found significant positive correlations between physical anhedonia scores and brain activity in the left middle temporal gyrus. Marginally significant correlations were also found between magical ideation subscale scores and activation in the medial frontal gyrus. For the empathy condition, positive correlations were found between social anhedonia scores and brain activity in the right cuneus and the middle temporal gyrus. The correlation between the MIS scores and brain activity in the right cuneus reached trend significance (see **Table 3**).

Discussion

In the present study, we adopted a comic strips functional imaging task to explore the brain regions involved in the

TABLE 2 | Brain activations associated with ToM and Empathy conditions.

	All participants ($n = 56$)					
	BA	Coordinate			Cluster	Peak
		x	*y*	*z*	size	(Z)
TOM MINUS PHYSICAL CAUSALITY						
Cuneus	BA17/18	18	−102	12	207	5.64
Precuneus/posterior cingulate	BA7/31	−3	−54	42	466	5.05
Cuneus	BA17	−9	−102	9	209	4.89
Middle temporal/precuneus	BA 19/39	−39	−78	42	285	4.59
Middle temporal gyrus	BA21	54	0	−27	106	4.32
Superior frontal gyrus, extending to cingulate	BA8/32	−18	33	42	75	4.19
Temporal-parietal junction	BA 13/22/39	48	−45	15	300	4.06
EMPATHY MINUS PHYSICAL CAUSALITY						
Cuneus/lingual gyrus	BA 18	−18	−105	3	84	5.48
Precuneus/posterior cingulate	BA7/31	0	−57	33	183	5.14
Cuneus	BA 18	21	−105	6	50	4.66
Middle temporal gyrus	BA 21/38	54	6	−27	90	4.25
Middle temporal gyrus	BA39	60	−66	18	67	3.89
CONJUNCTION ANALYSIS						
Cuneus	BA17/18	18	−105	9	99	6.86
Precuneus/posterior cingulate	BA7/31	0	−57	36	251	6.65
Cuneus	BA17/18	−15	−105	6	106	6.51
Middle temporal gyrus	BA 21/38	54	6	−27	100	5.95
Temporal-parietal junction	BA 39	−51	−72	27	107	5.53
Temporal-parietal junction	BA 39	54	−66	21	105	5.21
Middle temporal gyrus	BA 21/38	−54	−6	−21	22	5.05
(TOM−PHYSICAL CAUSALITY) MINUS (EMPATHY−PHYSICAL CAUSALITY)						
Temporal-parietal junction	BA 39	−42	−72	39	94	4.10
Cuneus/lingual gyrus	BA17/18	−3	−93	6	253	3.89
(EMPATHY−PHYSICAL CAUSALITY) MINUS (TOM−PHYSICAL CAUSALITY)						
No significant cluster						

One sample t-tests were conducted for Theory of Mind (ToM) and Empathy conditions, respectively. Threshold was set at $p < 0.001$, cluster size > 50 voxels. For the conjunction analysis, the threshold was set at $p < 0.05$, family-wise error correction. ToM, Theory of Mind; BA, Brodmann Area.

mentalizing process of ToM and empathy. We found several brain regions related to the process of inferring others' beliefs, including the TPJ, the middle temporal gyrus, the medial prefrontal cortex, the cuneus and the precuneus. We found that similar brain regions, namely, the cuneus, the precuneus and the middle temporal gyrus, were also activated when inferring the emotional state of others. By using conjunction analysis, we found regions such as the bilateral TPJ, the middle temporal gyrus and the cuneus to be activated in both conditions. In addition, we explored the associations between schizotypal traits and brain activities in these clusters. The results showed that social anhedonia scores, a negative dimension of schizotypy, had negative correlations with self-report empathy, but they were positively correlated with brain activity of the cuneus, the middle temporal gyrus and the TPJ, which are brain regions involved in ToM/empathy. For positive schizotypal traits, scores on the magical ideation subscale of the Chapman scales were negatively correlated with brain activity of the medial prefrontal cortex.

Key brain regions involved in the attribution of mental states, the so-called "social brain," include the medial prefrontal gyrus, the posterior STS/TPJ, the middle temporal gyrus, the anterior cingulate and the anterior insula (Blakemore, 2008). Adopting the comic strips task, Vollm et al. (2006) found that the medial prefrontal gyrus, the TPJ and the temporal pole were activated in both ToM and empathy processing tasks and suggested that both processes rely on the brain network associated with making inferences of others' mental states. The posterior STS/TPJ integrates information from the external environment and internal sensory and perceptual information and plays an important role in self-other distinction (Abu-Akel and Shamay-Tsoory, 2011). Others have also suggested that the TPJ is selectively activated in the attribution of mental states and plays a specific and independent role in the prediction of the behavior of others (Saxe and Wexler, 2005; Carter et al., 2012). In our study, both the ToM and empathy tasks required participants to infer the intentions of the character in the comic strips and choose the most appropriate ending of the story. As expected,

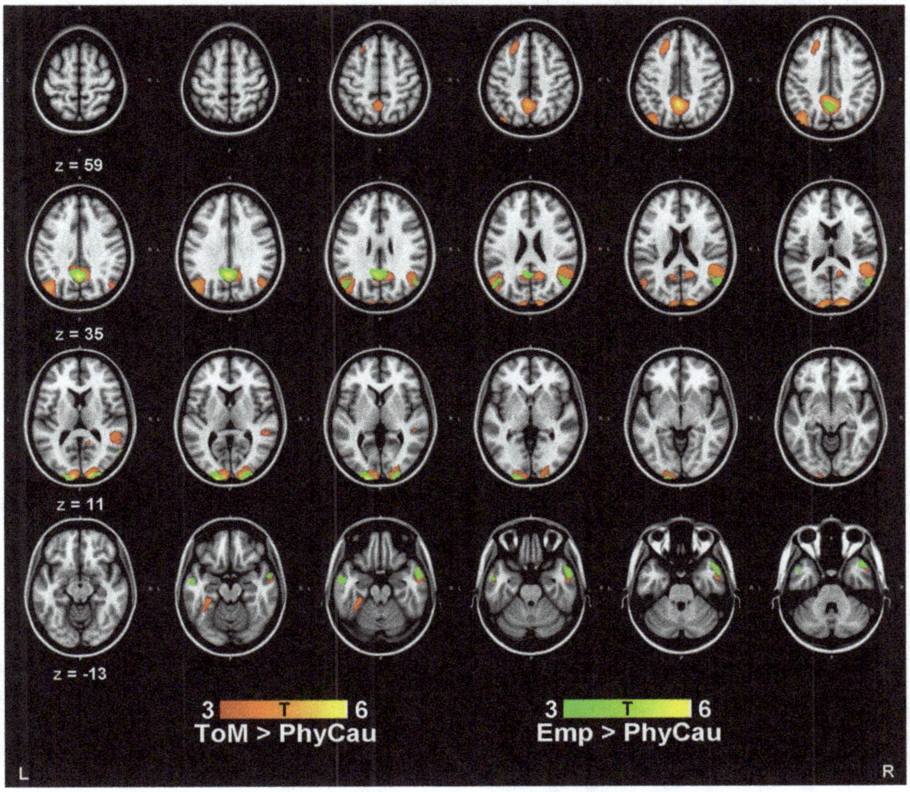

FIGURE 1 | The Brain activations associated with the ToM and Empathy conditions. Compared to the control condition (physical causality with one character), increased brain activity were found in bilateral cuneus, bilateral middle temporal gyrus, left precuneus, left superior frontal cortex and the right TPJ during the ToM blocks. For the empathy condition, increased brain activations were found in bilateral cuneus, left precuneus and also the right middle temporal gyrus. One sample *t*-tests were conducted for ToM and Empathy conditions, respectively. Threshold was set at $p < 0.001$, cluster size >50 voxels.

we found increased brain activation in the bilateral TPJ (BA39) and the middle temporal gyrus (BA21/38) during the ToM and empathy conditions compared to the physical causality blocks. At the same time, we also found increased activation in the middle occipital gyrus (cuneus, BA18) in the conjunction analysis, which has also been reported previously (Vollm et al., 2006).

Increased activation in the posteromedial regions, including the posterior cingulate and the precuneus, was consistently found under both ToM and empathy conditions in our study. These findings are consistent with previous studies on mentalizing tasks (Vollm et al., 2006; Abu-Akel and Shamay-Tsoory, 2011). The precuneus is involved in self-processing, mental imaginary as well as episodic memory retrieval (Cavanna and Trimble, 2006) and all these processes might be related to inferring the intention of others. For example, during the mentalizing task, participants needed to imagine the scene or story of the characters in the comic strip and infer their emotional states. Abu-Akel and Shamay-Tsoory (2011) have proposed a model to explain the neuroanatomical basis of ToM, in which the posterior cingulate and the precuneus are involved in representing and distinguishing self from the mental states of others.

Compared to the empathy condition, increased activation in the temporal-parietal junction and the cuneus were found during the ToM condition. This difference might be related to the difference in difficulty of the ToM and empathy conditions. In the present study, the mean accuracy of the ToM and empathy condition was 0.80 and 0.94, respectively. The difference in accuracy might be a reflection of the difficulty of the ToM condition.

Consistent with previous findings, we found that a higher level of negative schizotypy was correlated with lower scores on the IRI scale (Henry et al., 2008; Wang et al., 2013a). With or without gender as covariate, we found significant correlations between negative schizotypy (social or physical anhedonia) and IRI fantasy/empathic concern scores, suggesting that individuals with higher social or physical anhedonia scores had poorer self-report empathic ability. As components of social cognition, ToM and empathy play important roles in social functioning (Schmidt et al., 2011). Our results suggest that schizotypy, especially the negative dimension of schizotypy, is associated with poorer social cognition, which may explain the deficits in social functioning in individuals with high-risk of developing schizophrenia and individuals with schizotypal traits, which is consistent with previous studies (Addington et al., 2011; Blanchard et al., 2011; Wang et al., 2013b).

TABLE 3 | The correlations between schizotypy and IRI, percent signal change.

	Correlation without covariate				Correlation with gender as covariate			
	CSAS	**CPAS**	**PAS**	**MIS**	**CSAS**	**CPAS**	**PAS**	**MIS**
IRI SCALE								
PD	0.19 (0.085)	0.18 (0.090)	0.06	**0.30***	**0.26***	**0.24***	0.11	**0.23***
PT	−0.06	0.02	0.02	0.01	−0.06	0.01	0.01	0.03
FA	−0.18 (0.097)	**−0.30***	−0.04	**0.30***	−0.16	**−0.30***	−0.03	**0.26***
EC	**−0.24***	**−0.34****	−0.06	0.09	**−0.23***	**−0.34****	−0.05	0.06
% SIGNAL CHANGE OF ROIS (CONTRAST, COORDINATES X, Y, Z)								
Cuneus (ToM, 18, −102, 12)	0.20 (0.075)	0.06	0.09	−0.05	0.18 (0.090)	0.05	0.08	0.00
Temporal-parietal junction (ToM, 48, −45, 15)	**0.27***	0.09	0.14	0.04	**0.27***	0.09	0.14	0.04
Middle temporal gyrus (ToM, 54, 0, −27)	**0.23***	0.05	0.13	0.04	**0.23***	0.05	0.13	0.04
Precuneus (ToM, −3, −54, 42)	0.15	0.13	0.06	−0.09	0.15	0.13	0.05	−0.07
Cuneus (ToM, −9, −102, 9)	−0.01	−0.03	0.02	−0.04	−0.02	−0.04	0.00	0.00
Superior frontal gyrus (ToM, −18, 33, 42)	0.21 (0.063)	0.09	−0.03	−0.22 (0.051)	0.20 (0.068)	0.09	−0.03	−0.21 (0.058)
Middle temporal gyrus (ToM, −39, −78, 42)	**0.24***	**0.23***	0.05	−0.11	**0.24***	**0.23***	0.05	−0.11
Precuneus (EMP, 0, −57, 33)	0.09	0.01	0.13	−0.05	0.09	0.02	0.14	−0.07
Cuneus (EMP, 21, −105, 6)	**0.23***	0.13	0.01	0.02	**0.23***	0.13	0.00	0.04
Middle temporal gyrus (EMP, 54, 6, −27)	0.14	0.07	0.15	0.11	0.17	0.09	0.18 (0.097)	0.06
Middle temporal gyrus (EMP, 60, −66, 18)	**0.22***	−0.05	0.13	0.08	0.22 (0.051)	−0.05	0.13	0.08
Cuneus (EMP, −18, −105, 3)	−0.06	−0.19 (0.083)	0.14	0.21 (0.061)	−0.06	−0.18 (0.089)	0.15	0.20 (0.070)

*Correlation and partial correlations with gender as covariate were conducted, threshold was set as p < 0.05 one-tailed. IRI, The Interpersonal Reactivity Index; PD, personal distress; PT, perspective taking; FA, fantasy; EC, empathic concern. CSAS, Chinese version of social anhedonia scale; CPAS, Chinese version of physical anhedonia scale; PAS, Chinese version of perceptual aberration scale; MIS, Chinese version of magical ideation scale; ToM, Theory of Mind; EMP, Empathy. *p < 0.05; **p < 0.01. The p-values are presented in parentheses were between 0.05 and 0.10. Values in bold indicate that they are statistical significant.*

Most interestingly, we extracted the percentage signal change of the activated brain regions and calculated the correlations with both positive and negative schizotypy traits. We found that social anhedonia was positively correlated with brain activity in several regions involved in ToM/empathy processing, including the bilateral middle temporal gyrus, the medial frontal gyrus and the right TPJ. In a previous study that adopted a similar task, Benedetti et al. (2009) found that patients with schizophrenia showed higher brain activation in their temporal and frontal lobes. Although reduced brain activities has been found in the frontal, temporal and parietal lobes of patients with schizophrenia in different functional imaging studies, an inverse pattern of brain activation has also been reported in high-risk populations. For example, increased activity was found in a visual imaging ToM task in individuals with high psychosis proneness measured by the Community Assessment of Psychic Experiences Questionnaire (CAPE) (Modinos et al., 2010). Using resting state fMRI techniques, researchers have also found positive correlations between SPQ scores and visual network in adolescents (Lagioia et al., 2010). Taken together, we believe that the increased brain activation observed in high risk populations may represent some form of compensatory or protective mechanism, which could be a valuable target for future studies in psychosis development.

We acknowledge several limitations in the present study. First, for the behavioral tasks that captured mental state attribution, we only used a self-report scale as there is a lack of appropriate behavioral paradigms suitable for young adults with good validity. Secondly, for the imaging data analysis, no stringent correction for multiple comparisons was used. Nevertheless, it should be pointed out that the threshold was set at $p < 0.001$ and cluster size was more than 50 voxels, which corresponded to a cluster level of $p < 0.01$ (AlphaSim correction for multiple comparison). It should also be noted that we did not adopt multiple comparison adjustment for the correlation analyses between the percentage signal change and schizotypy scores on the Chapman scales, and so the results would need to be considered cautiously. Thirdly, our findings were limited to healthy individuals with schizotypal traits. Finally, the comic strips task does not isolate the individual subcomponents of ToM and empathy. For example, empathy is considered to consist of components such as affect sharing, perspective taking, and understanding others' situation (Neumann et al., 2013). Further research that uses a modified version of the comics strips task to examine the relationships between schizotypy and brain activation under different empathy conditions is needed.

In conclusion, our results led us to postulate that negative schizotypy may play an important role in social cognition processing, such as mentalizing, which may further influence an individual's social functioning. The inverse correlation pattern between brain activity and positive and negative schizotypy strengthens the idea that the multidimensional structure of schizotypy is complex and should be examined more systematically in future studies.

Acknowledgments

This study was supported by a grant from the "Strategic Priority Research Program (B)" of the Chinese Academy of Sciences (XDB02030002), the National Science Fund China (81088001, 91132701), the Beijing Training Project for the Leading Talents in S & T (Z151100000315020), and a grant from the CAS/SAFEA International Partnership Program for Creative Research Teams (Y2CX131003). YW was supported by a National Science Fund China (31400884) and a Scientific Foundation of Institute of Psychology, Chinese Academy of Sciences, No. Y3CX161005.

References

Abu-Akel, A., and Shamay-Tsoory, S. (2011). Neuroanatomical and neurochemical bases of theory of mind. *Neuropsychologia* 49, 2971–2984. doi: 10.1016/j.neuropsychologia.2011.07.012

Addington, J., Cornblatt, B. A., Cadenhead, K. S., Cannon, T. D., McGlashan, T. H., Perkins, D. O., et al. (2011). At clinical high risk for psychosis: outcome for nonconverters. *Am. J. Psychiatry* 168, 800–805. doi: 10.1176/appi.ajp.2011.10081191

Aldebot Sacks, S., Weisman De Mamani, A. G., and Garcia, C. P. (2012). Associations between cognitive biases and domains of schizotypy in a non-clinical sample. *Psychiatry Res.* 196, 115–122. doi: 10.1016/j.psychres.2011.09.019

Annett, M. (1970). A classification of hand preference by association analysis. *Br. J. Psychol.* 61, 303–321. doi: 10.1111/j.2044-8295.1970.tb01248.x

Barragan, M., Laurens, K. R., Navarro, J. B., and Obiols, J. E. (2011). 'Theory of Mind', psychotic-like experiences and psychometric schizotypy in adolescents from the general population. *Psychiatry Res.* 186, 225–231. doi: 10.1016/j.psychres.2010.07.051

Beck, A. T., Ward, C. H., Mendelson, M., Mock, J., and Erbaugh, J. (1961). An inventory for measuring depression. *Arch. Gen. Psychiatry* 4, 561–571.

Benedetti, F., Bernasconi, A., Bosia, M., Cavallaro, R., Dallaspezia, S., Falini, A., et al. (2009). Functional and structural brain correlates of theory of mind and empathy deficits in schizophrenia. *Schizophr. Res.* 114, 154–160. doi: 10.1016/j.schres.2009.06.021

Blakemore, S. J. (2008). The social brain in adolescence. *Nat. Rev. Neurosci.* 9, 267–277. doi: 10.1038/nrn2353

Blanchard, J. J., Collins, L. M., Aghevli, M., Leung, W. W., and Cohen, A. S. (2011). Social anhedonia and schizotypy in a community sample: the Maryland longitudinal study of schizotypy. *Schizophr. Bull.* 37, 587–602. doi: 10.1093/schbul/sbp107

Bora, E., and Pantelis, C. (2013). Theory of mind impairments in first-episode psychosis, individuals at ultra-high risk for psychosis and in first-degree relatives of schizophrenia: systematic review and meta-analysis. *Schizophr. Res.* 144, 31–36. doi: 10.1016/j.schres.2012.12.013

Bora, E., Yucel, M., and Pantelis, C. (2009). Theory of mind impairment in schizophrenia: meta-analysis. *Schizophr. Res.* 109, 1–9. doi: 10.1016/j.schres.2008.12.020

Bosia, M., Riccaboni, R., and Poletti, S. (2012). Neurofunctional correlates of theory of mind deficits in schizophrenia. *Curr. Top. Med. Chem.* 12, 2284–2302. doi: 10.2174/156802612805289917

Brune, M., Ozgurdal, S., Ansorge, N., Von Reventlow, H. G., Peters, S., Nicolas, V., et al. (2011). An fMRI study of "theory of mind" in at-risk states of psychosis: comparison with manifest schizophrenia and healthy controls. *Neuroimage* 55, 329–337. doi: 10.1016/j.neuroimage.2010.12.018

Brunet-Gouet, E., and Decety, J. (2006). Social brain dysfunctions in schizophrenia: a review of neuroimaging studies. *Psychiatry Res.* 148, 75–92. doi: 10.1016/j.pscychresns.2006.05.001

Carter, R. M., Bowling, D. L., Reeck, C., and Huettel, S. A. (2012). A distinct role of the temporal-parietal junction in predicting socially guided decisions. *Science* 337, 109–111. doi: 10.1126/science.1219681

Cavanna, A. E., and Trimble, M. R. (2006). The precuneus: a review of its functional anatomy and behavioural correlates. *Brain* 129, 564–583. doi: 10.1093/brain/awl004

Chan, C. Y. (1986). *The Relations between Age, Sex-role, Orientation of Human and Empathy.* Taipei: Master, National Chengchi University.

Chapman, J. P., Chapman, L. J., and Kwapil, T. R. (1995). "Scales for the measurement of schizotypy," in *Schizotypal Personality*, eds A. Raine, T. Lencz, and S. A. Mednick (New York, NY: Cambridge University Press), 79–109.

Davis, M. H. (1983). Measuring individual differences in empathy: evidence for a multidimensional approach. *J. Pers. Soc. Psychol.* 44, 113–126. doi: 10.1037/0022-3514.44.1.113

Ettinger, U., Meyhofer, I., Steffens, M., Wagner, M., and Koutsouleris, N. (2014). Genetics, cognition, and neurobiology of schizotypal personality: a review of the overlap with schizophrenia. *Front. Psychiatry* 5:18. doi: 10.3389/fpsyt.2014.00018

Fernyhough, C., Jones, S. R., Whittle, C., Waterhouse, J., and Bentall, R. P. (2008). Theory of mind, schizotypy, and persecutory ideation in young adults. *Cogn. Neuropsychiatry* 13, 233–249. doi: 10.1080/13546800801936516

Frith, C., and Frith, U. (2005). Theory of mind. *Curr. Biol.* 15, R644–R645. doi: 10.1016/j.cub.2005.08.041

Gong, Y. X., and Dai, X. Y. (1984). Application of the short forms of Wechsler Intelligence Scale. *J. Cen. South Univ. Med. Sci.* 4, 393–400.

Gooding, D. C., and Pflum, M. J. (2011). Theory of Mind and psychometric schizotypy. *Psychiatry Res.* 188, 217–223. doi: 10.1016/j.psychres.2011.04.029

Green, M. F., Penn, D. L., Bentall, R., Carpenter, W. T., Gaebel, W., Gur, R. C., et al. (2008). Social cognition in schizophrenia: an NIMH workshop on definitions, assessment, and research opportunities. *Schizophrenia Bull.* 34, 1211–1220. doi: 10.1093/schbul/sbm145

Henry, J. D., Bailey, P. E., and Rendell, P. G. (2008). Empathy, social functioning and schizotypy. *Psychiatry Res.* 160, 15–22. doi: 10.1016/j.psychres.2007.04.014

Hooker, C. I., Bruce, L., Lincoln, S. H., Fisher, M., and Vinogradov, S. (2011). Theory of mind skills are related to gray matter volume in the ventromedial prefrontal cortex in schizophrenia. *Biol. Psychiatry* 70, 1169–1178. doi: 10.1016/j.biopsych.2011.07.027

Jahshan, C. S., and Sergi, M. J. (2007). Theory of mind, neurocognition, and functional status in schizotypy. *Schizophr. Res.* 89, 278–286. doi: 10.1016/j.schres.2006.09.004

Koelkebeck, K., Hirao, K., Miyata, J., Kawada, R., Saze, T., Dannlowski, U., et al. (2013). Impact of gray matter reductions on theory of mind abilities in patients with schizophrenia. *Soc. Neurosci.* 8, 631–639. doi: 10.1080/17470919.2013.837094

Lagioia, A., Van De Ville, D., Debbane, M., Lazeyras, F., and Eliez, S. (2010). Adolescent resting state networks and their associations with schizotypal trait expression. *Front. Syst. Neurosci.* 4:35. doi: 10.3389/fnsys.2010.00035

Matthew, B., Jean-Luc, A., Romain, V., and Jean-Baptiste, P. (2002). "Region of interest analysis using an SPM toolbox [abstract]," in *Presented at the 8th International Conference on Functional Mapping of the Human Brain*, Vol. 16 (Sendai). Available on CD-ROM in NeuroImage.

McCleery, A., Divilbiss, M., St-Hilaire, A., Aakre, J. M., Seghers, J. P., Bell, E. K., et al. (2012). Predicting social functioning in schizotypy: an investigation of the relative contributions of theory of mind and mood. *J. Nerv. Ment. Dis.* 200, 147–152. doi: 10.1097/NMD.0b013e3182439533

Modinos, G., Renken, R., Shamay-Tsoory, S. G., Ormel, J., and Aleman, A. (2010). Neurobiological correlates of theory of mind in psychosis proneness. *Neuropsychologia* 48, 3715–3724. doi: 10.1016/j.neuropsychologia.2010.09.030

Morrison, S. C., Brown, L. A., and Cohen, A. S. (2013). A multidimensional assessment of social cognition in psychometrically defined schizotypy. *Psychiatry Res.* 210, 1014–1019. doi: 10.1016/j.psychres.2013.08.020

Nelson, M. T., Seal, M. L., Pantelis, C., and Phillips, L. J. (2013). Evidence of a dimensional relationship between schizotypy and schizophrenia: a systematic review. *Neurosci. Biobehav. Rev.* 37, 317–327. doi: 10.1016/j.neubiorev.2013.01.004

Neumann, D. L., Boyle, G. J., and Chan, R. C. K. (2013). Empathy towards individuals of the same and different ethnicity when depicted in negative and positive contexts. *Pers. Individ. Dif.* 55, 8–13. doi: 10.1016/j.paid.2013.01.022

Neumann, D. L., Chan, R. C. K., Boyle, G. J., Wang, Y., and Westbury, H. R. (2014). "Self-report, behavioral, and neuroscientific approaches to measuring empathy: a multidisciplinary perspective," in *Measurement of Personality and Social Psychological Constructs*, eds G. J. Boyle and D. H. Saklofske (Chennai: Elsevier), 257–289.

Pflum, M. J., Gooding, D. C., and White, H. J. (2013). Hint, hint: theory of mind performance in schizotypal individuals. *J. Nerv. Ment. Dis.* 201, 394–399. doi: 10.1097/NMD.0b013e31828e1016

Pickup, G. J. (2006). Theory of mind and its relation to schizotypy. *Cogn. Neuropsychiatry* 11, 177–192. doi: 10.1080/13546800444000236

Premack, D., and Woodruff, G. (1978). Does the chimpanzee have a theory of mind? *Behav. Brain Sci.* 1, 515–526. doi: 10.1017/S0140525X00076512

Raine, A. (1991). The SPQ: a scale for the assessment of schizotypal personality based on DSM-III-R criteria. *Schizophr. Bull.* 17, 555–564.

Saxe, R., and Wexler, A. (2005). Making sense of another mind: the role of the right temporo-parietal junction. *Neuropsychologia* 43, 1391–1399. doi: 10.1016/j.neuropsychologia.2005.02.013

Schmidt, S. J., Mueller, D. R., and Roder, V. (2011). Social cognition as a mediator variable between neurocognition and functional outcome in schizophrenia: empirical review and new results by structural equation modeling. *Schizophr. Bull.* 37(Suppl. 2), S41–S54. doi: 10.1093/schbul/sbr079

Sebastian, C. L., Fontaine, N. M., Bird, G., Blakemore, S. J., Brito, S. A., McCrory, E. J., et al. (2012). Neural processing associated with cognitive and affective Theory of Mind in adolescents and adults. *Soc. Cogn. Affect. Neurosci.* 7, 53–63. doi: 10.1093/scan/nsr023

Shamay-Tsoory, S. G., Shur, S., Barcai-Goodman, L., Medlovich, S., Harari, H., and Levkovitz, Y. (2007). Dissociation of cognitive from affective components of theory of mind in schizophrenia. *Psychiatry Res.* 149, 11–23. doi: 10.1016/j.psychres.2005.10.018

Sprong, M., Schothorst, P., Vos, E., Hox, J., and Van Engeland, H. (2007). Theory of mind in schizophrenia: meta-analysis. *Br. J. Psychiatry* 191, 5–13. doi: 10.1192/bjp.bp.107.035899

Vollm, B. A., Taylor, A. N., Richardson, P., Corcoran, R., Stirling, J., McKie, S., et al. (2006). Neuronal correlates of theory of mind and empathy: a functional magnetic resonance imaging study in a nonverbal task. *Neuroimage* 29, 90–98. doi: 10.1016/j.neuroimage.2005.07.022

Wang, Y., Neumann, D. L., Shum, D. H., Liu, W. H., Shi, H. S., Yan, C., et al. (2013a). Cognitive empathy partially mediates the association between negative schizotypy traits and social functioning. *Psychiatry Res.* 210, 62–68. doi: 10.1016/j.psychres.2013.03.015

Wang, Y., Neumann, D., Shum, D. H., and Chan, R. C. (2012). A cross-validation study of clustering of schizotypy using a non-clinical Chinese sample. *Psychiatry Res.* 200, 55–58. doi: 10.1016/j.psychres.2012.03.026

Wang, Y., Yeh, Y. H., Tsang, S. M., Liu, W. H., Shi, H. S., Li, Z., et al. (2013b). Social functioning in Chinese college students with and without schizotypal personality traits: an exploratory study of the Chinese version of the First Episode Social Functioning Scale. *PLoS ONE* 8:e61115. doi: 10.1371/journal.pone.0061115

Conflict of Interest Statement: The authors declare that the research was conducted in the absence of any commercial or financial relationships that could be construed as a potential conflict of interest.

16

Neural Substrates of Sexual Desire in Individuals with Problematic Hypersexual Behavior

Edited by:
Morten L. Kringelbach,
University of Oxford, UK and
University of Aarhus, Denmark, UK

***Correspondence:**
Jin-Hun Sohn
jhsohn@cnu.ac.kr

*Ji-Woo Seok and Jin-Hun Sohn **

Department of Psychology, Brain Research Institute, Chungnam National University, Daejeon, South Korea

Studies on the characteristics of individuals with hypersexual disorder have been accumulating due to increasing concerns about problematic hypersexual behavior (PHB). Currently, relatively little is known about the underlying behavioral and neural mechanisms of sexual desire. Our study aimed to investigate the neural correlates of sexual desire with event-related functional magnetic resonance imaging (fMRI). Twenty-three individuals with PHB and 22 age-matched healthy controls were scanned while they passively viewed sexual and nonsexual stimuli. The subjects' levels of sexual desire were assessed in response to each sexual stimulus. Relative to controls, individuals with PHB experienced more frequent and enhanced sexual desire during exposure to sexual stimuli. Greater activation was observed in the caudate nucleus, inferior parietal lobe, dorsal anterior cingulate gyrus, thalamus, and dorsolateral prefrontal cortex in the PHB group than in the control group. In addition, the hemodynamic patterns in the activated areas differed between the groups. Consistent with the findings of brain imaging studies of substance and behavior addiction, individuals with the behavioral characteristics of PHB and enhanced desire exhibited altered activation in the prefrontal cortex and subcortical regions. In conclusion, our results will help to characterize the behaviors and associated neural mechanisms of individuals with PHB.

Keywords: problematic hypersexual behavior, sexual desire, functional magnetic resonance imaging, dorsolateral prefrontal cortex, hemodynamic response

INTRODUCTION

Problematic hypersexual behavior (PHB) is defined as the continuous participation in repeated sex acts with no control over excessive sexual compulsivity and behavior despite the awareness of the associated negative outcomes (Goodman, 1993; Carnes, 2001, 2013). Those who suffer from PHB can experience extreme difficulties in their family relationships and job performance. In addition, they are at greater risk for contracting sexually transmitted diseases or experiencing unwanted pregnancies from promiscuous sexual relations (Schneider and Schneider, 1991; Kuzma and Black, 2008). In the US, 3–6% of the community and college students have PHB (Coleman, 1992; Black, 2000; Seegers, 2003). In Korea, approximately 2% of all college students have PHB (Kim and Kwak, 2011). Due to its high prevalence and related problems, the associated risks are increasingly recognized in society as the incidence of PHB appears to be growing.

Although the seriousness of PHB is now recognized, it was not included in the DSM-5 (American Psychiatric Association, 2013) Debates are ongoing as to whether hypersexual disorder should be classified as a disease; therefore, there is no consensus on its definition, classification, or diagnostic criteria. This reflects the difficulties in establishing a clear classification standard due to the lack of objective and empirical studies on the factors related to hypersexuality disorder.

Although, the classification of PHB as a disease is still controversial, it has been proposed that excessive sexual activity should be classified as a category of addictive disorders because PHB includes symptoms that are similar to other forms of addiction (Goodman, 2001; Kor et al., 2013). Enhanced desire is strongly related to the clinically relevant aspects of addictive disorders. Imaging studies have shown that the function of brain regions that are involved in desire is altered in those with substance addiction (Garavan et al., 2000; Tapert et al., 2003; Franklin et al., 2007; McClernon et al., 2009). Behavioral addictions, such as gambling, internet gaming, and sexual behavior, that do not involve the direct intake of drugs also involve a heightened desire that seems to be related to altered functions in relevant brain regions (Crockford et al., 2005; Ko et al., 2009; Kühn and Gallinat, 2014; Voon et al., 2014).

Brain imaging studies of desire in substance addiction and behavioral addiction have shown functional changes in the prefrontal cortex (PFC) and subcortical reward circuits in subjects with these disorders (Goldstein and Volkow, 2011). In particular, these studies have identified the key involvement of the PFC in addiction, both through its regulation of limbic reward regions and its involvement in the motivational aspects of repetitive substance use and compulsive behavior. The disrupted functioning of the PFC leads to impairments in response inhibition and salience attribution, such as the attribution of inappropriately excessive salience to an addictive cue, as in substance and addicted behaviors, and a decreased desire for normal rewarding stimuli (Goldman-Rakic and Leung, 2002; Goldstein and Volkow, 2011).

Consistent with these results, the results of a neuroimaging study on PHBs suggested that individuals with PHBs have greater subjective sexual desire compared to healthy controls and that the enhanced desire is associated with different patterns of neural responses in the dorsal anterior cingulate-ventral striatal-amygdala functional network (Voon et al., 2014). In a brain structure and functional connectivity study, Kühn and Gallinat (2014) demonstrated that frequent pornography exposure is associated with altered brain structure and functioning in PFC areas and might lead to a tendency to search for novel and more extreme sexual material.

These studies provide evidence that heightened desire and the functional abnormalities implicated in desire are also involved in PHB, even though the behavior itself does not induce neurotoxic effects.

Unfortunately, the empirical data on sexual desire-associated neural responses in individuals with PHB are insufficient. Previous studies on the brain mechanisms underlying the processing of sexual desire in individuals with PHB have used conventional block paradigms during functional magnetic resonance imaging (fMRI) and a relatively prolonged exposure to erotic stimuli. In studies of sexual desire, the presentation duration appears to be important from a methodological point of view and because of differences in information processing (Bühler et al., 2008). In block designs, the duration of stimulus presentation is prolonged, and the occurrence of continuous stimuli in a block is completely predictable (Zarahn et al., 1997). Therefore, block designs likely activate areas that are associated with cognitive processes, such as sustained attention, top-down control, and the inhibition of sexual arousal. This could lead to reduced emotional involvement and therefore change the underlying neural activity (Schafer et al., 2005). Methodologically, event-related designs are inferior to conventional block designs for detecting activated brain areas, while they are superior for estimating hemodynamic response function (Birn et al., 2002).

Therefore, the objectives of this study were to (1) replicate previous behavioral findings of heightened sexual desire in individuals with PHBs, (2) identify the changes in brain function in regions known to be associated with enhanced desire, and (3) understand the differences in the hemodynamic responses of those brain areas over time in individuals with PHBs by using event-related fMRI. We hypothesized that individuals with PHBs are more likely to show greater sexual desire compared to healthy controls and that brain regions, such as the PFC and subcortical reward circuits, show altered activity and hemodynamic responses compared to healthy controls.

METHODS

Participants

The present study included 23 heterosexual male participants in the PHB group [mean age = 26.12, standard deviation (SD) = 4.11 years] and 22 heterosexual male participants in the control group (mean age = 26.27, *SD* = 3.39 years). Approximately 70 potential participants were recruited from treatment facilities for problematic sexual behavior and Sex Addiction Anonymous meetings. The inclusion criteria were based on the PHB diagnostic criteria of previous studies (Table S1; Carnes et al., 2010; Kafka, 2010). The exclusion criteria were the following: age over 45 or under 18; a serious psychiatric disorder, such as alcohol use disorder, gambling disorder, major depressive disorder, bipolar disorder, or obsessive-compulsive disorder; currently taking medication; a history of serious head injury; homosexuality; a criminal record; or ineligibility for imaging (i.e., having a metal in his body, severe astigmatism, or claustrophobia). The clinicians conducted clinical interviews of all of the potential subjects, and a final group of 23 males who met the inclusion criteria and not the exclusion criteria were selected for the PHB group. For the control group, 22 participants with demographic characteristics (age, gender, education level, and income level) that matched the PHB group were selected. All of the participants provided written informed consents after the contents of the present study were explained to them. The Chungnam National University Institutional Review Board approved the experimental and consent procedures (approval number: 201309-SB-003-01). All of the participants received financial compensation (150 dollars) for their participation.

Measurement Instruments

The participants completed a survey containing questions on their demographic characteristics and sexual activities for the previous 6 months and standardized scales, such as the Barratt Impulsiveness Scale-11 (Patton et al., 1995), Buss-Perry Aggression questionnaire (Buss and Perry, 1992), Beck Depression Inventory (Beck et al., 1996), Beck Anxiety Inventory (Beck et al., 1996), Sexual Addiction Screening Test-R (SAST-R; Carnes et al., 2010), and Hypersexual Behavior Inventory (HBI; Reid et al., 2011; **Table 1**). The questions on sexual behavior were age of first sexual intercourse and current sexual relationship status. An *exclusive sexual situation* was defined as a relationship in which only two individuals engage in sexual intercourse exclusively with each other. A *nonexclusive sexual relationship* was defined as the maintaining of multiple sexual relationships with several different sexual partners without maintaining any sort of intimacy in the relationship.

The questions on sexual activity-related characteristics included the frequency of sexual intercourse per week, the frequency of masturbation per week, the frequency of viewing pornography per week, and the number of total sexual partners in the past 6 months. Furthermore, the SAST-R (Carnes et al., 2010) and HBI (Reid et al., 2011) were used to assess the degree of PHB in the participants. The SAST-R consists of 20 questions designed to assess the degree of sexual addiction. The score ranges from 0 to 20 points, with higher scores indicating more severe sexual addiction. The HBI is comprised of 19 questions, and the score ranges from 19 to 95. A total score of 53 or higher is indicative of a hypersexual disorder. The internal consistencies (Cronbach's α coefficient) of the SAST-R and HBI are 0.91 and 0.96, respectively (Carnes et al., 2010; Reid et al., 2011).

TABLE 1 | Subject characteristics.

	Controls ($n = 22$)	Individuals with PHB ($n = 23$)	*T*-values
Age	26.3 (3.4)	26.1 (4.1)	
Marital Status[a]			
Single	50.0	47.8	
In a relationship	41.0	43.5	
Engaged/Married	9.0	8.7	
Age of first sexual intercourse	20.3 (3.7)	16.7 (5.9)	2.44*
Sexual Relationship Status[a]			
Exclusive	50.0	30.4	
Nonexclusive	13.6	56.5	
Not sexually active	36.4	13.1	
Number of sex partners[b]	2.5 (3.5)	20.9 (27.5)	3.11**
Frequency of sexual intercourse per week[b]	0.5 (0.7)	3.7 (2.6)	5.58***
Frequency of masturbation per week[b]	1.7 (0.9)	5.1 (3.2)	4.80***
Frequency of viewing pornography per week[b]	2.3 (0.6)	5.5 (2.7)	5.42***
Barratt Impulsiveness Scale-11 Score	50.9 (5.5)	52.6 (6.9)	0.91
Buss-Perry Aggression questionnaire Score	37.4 (6.9)	51.5 (16.6)	3.68**
Beck depression inventory score	5.3 (1.6)	7.5 (4.8)	1.53
Beck anxiety inventory score	7.3 (6.4)	8.5 (8.3)	2.04*
Sexual addiction screening test-R score	0.5 (0.9)	11.3 (3.3)	14.82***
Hypersexual behavior inventory score	26.9 (13.5)	54.4 (7.3)	8.55***

PHB, Problematic Hypersexual Behavior.
[a] *Data are represented as percentage.*
[b] *During 6 months; Data are represented as means (standard deviation).*
$^{*}p < 0.05$, $^{**}p < 0.01$, $^{***}p < 0.001$.

Experimental Stimuli and Experimental Paradigm

A prestudy was conducted on 130 men with normal sexual functions who did not participate in the fMRI experiment in order to select the sexual and nonsexual stimuli for the fMRI study (File S1). The visual stimuli consisted of 20 photos that were collected from the International Affective Picture System (6 photos; Lang et al., 2008) and Internet websites (14 photos). The sexual stimuli consisted of photographs depicting naked women and sexual activity. In addition, 20 photos that did not induce any sexual desire were chosen as the nonsexual stimuli. They were matched with the sexual stimuli for their level of pleasantness. The nonsexual stimuli displayed highly arousing scenes, such as water sport activities, celebration of a winning victory, and skiing. These stimuli were chosen in order to identify the brain activity that was solely related to sexual desire by ruling out activity that resulted from feelings of pleasantness and general arousal.

For the fMRI experimental paradigm, brief instructions about the experiment were given for 6 s at the beginning of the experiment, which was followed by the random presentation of either sexual or nonsexual stimuli for 5 s each. Each interstimulus interval was 7–13 s (average, 10 s) to help the participant to return to their baseline state. To keep the participants focused on the stimuli, they were asked to press the response button when an unexpected target was presented for approximately 500 ms for a total of 12 times during any interval. The total time required for the experiment was 8 min and 48 s (**Figure 1**).

After completing the fMRI experiment, the participants watched the same stimuli that were presented in the fMRI experiment, and they were required to respond to the following three questions for a psychological assessment. First, they were asked to respond "yes" or "no" when asked whether they felt sexual desire when they visualized each stimulus. Second, they were required to rate their sexual desire on a five-point Likert scale ranging from 1 (least intense) to 5 (most intense). Third, the participants' subjective ratings on the dimensions of valence and arousal to each stimulus were determined according to a seven-point Likert scale. The ratings were formulated on two dimensions. Valence, which was positive or negative, ranged from very negative at 1 to very positive at 7, and emotional arousal ranged from calm at 1 to excited/aroused at 7. Finally, the participants were required to report any other emotions that they experienced besides sexual desire during their exposure to each stimulus.

Image Acquisition

Image acquisition was performed with a 3.0 T Philips magnetic resonance scanner (Philips Healthcare, Best, The Netherlands).

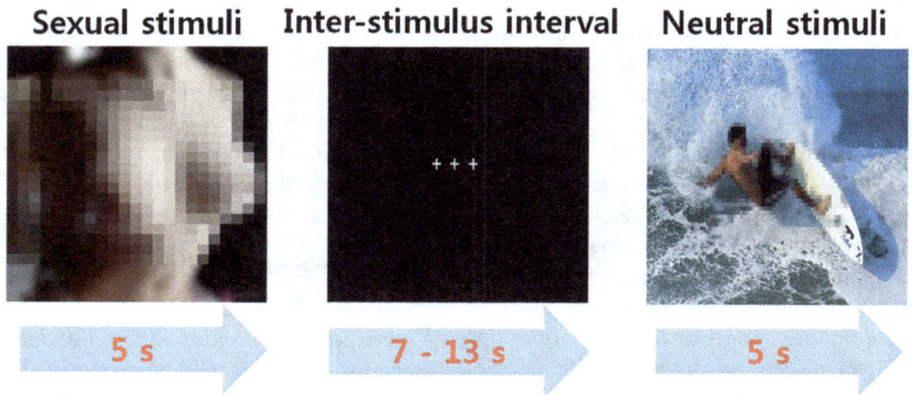

FIGURE 1 | The event-related paradigm for sexual desire.

A single-shot echo-planar imaging fMRI scanning method [imaging variables: repetition time (TR) = 2,000 ms, echo time (TE) = 28 ms, slice thickness = 5 mm with no gap, matrix = 64 × 64, field of view (FOV) = 24 × 24 cm, flip angle = 80°, and in-plane resolution = 3.75 mm] was used to acquire 35 continuous slices of blood oxygen level-dependent (BOLD) images. T1-weighted anatomical images were obtained with a 3-dimensional fluid-attenuated inversion recovery sequence (*TR* = 280, *TE* = 14 ms, flip angle = 60°, *FOV* = 24 × 24 cm, matrix = 256 × 256, and slice thickness = 4 mm).

Statistical Analyses

In order to investigate the behavioral and neural responses that were based solely on sexual desire, the imaging and psychological data for the three pictures that induced other emotions, such as disgust, anger, or surprise, other than sexual arousal were excluded from the data analysis. Independent *t*-tests of the frequencies and intensities of sexual desire between the two groups were performed using SPSS 22 (IBM Corporation, Armonk, NY, USA). The frequency of sexual desire was considered the number of stimuli for which each participant experienced sexual desire from among the total 20 sexual stimuli, and the intensity of sexual arousal was the average level of subjective sexual desire for the 20 erotic pictures.

SPM8 (Wellcome Department of Imaging Neuroscience, London, UK) was used to analyze the fMRI data. In the preprocessing stage, MRI image acquisition was performed in the following order: slice-timing correction for interleaved acquisition, motion correction, and spatial normalization onto a standard template provided by the Montreal Neurological Institute (MNI). Subsequently, the normalized images were smoothed with an 8-mm Gaussian kernel.

After completing the preprocessing, design matrices with two conditions (sexual condition and nonsexual condition) were created for each participant to identify the areas with sexual desire-related activation. Individual first-level analyses of the comparisons of sexual condition minus nonsexual condition were used for a random effects analysis, and mean images were created for each subject. One-sample *t*-tests on the mean images were used to assess the significant group effects in each group in the contrast images created in the individual analyses. Two-sample *t*-tests were conducted to identify the differences between the two groups for the brain responses in the sexual condition relative to the nonsexual condition. Additionally, correlational analyses were conducted only in the PHB group to determine the regions of activation that correlated with the severity of hypersexuality according to the SAST-R. Because the variance of the questionnaire scores might have been too low to reveal more significant correlations in the control group, correlational analyses were not conducted in the control group. P values less than 0.05 (False Discovery Rate, corrected, cluster size ≥ 20) or 0.001 (uncorrected, cluster size ≥ 20) were considered significant for brain activity as these levels are generally accepted in fMRI studies. All of the coordinates of the activated voxels are shown as MNI coordinates in **Tables 3, 4**.

The percent signal change was extracted from the Regions of Interest (ROIs) based on the results of the between-group and correlation analyses [i.e., bilateral thalamus, right dorsolateral prefrontal cortex (DLPFC), left caudate nucleus, right supramarginal gyrus, and right dorsal anterior cingulate gyrus] with MarsBaR (http://www.sourceforge.net/projects/marsbar). The ROIs were created by placing a 5-mm sphere around the coordinates reported in **Tables 3, 4**. In order to examine the temporal characteristics of the hemodynamic responses, the BOLD signal time course was also extracted from the ROIs during the presentation of each sexual stimulus (total of 12 s; 5 s and 7 s thereafter) for all of the participants. The time courses were then averaged across the participants in each group.

As a follow-up test of correlation to calculate the correlation coefficient, the relationships between the scores on the SAST-R and HBI and the percent signal changes in the ROIs based on the results of the correlation analysis (**Table 4**) were analyzed in the PHB group with SPSS 22.

RESULTS

Results of the Psychological Assessments

Of the 20 healthy control subjects, only two reported other emotions besides sexual arousal in response to the three sexual

TABLE 2 | Psychological assessment results.

	Controls ($n = 22$)	Individuals with PHB ($n = 23$)	t
Frequency of sexual desire (%)[a]	50.2 (36.7)	81.6 (28.0)	3.23**
Intensity of sexual desire[b]	0.5 (0.5)	2.6 (0.5)	14.30***
Valence	4.45 (1.41)	4.51 (1.45)	0.14
Arousal	3.53 (1.72)	3.69 (1.70)	0.30

PHB, Problematic Hypersexual Behavior.
*Data are represented as means (standard deviation); **$p < 0.01$, ***$p < 0.001$.*
[a]Represented as percentage of sexual stimuli that evoked sexual desire among 20 erotic pictures.
[b]Degree of sexual desire triggered by the sexual cues on a five-point Likert scale.

stimuli. One participant in the control group reported that two sexual stimuli among the 20 sexual stimuli induced disgust and anger, while the other participant in the control group rated that one sexual picture induced surprise. The three sexual pictures that induced feelings other than sexual arousal were excluded from the data analysis.

An independent t-test indicated no group differences in the dimensions of valence and arousal in response to sexual cues [valence: $t_{(43)} = 0.14$, $p > 0.05$, Cohen's $d = 0.042$; arousal: $t_{(43)} = 0.30$, $p > 0.05$, Cohen's $d = 0.089$]. Additionally, the percentage of sexual stimuli among the 20 erotic pictures that evoked sexual desire showed that the PHB group felt sexual desire more frequently than the control group during exposure to sexual stimuli [$t_{(43)} = 3.23$, $p < 0.01$, Cohen's $d = 0.960$]. The intensity of sexual arousal showed that the PHB group experienced more intense sexual arousal than the control group in response to sexually stimulating photos [$t_{(43)} = 14.3$, $p < 0.001$, Cohen's $d = 4.26$]. The results of the psychological assessments are shown in **Table 2**.

fMRI Results

In the PHB group, activation was observed in the bilateral middle/inferior frontal gyri [Brodmann area (BA) 9], cuneus/precuneus (BA 7, 18, and 19), striatum, thalamus, and cingulate gyri (BA 24 and 32) in response to sexual stimuli compared with nonsexual stimuli. In the control group, activation was displayed in the bilateral middle/inferior frontal gyri (BA 9), cuneus/precuneus (BA 7, 18, and 19), striatum, thalamus, and left cingulate gyrus (BA 24) (corrected False Discovery Rate, $p < 0.05$).

In the between-group analysis, the PHB group exhibited greater activation in the right dorsal anterior cingulate cortex (dACC; BA 24 and 32), bilateral thalami, left caudate nucleus, right DLPFC (BA 9, 46), and right supramarginal gyrus (BA 40) relative to the activation in the control group during exposure to sexual stimuli compared with nonsexual stimuli. No brain regions in the control group showed greater activation than in the PHB group. All of the coordinates for the activated voxels are shown as MNI coordinates in **Tables 3, 4. Figure 2** shows the percent signal changes in the control and PHB groups in each experimental condition (that is, sexual and nonsexual conditions) for the selected ROIs, and **Figure 3** displays the mean time series for each group of the percent signal changes at each time point in the ROIs during the presentation of each sexual stimulus (total of 12 s; 5 and 7 s thereafter) based on the results of the between group analysis.

The correlation analysis of the regions that were related to the SAST-R score demonstrated that the right thalamus and DLPFC (BA 9) were correlated with the SAST-R scores ($p < 0.001$, uncorrected) in the PHB group during the exposure to sexual stimuli, as shown in **Table 4**. The results of the follow-up analysis showed that the percent signal change that was extracted from the right thalamus and DLPFC correlated significantly with the severity of hypersexuality, as shown in **Figure 4**. The percent signal changes in the right thalamus and right DLPFC correlated positively with the SAST-R scores in the PHB group during exposure to sexual stimuli (right thalamus: $r = 0.74$, $n = 23$, $p < 0.01$; right DLPFC: $r = 0.63$, $n = 23$, $p < 0.01$). In addition, the percent signal changes in the right DLPFC and right thalamus

TABLE 3 | Brain regions identified by the group analysis.

Brain regions	P	No. of Voxels in cluster	Cluster z Score	x, y, z MNI coordinates		
INDIVIDUALS WITH PHB < CONTROLS						
No region						
INDIVIDUALS WITH PHB > CONTROLS						
Bilateral thalamus	0.034	129	4.25	6	−36	4
Right dorsolateral prefrontal	0.035	190	3.75	56	10	22
cortex	0.041		3.42	54	16	14
(BA 9, 46)	0.042	22	3.32	46	16	26
Right supramarginal gyrus	0.037	78	3.56	50	−42	32
(BA 40)	0.049		3.01	42	−38	32
Right dorsal cingulate gyrus	0.037	79	3.54	24	16	34
(BA 24, 32)	0.043		3.28	16	10	40
Left caudate nucleus	0.038	53	3.51	−38	−32	2

MNI, Montreal Neurological Institute; PHB, Problematic Hypersexual Behavior; BA, Brodmann area.
Comparison of brain activation between the two groups (PHB group vs. control group) during the sexual condition compared to the nonsexual condition (corrected False Discovery Rate, $p < 0.05$).

TABLE 4 | Brain regions identified in the correlational analysis in the PHB group during exposure to sexual stimuli.

Brain region	p	No. of Voxels in cluster	Cluster z Score	x, y, z MNI coordinates		
Right thalamus	0.001	80	4.25	4	−32	6
Right dorsolateral prefrontal cortex	0.001	22	3.77	56	8	22

PHB, Problematic Hypersexual Behavior; MNI, Montreal Neurological Institute.
Brain regions significantly correlated with Sexual Addiction Screening Test-R (SAST-R) scores during the sexual condition in the PHB group ($p < 0.001$, uncorrected).

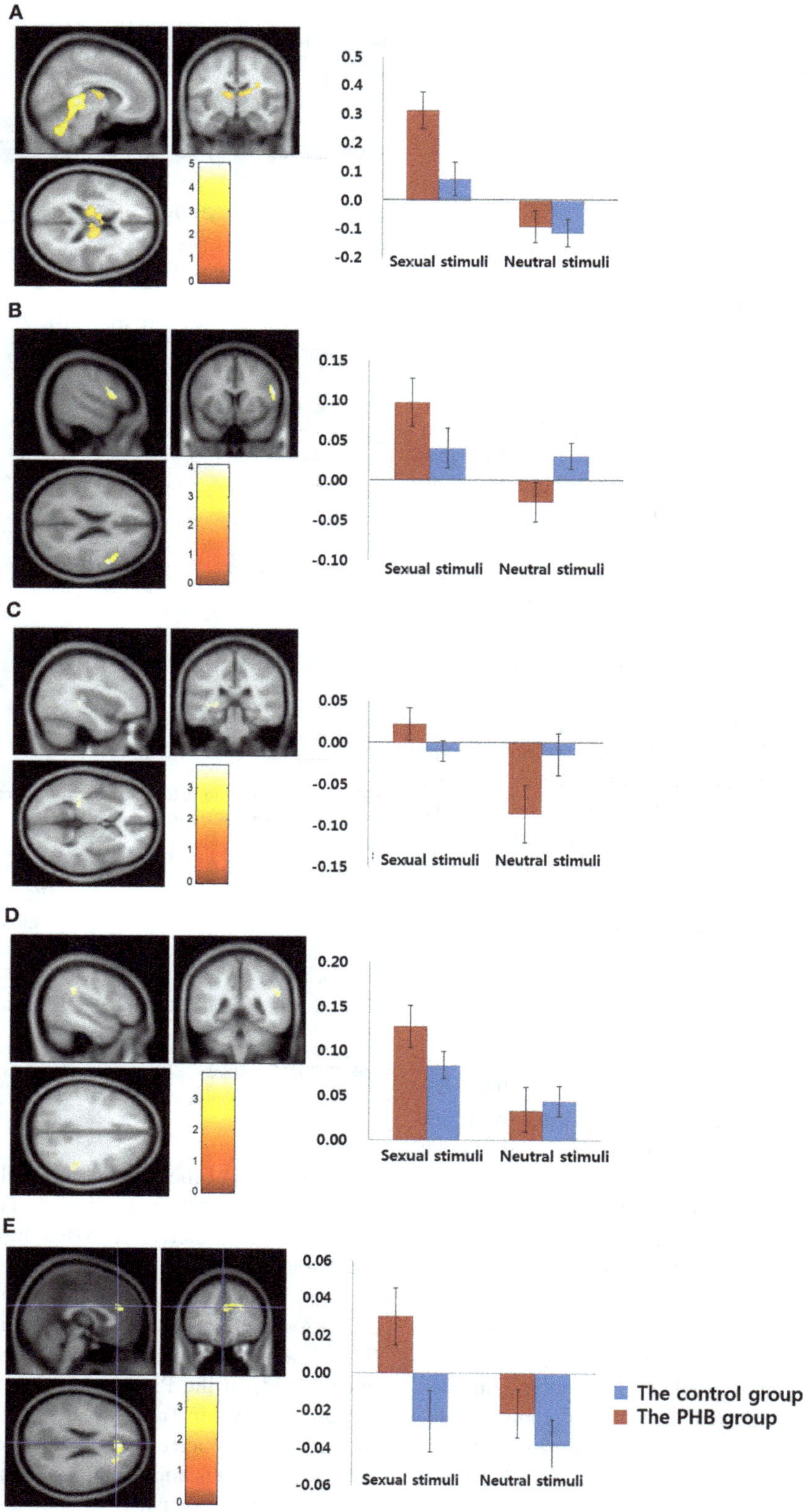

FIGURE 2 | Results of the between-group analysis. (A) Bilateral thalamus (MNI coordinate; $x = 6$, $y = -36$, $z = 4$) **(B)** Right dorsolateral prefrontal cortex (MNI coordinate; $x = 56$, $y = 10$, $z = 22$) **(C)** Left caudate nucleus (MNI coordinate; $x = -38$, $y = -32$, $z = 2$) **(D)** Right supramarginal gyrus (MNI coordinate; $x = 50$, $y = -42$, $z = 32$) **(E)** Right dorsal anterior cingulate gyrus (MNI coordinate; $x = 24$, $y = -16$, $z = 34$). Results of the comparisons of activation in sexual stimuli minus nonsexual stimuli between the PHB and control groups ($p < 0.05$, False Discovery Rate, corrected). The control group and the PHB group are represented as blue and red, respectively. The y-axis shows the percent signal change and the error bars represents Standard Error of the Mean.

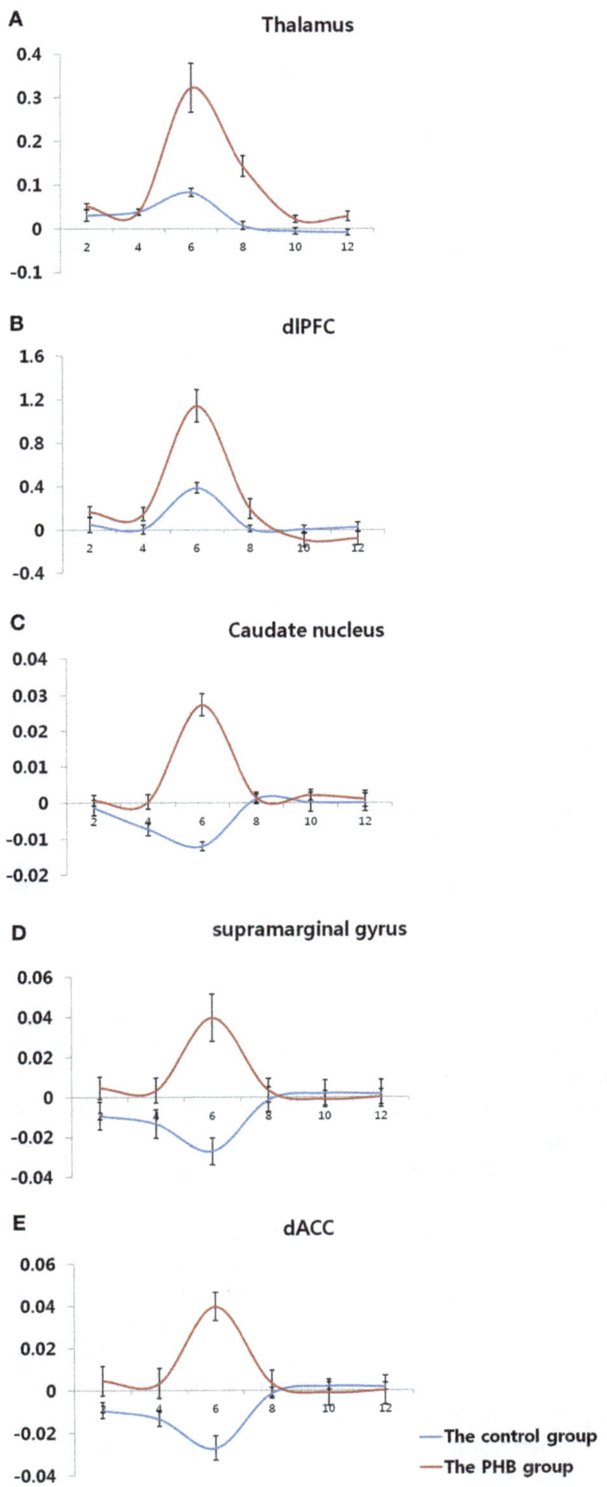

FIGURE 3 | Time course of the hemodynamic responses in each region of interest. (A) Bilateral thalamus (MNI coordinate; $x = 6$, $y = -36$, $z = 4$) **(B)** Right dorsolateral prefrontal cortex (MNI coordinate; $x = 56$, $y = 10$, $z = 22$) **(C)** Left caudate nucleus (MNI coordinate; $x = -38$, $y = -32$, $z = 2$) **(D)** Right supramarginal gyrus (MNI coordinate; $x = 50$, $y = -42$, $z = 32$) **(E)** Right dorsal anterior cingulate gyrus (MNI coordinate; $x = 24$, $y = -16$, $z = 34$). The y-axis and x-axis display the percent signal change and time (s), respectively, and the error bars represent the Standard Error of the Mean.

were positively related to the HBI scores in the PHB group (right thalamus: $r = 0.65$, $n = 23$, $p < 0.01$; right DLPFC: $r = 0.53$, $n = 23$, $p < 0.01$), as shown in **Figure 4**.

DISCUSSION

The present study examined whether there was a difference in the levels of sexual desire between individuals with PHB and healthy controls and, if so, whether this difference was related to functional alterations in the neural substrates of sexual desire in these individuals. As predicted, the PHB group showed significantly heightened levels of sexual desire and altered activation in the PFC and subcortical areas compared to controls. These results suggested that the functional changes in the neural circuitry that mediates cue-induced desire for sexual behavior were similar to those in response to cue presentation in individuals with substance addiction or behavioral addiction (Garavan et al., 2000; Tapert et al., 2003; Crockford et al., 2005; Franklin et al., 2007; Ko et al., 2009; McClernon et al., 2009). Voon et al. (2014) reported abnormal desire and functional changes in regions associated with heightened desire in individuals with compulsive sexual behavior. We replicated and extended these results by investigating the times series of the activation during the total 12 s in the areas associated with sexual desire.

As hypothesized, the analyses of the results of the psychological assessments showed that the PHB group exhibited more frequent sexual desire than the control group during exposure to sexual stimuli, which suggested that this group had a lower threshold for sexual desire. When sexual desire was induced, the PHB group showed a higher intensity of sexual desire than the control group did. This result was consistent with previous findings on individuals with PHB group (Laier et al., 2013; Laier and Brand, 2014; Voon et al., 2014), especially demonstrate that the desire for pornography might play a key role in cybersex addiction.

The results on the brain responses to sexual stimuli dovetail nicely with previous neuroimaging findings that indicated that activity is observed in the brain regions involved in sexual wanting or motivation/anticipation, as well as sexual liking or arousal/consummation, when all of the participants are exposed to sexual stimuli (Georgiadis and Kringelbach, 2012). The results of the group comparisons of the brain imaging revealed altered activation in the right DLPFC (BA 9) and subcortical regions, including the right dACC (BA 24 and 32), left caudate nucleus, right supramarginal gyrus (BA 40), and right thalamus, and these alterations might be associated with the behavioral characteristics of the PHB group. In addition to brain activation, we examined a time series of the hemodynamic responses in these areas during and after the arousal of sexual desire in these areas.

Among these regions, the left caudate nucleus and right ACC (BA 24 and 32) and the right DLPFC are assumed to be associated with the motivational component of sexual desire. The involvement of the caudate nucleus in motivation and reward processing might account for its response to sexual stimuli (Delgado, 2007). The dorsal striatum is activated during reward anticipation (Delgado, 2007), which possibly reflects the

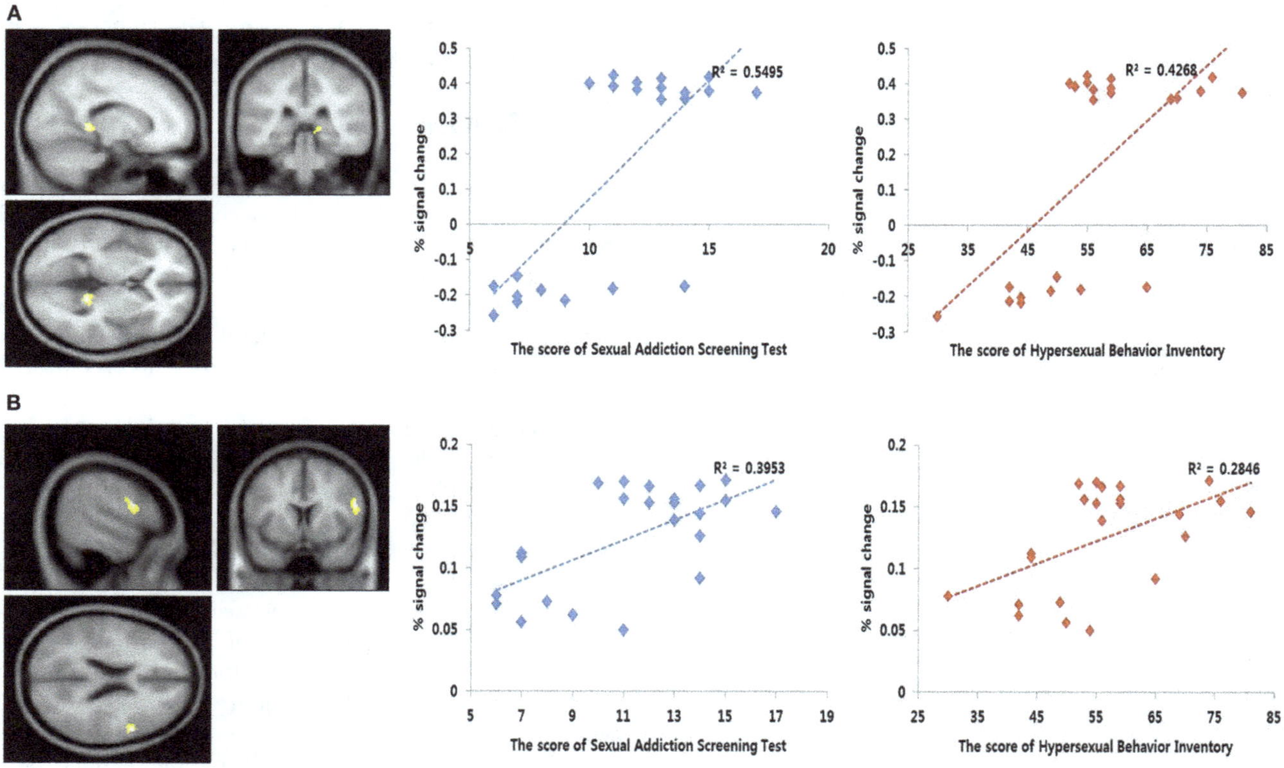

FIGURE 4 | Results of the correlation analysis. Left, functional magnetic resonance imaging (fMRI) correlational analysis. The regions showing significant correlation between the brain activity during sexual desire and the Sexual Addiction Screening Test-R (SAST-R) scores ($p < 0.001$, uncorrected). Right, linear relationship between the percent signal changes extracted from each area and sexual severity scores [i.e., SAST-R and Hypersexual Behavior Inventory (HBI) scores]. The x-axis shows the sexual severity scores, and the y-axis represents the percent signal change. **(A)** Bilateral thalamus (MNI coordinate; $x = 4$, $y = -32$, $z = 6$) **(B)** Right dorsolateral prefrontal cortex (MNI coordinate; $x = 56$, $y = 8$, $z = 22$).

desire that is associated with such anticipation. In a study of the neural responses associated with pornography consumption, frequent activation as a result of pornography exposure might result in the wearing down and downregulation of the striatum, including the caudate nucleus, in healthy controls (Kühn and Gallinat, 2014). However, in the current study, greater activation was observed in the caudate nucleus in the PHB group, even though the PHB group watched pornography more often. These differences between the results of the present study and those of Kühn and Gallinat (2014) might be explained by the difference in the participants. That is, in contrast to the use of healthy male adults in the previous study, our study was conducted on individuals with PHB. Accumulating evidence suggests that the caudate nucleus is important for stimulus-response habit learning and the maintenance of addictive behavior (Vanderschuren and Everitt, 2005). The activation of the caudate nucleus in this study might suggest that sexual cue-reactivity is established after repeated exposure to sexual experience.

The dACC is known to be related to the motivational mechanisms of sexual desire (Redouté et al., 2000; Arnow et al., 2002; Hamann et al., 2004; Ferretti et al., 2005; Ponseti et al., 2006; Paul et al., 2008). Our findings of dACC activation suggest that it has a role in sexual desire, and these results were similar to those of a study on desire-related neural activity in subjects with compulsive sexual behaviors (Voon et al., 2014). In addition, the dACC is known to be important in the initial processing of goal-oriented behavior by engaging in conflict monitoring between the urge for behavioral expression and the suppression of that urge (Devinsky et al., 1995; Arnow et al., 2002; Karama et al., 2002; Moulier et al., 2006; Safron et al., 2007). Neuroanatomically, the dACC projects to the DLPFC and parietal lobe (Devinsky et al., 1995; Pizzagalli et al., 2001). In this study, the activation in the dACC in the PHB group might reflect internal conflict between the urge to express sexual impulses as actions and the urge to suppress the impulses due to situational factors during the presentation of sexual stimuli.

The activation of the supramarginal gyrus is associated with increased attention to targets that are perceived as sexual cues (Redouté et al., 2000; Stoléru et al., 2012). Previous studies have proposed that the increased attention to sexual stimuli plays an important role in maintaining sexual desire (Barlow, 1986; Janssen and Everaerd, 1993) and is related to sexual sensation seeking (Kagerer et al., 2014). In the current study, the supramarginal activation could reflect the greater attention that was paid by PHB subjects to sexual stimuli and that could result in the higher levels of sexual desire compared with the control group.

Among the regions that were significantly activated in the between group results, the DLPFC and thalamus directly correlated with the severity of sexual addiction in the PHB subjects. We observed greater thalamus activation, which was in line with previous findings of studies on sexual arousal (Redouté et al., 2000; Moulier et al., 2006). According to previous studies on sexual desire, the activation of the thalamus is related to the physiological responses (i.e., readiness for sexual activity) that are induced by sexual desire and is positively correlated with penile erection (MacLean and Ploog, 1962; Redouté et al., 2000; Moulier et al., 2006). Interestingly, we also found a higher and wider hemodynamic pattern in the thalamus compared with that in controls. This higher and wider hemodynamic response might indicate that sexual arousal was stronger and prolonged in the individuals with PHB.

Similar to the findings of studies on neural activity in individuals with addiction during cue-induced desire, we found altered PFC function in the PHB group. The PFC plays a critical role in future planning and working memory (Bonson et al., 2002). Neuroanatomically, the PFC is interconnected to various areas, including the dACC, caudate nucleus, and parietal lobe (Devinsky et al., 1995; Pizzagalli et al., 2001; Goldman-Rakic and Leung, 2002). Previous studies on addiction have demonstrated that dysfunction of this network, including the PFC, is related to the PFC's regulation of limbic reward regions and its involvement in higher-order executive function, including self-control, salience attribution, and awareness (Goldman-Rakic and Leung, 2002; Feil et al., 2010; Goldstein and Volkow, 2011; Kühn and Gallinat, 2014). In particular, these studies have identified the disrupted function of DLPFC as an impairment in salience attribution, which results in symptoms, such as the abnormally increased sensitivity to an addictive cue as in substance and addicted behaviors and decreased interest to normal-rewarding stimuli (Goldman-Rakic and Leung, 2002; Goldstein and Volkow, 2011). In the current study, the observation of greater DLPFC activation in the PHB group compared to the control group might reflect excessive salience attribution to sexual cues.

In summary, the PHB group showed greater sexual desire that was associated with altered brain activity. These findings indicate that the PHB group might pay excessive attention to sexual stimuli and that it might have an automatic response because the conditional response to sexual stimuli could not be mediated properly. The limitations of the present study were as follows. First, the race of the subjects was Asian. Second, this study involved only heterosexual male subjects, and future studies involving females and homosexual male subjects should be helpful in better understanding PHB. PHB subjects with co-occurring mental disorders were not enrolled in the present study, thus ensuring the investigation of neural dysfunction based solely on PHB. However, according to a study by Weiss (2004), 28% of males with PHB suffer from major depressive disorder. Taking these factors together limit the generalizability of the study results to the broader universal population. Finally, the two groups may have differed with respect to self-awareness and/or emotional sensitivity due to the treatment of the PHB participants. We tried to decrease the differences between the control and PHB groups by matching for important demographic variables, including age, education level, and handedness, for comparison purposes and by applying strict exclusion criteria, such as the presence of psychiatric disorders and the current use of psychotropic medication, to both groups. Next, we plan to examine how variables that are related to treatment period or treatment type affect the emotional responses, including responses to sexual cues, of individuals with PHB.

Despite these limitations, the results of this study contribute significantly to the literature and have significant implications for future research. We identified specific brain regions that were directly associated with sexual desire and the temporal changes in the activities of these regions among subjects with PHB. Like brain imaging studies on substance and behavior addiction, PHB was related to functional changes in the PFC and subcortical areas, even without the neurotoxicity of drugs. Our results are therefore useful for characterizing the behaviors and associated neural mechanisms of individuals with PHB, and go a step beyond the descriptions of characteristics as in previous studies.

FUNDING

This work was supported by the Korea Basic Science Institute (No. E35600) and research fund of 2014 Chungnam National University.

ACKNOWLEDGMENTS

The authors would like to thank Korea Basic Science Institute for allowing this study to be conducted at the Department of Human Imaging Center by using 3T MRI scanner (Phillips).

REFERENCES

American Psychiatric Association (2013). *Diagnostic and Statistical Manual of Mental Disorders, 5th Edn*. Arlington, VA: American Psychiatric Publishing.

Arnow, B. A., Desmond, J. E., Banner, L. L., Glover, G. H., Solomon, A., Polan, M. L., et al. (2002). Brain activation and sexual arousal in healthy, heterosexual males. *Brain* 125, 1014–1023. doi: 10.1093/brain/awf108

Barlow, D. H. (1986). Causes of sexual dysfunction: the role of anxiety and cognitive interference. *J. Consult. Clin. Psychol.* 54, 140–148. doi: 10.1037/0022-006X.54.2.140

Beck, A. T., Steer, R. A., and Brown, G. K. (1996). *Beck Depression Inventory-II*. San Antonio, TX: Psychological Corporation.

Birn, R. M., Cox, R. W., and Bandettini, P. A. (2002). Detection versus estimation in event-related fMRI: choosing the optimal stimulus timing. *Neuroimage* 15, 252–264. doi: 10.1006/nimg.2001.0964

Black, D. W. (2000). The epidemiology and phenomenology of compulsive sexual behavior. *CNS Spectr.* 5, 26–72. doi: 10.1017/S1092852900012645

Bonson, K. R., Grant, S. J., Contoreggi, C. S., Links, J. M., Metcalfe, J., Weyl, H. L., et al. (2002). Neural systems and cue-induced cocaine craving. *Neuropsychopharmacology* 26, 376–386. doi: 10.1016/S0893-133X(01)00371-2

Bühler, M., Vollstädt-Klein, S., Klemen, J., and Smolka, M. N. (2008). Does erotic stimulus presentation design affect brain activation patterns? Event-related vs. blocked fMRI designs. *Behav. Brain Funct.* 4:30. doi: 10.1186/1744-9081-4-30

Buss, A. H., and Perry, M. (1992). The aggression questionnaire. *J. Pers. Soc. Psychol.* 63, 452–459. doi: 10.1037/0022-3514.63.3.452

Carnes, P. (2013). *Contrary to Love: Helping the Sexual Addict.* Center City, MN: Hazelden Publishing.

Carnes, P., Green, B., and Carnes, S. (2010). The same yet different: refocusing the Sexual Addiction Screening Test (SAST) to reflect orientation and gender. *Sex. Addict. Compuls.* 17, 7–30. doi: 10.1080/10720161003604087

Carnes, P. J. (2001). *Out of the Shadows: Understanding Sexual Addiction.* Center City, MN: Hazelden Publishing.

Coleman, E. (1992). Is your patient suffering from compulsive sexual behavior? *Psychiatr. Ann.* 22, 320–325. doi: 10.3928/0048-5713-19920601-09

Crockford, D. N., Goodyear, B., Edwards, J., Quickfall, J., and el-Guebaly, N. (2005). Cue-induced brain activity in pathological gamblers. *Biol. Psychiatry* 58, 787–795. doi: 10.1016/j.biopsych.2005.04.037

Delgado, M. R. (2007). Reward-related responses in the human striatum. *Ann. N.Y. Acad. Sci.* 1104, 70–88. doi: 10.1196/annals.1390.002

Devinsky, O., Morrell, M. J., and Vogt, B. A. (1995). Contributions of anterior cingulate cortex to behaviour. *Brain* 118, 279–306. doi: 10.1093/brain/118.1.279

Feil, J., Sheppard, D., Fitzgerald, P. B., Yücel, M., Lubman, D. I., and Bradshaw, J. L. (2010). Addiction, compulsive drug seeking, and the role of frontostriatal mechanisms in regulating inhibitory control. *Neurosci. Biobehav. Rev.* 35, 248–275. doi: 10.1016/j.neubiorev.2010.03.001

Ferretti, A., Caulo, M., Del Gratta, C., Di Matteo, R., Merla, A., Montorsi, F., et al. (2005). Dynamics of male sexual arousal: distinct components of brain activation revealed by fMRI. *Neuroimage* 26, 1086–1096. doi: 10.1016/j.neuroimage.2005.03.025

Franklin, T. R., Wang, Z., Wang, J., Sciortino, N., Harper, D., Li, Y., et al. (2007). Limbic activation to cigarette smoking cues independent of nicotine withdrawal: a perfusion fMRI study. *Neuropsychopharmacology* 32, 2301–2309. doi: 10.1038/sj.npp.1301371

Garavan, H., Pankiewicz, J., Bloom, A., Cho, J. K., Sperry, L., Ross, T. J., et al. (2000). Cue-induced cocaine craving: neuroanatomical specificity for drug users and drug stimuli. *Am. J. Psychiatry* 157, 1789–1798. doi: 10.1176/appi.ajp.157.11.1789

Georgiadis, J. R., and Kringelbach, M. L. (2012). The human sexual response cycle: brain imaging evidence linking sex to other pleasures. *Prog. Neurobiol.* 98, 49–81. doi: 10.1016/j.pneurobio.2012.05.004

Goldman-Rakic, P. S., and Leung, H. C. (2002). "Functional architecture of the dorsolateral prefrontal cortex in monkeys and humans," in *Principles of Frontal Lobe Function*, eds D. T. Stuss and R. T. Knight (New York, NY: Oxford University Press), 85–95.

Goldstein, R. Z., and Volkow, N. D. (2011). Dysfunction of the prefrontal cortex in addiction: neuroimaging findings and clinical implications. *Nat. Rev. Neurosci.* 12, 652–669. doi: 10.1038/nrn3119

Goodman, A. (1993). Diagnosis and treatment of sexual addiction. *J. Sex Marital Ther.* 19, 225–251. doi: 10.1080/00926239308404908

Goodman, A. (2001). What's in a name? Terminology for designating a syndrome of driven sexual behavior. *Sexual Addict. Compuls.* 8, 191–213. doi: 10.1080/107201601753459919

Hamann, S., Herman, R. A., Nolan, C. L., and Wallen, K. (2004). Men and women differ in amygdala response to visual sexual stimuli. *Nat. Neurosci.* 7, 411–416. doi: 10.1038/nn1208

Janssen, E., and Everaerd, W. (1993). Determinants of male sexual arousal. *Ann. Rev. Sex Res.* 4, 211–245. doi: 10.1080/10532528.1993.10559888

Kafka, M. P. (2010). Hypersexual disorder: a proposed diagnosis for DSM-V. *Arch. Sex. Behav.* 39, 377–400. doi: 10.1007/s10508-009-9574-7

Kagerer, S., Wehrum, S., Klucken, T., Walter, B., Vaitl, D., and Stark, R. (2014). Sex attracts: investigating individual differences in attentional bias to sexual stimuli. *PLoS ONE* 9:e107795. doi: 10.1371/journal.pone.0107795

Karama, S., Lecours, A. R., Leroux, J. M., Bourgouin, P., Beaudoin, G., Joubert, S., et al. (2002). Areas of brain activation in males and females during viewing of erotic film excerpts. *Hum. Brain Mapp*, 16, 1–13. doi: 10.1002/hbm.10014

Kim, M., and Kwak, J. B. (2011). Youth cybersex addiction in the digital media era. *J. Humanit.* 29, 283–326.

Ko, C. H., Liu, G. C., Hsiao, S., Yen, J. Y., Yang, M. J., Lin, W. C., et al. (2009). Brain activities associated with gaming urge of online gaming addiction. *J. Psychiatr. Res.* 43, 739–747. doi: 10.1016/j.jpsychires.2008.09.012

Kor, A., Fogel, Y., Reid, R. C., and Potenza, M. N. (2013). Should hypersexual disorder be classified as an addiction? *Sex. Addict. Compuls.* 20, 27–47. doi: 10.1080/10720162.2013.768132

Kühn, S., and Gallinat, J. (2014). Brain structure and functional connectivity associated with pornography consumption: the brain on porn. *JAMA Psychiatry* 71, 827–834. doi: 10.1001/jamapsychiatry.2014.93

Kuzma, J. M., and Black, D. W. (2008). Epidemiology, prevalence, and natural history of compulsive sexual behavior. *Psychiatr. Clin. North Am.* 31, 603–611. doi: 10.1016/j.psc.2008.06.005

Laier, C., and Brand, M. (2014). Empirical evidence and theoretical considerations on factors contributing to cybersex addiction from a cognitive-behavioral view. *Sex. Addict. Compuls.* 21, 305–321. doi: 10.1080/10720162.2014.970722

Laier, C., Pawlikowski, M., Pekal, J., Schulte, F. P., and Brand, M. (2013). Cybersex addiction: experienced sexual arousal when watching pornography and not real-life sexual contacts makes the difference. *J. Behav. Addict.* 2, 100–107. doi: 10.1556/JBA.2.2013.002

Lang, P. J., Bradley, M. M., and Cuthbert, B. N. (2008). *International Affective Picture System (IAPS): Affective Ratings of Pictures and Instruction Manual.* Technical Report A-8. Gainesville, FL: University of Florida.

MacLean, P. D., and Ploog, D. W. (1962). Cerebral representation of penile erection. *J. Neurophysiol.* 25, 29–55.

McClernon, F. J., Kozink, R. V., Lutz, A. M., and Rose, J. E. (2009). 24-h smoking abstinence potentiates fMRI-BOLD activation to smoking cues in cerebral cortex and dorsal striatum. *Psychopharmacology* 204, 25–35. doi: 10.1007/s00213-008-1436-9

Moulier, V., Mouras, H., Pélégrini-Issac, M., Glutron, D., Rouxel, R., Grandjean, B., et al. (2006). Neuroanatomical correlates of penile erection evoked by photographic stimuli in human males. *Neuroimage* 33, 689–699. doi: 10.1016/j.neuroimage.2006.06.037

Patton, J. H., Stanford, M. S., and Barratt, E. S. (1995). Factor structure of the Barratt Impulsiveness Scale. *J. Clin. Psychol.* 51, 768–774.

Paul, T., Schiffer, B., Zwarg, T., Krüger, T. H., Karama, S., Schedlowski, M., et al. (2008). Brain response to visual sexual stimuli in heterosexual and homosexual males. *Hum. Brain Mapp.* 29, 726–735. doi: 10.1002/hbm.20435

Pizzagalli, D., Pascual-Marqui, R. D., Nitschke, J. B., Oakes, T. R., Larson, C. L., Abercrombie, H. C., et al. (2001). Anterior cingulate activity as a predictor of degree of treatment response in major depression: evidence from brain electrical tomography analysis. *Am. J. Psychiatry* 158, 405–415. doi: 10.1176/appi.ajp.158.3.405

Ponseti, J., Bosinski, H. A., Wolff, S., Peller, M., Jansen, O., Mehdorn, H. M., et al. (2006). A functional endophenotype for sexual orientation in humans. *Neuroimage* 33, 825–833. doi: 10.1016/j.neuroimage.2006.08.002

Redouté, J., Stoléru, S., Grégoire, M. C., Costes, N., Cinotti, L., Lavenne, F., et al. (2000). Brain processing of visual sexual stimuli in human males. *Hum. Brain Mapp.* 11, 162–177. doi: 10.1002/1097-0193(200011)11:3<162::AID-HBM30>3.0.CO;2-A

Reid, R. C., Garos, S., and Carpenter, B. N. (2011). Reliability, validity, and psychometric development of the Hypersexual Behavior Inventory in an outpatient sample of men. *Sex. Addict. Compuls.* 18, 30–51. doi: 10.1080/10720162.2011.555709

Safron, A., Barch, B., Bailey, J. M., Gitelman, D. R., Parrish, T. B., and Reber, P. J. (2007). Neural correlates of sexual arousal in homosexual and heterosexual men. *Behav. Neurosci.* 121, 237–248. doi: 10.1037/0735-7044.121.2.237

Schafer, A., Schienle, A., and Vaitl, D. (2005). Stimulus type and design influence hemodynamic responses towards visual disgust and fear elicitors. *Int. J. Psychophysiol.* 57, 53–59. doi: 10.1016/j.ijpsycho.2005.01.011

Schneider, J. P., and Schneider, B. (1991). *Sex, Lies, And Forgiveness: Couples Speaking Out On Healing From Sex Addiction.* Center City, MN: Hazeldon Publishing.

Seegers, J. A. (2003). The prevalence of sexual addiction symptoms on the college campus. *Sex. Addict. Compuls.* 10, 247–258. doi: 10.1080/713775413

Stoléru, S., Fonteille, V., Cornélis, C., Joyal, C., and Moulier, V. (2012). Functional neuroimaging studies of sexual arousal and orgasm in healthy men and women: a review and meta-analysis. *Neurosci. Biobehav. Rev.* 36, 1481–1509. doi: 10.1016/j.neubiorev.2012.03.006

Tapert, S. F., Cheung, E. H., Brown, G. G., Frank, L. R., Paulus, M. P., Schweinsburg, A. D., et al. (2003). Neural response to alcohol stimuli in adolescents with alcohol use disorder. *Arch. Gen. Psychiatry* 60, 727–735. doi: 10.1001/archpsyc.60.7.727

Vanderschuren, L. J., and Everitt, B. J. (2005). Behavioral and neural mechanisms of compulsive drug seeking. *Eur. J. Pharmacol.* 526, 77–88. doi: 10.1016/j.ejphar.2005.09.037

Voon, V., Mole, T. B., Banca, P., Porter, L., Morris, L., Mitchell, S., et al. (2014). Neural correlates of sexual cue reactivity in individuals with and without compulsive sexual behaviours. *PLoS ONE* 9:e102419. doi: 10.1371/journal.pone.0102419

Weiss, D. (2004). The prevalence of depression in male sex addicts residing in the United States. *Sex. Addict. Compulsivity* 11, 57–69. doi: 10.1080/10720160490458247

Zarahn, E., Aguirre, G., and D'Esposito, M. (1997). A trial-based experimental design for fMRI. *Neuroimage* 6, 122–138. doi: 10.1006/nimg.1997.0279

Conflict of Interest Statement: The authors declare that the research was conducted in the absence of any commercial or financial relationships that could be construed as a potential conflict of interest.

17

Hoarders only Discount Consumables and are more Patient for Money

Edited by:
Matthias Brand,
University of Duisburg-Essen, Germany

***Correspondence:**
Stephanie D. Preston
prestos@umich.edu

†Present address:
Andrea M. Angott,
SciMed Solutions, Durham, NC, USA

Brian D. Vickers, Stephanie D. Preston*, Richard Gonzalez and Andrea M. Angott†

Department of Psychology, University of Michigan, Ann Arbor, MI, USA

Individuals with hoarding disorder (HD) excessively acquire and retain goods while also exhibiting characteristics of impulsivity and addiction. However, HD individuals do not always perform impulsively in experiments, they do not appear interested in money, and they exhibit many features of risk-aversion and future-planning. To examine impulsivity in HD, we compared validated community participants high and low in hoarding tendencies on questionnaire measures of hoarding and impulsivity as well as a standard experimental measure of impulsivity (intertemporal discounting) that was modified to compare decisions about money, pens, and snacks. Common discounting effects were replicated. Compared to the low hoarding group, the high hoarding group was more impatient for consumables (pens and snacks) but they were more patient for money. This increased patience for money in high hoarding individuals is in contrast to all other studies on discounting in disordered populations, but consistent with the phenomenology of HD. HD does not appear to be driven by a fundamental inability to wait, but rather a specific, potent desire for consumable rewards.

Keywords: hoarding disorder, discounting, impulsivity, addiction, consumption

INTRODUCTION

Individuals with hoarding disorder (HD) are characterized by their excessive acquisition and retention of goods with limited or no value, leading to significantly cluttered living spaces that cannot be used for their original purpose, and significant associated distress and life impairment (Frost and Hartl, 1996). HD now occupies its own diagnostic category in the DSM-V under the OCD and related disorders section (American Psychological Association [APA], 2013), but it is often comorbid with other impulsive-compulsive disorders, including OCD, compulsive buying, gambling, and trichotillomania (Samuels et al., 2002; Frost et al., 2011), leading some to characterize it as one of an extended family of compulsive–impulsive spectrum disorders (e.g., see McElroy et al., 1995). HD also shares many features with addiction, which is also considered by many to be a disorder of impulsivity (reviewed in Bickel and Marsch, 2001; Perry and Carroll, 2008; Odum, 2011). Like addiction, HD involves prioritizing rewarding items over other important life priorities like safety, shelter, and social relationships; it is associated with neural changes in the mesolimbocortical system (reviewed in Wang et al., 2012); and it is difficult to remit even if there are some promising treatment options (Tolin et al., 2015). Thus, despite now occupying its own diagnostic category, transdiagnostic approaches need to continue to understand the role of impulsivity in HD (e.g., Tolin and Villavicencio, 2011; Rasmussen et al., 2013; Timpano et al., 2013).

There is empirical evidence that HD individuals are more impulsive than comparison individuals (comparison groups range across studies from typical community samples to clinical groups with and without hoarding symptoms). However, the evidence is more consistent when individual differences measures are used than when experimental tasks are used. This inconsistency likely reflects the fact that there are multiple, distinct constructs associated with impulsivity including risk seeking, present-focus, response inhibition, loss of control, and delay discounting (see Perry and Carroll, 2008). HD individuals scored more highly on multiple impulsive action and inattention individual difference survey measures (Grisham et al., 2007; Tolin and Villavicencio, 2011; Timpano et al., 2013). They were also more impulsive on a signal detection task despite performing the task more slowly (Grisham et al., 2007) and they had poorer response inhibition on this task, but this appears to be because the HD participants were older than the control participants (Rasmussen et al., 2013). In one study, HD individuals preferred the larger, more immediate reward on the Iowa Gambling Task (Lawrence et al., 2006), but they performed like controls in two other studies using the same task (Grisham et al., 2007; Tolin and Villavicencio, 2011). Thus, evidence for impulsivity in HD is more questionable to date for experimental data, and research has yet to compare HD individuals to controls on a common experimental measure of impulsivity in behavioral economics—the intertemporal discounting task (ITD).

Beyond experimental inconsistencies linking HD to impulsivity, multiple facts question the assumption that HD individuals do have a domain-general problem with impulsivity. HD individuals do not impulsively acquire or keep money and, in fact, they use money especially frugally to obtain goods (Samuels et al., 2008; Frost et al., 2009). The documented paranoid personality traits in HD and their excessive fear of events like home break-ins (Samuels et al., 2008), as well as their indecision and perfectionism (Frost and Gross, 1993), are also characteristics that are more associated with risk-aversion and a future-focus that is unlike that associated with addiction or trait impulsivity (Loewenstein et al., 2001). The goal of hoarding behavior *per se* can also be construed as fundamentally risk-avoidant and future-oriented, as individuals acquire and protect resources that they think they may need later (Frost and Hartl, 1996)—much like the way food-storing animals create, maintain, and protect hoards of food to prepare for future scarcities (Preston and Jacobs, 2001, 2005; Preston, 2013). The hoarding in HD also results in significant interpersonal conflict, discomfort, and difficulty using living spaces (Frost et al., 2000), which could be construed as a short term pain that is being suffered in order to provide a long-term benefit or protection from risk—again unlike impulsivity. Thus, from a global perspective, hoarding behavior actually bears many hallmarks of extreme patience, at least regarding the ultimate goal of the behavior. HD individuals may simply report fears about future needs to mask an irrational impulse to acquire; however, it is also possible that their impulsiveness is a proximate mechanism by which HD individuals achieve a genuine, ultimate goal to provide for the future.

Taken together, impulsiveness in HD needs to be examined empirically, across domains, particularly using the standard, accepted laboratory task for measuring impulsivity in the addiction literature—the ITD. On a typical ITD trial, participants are asked to make a forced choice between accepting a smaller quantity of a reward sooner (e.g., $5 today) vs. a larger quantity of the reward later (e.g., $12 in a month). The exact quantities of the reward sooner vs. later and the precise latency that participants have to wait for each option are systematically altered over many otherwise identical trials so that a "discounting rate" can be calculated per person, over time, representing the degree to which they are susceptible to prefer a smaller amount when delivered sooner—the operationalization of impulsivity.

The current study compared individuals with high and low hoarding tendencies on their intertemporal discounting for goods, food, and money. Most hoarding studies only examine the degree to which individuals acquire or fail to discard material goods; however, we included food because we were interested in the degree to which hoarding reflects an evolved, adaptive food-storing instinct shared with other species (Preston, 2013). We also included money not only because it is the typical unit of reward for ITD tasks in behavioral economics, but also because we hypothesized that high hoarding participants would not be uniformly impulsive, based on anecdotal reports and case studies suggesting that HD individuals are not interested in money *per se*. It is also useful for the large ITD literature to realize that not all individuals are highly motivated by money, which is almost always the only reward provided or compared in behavioral economic studies. Based on our evolutionary view and the phenomenological reports of HD, we predicted that high hoarding individuals would be impulsive for goods and food (pens and snacks), but not money.

MATERIALS AND METHODS

Participants

In order to ensure a broad distribution of hoarding tendencies, participants were recruited using two different advertisements for a decision making study, one that specifically asked for participants who would consider themselves "packrats" and another that did not specify. Of the 38 participants, 27 were community members of any adult age who were compensated $10 for participation (16 high hoarding from the packrat advertisement and 11 low hoarding from the unspecified advertisement). The remaining 11 participants were recruited and compensated with course credit through the university psychology pool (three high hoarding, eight low hoarding). All participants were female, which is common in HD studies (e.g., Frost and Gross, 1993) and practical, given a strong bias for females to respond to community advertisements looking for "packrats" (hereafter referred to as the "high hoarding" group when not discussing the advertisement itself).

This was a study of individual differences rather than the clinical diagnostic category of HD. As such, participants were not given an official clinical interview or diagnosis and they are not referred to here as hoarders or individuals with HD. Instead, we placed participants into high and low hoarding groups based on their response to the advertisements and a validated clinical instrument with high specificity and sensitivity for detecting hoarding with scores >14 on the Hoarding Rating Scale (HRS) (Tolin et al., 2010). The HRS is typically administered in a clinical setting using an interview format, but we have adapted it into an easy-to-administer self-report questionnaire that reliably demonstrates individual differences in the non-clinical population, which also correlate with other individual difference measures that are commonly elevated in HD and with a longer published, validated hoarding questionnaires [i.e., the Savings Inventory-Revised (SI-R); Frost et al., 2004] (see, Wang et al., 2012). To ensure a clear distinction between low and high hoarding participants, rather than just split participants by the advertisement they responded to or whether their HRS scores were above or below of 14, we allowed participants to be placed into the high hoarding group regardless of which advertisement they responded to if they had an HRS scores > 19 (median = 27.00, mean = 26.74, SD = 4.96; n = 19, mean age = 35.05, SD = 17.42) and we allowed participants to be placed into the low hoarding group, regardless of which ad they responded to, if they had an HRS score < 13 (median = 4.00, mean = 4.53, SD = 4.03; n = 19, mean age = 48.21, SD = 15.20). Participants with HRS scores between 13 and 19 were excluded. The two groups did differ statistically in age, $t(36) = 2.48$, $p = 0.018$, $\eta_p^2 = 0.146$, but in the direction opposite to the predicted confound, as usually HD individuals are older but our high hoarding individuals were younger than our low hoarding individuals. Age was used as a factor in analysis (below) and did not influence the results. High and low hoarding participants did not differ statistically on income, based on results from the Happiness Spending Inventory (Dunn et al., 2008) that we administered for another study completed by the same participants, $t(36) = 1.04$, $p = 0.306$.

Participants were consented and tested individually in the laboratory using MediaLab (Jarvis, 2006) on a Dell desktop PC. All participants were consented and debriefed in writing and in person; all procedures were approved by the Institutional Review Board of the University of Michigan.

Intertemporal Discounting Task

The ITD task used in this study consisted of three blocks (order randomized) of intertemporal choices about money, pens, or snacks. Units were equilibrated across domains as money was listed in whole dollars and pen and snack choices were worth approximately one dollar each. Participants selected their favorite pen or snack from an array, and all choices thereafter used their chosen item to ensure task interest (e.g., Easy Touch or Precise Gel pens; M&M or Oreo snacks). Each block consisted of 45 choices between a smaller reward (x_1) sooner (t_1) or a larger reward (x_2) later (t_2) (see **Table 1**). Reward quantities (0–85) and delays (now to 135 days from now) varied across trials.

Before each block participants would select their most preferred stimulus for that domain (e.g., Easy Touch vs. Precise Gel pens in the pen domain). Then, each trial would show them a choice between a smaller amount of their selected item sooner or a larger amount of that same item later, such as 3 Easy Touch pens today or 12 Easy Touch pens in 19 days. The task was self-paced including the length of the break between each of the three blocks. The task within each domain included nine trials used in a prior ITD study of addiction (Kirby et al., 1999), plus 36 more trials that we added to measure responses to smaller and larger quantities and shorter and longer delays than was previously included (described in full below), and to systematically investigate different aspects of the choice attributes. This led to a total of 135 trials for each participant.

Additional trial types were included to expand upon results in four ways. A set of trials at small x_1, x_2 values was included to test whether discounting effects are present even for relatively small amounts. Another set of trials systematically varied time and quantity to more precisely estimate how changes in time and quantity influence choice. The final two types of trials investigated whether high or low hoarding participants were more likely to violate assumptions of typical discounting models. Exponential discounting assumes a steadily decreasing likelihood of choosing the larger later (LL) option as the time to acquire it increases at a rate proportional to $\frac{1}{1+t}$, where t is time. Power utility is based on the fact that people value increasing amounts less (i.e., diminishing utility); power utility requires that if amounts are both multiplied by a constant, then choices should not change (see **Table 2** for a summary of the specific trials). Because the present study used amounts in three different domains (money, pens, snacks) it is important to distinguish whether patterns of choice are due to changes in the utility of the amount or to changes in the discounting of time. Different discounting patterns could arise when comparing, say, choices for money and choices for pens, not because participants discount time differentially in those two domains but because they value increments in the amounts differentially. The ability to separate utility from discounting comes from our design where we systematically manipulate elements of the amounts and time in each trial.

Psychopathological Symptoms

After the ITD, participants completed psychopathology inventories that could be correlated with differences in impulsivity emerging from the task, including the HRS, SI-R, Obsessive Compulsive Inventory-Revised (OCI-R; Foa et al., 2002), Barratt Impulsivity Scale (BIS; Patton and Stanford, 1995), Beck Anxiety Inventory (BAI; Beck et al., 1988a), and Beck Depression Inventory II (BDI; Beck et al., 1988b). All survey measures were administered after the ITD task to avoid priming participants with issues related to their psychopathology before the task.

Analysis

To assess overall discounting, the more impulsive, SS responses were recoded as 0 and the more patient, LL responses were recoded as 1. Results are presented in terms of the proportion of LL choices, representing the degree of patience or willingness to wait longer for the larger reward. But as is common in the behavioral economics literature, any time a participant or group is referred to as having a higher or steeper discount rate, that

TABLE 1 | Trials in the Intertemporal Discounting Task (ITD), sorted by trial type.

Trial type	Options				Analysis Subsection			
	x_1	t_1	x_2	t_2	Increasing the later reward	Increasing the reward and delay	Exponential discounting	Power utility function
Small quantities, now or later								
	1	0	2	16	1			
	1	0	4	16	1			
	1	0	6	16	1			
	1	0	8	16	1			
	1	0	10	16	1			
	0	0	1	7				
	3	0	12	19				
	5	0	8	7				
	10	0	30	40				
Moderate quantities, now or later								
	14	0	25	4		1		
	19	0	25	38		2		
	24	0	35	14		3		
	27	0	50	6		4		
	34	0	50	15		5		
	40	0	55	47		6		
	41	0	75	5		7		
	54	0	80	15		8		
	55	0	75	46		9		
Moderate quantities, now or later (original Kirby items)								
	14	0	25	19		1		
	19	0	25	53		2	1	
	24	0	35	29		3		
	27	0	50	21		4	3	
	34	0	50	30		5		
	40	0	55	62		6		
	41	0	75	20		7		
	54	0	80	30		8		
	55	0	75	61		9	2	
Moderate quantities, now or much later								
	14	0	25	79		1		
	19	0	25	113		2		
	24	0	35	89		3		
	27	0	50	81		4		
	34	0	50	90		5		
	40	0	55	122		6		
	41	0	75	80		7		
	54	0	80	90		8		
	55	0	75	121		9		
Larger quantities, all delayed								
	44	32	60	93				1
	55	32	75	93			2	1
	66	32	90	93				1
	32	28	44	90				2
	48	28	66	90				2
	19	20	25	73			1	
	27	15	50	36			3	
	40	28	55	29				
	69	44	85	135				

Options denoted as in the text with x_1 representing the smaller amount, t_1 the sooner time, x_2 the larger amount, and t_2 the later time; all choices were presented as pairs of (x_1, t_1 vs. x_2, t_2). Original Kirby items were taken from Kirby et al. (1999). Trials with very small quantities offered now or after a delay were added to their set as were trials that offered their moderate reward amounts with a smaller or a larger delay than they used. New items were added to test specific functional forms and to separate delay from amount. The separate subsections of analysis are presented in the final four columns, with numbers depicting which trials (rows) were relevant for that comparison.

TABLE 2 | Subcategories of trials added to examine different attributes of discounting.

Subcategory	Trials	Variables		
		Manipulated	Fixed	Test
Later reward	5	x_2	x_1, t_1, t_2	Increasing later reward from small x_2
Delay and moderate reward amounts	27	t_2	t_1; x_1, x_2	Increasing longer delay
Adding a constant to Time	6	t_1, t_2	x_1, x_2	Increasing time by the same amount for both ts; Exponential discounting
Multiplying amounts by constant	5	x_1, x_2	t_1, t_2	Increasing amount by the same amount for both xs; power utility

Each subcategory is listed below with the number of trials per domain, which variables were manipulated vs. held constant, and the attribute of interest. x_1, smaller amount, x_2, larger amount, t_1, sooner time, t_2, later time.

means that they value the more patient LL option less in favor of the more impulsive SS option.

All contrasts used the following model except where noted: a logistic curve was fit using a logistic hierarchical linear model (HLM) including fixed factors for group (low hoarding = 0; high hoarding = 1), domain (money, pen, snack), their interaction, and a random factor for each participant's intercept. Planned contrasts compared discounting money vs. consumables (pens and snacks together) (2, −1, −1) and pens vs. snacks (0, 1, −1). All discounting results remained after separately controlling for age or participant population (community vs. psychology pool), but a few small shifts in result thresholds are noted below under individual difference correlations.

RESULTS

Analyses are organized by comparing overall discounting rates first, followed by the specific tests for the degree to which choices were influenced by delay and quantity, followed by tests to examine behavioral consistency with both exponential and power law forms of discounting (defined below).

Overall Discounting

Overall rates of discounting were not different in the two groups, $\chi^2(1) = 1.35$, $p = 0.25$, but they did differ by domain, $\chi^2(2) = 7.97$, $p = 0.021$, and the two interacted, $\chi^2(2) = 105.76$, $p < 0.001$. Money was discounted less than consumables overall, odds ratio (OR) = 1.10, $z = 2.76$, $p = 0.006$, and the difference in discounting money compared to pens and snacks was 61% larger in high hoarding than low hoarding participants, money vs. consumables contrast by group: $OR = 1.61$, $z = 10.17$, $p < 0.001$. This interaction was due to high hoarding individuals discounting pens and snacks more steeply than low hoarders and money less steeply than low hoarders, and low hoarders discounting all three domains at similar levels. The contrast between pens and snacks was also marginally larger in high than low hoarders, $OR = 0.86$, $z = -1.78$, $p = 0.075$, with high hoarders responding more impulsively for pens than for snacks, $OR = 0.85$, $z = -2.81$, $p = 0.005$, and low hoarders again treating them similarly, $OR = 0.98$, $z = -0.35$, $p = 0.729$ (see **Figure 1A**). These main effects and interactions were consistent across the subsets of trial types reported below and so are not re-presented in each subsection.

Effect of the Later Reward Amount with a Fixed Early Reward and Delay

This subset of trials examined the effect on choice of increasing the larger amount (x_2 = 2, 4, 6, 8, 10) while fixing the smaller amount ($x_1 = 1$) and fixing the delay periods ($t_1 = 0$, $t_2 = 16$ days). The logistic HLM with a centered x_2 parameter found that people generally waited longer as the amounts increased, x_2 effect: $OR = 1.33$, $z = 4.95$, $p < 0.001$, and this effect did not differ between high and low hoarding individuals, $OR = 1.03$, $z = 0.37$, $p = 0.711$. As with the overall discounting effects above, as later quantities increased people were still more patient for money than for consumables, domain effect: $\chi^2(2) = 7.30$, $p = 0.026$; money vs. consumables: $OR = 1.24$, $z = 2.00$, $p = 0.046$, and waited marginally longer for more pens than for more snacks, $OR = 0.71$, $z = -1.86$, $p = 0.063$. At these low reward values, there was no omnibus group difference between money and consumables, group by money vs. consumables: $OR = 1.22$, $z = 1.29$, $p = 0.196$, but high hoarding individuals were more impulsive for snacks than pens while low hoarding individuals were more impulsive for pens than snacks, group by pens vs. snacks: $OR = 2.13$, $z = 2.97$, $p = 0.003$. These slopes across values of x_2 did not significantly interact by domain and group, x_2 by domain by group interaction, $\chi^2(2) = 0.70$, $p = 0.704$. Thus, small and increasing quantities of the larger, later reward (holding the three terms x_1, t_1, and t_2 fixed) reveals no difference in impulsivity for money compared to consumables as x_2 increases, and at these small amounts high hoarding individuals actually wait longer to acquire more pens than snacks compared to controls (see **Figure 1B**).

Effect of the Delay and Moderate Reward Amounts with a Fixed Initial Time (Now)

A second subset of trials compared choices between nine original trials (Kirby et al., 1999) to two identical types that varied t_2 to be earlier or later than the original one. The initial time was fixed to deliver immediate reward ($t_1 = 0$), and the early

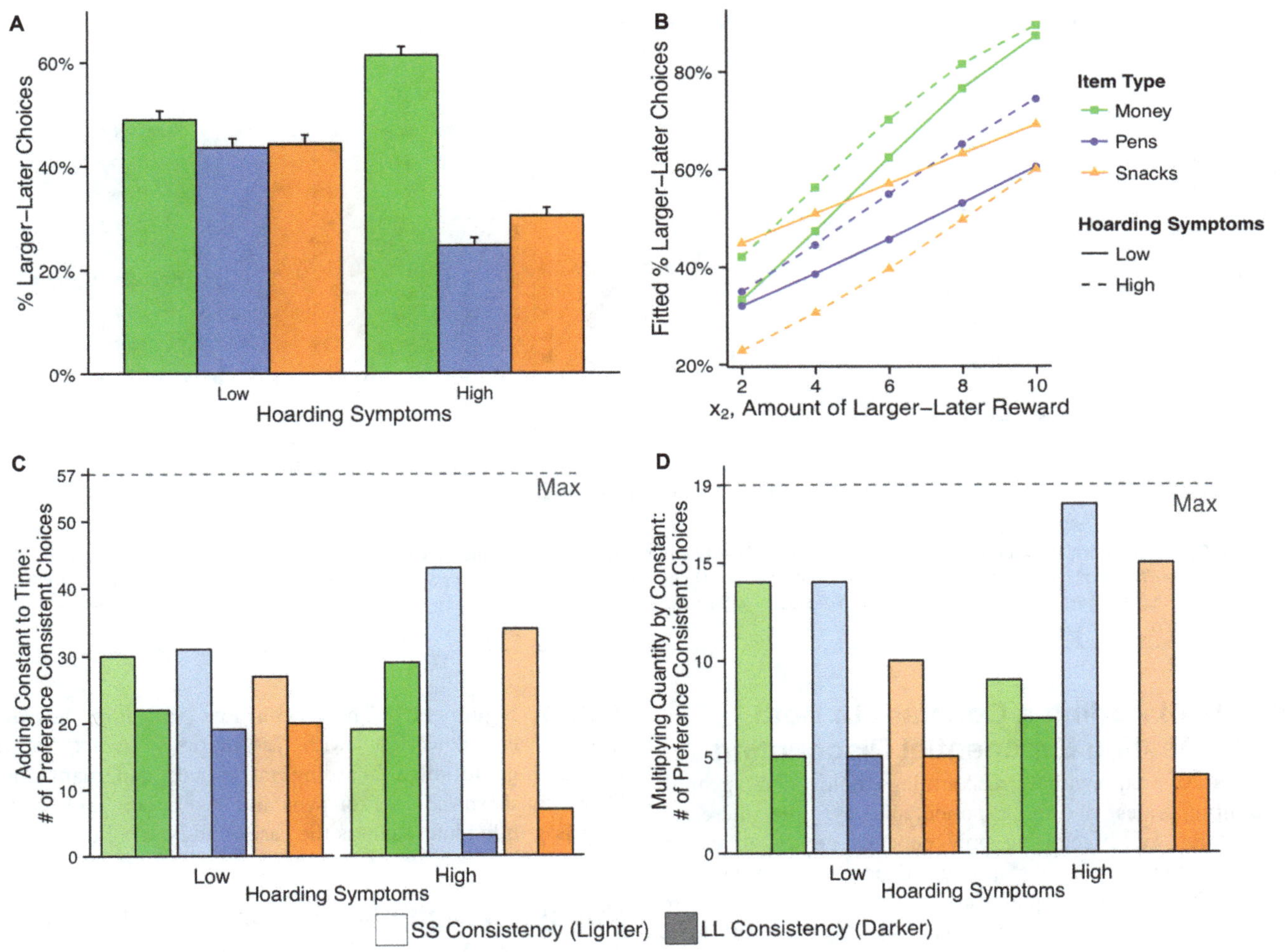

FIGURE 1 | Intertemporal discounting responses by group (high hoarding vs. low hoarding individuals) and domain (money, pens, snacks). Percent of participants choosing the larger-later (LL) option overall **(A)**; effects of the increasing later reward amount with a fixed early reward and delay **(B)**; effects of adding a constant to both times **(C)**; effects of a constant multiplier **(D)**. In all plots, choices for money are represented with green coloration, pens in blue, and snacks in orange. For **(B)**, low hoarding individuals are represented by solid lines and high hoarding individuals are represented by dashed lines. For **(C,D)**, the number of times participants made consistent SS choices are in the lighter shade and the number of times participants made consistent LL choices are in the darker shade.

and later reward were moderately sized and fixed within sets of three choices (e.g., $x_1 = 24$, $x_2 = 35$) (see **Table 1**). HLM analyses compared the effect of the delay within sets of three trials (original t_2, earlier t_2, later t_2) and the effect of the total amount of reward across the nine sets of three trials. A parameter was added to the HLM for t_2, ordering each of the nine triplets by their mean x_1, x_2 amounts to assess quantity effects with a centered linear "quantity contrast." This analysis complements the previous one by changing which variable was manipulated while leaving the others constant. Previously we only varied the second quantity and this time we only varied the length of the larger delay interval while holding the other three parameters fixed.

As the t_2 delay increased, participants generally became increasingly impatient for money compared to consumables, t_2 by money vs. consumables: $OR = 0.99$, $z = -4.47$, $p < 0.001$, and more impatient for pens than snacks, t_2 by domain omnibus: $\chi^2(2) = 26.85$, $p < 0.001$; t_2 by pens vs. snacks: $OR = 0.994$, $z = -2.54$, $p = 0.011$. But looking separately at each group, only low hoarding individuals showed this increasing impatience with longer delays for money and pens, t_2 by group by domain: $\chi^2(2) = 11.77$, $p = 0.003$; t_2 by domain in high hoarding individuals: $\chi^2(2) = 0.37$, $p = 0.831$; t_2 by domain in low hoarding individuals: $\chi^2(2) = 27.03$, $p < 0.001$; t_2 by money vs. consumables in low hoarding individuals: $OR = 0.993$, $z = -4.48$, $p < 0.001$; t_2 by pen vs. snack in low hoarding individuals: $OR = 0.994$, $z = -2.55$, $p = 0.011$. There were no effects of the amount of moderate reward or any other effects in this model, χ^2s < 2.55, $ps > 0.115$ (see **Figure 2**). Therefore, low hoarding individuals had high discount rates for money compared to consumables (i.e., would only choose LL after short delays for money) but high hoarding individuals had similar discount rates for both money and consumables as t_2 increases.

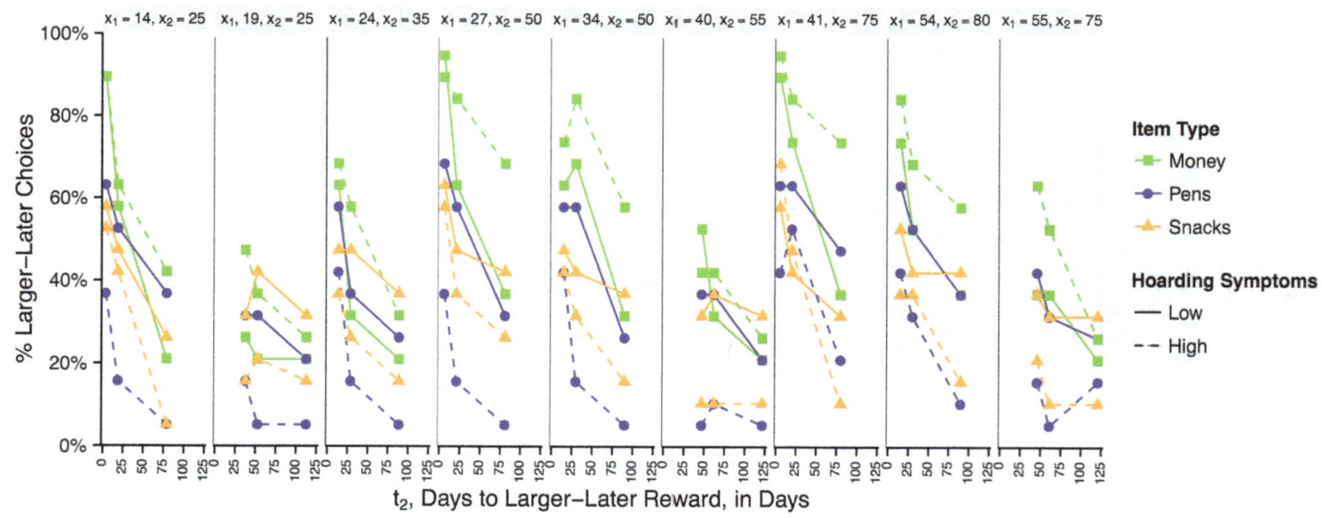

FIGURE 2 | Intertemporal discounting responses for effects of delay and moderate reward amounts with a fixed initial time (now). The percent of participants choosing the LL option overall split by smaller-sooner (x_1) and larger-later (x_2) reward amounts, which are listed above plots. Choices for money are represented with green lines, pens in blue, and snacks in orange. Low hoarding incividuals are represented by solid lines and high hoarding individuals are represented by dashed lines.

Effects of Adding a Constant to Both Times: Testing Exponential Discounting

Theories of exponential discounting hold that people's discounting rates decline exponentially as time increases, and the rate of discounting only depends on the difference in time between the two points. Exponential discounting assumes that with fixed quantities, delaying both t_1 and t_2 by the same constant will not alter choices. To assess the fit of exponential curves, crosstabs were created in the form (x_1, t_1 vs. x_2, t_2) compared to (x_1, $t_1 + k$ vs. x_2, $t_2 + k$), where k is a constant.

The number of preference reversals were summed over the three trial pairs (i.e., 0, 1, 2, or 3 preference reversals) and compared with a Poisson HLM, but this time using the number of preference reversals as the dependent variable. The original trials involved moderate reward amounts (19–75 items) offered immediately (0 days) or after a moderate to large delay (21–93 days), and to these trials a corresponding constant of 15, 20, or 32 days was added to both the early and the later option.

Overall, choices were consistent across groups and domains, $\chi^2(1)$s < 0.348, $ps > 0.50$. Within each domain, there was also no difference in the number of consistent compared to inconsistent choices between the low and high hoarding groups, $zs < 0.20$, $ps > 0.60$. In line with the high hoarding group's general consummatory impulsiveness, high hoarding individuals predominantly made consistently impulsive choices for pens and snacks (about eight times more often SS–SS than LL–LL) but chose more often to be consistently patient for money (50% more LL–LL than SS–SS). The low hoarding individuals, instead, were biased to be somewhat impulsive for all three domains, choosing SS–SS about 50% more often than LL–LL for pens, snacks, and money (see **Table 3**; **Figure 1C**). Thus, both low and high hoarding groups were consistent with assumptions of exponential discounting, but high hoarding individuals had many more SS–SS consistent choices for pens and snacks compared to low hoarding individuals, as was the case in the overall discounting rates.

Effects of Multiplying a Constant by Both Amounts: Testing the Power Utility Function

The power utility function can produce effects that may be similar to discounting. If people have different utilities for, say, money and pens, then we may incorrectly attribute the difference to discounting rather than utility. Power utility assumes that when both times in the same trial are multiplied by a constant, k, the preferences will not change.

We compared trials that were identical except for a constant k multiplier that was applied to both smaller (x_1) and larger (x_2) reward amounts; e.g., (x_1, t_1 vs. x_2, t_2) compared to ($k \bullet x_1$, t_1 vs. $k \bullet x_2$, t_2). These trials all involved larger quantities of items in both smaller and larger positions (i.e., from 32 to 90) offered at two delays that were both displaced in time and never immediate (32 vs. 93 days or 29 vs. 90 days). This set of trials included one pair and one triplet. The trial pair used $k = 1.38$ with x_1, x_2 pairs of (32, 44) and (48, 66). The triplet used $k = 1.36$ with x_1, x_2 pairs of (44, 60), (55, 75), and (66, 90). Again, the Poisson test was used to compare the number of preference reversals for each domain (0, 1, 2, or 3 of the possible 3 reversals from SS to LL or from LL to SS). Supporting the power utility function, choices on these trials were consistent in both low and high hoarding groups, across domains, $\chi^2(1) < 1.96$, $ps > 0.373$. Within each

TABLE 3 | Cross-tabulations by group and domain for tests of exponential discounting, with a constant added to both times with (x_1, t_1 vs. x_2, t_2) compared to ($x_1, t_1 + k$ vs. x_2, t_2+k).

Low hoarding individuals, money			High hoarding individuals, money		
	$(x_1, t_1 + k)$ vs. $(x_2, t_2 + k)$			$(x_1, t_1 + k)$ vs. $(x_2, t_2 + k)$	
(x_1, t_1) vs. (x_2, t_2)	SS	LL	(x_1, t_1) vs. (x_2, t_2)	SS	LL
SS	30	4	SS	19	5
LL	1	22	LL	4	29
Low hoarding individuals, pens			**High hoarding individuals, pens**		
	$(x_1, t_1 + k)$ vs. $(x_2, t_2 + k)$			$(x_1, t_1 + k)$ vs. $(x_2, t_2 + k)$	
(x_1, t_1) vs. (x_2, t_2)	SS	LL	(x_1, t_1) vs. (x_2, t_2)	SS	LL
SS	31	3	SS	43	9
LL	4	19	LL	2	3
Low hoarding individuals, snacks			**High hoarding individuals, snacks**		
	$(x_1, t_1 + k)$ vs. $(x_2, t_2 + k)$			$(x_1, t_1 + k)$ vs. $(x_2, t_2 + k)$	
(x_1, t_1) vs. (x_2, t_2)	SS	LL	(x_1, t_1) vs. (x_2, t_2)	SS	LL
SS	27	7	SS	34	10
LL	3	20	LL	6	7

Each 2 × 2 Table is based on three trials per participant (each 2 × 2 table has 57 entries).

TABLE 4 | Cross-tabulations by group and domain for tests of the power utility function, with a constant added to both amounts with (x_1, t_1 vs. x_2, t_2) compared to ($k \bullet x_1, t_1$ vs. $k \bullet x_2, t_2$).

Low hoarding individuals, money			High hoarding individuals, money		
	$(k \bullet x_1, t_1)$ vs. $(k \bullet x_2, t_2)$			$(k \bullet x_1, t_1)$ vs. $(k \bullet x_2, t_2)$	
(x_1, t_1) vs. (x_2, t_2)	SS	LL	(x_1, t_1) vs. (x_2, t_2)	SS	LL
SS	14	0	SS	9	2
LL	0	5	LL	1	7
Low hoarding individuals, pens			**High hoarding individuals, pens**		
	$(k \bullet x_1, t_1)$ vs. $(k \bullet x_2, t_2)$			$(k \bullet x_1, t_1)$ vs. $(k \bullet x_2, t_2)$	
(x_1, t_1) vs. (x_2, t_2)	SS	LL	(x_1, t_1) vs. (x_2, t_2)	SS	LL
SS	14	0	SS	18	0
LL	0	5	LL	1	0
Low hoarding individuals, snacks			**High hoarding individuals, snacks**		
	$(k \bullet x_1, t_1)$ vs. $(k \bullet x_2, t_2)$			$(k \bullet x_1, t_1)$ vs. $(k \bullet x_2, t_2)$	
(x_1, t_1) vs. (x_2, t_2)	SS	LL	(x_1, t_1) vs. (x_2, t_2)	SS	LL
SS	10	4	SS	15	0
LL	0	5	LL	0	4

Consistent preferences are demonstrated by higher values in SS/SS and LL/LL cells (diagonals in quadrants one and three), indicating that participants decided similarly in the original decision and the k shifted version. This trial type included one pair and one triplet but to avoid overlapping choices from the triplet only the pair is presented here.

domain, there was also no difference in the number of preference reversals between low and high hoarding groups, $zs < |1.20|$, $ps > 0.250$. The nature of the consistent choices in this set of trials was similar to that of the prior section, with high hoarding individuals being overwhelmingly, consistently impatient for pens and snacks (SS–SS, with actually no LL–LL choices for high hoarding individuals deciding about pens), but more often consistently patient for money. Conversely, the low hoarding group was biased to be consistent in all three domains by being two to three times more impatient than patient (see **Table 4**; **Figure 1D**).

Individual Differences Measures

As a complementary analysis to the group-level analysis above, we also investigated whether continuous, individual-level variation in the degree to which participants exhibited hoarding, impulsivity, and psychopathological tendencies correlated with their main outcome variable from the discounting analysis reported above. For each person we correlated their individual difference data across all of the scales with the degree to which they were more patient for money than consumables by subtracting their pooled LL choices for both pens and snacks from their percent of LL choices for money. This produced a variable ranging from +1 (100% choices for money and 0% choices for pens and snacks) to −1 (0% choices for money and 100% LL choices for pens and snacks), with the zero point representing similar proportions for money and consumables. Consistent with the group-level effects above—where high hoarding individuals were more patient for money than consumables—this behavior was also significantly correlated with the continuous, individual difference measures across the whole sample including all hoarding scales (HRS, SI-R Clutter, SI-R Difficulty Discarding, SI-R Acquisition, OCI-R Hoarding), $rs(36) > 0.33$, $ps \leq 0.05$, $\eta_p^2 s > 0.10$, and the BIS Attentional Impulsivity subscale, $r(36) = 0.40$, $p = 0.012$, $\eta_p^2 = 0.16$ (see **Table 5**). Even after controlling for age and population (community vs. or psychology pool) all results remained except that scores from the pre-screening administration of the HRS became marginal in both cases and the correlations with SI-R acquisition dropped to the marginal level, $ts(35) > 1.77$, $ps < 0.09$, $\eta_p^2 s > 0.08$.

DISCUSSION

Using a modified version of a standard impulsivity task from behavioral economics, we found reliable evidence across multiple measures and analysis strategies that people with problematic hoarding tendencies are actually more patient than people with low hoarding tendencies for money, but they are indeed less patient for consumable goods, particularly pens. The high hoarding group's greater patience for money suggests that they do not have a domain-general problem with impulsivity as has been suggested for addiction (e.g., Odum, 2011), and that they do possess the cognitive capacity to save or wait for larger reward.

To our knowledge, this is the first time a disordered population has demonstrated greater patience for money compared to controls, or to have shown discounting rates for money that are inversely correlated with discounting for consumable rewards. Extensive prior research finds that impaired populations—including those addicted to heroin, cocaine, alcohol, cigarettes, food and gambling—discount their drug of choice more steeply than money while also discounting money more steeply than controls, even compared to ex-users (see reviews in Bickel and Marsch, 2001; Perry and Carroll, 2008). The fact that drugs are usually discounted more steeply than money is attributed to the more direct impact of consumables on the biological reward system, with many studies finding greater discounting for consumables like food, candy, or beer compared to money, even in non-disordered populations (Odum and Rainaud, 2003; Odum et al., 2006; Estle et al., 2007). We replicated this overall effect of greater discounting for consumables, but also found that participants with low tendencies to hoard treated the three domains more similarly to one another. However, the group with high hoarding tendencies discounted money less steeply and discounted consumables more steeply than controls. Thus, domain-specific discounting rates may be more powerful in populations with a focused desire. This differential treatment of money by individuals with high hoarding tendencies does accord with their real-world apparent lack of interest in making and accumulating money and their frugal use of it to obtain desired goods (Frost et al., 2009).

Our results also suggest that the delay impacts choice more than the quantity, particularly for rewards that are offered "now." The participants with high hoarding tendencies were particularly prone to impulsively obtain pens—even more so than snacks—again attesting to their domain-specific interest in goods *per se*. This is particularly interesting in light of prior studies across domains that presumed that drugs of abuse and food are discounted more steeply than money because they can be consumed (and, thus, activate the biological reward system more strongly). For the participants with high hoarding tendencies, pens are their desired item of choice and they appear to strongly drive the choice system despite not being literal consummatory reward. However, paradoxically, the individuals with high hoarding tendencies did prefer a single snack delivered immediately over more snacks delivered later while being willing to wait for a delay from now to accumulate more than one pen; they also generally preferred multiple pens immediately over more pens later. Such reversals perhaps make sense if you either consider that only single snacks can be consumed immediately (and thus have a greater appeal to people with hoarding tendencies only in cases when $t_1 = 0$) or if wanting to accumulate material goods takes a non-linear function that eventually curves downward, whereby more pens is better but there are limits to how many you could need or how many in the short term could satisfy the desire. Regardless, these complexities attest to the need for future ITD work to include a broad range of relevant units and delays to capture important biologically-relevant stages of the process and units of interest (see also Odum et al., 2006).

The particular impatience of high hoarding individuals for immediate consumables suggests that the "incentive salience" (cf., Berridge and Robinson, 2003) of goods is what makes the items difficult for these people to resist (see an overview of the biological mechanisms for cross-domain reward in Preston et al., 2014). Similarly, in a prior study, neural activity in the nucleus accumbens—the region associated with the motivation to acquire rewarding drugs—increased during the acquisition of goods to the extent that participants reported real-world problems with hoarding (Wang et al., 2012). This rewarding property of goods for people with HD, but not for money, has been underappreciated—with most theories focusing on their indecision or fear of making mistakes (e.g., see Frost and Hartl, 1996). Perhaps fear can potentiate

TABLE 5 | Correlations of psychopathology measures with the main effect of the intertemporal discounting task (ITD).

Scale	% LL Difference Money – Snack and Pen	
	r	*p*
Hoarding scales		
HRS pre-screen	0.33	0.04*
HRS post	0.37	0.02*
SIR clutter	0.35	0.03*
SIR difficulty discarding	0.39	0.02*
SIR acquire	0.36	0.03*
OCI-R hoarding	0.36	0.03*
Non-hoarding psychopathology scales		
BAI	0.13	0.44
BDI	0.27	0.10ᵗ
STAIT	0.13	0.44
Impulsivity subscales		
BIS attention	0.40	0.01*
BIS motor	0.15	0.38
BIS non-planning	0.16	0.35

*High hoarding individuals discounted money less and consumables (pens and snacks) more than low hoarding individuals, so individual differences measures were correlated with the difference score of the % larger-later (LL) decisions for money minus pens and snacks. All correlations have df = 36. HRS, Hoarding Rating Scale. SIR, Savings Inventory Revised. OCI-R, Obsessive Compulsive Inventory, Revised. BAI, Beck Anxiety Inventory. BDI, Beck Depression Inventory. BIS, Behavioral Impulsivity Scale. STAIT, State Trait Anxiety Inventory, State. *p < 0.05, ᵗp < 0.10.*

a proximate motivation toward goods to alleviate future uncertainty, to provide comfort in the absence of rewarding social bonds, or to provide literal, physical protection (Preston, 2013).

Multiple facts suggest that our task and results are valid. Unlike in some other experimental tests of HD and impulsivity, we did not find null effects and we replicated most standard discounting effects, including greater patience for increasing later reward and greater impatience for immediate, early reward and for consumables over money. We also replicated our results from the two group comparison of high vs. low hoarding individuals with continuously-varying individual difference correlations across the whole sample; these correlations also replicate a prior study that found greater attentional impulsivity in HD (Tolin and Villavicencio, 2011). Our results also remained similar after controlling for age and recruitment method (community or psychology pool). Moreover, our results affirmed the assumptions of exponential discounting and the power utility function, particularly in low hoarding participants. The individuals with high hoarding tendencies did tend to be consistent for consumables when a constant was added to both delays (which does not violate exponential discounting), but only because they preferred smaller amounts of pens or snacks offered immediately while preferring the larger quantity when the two time periods were shifted away from "now," which is consistent with the known potency of immediately available reward.

In addition to replicating many common findings in the delay discounting literature, our task and trial design used an enhanced version of a standard set of delay discounting items (Kirby et al., 1999) with items that allowed us to test for specific forms of discounting. For instance, exponential discounting requires that if a person chooses (x_1, t_1) over (x_2, t_2) then they should choose (x_1, $t_1 + k$) over (x_2, $t_2 + k$). Evidence of preference reversals across such a pair rejects exponential discounting without requiring that we estimate parameter values (see Krantz et al., 1971, for an explanation of this approach). This approach allows us to determine whether exponential discounting holds across money, pens, and snacks, and whether it holds equally in the two groups. We opted not to perform non-linear parameter estimation because it would be difficult to compare across three domains. For example, if we fit a hyperbolic discounting function and observed differences across the three domains in the discounting parameter, we would not be able to determine whether the different parameters actually resulted from differences in discounting across the domains or from a confounding difference in utility (e.g., because a pack of cookies really isn't worth an exact dollar or means something different when you have 5 packs or 35 packs compared to 1). The approach adopted in this study tailored the trial types to study different aspects of the decision while making fewer assumptions about the domains and using statistically powered but simple tests that allow us to compare groups and domains. A more careful simultaneous assessment of discounting vs. utility functions across domains is beyond the scope of this project, but should also be investigated.

Despite the novelty and consistency of our results, there are some limitations. Our choices were not incentivized with real rewards and our high hoarding group was identified through self-report, which was followed up with a validated clinical questionnaire rather than a structured clinical interview. However, ITD procedures are known to produce similar results whether the rewards are hypothetical or real (Johnson and Bickel, 2002; Madden et al., 2003) and hoarding should be thought of as a continuously varying individual difference and not just a present or absent psychopathology (reviewed in Preston et al., 2009; Preston, 2013). One must also not assume that greater attentional impulsivity and ITD discounting for goods should be extended to other forms of impulsivity that we did not measure, or other aspects of HD such as discarding problems. In clinical samples up to 60% of hoarding patients meet the criteria for compulsive buying (e.g., Frost et al., 2002), so it is possible that this impulsiveness for consumable reward explains the compulsive buying and acquisition of free items in HD, but we need to determine empirically which if any other forms of impulsiveness are disordered in HD. A large, systematic study that compares all forms of impulsivity within participants and across groups and domains is still needed.

A trans-diagnostic, symptom-based approach to HD that generously includes both empirically validated tasks and individual difference measures can help us understand the underlying problems that promote HD. This approach can also help us understand the potential link between

HD and other related phenomena like impulse-control disorders and addiction, which is currently poorly understood and likely prevents us from being maximally effective in treating HD.

AUTHOR CONTRIBUTIONS

SP developed the study concept. SP, RG, and AA designed the study. SP and AA oversaw subject recruitment and testing. BV performed data analysis under the supervision of SP and RG. SP and BV drafted the paper, and all authors provided revisions and approved the final version of the paper for submission.

ACKNOWLEDGMENTS

Research was supported by a grant from the University of Michigan Office for the Vice President for Research (OVPR) to SP. Thanks to Jenny Porter, Jacqueline Rau, David Chester, Aleah Burson, Chris Boffi, and Lauren Oglevee for assistance.

REFERENCES

American Psychological Association [APA] (2013). *Diagnostic and Statistical Manual of Mental Disorders*, 5th Edn. Arlington, VA: American Psychiatric Publishing.

Beck, A. T., Epstein, N., Brown, G., and Steer, R. A. (1988a). An inventory for measuring clinical anxiety: psychometric properties. *J. Consult. Clin. Psychol.* 56, 893–897. doi: 10.1037/0022-006X.56.6.893

Beck, A. T., Steer, R. A., and Garbin, M. G. (1988b). Psychometric properties of the Beck Depression Inventory: twenty-five years of evaluation. *Clin. Psychol. Rev.* 8, 77–100. doi: 10.1016/0272-7358(88)90050-5

Berridge, K. C., and Robinson, T. E. (2003). Parsing reward. *Trends Neurosci.* 26, 507–513. doi: 10.1016/S0166-2236(03)00233-9

Bickel, W. K., and Marsch, L. A. (2001). Toward a behavioral economic understanding of drug dependence: delay discounting processes. *Addiction* 96, 73–86. doi: 10.1046/j.1360-0443.2001.961736.x

Dunn, E. W., Aknin, L. B., and Norton, M. I. (2008). Spending money on others promotes happiness. *Science* 319, 1687–1688. doi: 10.1126/science.1150952

Estle, S. J., Green, L., Myerson, J., and Holt, D. D. (2007). Discounting of monetary and directly consumable rewards. *Psychol. Sci.* 18, 58–63. doi: 10.1111/j.1467-9280.2007.01849.x

Foa, E. B., Huppert, J. D., Leiberg, S., Langner, R., Kichic, R., Hajcak, G., et al. (2002). The obsessive-compulsive inventory: development and validation of a short version. *Psychol. Assess.* 14, 485–496. doi: 10.1037/1040-3590.14.4.485

Frost, R. O., and Gross, R. C. (1993). The hoarding of possessions. *Behav. Res. Ther.* 31, 367–381. doi: 10.1016/0005-7967(93)90094-B

Frost, R. O., and Hartl, T. L. (1996). A cognitive-behavioral model of compulsive hoarding. *Behav. Res. Ther.* 34, 341–350. doi: 10.1016/0005-7967(95)00071-2

Frost, R. O., Steketee, G., and Grisham, J. (2004). Measurement of compulsive hoarding: saving inventory-revised. *Behav. Res. Ther.* 42, 1163–1182. doi: 10.1016/j.brat.2003.07.006

Frost, R. O., Steketee, G., and Tolin, D. F. (2011). Comorbidity in hoarding disorder. *Depress. Anxiety* 28, 876–884. doi: 10.1002/da.20861

Frost, R. O., Steketee, G., and Williams, L. (2000). Hoarding: a community health problem. *Health Soc. Care Community* 8, 229–234. doi: 10.1046/j.1365-2524.2000.00245.x

Frost, R. O., Steketee, G., and Williams, L. (2002). Compulsive buying, compulsive hoarding, and obsessive-compulsive disorder. *Behav. Ther.* 33, 201–214. doi: 10.1016/S0005-7894(02)80025-9

Frost, R. O., Tolin, D. F., Steketee, G., Fitch, K. E., and Selbo-Bruns, A. (2009). Excessive acquisition in hoarding. *J. Anxiety Disord.* 23, 632–639. doi: 10.1016/j.janxdis.2009.01.013

Grisham, J. R., Brown, T. A., Savage, C. R., Steketee, G., and Barlow, D. H. (2007). Neuropsychological impairment associated with compulsive hoarding. *Behav. Res. Ther.* 45, 1471–1483. doi: 10.1016/j.brat.2006.12.008

Jarvis, B. G. (2006). *MediaLab (Version 2006.2.40)*. New York, NY: Empirisoft Corporation.

Johnson, M. W., and Bickel, W. K. (2002). Within-subject comparison of real and hypothetical money rewards in delay discounting. *J. Exp. Anal. Behav.* 77, 129–146. doi: 10.1901/jeab.2002.77-129

Kirby, K. N., Petry, N. M., and Bickel, W. K. (1999). Heroin addicts have higher discount rates for delayed rewards than non-drug-using controls. *J. Exp. Psychol. Gen.* 128, 78–87. doi: 10.1037/0096-3445.128.1.78

Krantz, D., Luce, R. D., Suppes, P., and Tversky, A. (1971). *Foundations of Measurement: Additive and Polynomial Representations*, Vol. 1. New York, NY: Academic Press.

Lawrence, N. S., Wooderson, S., Mataix-Cols, D., David, R., Speckens, A., and Phillips, M. L. (2006). Decision making and set shifting impairments are associated with distinct symptom dimensions in obsessive-compulsive disorder. *Neuropsychology* 20, 409–419. doi: 10.1037/0894-4105.20.4.409

Loewenstein, G. F., Weber, E. U., Hsee, C. K., and Welch, N. (2001). Risk as feelings. *Psychol. Bull.* 127, 267–286. doi: 10.1037/0033-2909.127.2.267

Madden, G. J., Begotka, A. M., Raiff, B. R., and Kastern, L. L. (2003). Delay discounting of real and hypothetical rewards. *Exp. Clin. Psychopharmacol.* 11, 139–145. doi: 10.1037/1064-1297.11.2.139

McElroy, S. L., Keck, P. E. Jr., and Phillips, K. A. (1995). Kleptomania, compulsive buying, and binge-eating disorder. *J. Clin. Psychiatry* 56, 14–26.

Odum, A. L. (2011). Delay discounting: trait variable? *Behav. Process.* 87, 1–9. doi: 10.1016/j.beproc.2011.02.007

Odum, A. L., Baumann, A. A. L., and Rimington, D. D. (2006). Discounting of delayed hypothetical money and food: effects of amount. *Behav. Process.* 73, 278–284. doi: 10.1016/j.beproc.2006.06.008

Odum, A. L., and Rainaud, C. P. (2003). Discounting of delayed hypothetical money, alcohol, and food. *Behav. Process.* 64, 305–313. doi: 10.1016/S0376-6357(03)00145-1

Patton, J. H., and Stanford, M. S. (1995). Factor structure of the Barratt impulsiveness scale. *J. Clin. Psychol.* 51, 768–774. doi: 10.1002/1097-4679(199511)51:6<768::AID-JCLP2270510607>3.0.CO;2-1

Perry, J. L., and Carroll, M. E. (2008). The role of impulsive behavior in drug abuse. *Psychopharmacology* 200, 1–26. doi: 10.1007/s00213-008-1173-0

Preston, S. D. (2013). "Hoarding in animals: the argument for a homology," in *The Oxford Handbook of Hoarding and Acquiring*, eds R. O. Frost and G. Steketee (London: Oxford University Press).

Preston, S. D., and Jacobs, L. F. (2001). Conspecific pilferage but not presence affects Merriam's kangaroo rat cache strategy. *Behav. Ecol.* 12, 517–523. doi: 10.1093/beheco/12.5.517

Preston, S. D., and Jacobs, L. F. (2005). Cache decision making: the effects of competition on cache decisions in Merriam's kangaroo rat. *J. Comp. Psychol.* 119, 187–196. doi: 10.1037/0735-7036.119.2.187

Preston, S. D., Kringelbach, M. L., and Knutson, B. (2014). *The Interdisciplinary Science of Consumption*. Cambridge, MA: MIT Press.

Preston, S. D., Muroff, J. R., and Wengrovitz, S. M. (2009). Investigating the mechanisms of hoarding from an experimental perspective. *Depress. Anxiety* 26, 425–437. doi: 10.1002/da.20417

Rasmussen, J. L., Brown, T. A., Steketee, G. S., and Barlow, D. H. (2013). Impulsivity in hoarding. *J. Obsessive Compuls. Relat. Disord.* 2, 183–191. doi: 10.1016/j.jocrd.2013.02.004

Samuels, J., Bienvenu, O. J. III, Riddle, M. A., Cullen, B. A., Grados, M. A., Liang, K. Y., et al. (2002). Hoarding in obsessive compulsive disorder: results from a case-control study. *Behav. Res. Ther.* 40, 517–528. doi: 10.1016/S0005-7967(01)00026-2

Samuels, J. F., Bienvenu, O. J., Grados, M. A., Cullen, B., Riddle, M. A., Liang, K. Y., et al. (2008). Prevalence and correlates of hoarding behavior in a community-based sample. *Behav. Res. Ther.* 46, 836–844. doi: 10.1016/j.brat.2008.04.004

Timpano, K. R., Rasmussen, J., Exner, C., Rief, W., Schmidt, N. B., and Wilhelm, S. (2013). Hoarding and the multi-faceted construct of impulsivity: a cross-cultural investigation. *J. Psychiatr. Res.* 47, 363–370. doi: 10.1016/j.jpsychires.2012.10.017

Tolin, D. F., Frost, R. O., and Steketee, G. (2010). A brief interview for assessing compulsive hoarding: the Hoarding Rating Scale-Interview. *Psychiatry Res.* 178, 147–152. doi: 10.1016/j.psychres.2009.05.001

Tolin, D. F., Frost, R. O., Steketee, G., and Muroff, J. (2015). Cognitive behavioral therapy for hoarding disorder: a meta-analysis. *Depress. Anxiety* 32, 158–166. doi: 10.1002/da.22327

Tolin, D. F., and Villavicencio, A. (2011). Inattention, but not OCD, predicts the core features of Hoarding Disorder. *Behav. Res. Ther.* 49, 120–125. doi: 10.1016/j.brat.2010.12.002

Wang, J. M., Seidler, R. D., Hall, J. L., and Preston, S. D. (2012). The neural bases of acquisitiveness: decisions to acquire and discard everyday goods differ across frames, items, and individuals. *Neuropsychologia* 50, 939–948. doi: 10.1016/j.neuropsychologia.2012.01.033

Conflict of Interest Statement: The authors declare that the research was conducted in the absence of any commercial or financial relationships that could be construed as a potential conflict of interest.

18

Anticipatory Pleasure Predicts Effective Connectivity in the Mesolimbic System

Edited by:
Israel Liberzon,
University of Michigan, USA

***Correspondence:**
Raymond C. K. Chan,
Neuropsychology and Applied
Cognitive Neuroscience Laboratory,
Key Laboratory of Mental Health,
Institute of Psychology, Chinese
Academy of Sciences, Room 526,
South Block, 16 Lincui Road,
Beijing 100101, China
rckchan@psych.ac.cn

Zhi Li[1,2]*, Chao Yan*[3]*, Wei-Zhen Xie*[4]*, Ke Li*[5]*, Ya-Wei Zeng*[5]*, Zhen Jin*[5]*, Eric F. C. Cheung*[6] *and Raymond C. K. Chan*[1]*

[1] Neuropsychology and Applied Cognitive Neuroscience Laboratory, Key Laboratory of Mental Health, Institute of Psychology, Chinese Academy of Sciences, Beijing, China, [2] The University of Chinese Academy of Sciences, Beijing, China, [3] Key Laboratory of Brain Functional Genomics (MOE and STCSM), School of Psychology and Cognitive Science, East China Normal University, Shanghai, China, [4] Department of Psychology, University of California, Riverside, CA, USA, [5] MRI Center, Hospital 306 of PLA, Beijing, China, [6] Castle Peak Hospital, Hong Kong Special Administrative Region, Tuen Mun, China

Convergent evidence suggests the important role of the mesolimbic pathway in anticipating monetary rewards. However, the underlying mechanism of how the sub-regions interact with each other is still not clearly understood. Using dynamic causal modeling, we constructed a reward-related network for anticipating monetary reward using the Monetary Incentive Delay Task. Twenty-six healthy adolescents (Female/Male = 11/15; age = 18.69 ± 1.35 years; education = 12 ± 1.58 years) participated in the present study. The best-fit network involved the right substantia nigra/ventral tegmental area (SN/VTA), the right nucleus accumbens (NAcc) and the right thalamus, which were all activated during anticipation of monetary gain and loss. The SN/VTA directly activates the NAcc and the thalamus. More importantly, monetary gain modulated the connectivity from the SN/VTA to the NAcc and this was significantly correlated with subjective anticipatory pleasure ($r = 0.649$, $p < 0.001$). Our findings suggest that activity in the mesolimbic pathway during the anticipation of monetary reward could to some extent be predicted by subjective anticipatory pleasure.

Keywords: hedonic capacity, monetary reward, dynamic causal modeling, anticipatory pleasure

Introduction

Deficits in hedonic capacity, namely anhedonia, are often found in patients with schizophrenia, bipolar disorder, major depression, substance addiction, anxiety, and eating disorders (Shankman et al., 2014). Traditional symptom-based psychiatric diagnosis may not be able to capture these underlying features that cut across diagnostic entities. The recently proposed Research Domain Criteria (RDoC) aims to address this problem (Cuthbert, 2014; Cuthbert and Workgrp, 2014). The RDoC suggests researchers to focus on elemental cognitive and emotional functions, such as hedonic capacity, using various approaches ranging from behavioral performance, through brain circuits, to genes (NIMH, 2008). The Monetary Incentive Delay (MID) task (Knutson et al., 2000) and the Temporal Experience of Pleasure Scale (TEPS; Gard et al., 2006) have been suggested as appropriate instruments to examine the two components of hedonic experience, namely anticipatory and consummatory pleasure. Converging evidence suggests that the nucleus accumbens (NAcc) is a vital hedonic hotspot in anticipatory pleasure (Kringelbach and Berridge, 2009; Berridge and Kringelbach, 2013). Using the MID task, activation of the NAcc has been observed during anticipation of secondary rewards (Knutson et al., 2000, 2001). Similar results have been reported in anticipation of primary rewards, such as sucrose solution (O'Doherty et al., 2002) and social rewards (Kohls et al., 2013). The NAcc appears to play a key role in integrating information from the midbrain, the limbic system and the frontal cortex to facilitate appropriate choice and goal-directed behavior (Camara et al., 2009). The substantia nigra/ventral tegmental area (SN/VTA) also plays an important role in reward processing (Horvitz, 2000; Duezel et al., 2009). Anticipation of primary and secondary rewards, taste (O'Doherty et al., 2002), money (Breiter et al., 2001), and happy faces (Aharon et al., 2001) activates the SN/VTA. Lastly, the thalamus also plays a role in hedonic experience. Previous studies have reported activation of the thalamus in anticipation of rewards (Knutson et al., 2000, 2001; Knutson and Greer, 2008). The thalamus integrates messages from the emotional, cognitive, and motor cortices and relays information to the frontal cortex to formulate goal-directed behavior (Haber and Calzavara, 2009). In addition, the thalamus also appears to be important in retrospective and prospective coding for predicted reward (Komura et al., 2001). The NAcc-nigra-thalamic circuit is involved in the regulatory function of the thalamus in reward processing (Montaron et al., 1996). Our study (Chan et al., in press), adopting the modified MID task, showed that anticipation of monetary gain activated the NAcc, the globus pallidus and the thalamus, whereas anticipation of monetary loss activated the NAcc, the thalamus and the SN/VTA. These findings further support the important roles of the SN/VTA, the NAcc and the thalamus during anticipation of rewards.

Although the functional connectivity between the NAcc, the SN/VTA and the thalamus have been a focus of recent studies in hedonic capacity (Camara et al., 2009; Haber and Calzavara, 2009; Cauda et al., 2011), to the best of our knowledge, few studies had examined the relationships between these three regions, especially the interaction between the SN/VTA and the NAcc during anticipation of rewards. Some studies have used dynamic causal modeling (DCM) to investigate reward related circuits (Alexander and Brown, 2010; Veldhuizen et al., 2011; Gonen et al., 2012; Cho et al., 2013; Yu et al., 2013). Using DCM, Veldhuizen et al. (2011) found that the anterior insular represents breaches of taste identity by receiving afferent connectivity from the ventral striatum and the inferior parietal cortex. Furthermore, by reciprocal connectivity from the amygdala, the ventral striatum plays a role in anticipating the attractability of human faces (Yu et al., 2013). Gonen et al. (2012) found that the VTA and the NAcc are related to the behavioral activation system and the NAcc represents the reward by cooperating with the dorsal medial prefrontal cortex. In addition, brain activity in the substantia nigra was found to be capable of predicting dopamine release in the NAcc during the anticipation of rewards (Schott et al., 2008). These findings suggest the vital role of the VS, especially the NAcc, in the reward circuit. In addition, the SN/VTA may also be engaged during the anticipation of rewards. However, the causal relationship between the SN/VTA and the NAcc is still unknown. In the present study, we constructed nine dynamic causal models between the SN/VTA, the NAcc and the thalamus, which contained reciprocal pathways between the SN/VTA and the NAcc, and between the NAcc and the thalamus and a non-reciprocal pathway from the SN/VTA to the thalamus (**Figure 1**). Taking into account the complexity of the models, the connectivity from the thalamus to the SN/VTA was excluded from consideration because this anatomical connectivity is not as clear-cut as the other five. Moreover, we measured the subjective anticipatory and consummatory pleasure of participants and correlated them with the parameters of the best-fit model.

Given these and our previous work using the MID task, we examined the reward-related network for anticipating monetary reward. We hypothesized that (1) the NAcc, the SN/VTA and the thalamus would all be activated during anticipation of monetary gain and loss; (2) the SN/VTA would exert a direct effect on the NAcc whereas the thalamus would integrate information from the SN/VTA and the NAcc.

Materials and Methods

Participants

Twenty-six (11 females) healthy right-handed adolescents with a mean age of 18.6 years (sd $=$ 1.35), a mean duration of education of 12 years (sd $=$ 1.58) and a mean IQ estimate of 95.38 (sd $=$ 13.56) [estimated by the shot-form of the Chinese version of the Wechsler Adult Intelligence Scale-Revised (WAIS-R; Gong, 1992)] were recruited from the community. Exclusion criteria included: a personal or family history of mental illness, a history of head injury, and a history of substance abuse. The study was approved by the Ethics Committee of the Institute of Psychology, the Chinese Academy of Sciences. Written informed consents were obtained from all participants. Each participant was recompensed with 100 CNY (China yuan) and the monetary rewards they acquired in the MID task after the completion of the study.

Temporal Experience Pleasure Scale

The TEPS was designed to measure anticipatory and consummatory pleasure (Gard et al., 2006). We used the Chinese version of the TEPS which consists of 10 items with a six-point Likert scale measuring anticipatory pleasure and 10 items measuring consummatory pleasure (Chan et al., 2012). The items measuring anticipatory pleasure capture the pleasure experienced during the anticipation of positive events, such as "When I hear about a new movie starring my favorite actor, I can't wait to see it," whereas the items measuring consummatory pleasure capture the pleasure experienced during the consummation of positive events, such as "A hot cup of coffee or tea on a cold morning is very satisfying to me." Higher score on the TEPS indicates higher hedonic capacity. Both the original and the Chinese version of the TEPS have been shown to have satisfactory reliability and validity (Gard et al., 2006; Chan et al., 2012).

Monetary Incentive Delay Task (MID)

In this study, we used an abbreviated version of the MID task developed by Chan et al. (in press). A cue lasting 250 ms was

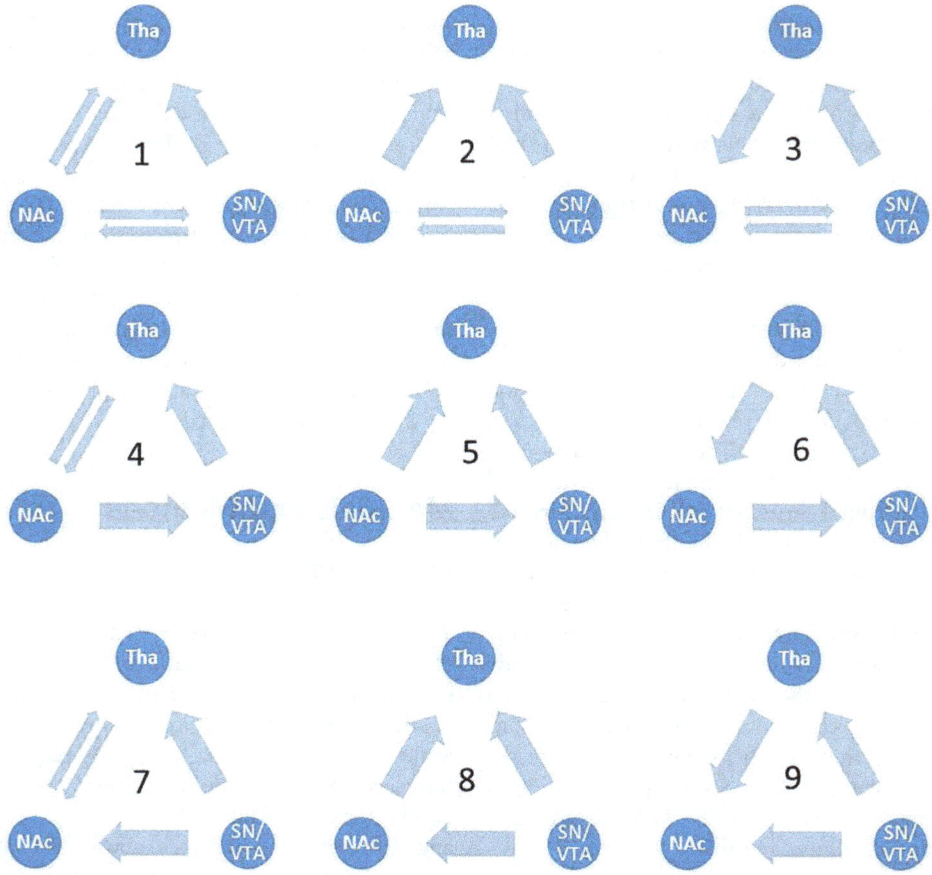

FIGURE 1 | Candidate dynamic causal models. All nine candidate models are shown. Model 1 contains reciprocal pathways between the substantia nigra/ventral tegmental area (SN/VTA) and the nucleus accumbens (NAcc), reciprocal pathways between the NAcc and the thalamus and a non-reciprocal pathway from the SN/VTA to the thalamus. External inputs, including anticipation of monetary gain and loss, initially impact the SN/VTA, followed by the NAcc and the thalamus.

presented on a projection screen which was reflected in a small mirror fixed on the head coil of the scanner, followed by the first interval and then a blue cross that the participants were asked to quickly hit by pressing a button. Then the second interval was presented which was followed by the monetary stimuli. The cues consisted of a triangle signifying the gain condition, a square signifying the loss condition and a circle signifying the neutral condition. In the gain condition, participants could gain five monetary points if the blue cross was hit. In the loss condition, participants would lose five monetary points if the blue cross was not hit. In the neutral condition, participants would gain or lose nothing whether the blue cross was hit or not. The duration of intervals were randomized to avoid participants from anticipating the blue cross and to maintain the duration of each trial at 12 s. In addition, the duration of the blue cross was jittered around 300 ms according to the performance of each participant to maintain the accuracy at about 66%. Participants were asked to perform two runs of the task. Each run contained 30 trials, 10 gain conditions, 10 loss conditions, 10 neutral conditions, and a blank screen lasting for 8 s presented in the first instance for a dummy scan. The order of the trials was pseudorandom across participants and different between the two runs. Participants were told that the final remuneration would be 100 CNY plus the monetary points they obtained in the task. The average hit rate, the reaction time by condition and the earnings are presented in Supplementary Table S1.

Functional MRI Data Collection

Imaging data were collected in a Siemens 3T Trio scanner with a 32-channel head coil at the MRI Centre of the 306 Hospital in Beijing. T2*-weighted echo planner ingredient sequence (TR = 2000 ms; TE = 30 ms; FOV = 210 mm; slices = 32; flip angle = 90°; image matrix = 64 × 64; voxel dimensions = 3.3 mm × 3.3 mm × 4 mm) was applied to acquire functional brain images. Then a high resolution T1 structure image was obtained with the sequence: TR = 2300 ms; TE = 3 ms; FOV = 256 mm; flip angle = 9°; image matrix = 256 × 256; voxel dimensions = 1 mm × 1 mm × 1 mm.

Functional MRI Data Processing

All the fMRI data were analyzed with the free software Statistical Parameter Mapping 8 (SPM8, Wellcome Trust Centre for

Neuroimaging, London, UK). Before pre-processing, the first four dummy scans were discarded. After slice timing correction, images were realigned to the twentieth slice of each TR. Then the mean EPI image was normalized to the single person template of the Montreal Neurological Institute. Finally all the images were smoothed with a Gaussian kernel of 5 mm full-width half-maximum.

Based on the canonical haemodynamic response function (HRF), only the three anticipatory events: the monetary gain, the monetary loss, and the neutral condition, were included in the general linear modeling. Besides, the six parameters of head movement generated in the realignment were included in the modeling as covariates. The contrast 'gain – neutral' was designed to examine brain activities in response to monetary gain, and the contrast 'loss – neutral' was designed to examine brain activities in response to monetary loss. The contrast 'all – neutral' referred to the general effect of monetary stimuli and was used in the DCM. The contrasts of each participant were included in a one-sample *t*-test which was set in the second-level analysis of the SPM8.

Since we aimed to examine the function of the SN/VTA, the NAcc, and the thalamus and their interaction during the anticipation of monetary stimuli, we analyzed brain activation with pre-defined regions of interest (ROI). The ROIs of the NAcc and the thalamus were selected from the Harvard-Oxford subcortical structure atlas. The ROI of the SN/VTA was adopted from a very high resolution subcortical probabilistic atlas which was quantified with a 7T structure MRI (Keuken et al., 2014). The three ROIs, were masked on the contrast 'gain – neutral' and the contrast 'loss – neutral' respectively. Small volume correction (SVC) within an 8-mm radius sphere was applied. The statistical threshold was set as familiar-wise-error (FWE) correction with $p < 0.05$.

TABLE 1 | Analysis of regions of interest (ROI) during the anticipation to monetary rewards.

Contrasts and areas	Side	*p*-value	Peak T	Coorinate (x,y,z)
All cues > Neutral cues				
Nucleus Accumbens (NAcc)	Right	<0.0001	10.46	6,6,−3
NAcc	Left	<0.0001	9.74	−6,6,−3
Substantia nigra/ventral tegmental area (SN/VTA)	Right	<0.0001	9.29	12,−24,−15
SN/VTA	Left	<0.0001	9.03	−9,−24,−15
Thalamus	Right	<0.0001	9.2	6,−3,−3
Thalamus	Left	<0.0001	9.18	−6,−3,−3
Gain cues > Neutral cues				
NAcc	Right	<0.0001	8.77	6,9,−3
NAcc	Left	<0.0001	8.35	−6,6,−6
SN/VTA	Right	<0.0001	8.62	9,−24,−15
SN/VTA	Left	<0.0001	8.35	−9,−24,−15
Thalamus	Right	<0.0001	8.25	6,−15,9
Thalamus	Left	<0.0001	8.81	−12,−18,15
Loss cues > Neutral cues				
NAcc	Right	<0.0001	11.67	6,6,−3
NAcc	Left	<0.0001	10.57	−6,6,−3
SN/VTA	Right	<0.0001	9.01	12,−21,−15
SN/VTA	Left	<0.0001	8.08	−9,−24,−15
Thalamus	Right	<0.0001	10.31	6,−3,−3
Thalamus	Left	<0.0001	9.34	−3,−9,6

The threshold was set as $p < 0.05$ with family-wise error (FWE) correction, small volume correction (SVC).

Dynamic Causal Modeling

Before the procedure, the time courses of the SN/VTA, the NAcc, and the thalamus were extracted from the contrast 'all – neutral' of all participants. The ROIs were defined as the overlaps between the masks used in the ROI analysis with an 8-mm radius sphere centered around the peak points activated in the SN/VTA, the NAcc, and the thalamus, respectively. The statistical threshold was set as uncorrected $p < 0.05$.

We constructed nine dynamic causal models. The complete model, Model 1, contained reciprocal connectivity between the SN/VTA and the NAcc, reciprocal connectivity between the NAcc and the thalamus, and a non-reciprocal connectivity from the SN/VTA to the thalamus. From Model 1, one or two connectivity was subtracted in different ways to form eight other models (**Figure 1**). The right SN/VTA, the right NAcc, and the right thalamus were included in the model for their stronger activations than their left- sided counterparts (**Table 1**). Using the SPM8, a HRF was constructed, which contained the event 'all,' 'gain,' and 'loss'. The event 'all' was defined as an input at the SN/VTA which is axiomatically considered a dopamine-rich region projecting to the terminals of the NAcc (Duezel et al., 2009; Haber and Knutson, 2010; Cauda et al., 2011). For the exploratory aim of this study and the unclear effect of valence to the connectivity of the reward circuit, the event 'gain' and 'loss' were, respectively, defined as perturbations to all the intrinsic connectivity, or the edges, of the models. A random-effect analysis of Bayesian Model Selection (BMS) was applied to identify the best-fit model with the highest exceedance probability (Friston et al., 2003; Stephan et al., 2010). Then the endogenous and perturbed parameters of the best-fit model were imported into the Predictive Analytics Software 18.0 (PASW 18.0) for significance testing. Bonferroni correction was applied to correct for multiple comparison. Finally, all the parameters were correlated with the total, the anticipatory and the consummatory subscale scores of the TEPS using Pearson Correlation.

Results

Regions of Interest Analysis

The bilateral NAcc, the bilateral SN/VTA and the bilateral thalamus were all significantly activated to the contrasts 'gain – neutral,' 'loss – neutral,' and 'all – neutral' (**Table 1**).

Dynamic Causal Modeling

The BMS identified Model 8 as the best-fit model with the highest exceedance probability during the anticipation of monetary stimuli (**Figures 2 and 3**). The endogenous connectivity of Model 8 contained two causal pathways from the SN/VTA to the NAcc

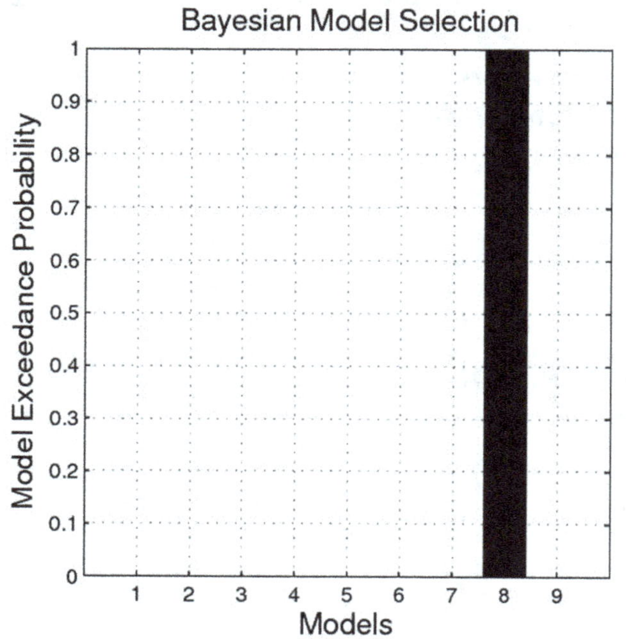

FIGURE 2 | Exceedance probability of each model. The exceedance probability of Model 8 is higher than the other eight models.

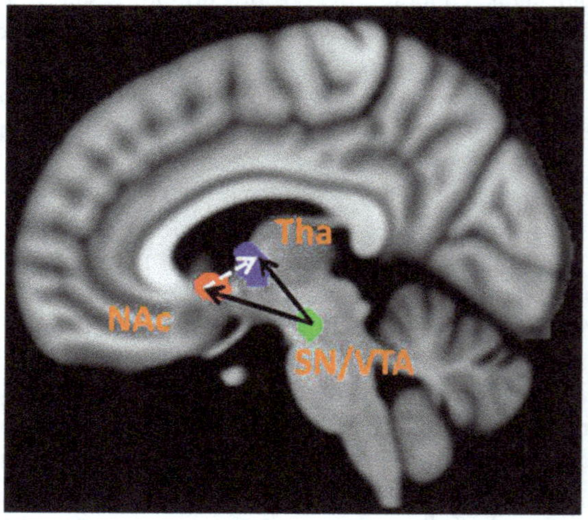

FIGURE 3 | Best-fit dynamic causal model. Model 8 is the best model in fitting the time series of the SN/VTA, the NAcc, and the thalamus. In Model 8, the SN/VTA projects two causal pathways to the NAcc and the thalamus, whereas the NAcc exerts a causal influence on the thalamus.

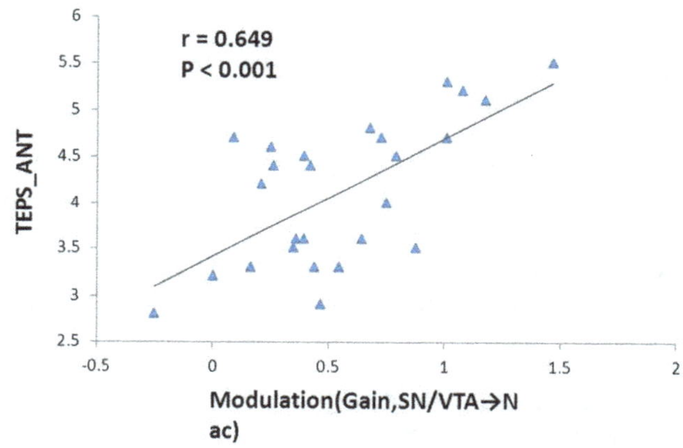

FIGURE 4 | Correlation between the effect of monetary gain on the mesolimbic pathway and anticipatory pleasure experience. Modulation of monetary gain on the causal connectivity from the SN/VTA to the NAcc positively correlates with anticipatory pleasure experience. The Pearson correlation coefficient remains significant after Bonferroni correction.

and to the thalamus, while the NAcc had a causal effect on the thalamus. Endogenous parameters of the pathway from the SN/VTA to the NAcc [$t(25) = 10.96$, $p < 0.001$] and to the thalamus [$t(25) = 8.42$, $p < 0.001$] were significant, while that from the NAcc to the thalamus was not [$t(25) = 1.27$, $p = 0.217$] (**Table 2**).

As for the modulation parameters caused by external experimental stimuli in the Model 8, both monetary 'gain' and 'loss' modulated the connectivity from the SN/VTA to the NAcc, from the SN/VTA to the thalamus and from the NAcc to the thalamus (**Table 2**).

Correlation between Subjective Pleasure Experience and Modeling Parameters

The mean total TEPS score of the participants was 78.18 ± 12.72, while the mean anticipatory and consummatory subscale scores were 41.78 ± 6.9 and 36.4 ± 7.39, respectively. We found significant positive correlation between the modulation by 'gain' events on the nigrostriatal pathway from the SN/VTA to the NAcc with anticipatory subscale score ($r = 0.649$, $p < 0.001$) and total score on the TEPS ($r = 0.555$, $p = 0.003$). The former correlation remained significant after Bonferroni correction (**Figure 4**).

TABLE 2 | Parameters of endogenous connections and modulation of the Model 8.

Path	Endogenous Connection	Modulation_gain	Modulation_loss
		Mean ± SEM	Mean ± SEM
SN/VTA→NAc	1.24 ± 0.15**	0.55 ± 0.08**	0.19 ± 0.04**
SN/VTA→Tha	1.96 ± 0.18**	0.28 ± 0.03**	0.17 ± 0.03**
NAc→Tha	0.09 ± 0.07	−0.26 ± 0.03**	−0.20 ± 0.03**

*SN/VTA, Substantia nigra/ventral tegmental area; Tha, Thalamus; NAc, Nucleus accumbens; **p < 0.01.*

Discussion

In the present study, using the MID Task, we observed activation of the SN/VTA, the NAcc, and the thalamus in healthy adolescents during anticipation of both monetary gain and loss. We found that the SN/VTA projects two causal pathways to the

NAcc and the thalamus. Importantly, the causal connection from the SN/VTA to the NAcc was strengthened by the anticipation of monetary gain. This modulation was also positively correlated with subjective pleasure ratings, especially anticipatory pleasure.

Consistent with results from previous fMRI studies (Knutson et al., 2000, 2001; Breiter et al., 2001; Zink et al., 2004), the NAcc is activated during anticipation of both reward and punishment in the present study. Earlier research in animals highlighted the role of the NAcc in reward anticipation, namely the "wanting" component of reward processing (Berridge and Robinson, 1998; Berridge, 2003). However, other animal studies had stressed the role of the NAcc in reward learning because local dopamine release was associated with novel stimuli and predictive cues indicating forthcoming reward or punishment (Schultz et al., 1997; Schultz, 2007). In human studies, the NAcc is conceptualized as a hedonic hotspot important in pleasure processing (Knutson and Greer, 2008; Kringelbach and Berridge, 2009). Knutson and Greer (2008) reviewed fMRI studies employing the MID task and suggested that the NAcc is involved in anticipating positive events and is associated with subjective pleasure and approaching behavior. Electrical stimulation of the NAcc in rodents and deep brain stimulation of the NAcc in humans both promote approaching behavior (Kringelbach and Berridge, 2009; Berridge and Kringelbach, 2013). Although a previous study had demonstrated that anticipation of reward rather than punishment activated the NAcc (Sabatinelli et al., 2007), activation of the NAcc had also been reported in anticipation of aversive stimuli in another study (Zink et al., 2004). Our findings lend support to the important role of NAcc in the processing of both salient information and pleasure during anticipation of rewards.

The role of the SN/VTA and the thalamus in reward processing is less controversial compared to the function of the NAcc discussed above. O'Doherty et al. (2002) found that the SN/VTA is activated during anticipation of glucose, whereas its role in anticipation of secondary rewards such as monetary stimuli is less clear. While Knutson et al. (2000, 2001) did not observe activation of the SN/VTA during anticipation of monetary stimuli, Breiter et al. (2001) identified activation in the VTA during anticipation of monetary rewards which was similar to our findings. Moreover, the VTA has been found to be activated in response to beautiful faces, which suggested that the midbrain may play an important role in positive social reward (Aharon et al., 2001). Activation of the SN/VTA to both monetary gain and loss identified in this study stresses the role of SN/VTA in reward processing.

Activation of the thalamus during anticipation of monetary gain and loss in the present study is consistent with results from a previous review (Knutson and Greer, 2008). While the thalamus is regarded as a center for information gathering and integration (Haber and Calzavara, 2009; Kohls et al., 2013), a previous study of electrical recording in rats suggested that the thalamus is also involved in retrospective and prospective coding to reward (Komura et al., 2001). In addition, the thalamus appears to be responsive to salient sensory information during the anticipation of incentives (Cho et al., 2013).

We also found a causal pathway from the SN/VTA to the NAcc during anticipation of monetary stimuli. To the best of our knowledge, few studies have investigated the causal relationship between the midbrain and the VS. A previous study on functional connectivity has reported that spontaneous activation of the NAcc correlated with reward-related brain circuits including the orbitofrontal cortex, the globus pallidus, the thalamus, the midbrain, the amygdala and the insular (Cauda et al., 2011). In addition, connectivity between the mesolimbic system and cortical areas appears to be altered in developmental conditions (Camara et al., 2009). The close relationship between mesolimbic connection and reward processing may be related to local dopaminergic metabolism. Schott et al. (2008) found that activation of the SN/VTA is associated with dopamine release in the NAcc. Moreover, Knutson and Gibbs (2007) identified that dopamine release in the NAcc activates postsynaptic D1 receptors which further induces activation in the NAcc during anticipation of reward. Both studies in functional connectivity and neurotransmitter stressed the role of mesolimbic connection in anticipation of positive events and pleasure, but the causal direction between the midbrain and the VS in this process is not clear. The causal connectivity from the SN/VTA to the NAcc identified in the present study is not only consistent with previous functional connectivity studies, but also provides new information regarding causal relationships in the mesolimbic pathway. Moreover, our findings support the role of the thalamus in integrating information from emotional, cognitive and motor cortical and subcortical areas to facilitate approaching and goal-directed behaviors (Haber and Calzavara, 2009; Haber and Knutson, 2010). In the best-fit model of our study, the SN/VTA projects an excitatory pathway to the thalamus, whereas the NAcc projects an inhibitory pathway to the thalamus. In another previous study which investigated brain circuits during anticipation of monetary incentives using DCM, Cho et al. (2013) found that the thalamus modulated the NAcc through the thalamus-to-NAcc and the thalamus-to-insula-to-NAcc connections which was different from our findings. We believe that the different findings may be related to the choice of the driven regions adopted. In the present study, the SN/VTA was chosen as the driven region, which is upstream to the dopaminergic complex in the NAcc (Schott et al., 2008; Duezel et al., 2009), whereas the thalamus was chosen as the driven region by Cho et al. (2013). However, a connection from the NAcc to the thalamus was also identified in Cho et al.'s (2013) study, which is similar to our findings. We found that both monetary 'gain' and 'loss' induced perturbation in all three connectivities in Model 8, namely the SN/VTA-to-thalamus connectivity, the SN/VTA-to-NAcc connectivity, and the NAcc-to-thalamus connectivity. In contrast to the study by Cho et al. (2013), which found different patterns of perturbation between monetary 'gain' and 'loss' in the thalamus-insula-NAcc circuit, our findings revealed a similar pattern regardless of valence in the SN/VTA-NAcc-thalamus network. The ROIs adopted and the driving ROI chosen may both cause the difference between the present and previous findings. The SN/VTA adopted here appears to play an elementary role in reward processing which may not be sensitive to the valence of the reward.

More interestingly, the modulation by monetary gain on the connectivity from the SN/VTA to the NAcc was correlated with anticipatory pleasure experience in the present study. The MID task and the TEPS are tools suggested by the RDoC for measuring anticipatory and consummatory pleasure in fMRI and behavioral paradigms, respectively, (NIMH, 2008), but few studies have investigated the underlying neural mechanism of the two instruments. People with schizophrenia spectrum disorders report dampened subjective anticipatory pleasure, while their consummatory pleasure is relatively preserved (Kring and Caponigro, 2010; Kring et al., 2011). In addition, previous studies have identified that people with schizophrenia showed reduced activation in the NAcc when anticipating monetary stimuli (Juckel et al., 2006, 2012; Walter et al., 2009). These results suggest that the two instruments seem to capture similar underlying neural mechanisms and our findings corroborated this in healthy adolescents. The connection from the SN/VTA to the NAcc in adolescents who reported higher anticipatory pleasure is more easily perturbed by positive events. This phenomenon may reflect inherent dopaminergic metabolism in the mesolimbic system and this hypothesis merits further research.

This study has several limitations. First, we only focused on the causal network in the mesolimbic system and did not investigate other important reward-related circuits such as the mesocortical system. The second limitation is that the adopted dopaminergic midbrain area is the SN rather than the VTA, but the boundary between the SN and the VTA in human is difficult to distinguish (Duezel et al., 2009). Furthermore, laterality was not taken into consideration in this study. We only focused on the right hemisphere which showed higher activation than the left. Finally, only nine models were tested in this study. Future identification of other relevant connectivity or models is needed.

Conclusion

Anticipation of both monetary gain and loss activated the NAcc and other reward-related areas, namely the SN/VTA and the thalamus. The SN/VTA projects causal pathways to the NAcc and the thalamus, while the thalamus integrates information from the SN/VTA and the NAcc. Anticipatory pleasure appears to predict the susceptibility of causal connection from the SN/VTA to the NAcc to positive events. The present findings also lend support to the applicability of the RDoC in research.

Acknowledgment

This study was supported by a grant from the "Strategic Priority Research Program (B)" of the Chinese Academy of Sciences (XDB02030002), the National Science Fund China (81088001, 91132701), the Beijing Training Project for Leading Talents in S&T (Z151100000315020).

References

Aharon, I., Etcoff, N., Ariely, D., Chabris, C. F., O'connor, E., and Breiter, H. C. (2001). Beautiful faces have variable reward value: fMRI and behavioral evidence. *Neuron* 32, 537–551. doi: 10.1016/S0896-6273(01)00491-3

Alexander, W. H., and Brown, J. W. (2010). Competition between learned reward and error outcome predictions in anterior cingulate cortex. *Neuroimage* 49, 3210–3218. doi: 10.1016/j.neuroimage.2009.11.065

Berridge, K. C. (2003). Pleasures of the brain. *Brain Cogn.* 52, 106–128. doi: 10.1016/S0278-2626(03)00014-9

Berridge, K. C., and Kringelbach, M. L. (2013). Neuroscience of affect: brain mechanisms of pleasure and displeasure. *Curr. Opin. Neurobiol.* 23, 294–303. doi: 10.1016/j.conb.2013.01.017

Berridge, K. C., and Robinson, T. E. (1998). What is the role of dopamine in reward: hedonic impact, reward learning, or incentive salience? *Brain Res. Rev.* 28, 309–369. doi: 10.1016/s0165-0173(98)00019-8

Breiter, H. C., Aharon, I., Kahneman, D., Dale, A., and Shizgal, P. (2001). Functional imaging of neural responses to expectancy and experience of monetary gains and losses. *Neuron* 30, 619–639. doi: 10.1016/S0896-6273(01)00303-8

Camara, E., Rodriguez-Fornells, A., Ye, Z., and Munte, T. F. (2009). Reward networks in the brain as captured by connectivity measures. *Front. Neurosci* 3:350–362. doi: 10.3389/neuro.01.034.2009

Cauda, F., Cavanna, A. E., D'agata, F., Sacco, K., Duca, S., and Geminiani, G. C. (2011). Functional connectivity and coactivation of the nucleus accumbens: a combined functional connectivity and structure-based meta-analysis. *J. Cognit. Neurosci.* 23, 2864–2877. doi: 10.1162/jocn.2011.21624

Chan, R. C. K., Li, Z., Li, K., Zeng, Y. W., Xie, W. Z., Yan, C., et al. (in press). Distinct processing of social and monetary rewards in late adolescents with trait anhedonia. *Neuropsychology*

Chan, R. C. K., Shi, Y. F., Lai, M. K., Wang, Y. N., Wang, Y., and Kring, A. M. (2012). The temporal experience of pleasure scale (TEPS): exploration and confirmation of factor structure in a healthy Chinese sample. *PLoS ONE* 7:e35352. doi: 10.1371/journal.pone.0035352

Cho, Y. T., Fromm, S., Guyer, A. E., Detloff, A., Pine, D. S., Fudge, J. L., et al. (2013). Nucleus accumbens, thalamus and insula connectivity during incentive anticipation in typical adults and adolescents. *Neuroimage* 66, 508–521. doi: 10.1016/j.neuroimage.2012.10.013

Cuthbert, B. N. (2014). The RDoC framework: facilitating transition from ICD/DSM to dimensional approaches that integrate neuroscience and psychopathology. *World Psychiatry* 13, 28–35. doi: 10.1002/wps.20087

Cuthbert, B. N., and Workgrp, N. R. (2014). The RDoC framework: continuing commentary. *World Psychiatry* 13, 196–197. doi: 10.1002/wps.20140

Duezel, E., Bunzeck, N., Guitart-Masip, M., Wittmann, B., Schott, B. H., and Tobler, P. N. (2009). Functional imaging of the human dopaminergic midbrain. *Trends Neurosci.* 32, 321–328. doi: 10.1016/j.tins.2009.02.005

Friston, K. J., Harrison, L., and Penny, W. (2003). Dynamic causal modelling. *Neuroimage* 19, 1273–1302. doi: 10.1016/S1053-8119(03)00202-7

Gard, D. E., Gard, M. G., Kring, A. M., and John, O. P. (2006). Anticipatory and consummatory components of the experience of pleasure: a scale development study. *J. Res. Pers.* 40, 1086–1102. doi: 10.1016/j.jrp.2005.11.001

Gonen, T., Admon, R., Podlipsky, I., and Hendler, T. (2012). From animal model to human brain networking: dynamic causal modeling of motivational systems. *J. Neurosci.* 32, 7218–7224. doi: 10.1523/JNEUROSCI.6188-11.2012

Gong, Y. X. (1992). *Manual of Wechsler Adult Intelligence Scale-Chinese Version*. Changsha: Chinese Map Press.

Haber, S. N., and Calzavara, R. (2009). The cortico-basal ganglia integrative network: the role of the thalamus. *Brain Res. Bull.* 78, 69–74. doi: 10.1016/j.brainresbull.2008.09.013

Haber, S. N., and Knutson, B. (2010). The reward circuit: linking primate anatomy and human imaging. *Neuropsychopharmacology* 35, 4–26. doi: 10.1038/npp.2009.129

Horvitz, J. C. (2000). Mesolimbocortical and nigrostriatal dopamine responses to salient non-reward events. *Neuroscience* 96, 651–656. doi: 10.1016/S0306-4522(00)00019-1

Juckel, G., Friedel, E., Koslowski, M., Witthaus, H., Oezguerdal, S., Gudlowski, Y., et al. (2012). Ventral striatal activation during reward processing in subjects with ultra-high risk for schizophrenia. *Neuropsychobiology* 66, 50–56. doi: 10.1159/000337130

Juckel, G., Schlagenhauf, F., Koslowski, M., Filonov, D., Wuestenberg, T., Villringer, A., et al. (2006). Dysfunction of ventral striatal reward prediction in schizophrenic patients treated with typical, not atypical, neuroleptics. *Psychopharmacology (Berl.)* 187, 222–228. doi: 10.1007/s00213-006-0405-4

Keuken, M. C., Bazin, P. L., Crown, L., Hootsmans, J., Laufer, A., Müller-Axt, C., et al. (2014). Quantifying inter-individual anatomical variability in the subcortex using 7 T structural MRI. *Neuroimage* 94, 40–46. doi: 10.1016/j.neuroimage.2014.03.032

Knutson, B., Fong, G. W., Adams, C. M., Varner, J. L., and Hommer, D. (2001). Dissociation of reward anticipation and outcome with event-related fMRI. *Neuroreport* 12, 3683–3687. doi: 10.1097/00001756-200112040-00016

Knutson, B., and Gibbs, S. E. B. (2007). Linking nucleus accumbens dopamine and blood oxygenation. *Psychopharmacology (Berl.)* 191, 813–822. doi: 10.1007/s00213-006-0686-7

Knutson, B., and Greer, S. M. (2008). Anticipatory affect: neural correlates and consequences for choice. *Philos. Trans. R Soc. Lond. B Biol. Sci.* 363, 3771–3786. doi: 10.1098/rstb.2008.0155

Knutson, B., Westdorp, A., Kaiser, E., and Hommer, D. (2000). FMRI visualization of brain activity during a monetary incentive delay task. *Neuroimage* 12, 20–27. doi: 10.1006/nimg.2000.0593

Kohls, G., Perino, M. T., Taylor, J. M., Madva, E. N., Cayless, S. J., Troiani, V., et al. (2013). The nucleus accumbens is involved in both the pursuit of social reward and the avoidance of social punishment. *Neuropsychologia* 51, 2062–2069. doi: 10.1016/j.neuropsychologia.2013.07.020

Komura, Y., Tamura, R., Uwano, T., Nishijo, H., Kaga, K., and Ono, T. (2001). Retrospective and prospective coding for predicted reward in the sensory thalamus. *Nature* 412, 546–549. doi: 10.1038/35087595

Kring, A. M., and Caponigro, J. M. (2010). Emotion in schizophrenia: where feeling meets thinking. *Curr. Dir. Psychol. Sci.* 19, 255–259. doi: 10.1177/0963721410377599

Kring, A. M., Gard, M. G., and Gard, D. E. (2011). Emotion deficits in schizophrenia: timing matters. *J. Abnorm. Psychol.* 120, 79–87. doi: 10.1037/a0021402

NIMH (2008). *Research Domain Criteria (RDoC)*. Available at: http://www.nimh.nih.gov/research-priorities/rdoc/index.shtml [accessed May 6, 2015].

O'Doherty, J. P., Deichmann, R., Critchley, H. D., and Dolan, R. J. (2002). Neural responses during anticipation of a primary taste reward. *Neuron* 33, 815–826. doi: 10.1016/S0896-6273(02)00603-7

Sabatinelli, D., Bradley, M. M., Lang, P. J., Costa, V. D., and Versace, F. (2007). Pleasure rather than salience activates human nucleus accumbens and medial prefrontal cortex. *J. Neurophysiol.* 98, 1374–1379. doi: 10.1152/jn.00230.2007

Schott, B. H., Minuzzi, L., Krebs, R. M., Elmenhorst, D., Lang, M., Winz, O. H., et al. (2008). Mesolimbic functional magnetic resonance imaging activations during reward anticipation correlate with reward-related ventral striatal dopamine release. *J. Neurosci.* 28, 14311–14319. doi: 10.1523/JNEUROSCI.2058-08.2008

Schultz, W. (2007). Behavioral dopamine signals. *Trends Neurosci.* 30, 203–210. doi: 10.1016/j.tins.2007.03.007

Schultz, W., Dayan, P., and Montague, P. R. (1997). A neural substrate of prediction and reward. *Science* 275, 1593–1599. doi: 10.1126/science.275.5306.1593

Shankman, S. A., Katz, A. C., Delizza, A. A., Sarapas, C., Gorka, S. M., and Campbell, M. L. (2014). "Chapter 1: the different facets of anhedonia and their associations with different psychopathologies," in: *Anhedonia: A Comprehensive Handbook*, ed. M. S. Ritsner (Dordrecht: Springer Science+Business Media).

Stephan, K. E., Penny, W. D., Moran, R. J., Den Ouden, H. E. M., Daunizeau, J., and Friston, K. J. (2010). Ten simple rules for dynamic causal modeling. *Neuroimage* 49, 3099–3109. doi: 10.1016/j.neuroimage.2009.11.015

Veldhuizen, M. G., Douglas, D., Aschenbrenner, K., Gitelman, D. R., and Small, D. M. (2011). The anterior insular cortex represents breaches of taste identity expectation. *J. Neurosci.* 31, 14735–14744. doi: 10.1523/JNEUROSCI.1502-11.2011

Walter, H., Kammerer, H., Frasch, K., Spitzer, M., and Abler, B. (2009). Altered reward functions in patients on atypical antipsychotic medication in line with the revised dopamine hypothesis of schizophrenia. *Psychopharmacology (Berl.)* 206, 121–132. doi: 10.1007/s00213-009-1586-4

Yu, H., Zhou, Z., and Zhou, X. (2013). The amygdalostriatal and corticostriatal effective connectivity in anticipation and evaluation of facial attractiveness. *Brain Cogn.* 82, 291–300. doi: 10.1016/j.bandc.2013.04.011

Zink, C. F., Pagnoni, G., Martin-Skurski, M. E., Chappelow, J. C., and Berns, G. S. (2004). Human striatal responses to monetary reward depend on saliency. *Neuron* 42, 509–517. doi: 10.1016/S0896-6273(04)00183-7

Conflict of Interest Statement: The authors declare that the research was conducted in the absence of any commercial or financial relationships that could be construed as a potential conflict of interest.

19

Impulsivity is Associated with Increased Metabolism in the Fronto-Insular Network in Parkinson's Disease

Edited by:
Morten L. Kringelbach,
University of Oxford, UK;
University of Aarhus, Denmark

***Correspondence:**
Masoud Tahmasian
masoud.tahmasian@uk-koeln.de

Masoud Tahmasian [1,2,3], Luisa Rochhausen [1], Franziska Maier [1], Kim L. Williamson [1], Alexander Drzezga [2], Lars Timmermann [1], Thilo Van Eimeren [1,2] and Carsten Eggers [1]*

[1] Department of Neurology, University Hospital of Cologne, Cologne, Germany, [2] Department of Nuclear Medicine, University Hospital of Cologne, Cologne, Germany, [3] Sleep Disorders Research Center, Kermanshah University of Medical Sciences (KUMS), Kermanshah, Iran

Various neuroimaging studies demonstrated that the fronto-insular network is implicated in impulsive behavior. We compared glucose metabolism (as a proxy measure of neural activity) among 24 patients with Parkinson's disease (PD) who presented with low or high levels of impulsivity based on the Barratt Impulsiveness Scale 11 (BIS) scores. Subjects underwent 18-fluorodeoxyglucose positron emission tomography (FDG-PET) and the voxel-wise group difference of FDG-metabolism was analyzed in Statistical Parametric Mapping (SPM8). Subsequently, we performed a partial correlation analysis between the FDG-metabolism and BIS scores, controlling for covariates (i.e., age, sex, severity of disease and levodopa equivalent daily doses). Voxel-wise group comparison revealed higher FDG-metabolism in the orbitofrontal cortex (OFC), anterior cingulate cortex (ACC), and right insula in patients with higher impulsivity scores. Moreover, there was a positive correlation between the FDG-metabolism and BIS scores. Our findings provide evidence that high impulsivity is associated with increased FDG-metabolism within the fronto-insular network in PD.

Keywords: impulsive behaviors, FDG-PET, orbitofrontal cortex, anterior cingulate cortex, insula

INTRODUCTION

Impulsivity is an umbrella term that covers "actions that are poorly conceived, prematurely expressed, unduly risky, or inappropriate to the situation and that often result in undesirable outcomes" (Evenden, 1999). Impulsivity is generally considered as a personality trait that is associated with self-control deficiency and several problematic behaviors such as aggression, risk-seeking behavior, driving violation and also suicide attempt (Owsley et al., 2003; Fineberg et al., 2014; Gvion et al., 2014). Impulsive behaviors can be observed in healthy individuals (Chamorro et al., 2012), drug-dependent individuals (Ersche et al., 2011; Qiu et al., 2013) or patients with neuropsychiatric disorders including bipolar mood disorders, borderline personality disorder and attention-deficit/hyperactivity disorder (Nandagopal et al., 2011; Cackowski et al., 2014; Sebastian et al., 2014; Fossati et al., 2015). In addition, high impulsivity is a risk factor for impulse control disorders (ICDs) that consist of serious behavioral symptoms such as pathological gambling, compulsive shopping, binge eating and hyper sexuality. Crucially, ICDs may develop due to overstimulation of the mesolimbic system by dopaminergic medication (Lee et al., 2010; Voon et al., 2011a,b; Probst and Van Eimeren, 2013). ICDs are common non-motor symptoms in Parkinson's disease (PD). For example, it has been shown that at least one form of ICDs was found in 13.6% of medicated PD patients (Weintraub et al., 2010). Moreover, the trait of impulsivity might be an important selection criterion for deep brain stimulation (DBS) of the subthalamic nucleus (STN), as DBS of the limbic part of the STN can reduce the activity of the inhibitory networks in PD (Jahanshahi, 2013). Thus, understanding the neural mechanisms of impulsivity in PD may lead to better treatment strategies in future.

Neuroimaging studies demonstrated that the fronto-insular network, including the orbitofrontal cortex (OFC), anterior cingulate cortex (ACC), medial prefrontal cortex (mPFC), dorsolateral prefrontal cortex (dlPFC), and insula, are involved in impulsive behavior in healthy controls (Matsuo et al., 2009a; Cho et al., 2013), patients with neuropsychiatric disorders (Antonucci et al., 2006; Matsuo et al., 2009b; Sebastian et al., 2014; Trost et al., 2014), high risk individuals for psychosis (Lee et al., 2013), and PD patients with ICDs (Cilia et al., 2008, 2011; Van Eimeren et al., 2010; Voon et al., 2011a; Biundo et al., 2015). In this study, we focused on impulsivity rather than ICDs to investigate the neural mechanisms underlying high level of impulsivity as a risk factor for developing ICDs in PD patients, while we controlled for age, gender, severity of disease, and levodopa equivalent daily dose (LEDD) for dopamine agonists. We hypothesized that PD patients with higher level of impulsivity have regional glucose metabolism alterations in the fronto-insular network, particularly in the OFC, ACC, and insula, which have been discussed to be associated with the inhibitory networks and impulsivity behaviors.

MATERIALS AND METHODS

Subjects

Twenty-four right-handed patients (mean age 66.29, SD 6.01) with idiopathic PD were recruited from the outpatient clinic of the Department of Neurology, University Hospital of Cologne. The study was approved and registered by the medical ethics board of the University Hospital of Cologne in line with Human Research Committee guidelines. All subjects provided informed consent in accordance with the standard protocol approvals (Nr.10-278). On every subject, medical history and neurological examination were performed. Patients fulfilled criteria for PD based on the United Kingdom Parkinson's Disease Society Brain Bank criteria (Hughes et al., 1992). Evaluation of motor symptoms was assessed with the Unified Parkinson's Disease Rating Scale (UPDRS) Part III (Fahn et al., 1987; Van Hilten et al., 1994) and severity of PD was assessed with Hoehn and Yahr (1967) staging in both the ON- and the OFF-state. The OFF-state reflects withdrawal from dopamine replacement therapy for at least 12 h or from controlled-released drugs, such as dopamine agonists, for at least 72 h. The ON-state was defined as patient's best response to 200 mg of levodopa after the OFF-state. Neuropsychological assessments were acquired in the regular daily medication ON-state. For subsequent analyses, the LEDD of dopamine agonists was calculated according to the guidelines of the German Neurological Society (Diener and Weimar, 2012). In addition, all patients were interviewed in a detailed survey that noted the side of onset and duration of disease since the first diagnoses. Two movement disorders specialists (C.E, L.T) assessed severity of PD. Our exclusion criteria were the following: (i) psychiatric comorbidities including depression (BDI-II score >19; Beck et al., 1996; Kühner et al., 2007), severe cognitive impairment or dementia (Mini Mental State *Exam* (MMSE) <27; Kessler et al., 2000); (ii) any other severe systemic diseases including cardiovascular diseases or diabetes mellitus; (iii) neurological diseases such as history of head trauma, stroke, brain tumor, epilepsy, or dyskinesia; and (iv) PD patients with diagnosis of ICDs.

Neuropsychological Assessment

The Barratt Impulsiveness Scale (BIS) is a self-report questionnaire to evaluate impulsivity, which consists of 30 four-point Likert-type items reflecting frequency of occurrence. The scale was filled out by all patients during their regular daily medication. The BIS can be divided into three sub-scores including attention, motor, and non-planning impulsiveness. Higher BIS scores reflect higher level of impulsivity (Patton et al., 1995).

Preprocessing and Analysis of FDG-PET Data

Preprocessing of fluorodeoxyglucose positron emission tomography (FDG-PET) images was carried out using Statistical Parametric Mapping (SPM8) (Wellcome Trust Center for Neuroimaging, London, UK) as described before Drzezga (2009), Eggers et al. (2014) and Tahmasian et al. (2015b). First, the scans were normalized to the standard stereotactical space using the standard PET template and then smoothed using a 6 mm full width at half maximum (FWHM) Gaussian filter.

FDG-PET Data Acquisition

As described previously (Eggers et al., 2009), a high-resolution 24-detector ring PET scanner (ECAT EXACT HRRT, Siemens CTI, Knoxville, TN, USA) with 207 transaxial image planes and 1.219 mm voxel size was used in this study. Images were acquired with subjects in resting position, with background noise reduced, and with light dimmed. After the injection of 370 MBq of 18F-fluorodeoxyglucose (FDG), cerebral glucose metabolism was measured, reflecting the regional neural activity. Arterialized venous blood sampling allowed absolute quantification for all participants. The imaging was performed in the 3-D mode and was subsequently reconstructed as well as corrected for random artifacts, head motion, attenuation and scatter. The resolution of the reconstructed images was almost isotropic with 2.2 mm

FWHM in the center and 2.5 mm FWHM at 10 cm off-axis. The FDG-PET measurement was performed with subjects in their regular medicated state (ON-state) to decrease head motion during scanning and to evaluate neural activity in a similar condition in terms of impulsivity in their daily routine.

Statistical Analyses

Following our hypothesis, we divided our patients into two groups based on their BIS scores according to the published standards i.e., patients with higher impulsivity (*BIS* > 65, $n = 8$) and lower impulsivity (BIS ≤ 65, $n = 16$; Voon et al., 2007; Stanford et al., 2009). For group comparisons of demographic and neuropsychiatric data, we carried out two-sample *t*-tests as a parametric test applied on normally distributed data, and Mann-Whitney U-tests as a nonparametric test for not normally distributed data and also Fisher's exact test for sex difference in the Statistical Package for Social Sciences, version 22 (SPSS). *P*-values less than 0.05 were considered statistically significant.

For group comparisons of FDG-PET data, a voxel-wise two-sample *t*-test in SPM8 was performed across the whole-brain, while PET images were normalized by the whole-brain FDG uptake values. The initial uncorrected threshold of 0.001 was applied for group comparison and results were reported as significant at *p*-value less than 0.05 with family-wise error (FWE) correction of the cluster-level. This analysis was controlled for covariates, including age, gender, severity of disease (UPDRS III OFF) and LEDD for dopamine agonists. We chose dopamine agonist LEDD instead of total LEDD because it has been shown that dopamine agonists change the activity of the OFC and rostral cingulate region in PD (Van Eimeren et al., 2009, 2010). Results with total LEDD as a covariate were highly similar (not shown). These analyses yielded a volume-of-interest (VOI) that showed significant metabolic changes in patients with higher impulsivity level compared to patients with lower impulsivity level. We chose the VOI based on significant metabolic changes in the whole brain voxel-wise group comparison to be independent from selection bias of *a-priori* defined regions. Subsequently, we extracted the absolute averaged FDG-metabolism within the mentioned VOI for each individual subject as applied previously in several neuroimaging studies (Matsuda et al., 2012; Tahmasian et al., 2013, 2015b; Wehrl et al., 2013; Klupp et al., 2014, 2015), then normalized those scores (FDG scores from the VOI divided to global uptake scores) and then performed independent *t*-test between groups using SPSS.

To detect the association between the FDG-metabolism and impulsivity, we performed a partial correlation analysis between the normalized averaged FDG-metabolism scores of the VOI and the total and sub-scores of BIS across all 24 patients in SPSS, controlling for covariates such as age, gender, severity of disease (UPDRS III OFF) and LEDD for dopamine agonists.

RESULTS

Demographic and Neuropsychological Data

Our sample consisted of 24 non-demented, non-depressed, non-ICD PD patients. Demographic information is summarized in **Table 1**. The mean total BIS for the patients with low level of impulsivity was 53.18 (SD 7.60; range 41–63) and for the patients with a high level of impulsivity was 70.37 (SD 4.17; range 65–79). Between groups, there were significant differences on the total and sub-scores of BIS, including attention, motor and non-planning ($p < 0.05$, **Table 1**). Group comparisons demonstrated no significant differences regarding the severity of disease and severity of motor symptoms. However, there was a significant difference between LEDD calculated only for dopamine agonists as suggested previously (Tomlinson et al., 2010). Hence, we controlled for the effects of dopamine agonists in further analyses. One should note that there was trend towards

TABLE 1 | Demographic and neuropsychological data ([a] = Mann-Whitney-Test, [b] = *t*-test, [c] = Fisher's exact test, degree of freedom was 22 for all group comparisons, results presented as mean ± SD).

	PD patients with lower impulsivity ($n = 16$)	PD patients with higher impulsivity ($n = 8$)	*p*-value
Sex (female/male)	6/10	2/6	0.667[c]
Age (year)	65 ± 6.59	68.88 ± 3.75	0.14[b]
Duration since diagnosis	7.41 ± 4.23	11.38 ± 5.21	0.054[b]
Hoehn und Yahr OFF	3 ± 0.89	2.62 ± 0.51	0.349[a]
Hoehn und Yahr ON	2.5 ± 1.03	2.25 ± 0.46	0.588[a]
UPDRS III OFF	35.06 ± 14.17	29.50 ± 5.15	0.177[b]
UPDRS III ON	24.19 ± 13.09	21.38 ± 6.34	0.759[a]
LEDD—total (mg)	600.94 ± 356.45	956.12 ± 475.51	0.051[b]
LEDD—dopamine agonists (mg)	180.62 ± 133.85	318.62 ± 181.68	0.046[b]
MMSE	28.69 ± 1.138	28.75 ± 1.275	0.928[a]
BIS—total	53.18 ± 7.60	70.37 ± 4.17	0.000[b]
BIS—attention	14.37 ± 2.80	18.375 ± 2.38	0.002[b]
BIS—motor impulsivity	19.00 ± 3.01	22.625 ± 2.32	0.007[b]
BIS—non-planning	19.81 ± 5.39	29.5 ± 3.92	0.000[b]

Abbreviations: BIS, barratt impulsiveness scale; LEDD, levodopa equivalent daily dose; MMSE, mini-mental state examination; PD, Parkinson's disease; SD, standard deviation; UPDRS, unified Parkinson's disease rating scale.

a significant group difference regarding the LEDD-total and duration of disease since diagnosis.

PD Patients with Higher Impulsivity Level Revealed Increased Glucose Metabolism in the Fronto-Insular Network

Voxel-wise two-sample *t*-test between groups demonstrated higher metabolism within the fronto-insular network including the OFC, medial-frontal gyrus, ACC and insula, mainly on the right hemisphere (based on Automated Anatomical Labeling atlas; Tzourio-Mazoyer et al., 2002) in subjects with higher impulsivity level compared to individuals with lower level of impulsivity ($p < 0.05$, FWE corrected; **Figure 1A**, **Table 2**). Moreover, patients with higher impulsivity revealed higher averaged FDG-metabolism using the group difference VOIs determined by SPM8 (mean ± SD = 2.28 ± 0.14 vs. 1.97 ± 0.10; **Figure 1B**). On the other hand, PD patients with higher level of impulsivity had significant decreased FDG-metabolism in the superior parietal gyrus and occipital cortex compared to PD patients with lower level of impulsivity ($p < 0.05$, FWE corrected, not shown).

Association between Impulsivity and Glucose Metabolism in the Fronto-Insular Network

We assessed the link between FDG-metabolism of the fronto-insular network and BIS scores. Results showed a positive correlation between the averaged FDG-metabolism and total BIS scores ($r = 0.761$, $p < 0.001$) across all patients (**Figure 2A**). Furthermore, significant positive correlations were found between the FDG-metabolism and BIS sub-score for attention ($r = 0.646$, $p < 0.05$), motor ($r = 0.506$, $p < 0.05$), and non-planning impulsivity ($r = 0.670$, $p < 0.001$; **Figures 2B–D**).

DISCUSSION

To assess the neural correlates of impulsivity in PD patients, we compared glucose metabolism of patients with higher impulsivity level and patients with lower impulsivity level. We found that patients with higher impulsivity level showed increased glucose metabolism within the fronto-insular network including the OFC, medial frontal gyrus, ACC, and right insula (**Figure 1**). Moreover, our findings demonstrated positive correlations between the averaged FDG-metabolism of those regions and BIS scores (i.e., total and sub-score for attention, motor, and non-planning impulsivity) across all patients (**Figure 2**). These results provide further evidence that higher impulsivity is linked with altered function of the fronto-insular network. Our findings are in line with previous reports indicating that high impulsivity is associated with structural and functional changes of regions associated with reward-related decision making and impulse control behavior including the OFC and ACC in healthy controls and individuals at ultra-high risk for psychosis (Horn et al., 2003; Brown et al., 2006; Cilia et al., 2008; Matsuo et al., 2009a; Cho et al., 2013; Lee et al., 2013). PD patients with higher level of impulsivity also demonstrated lower FDG-metabolism in the superior parietal gyrus and occipital cortex compared to other group. Based on our hypothesis we did not expect changes in these parieto-occipital regions. These findings might

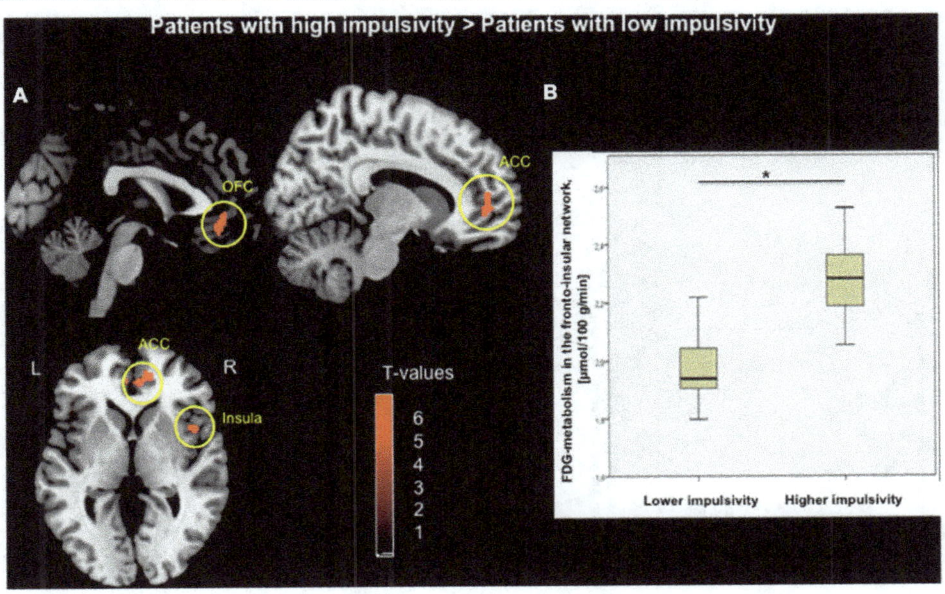

FIGURE 1 | (A) Voxel-wise group comparison of FDG-metabolism generated by independent *t*-test in SPM8. Red maps illustrate increased metabolism in PD patients with higher impulsivity compared to PD patients with lower impulsivity in the orbitofrontal cortex (OFC), anterior cingulate cortex (ACC), and right insula ($p < 0.05$, FWE corrected in cluster level, bars represent range of *t*-values). **(B)** Group difference based on the averaged FDG-metabolism of the fronto-insular network including the OFC, ACC, and insula within (*$p < 0.001$).

TABLE 2 | Voxel-wise group comparison *t*-test demonstrated increased metabolism in PD patients with higher impulsivity compared to PD patients with lower impulsivity.

Anatomical region	L/R	Cluster	*p*-value (FWE-corrected)	*T*-score	Peak coordinates (MNI)
Orbitofrontal cortex	L	170	0.004	5.82	−2, 38, −10
Medial frontal gyrus	R	170	0.004	5.77	12, 48, 2
Anterior cingulate cortex	R	170	0.004	4.47	4, 44, 0
Insula-operculum	R	115	0.029	5.24	46, 2, 14
Insula	R	115	0.029	4.75	46, 10, 2

Abbreviations: FWE, family-wise error; MNI, Montreal Neurological Institute.

be additionally due to the increased FDG-metabolism in the fronto-insular network a secondary compensatory change of network activity.

Its worthy to note that FDG-PET imaging provides a quantitative measurement of regional metabolism within the synaptic terminals of the neuron-astrocyte functional unit. In detail, after injection of FDG, its tissue uptake increases in the active region, which correlates with the local metabolism of brain tissue. Hence, increase of glucose uptake provides indirect evidence of higher synaptic metabolism in a particular region (Lucignani and Nobili, 2010).

Neural Correlates of Impulsivity within the Fronto-Insular Network

Distinct brain regions are responsible for processing of reward-related learning, goal-directed actions, decision-making and the formation of habits (Schultz et al., 2000; Torregrossa et al., 2008). Among them, the OFC is involved in sensory and emotional integration, encoding the affective value of reinforcers and evaluation of the expected rewards/punishments of a decision. Therefore, the OFC has an important role in adaptive decision-making, guiding behavior, judgments, and behavioral regulation (Kringelbach, 2005; Torregrossa et al., 2008; Schoenbaum et al., 2011). Animal studies revealed that OFC lesions result in failure to assess the value of an outcome under changing conditions, improper inhibition of motor responses, devalue the reinforce, increase in habitual responding and increased premature responses (Torregrossa et al., 2008). Thus, it seems that activity of the OFC is essential for proper impulse control. Moreover, it has been shown that the association of the lateral PFC to both aggression and attentional impulsivity depends on OFC contribution (Gansler et al., 2011). In a functional neuroimaging (fMRI) study, Horn et al. (2003) applied

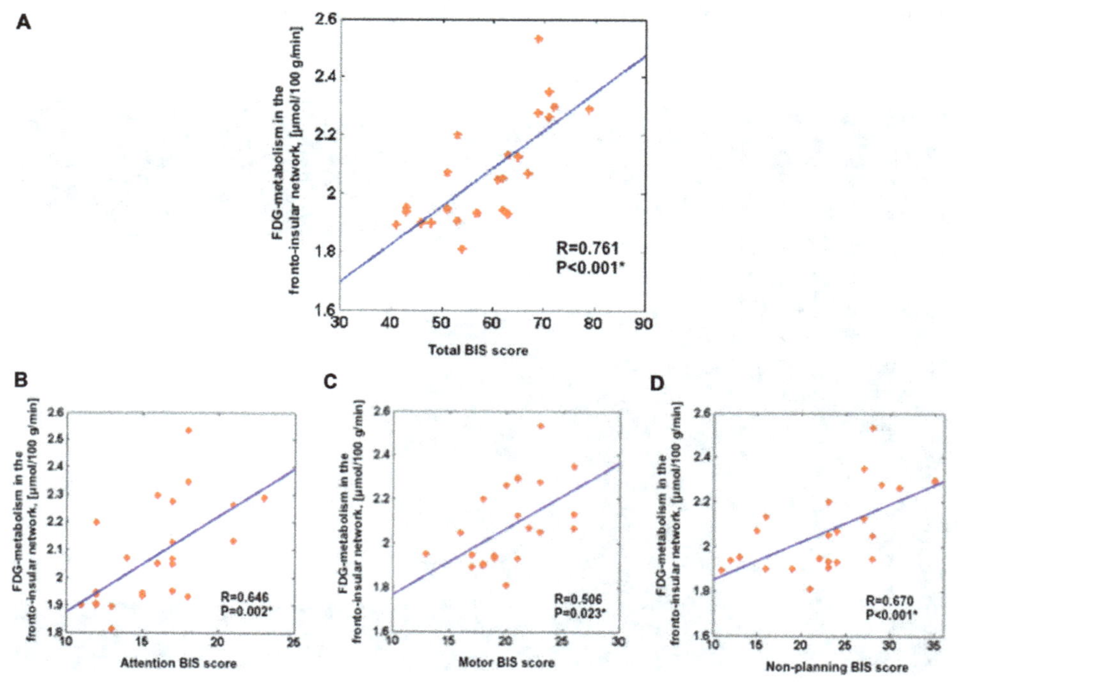

FIGURE 2 | Positive correlation between the averaged FDG-metabolism within the group comparison volume-of-interest (i.e., the fronto-insular network) extracted for each subject and the total BIS scores (A), attention BIS score (B), motor BIS score (C), non-planning BIS score (D). Partial correlations were performed across all 24 PD patients with additional covariates such as age, sex, severity of disease and LEDD for dopamine agonists; $^*p < 0.05$). BIS, Barratt Impulsiveness Scale; LEDD, levodopa equivalent daily dose.

Go/No-Go task. This task is often used to assess a participant's ability to sustain attention and inhibit responses. The authors demonstrated a significant activation in the anterior lateral OFC during the inhibition task. They showed that subjects with higher impulsivity activated the right inferior frontal gyrus, posterior lateral OFC and anterior insula (Horn et al., 2003). Similarly, our results support the idea that hyperactivity of the OFC is essential for proper inhibition in PD patients with high impulsivity.

The OFC has reciprocal connections with the ACC, which is involved in executive functions such as attention, inhibition and emotion regulation (Devinsky et al., 1995; Banks et al., 2007; Rushworth et al., 2007). Another fMRI study demonstrated that activation of several regions, including the ACC, was positively correlated with impulsivity level during inhibitory control paradigms, suggesting a regulatory role of ACC in modulating impulsive behaviors (Brown et al., 2006). Recently, Kerr et al. (2015) revealed that impulsivity was linked with higher activation of the ACC and amygdala during anticipation of the primary reward. In addition, impulsivity was negatively associated with functional connectivity between the ACC and amygdala (Kerr et al., 2015). Wilbertz et al. (2014) highlighted a link between urgency as an impulsivity subdomain and a network including the inferior frontal gyrus, anterior insula and dorsal ACC. Another Go/No-Go fMRI study revealed that subjects with internet gaming addiction had hyperactivity during No-Go trials in several brain regions including the left superior medial frontal gyrus, right ACC, right superior/middle frontal gyrus. Interestingly, activation of the superior medial frontal gyrus was positively associated with BIS-11, suggesting an association between impulsivity and impaired prefrontal impulse inhibition (Ding et al., 2014). Moreover, it has been reported that self-control and successful inhibition of impulsive behaviors, particularly motor impulsivity, and reactive aggression depends on the anterior insula activity (Dambacher et al., 2015).

Several studies highlighted the relationship between gray matter volume changes and the BIS scores in healthy controls and subjects at ultra-high risk for psychosis (Matsuo et al., 2009a; Cho et al., 2013; Lee et al., 2013). For example, Cho et al. (2013) found positive correlations between volume of mPFC, dlPFC, OFC, ACC and total, non-planning, and attention/cognitive BIS scores but not with motor impulsivity. Churchwell and Yurgelun-Todd (2013) found a positive linear association between anterior insula thickness and non-planning imulsivity, and both of them had negative correlations with age. Similarly, it has been demonstrated that patients with major depressive disorder, alcoholism, posttraumatic stress disorder, attention-deficit/hyperactivity disorder, antisocial personality disorder or bipolar disorder showed positive correlations between the left, right, and total OFC gray matter volume and BIS motor impulsivity scores and aggression (Antonucci et al., 2006). Our results are similar to these findings, as we found significant positive associations between the FDG-metabolism of the fronto-insular network and the total, non-planning, attention and motor impulsivity. On the other hand, Matsuo et al. (2009a) demonstrated that gray matter volumes of the bilateral OFC and left ACC were negatively correlated with the total BIS scores. More specifically, they found negative associations between the right OFC volume and non-planning impulsivity, and between the left OFC volume and motor impulsivity.

In the right fronto-insular cortex and anterior limbic area of the human brain there are large bipolar neurons so-called "von Economo neurons", particularly in the ACC and the anterior insula. These neurons are involved in empathy, social awareness, and self-control and their numbers are reduced in several neuropsychiatric disorders including fronto-temporal dementia, schizophrenia, bipolar disorder, addiction and ICDs (Allman et al., 2011a,b; Kim et al., 2012).

Taken together, the above-mentioned studies showed that the fronto-insular network is critically involved in impulsiveness. With regards to our findings of the increased metabolism within this network, it is possible to speculate that subjects with higher impulsivity scores need this network to be more active in order to inhibit their impulses, compared to subjects with lower impulsivity.

Impulsivity vs. Impulse Control Disorders

Although impulsivity is a natural behavior that can be controlled by inhibitory mechanisms in healthy individuals, it can be considered as a risk factor for ICDs in patients with PD (Cilia and Van Eimeren, 2011; Probst and Van Eimeren, 2013). Patients with ICDs such as pathological gambling, hypersexuality, and kleptomania have more compulsive characteristics resulting in failure to resist aggressive impulses (Weiss and Marsh, 2012; Fineberg et al., 2014). Although the neural systems for regulating impulsive, compulsive, and habitual behaviors have an overlapping regional pathophysiology (i.e., activation of the OFC), impulsivity and subdomains of ICDs have different pathophysiological mechanisms (Torregrossa et al., 2008; Leeman and Potenza, 2012). Accordingly, one should be aware that impulsivity and ICDs are conceptually and pathophysiologically distinct.

A recent study demonstrated that PD patients with ICDs had cortical thinning in fronto-striatal circuitry including the right superior OFC, left rostral middle frontal, bilateral caudal middle frontal region, corpus callosum, right accumbens, as well as an increase in the left amygdala. Moreover, they found a positive correlation between severity of impulsive symptoms and cortical thickness of left rostral middle frontal, inferior parietal, and supramarginal regions (Biundo et al., 2015).

Several fMRI studies revealed that dopamine agonist therapy mediates the ability of PD patients to control their impulses and may lead to high impulsivity and ICDs (Cilia et al., 2008; Van Eimeren et al., 2009, 2010; Ray and Strafella, 2010; Voon et al., 2011a; Weiss and Marsh, 2012; Napier et al., 2015). For example, it has been suggested that PD patients with pathological gambling have an ACC-striatal disconnection and also a hyperactivity in the OFC, hippocampus, amygdala, insula, and ventral pallidum, possibly associated with a drug-induced overstimulation of relatively preserved reward-related neuronal systems (Cilia et al., 2008, 2011).

Van Eimeren et al. (2010) demonstrated that in the lateral OFC, rostral cingulate zone, amygdala, and external pallidum, healthy controls had higher activity in response to dopamine agonist, while PD patients with pathological gambling showed a significant DA-induced reduction of activity. To control for the influence of dopamine agonists on the suggested relationship (Tahmasian et al., 2015a), we applied a partial correlation approach, which accounts separately for influences of medication (LEDD for dopamine agonists) on local FDG-metabolism. Furthermore, the results were also independent from age and sex.

Due to our results, we assume that higher activity of fronto-insular network is necessary in patients with higher impulsivity. In particular, patients with higher impulsivity level have self-control deficiency and tendency to do problematic risky behaviors (Owsley et al., 2003; Fineberg et al., 2014; Gvion et al., 2014). Thus, they need to inhibit their impulses more than subjects with lower impulsivity level. As mentioned above, patients with lesions or atrophy in the OFC and ACC show more impulsive, antisocial, and risky behaviors (Winstanley et al., 2004; Berlin et al., 2005; Matsuo et al., 2009a,b; Kerr et al., 2015). Taken together, we suggest that the observed increased activity in the inhibitory network (Van Eimeren et al., 2010) within the fronto-insular regions is necessary to allow an active inhibition of risk-related impulsive behaviors, particularly in patients with higher impulsivity (for review, see Seguin, 2004; Crews and Boettiger, 2009; Perry et al., 2011). One should note that our subjects had higher impulsivity and not ICDs diagnosis. Hence, future studies should systematically compare subjects with different levels of impulsivity vs. healthy subjects and patients with ICDs to provide explicit proof of this hypothesis.

LIMITATIONS

Our study has several limitations: (i) albeit the BIS scale is the most common tool to assess of impulsivity, it is a self-report and subjective questionnaire. Thus, it is not an objective assessment of impulsivity; (ii) it should be noted that our findings may be limited to moderate impulsivity level of our subjects and can not be generalized to ICDs in PD patients; (iii) the observed difference in glucose metabolism might be due to underlying mechanism including the different levels of von Economo neurons in the fronto-insular network, receptor availability or genetic difference across subjects but these data were not available for us to correct for their influence. In particular, gray matter volume difference is probably one of the most important confounding factors, but we did not have structural MRI data from these subjects to perform atrophy correction; and (iv) our sample size was rather small, particularly in patients with higher impulsivity level, we also did not include healthy control subjects or PD patients with ICDs. Future studies with larger sample size should consider atrophy correction and systematically compare healthy controls and PD patients with and without ICDs.

CONCLUSION

In summary, the current study provides evidence that PD patients with higher impulsivity level have increased glucose metabolism within the fronto-insular network compared to PD patients with lower impulsivity level. The data are consistent with several structural and fMRI studies, suggesting that the activity of fronto-insular network is essential for proper impulse inhibition, particularly in PD patients with higher impulsivity. Our findings shed new light on the neural correlates of impulsivity in PD.

ACKNOWLEDGMENTS

This study was supported by the German Research Foundation (KFO 219, TP10). We wish to thank all patients for their participation in the study. Furthermore, we thank the staff of the Departments of Neurology, University Hospital of Cologne and also Max Planck institute for Metabolism Research for their help in recruitment and data collection.

REFERENCES

Allman, J. M., Tetreault, N. A., Hakeem, A. Y., and Park, S. (2011a). The von economo neurons in apes and humans. *Am. J. Hum. Biol.* 23, 5–21. doi: 10.1002/ajhb.21136

Allman, J. M., Tetreault, N. A., Hakeem, A. Y., Manaye, K. F., Semendeferi, K., Erwin, J. M., et al. (2011b). The von economo neurons in the frontoinsular and anterior cingulate cortex. *Ann. N Y Acad. Sci.* 1225, 59–71. doi: 10.1111/j.1749-6632.2011.06011.x

Antonucci, A. S., Gansler, D. A., Tan, S., Bhadelia, R., Patz, S., and Fulwiler, C. (2006). Orbitofrontal correlates of aggression and impulsivity in psychiatric patients. *Psychiatry Res.* 147, 213–220. doi: 10.1016/j.pscychresns.2005.05.016

Banks, S. J., Eddy, K. T., Angstadt, M., Nathan, P. J., and Phan, K. L. (2007). Amygdala-frontal connectivity during emotion regulation. *Soc. Cogn. Affect. Neurosci.* 2, 303–312. doi: 10.1093/scan/nsm029

Beck, A. T., Steer, R. A., Ball, R., and Ranieri, W. (1996). Comparison of beck depression inventories -IA and -II in psychiatric outpatients. *J. Pers. Assess.* 67, 588–597. doi: 10.1207/s15327752jpa6703_13

Berlin, H. A., Rolls, E. T., and Iversen, S. D. (2005). Borderline personality disorder, impulsivity and the orbitofrontal cortex. *Am. J. Psychiatry* 162, 2360–2373. doi: 10.1176/appi.ajp.162.12.2360

Biundo, R., Weis, L., Facchini, S., Formento-Dojot, P., Vallelunga, A., Pilleri, M., et al. (2015). Patterns of cortical thickness associated with impulse control disorders in Parkinson's disease. *Mov. Disord.* 30, 688–695. doi: 10.1002/mds.26154

Brown, S. M., Manuck, S. B., Flory, J. D., and Hariri, A. R. (2006). Neural basis of individual differences in impulsivity: contributions of corticolimbic circuits for behavioral arousal and control. *Emotion* 6, 239–245. doi: 10.1037/1528-3542.6.2.239

Cackowski, S., Reitz, A. C., Ende, G., Kleindienst, N., Bohus, M., Schmahl, C., et al. (2014). Impact of stress on different components of impulsivity in borderline personality disorder. *Psychol. Med.* 44, 3329–3340. doi: 10.1017/s0033291714000427

Chamorro, J., Bernardi, S., Potenza, M. N., Grant, J. E., Marsh, R., Wang, S., et al. (2012). Impulsivity in the general population: a national study. *J. Psychiatr. Res.* 46, 994–1001. doi: 10.1016/j.jpsychires.2012.04.023

Cho, S. S., Pellecchia, G., Aminian, K., Ray, N., Segura, B., Obeso, I., et al. (2013). Morphometric correlation of impulsivity in medial prefrontal cortex. *Brain Topogr.* 26, 479–487. doi: 10.1007/s10548-012-0270-x

Churchwell, J. C., and Yurgelun-Todd, D. A. (2013). Age-related changes in insula cortical thickness and impulsivity: significance for emotional development and decision-making. *Dev. Cogn. Neurosci.* 6, 80–86. doi: 10.1016/j.dcn.2013.07.001

Cilia, R., Cho, S. S., Van Eimeren, T., Marotta, G., Siri, C., Ko, J. H., et al. (2011). Pathological gambling in patients with Parkinson's disease is associated with fronto-striatal disconnection: a path modeling analysis. *Mov. Disord.* 26, 225–233. doi: 10.1002/mds.23480

Cilia, R., Siri, C., Marotta, G., Isaias, I. U., De Gaspari, D., Canesi, M., et al. (2008). Functional abnormalities underlying pathological gambling in Parkinson's disease. *Arch. Neurol.* 65, 1604–1611. doi: 10.1001/archneur.65.12.1604

Cilia, R., and Van Eimeren, T. (2011). Impulse control disorders in Parkinson's disease: seeking a roadmap toward a better understanding. *Brain Struct. Funct.* 216, 289–299. doi: 10.1007/s00429-011-0314-0

Crews, F. T., and Boettiger, C. A. (2009). Impulsivity, frontal lobes and risk for addiction. *Pharmacol. Biochem. Behav.* 93, 237–247. doi: 10.1016/j.pbb.2009.04.018

Dambacher, F., Sack, A. T., Lobbestael, J., Arntz, A., Brugman, S., and Schuhmann, T. (2015). Out of control: evidence for anterior insula involvement in motor impulsivity and reactive aggression. *Soc. Cogn. Affect. Neurosci.* 10, 508–516. doi: 10.1093/scan/nsu077

Devinsky, O., Morrell, M. J., and Vogt, B. A. (1995). Contributions of anterior cingulate cortex to behaviour. *Brain* 118, 279–306. doi: 10.1093/brain/118.1.279

Diener, H. C., and Weimar, C. (2012). *Leitlinien für Diagnostik und Therapie in der Neurologie.* Stuttgart: Thieme Verlag.

Ding, W. N., Sun, J. H., Sun, Y. W., Chen, X., Zhou, Y., Zhuang, Z. G., et al. (2014). Trait impulsivity and impaired prefrontal impulse inhibition function in adolescents with internet gaming addiction revealed by a Go/No-Go fMRI study. *Behav. Brain Funct.* 10:20. doi: 10.1186/1744-9081-10-20

Drzezga, A. (2009). Diagnosis of Alzheimer's disease with [18F]PET in mild and asymptomatic stages. *Behav. Neurol.* 21, 101–115. doi: 10.3233/BEN-2009-0228

Eggers, C., Hilker, R., Burghaus, L., Schumacher, B., and Heiss, W. D. (2009). High resolution positron emission tomography demonstrates basal ganglia dysfunction in early Parkinson's disease. *J. Neurol. Sci.* 276, 27–30. doi: 10.1016/j.jns.2008.08.029

Eggers, C., Schwartz, F., Pedrosa, D. J., Kracht, L., and Timmermann, L. (2014). Parkinson's disease subtypes show a specific link between dopaminergic and glucose metabolism in the striatum. *PLoS One* 9:e96629. doi: 10.1371/journal.pone.0096629

Ersche, K. D., Barnes, A., Jones, P. S., Morein-Zamir, S., Robbins, T. W., and Bullmore, E. T. (2011). Abnormal structure of frontostriatal brain systems is associated with aspects of impulsivity and compulsivity in cocaine dependance. *Brain* 134, 2013–2024. doi: 10.1093/brain/awr138

Evenden, J. L. (1999). Varieties of impulsivity. *Psychopharmacology (Berl)* 146, 348–361. doi: 10.1007/pl00005481

Fahn, S., Elton, R., and Committee, U. D. (1987). "Unified Parkinson's disease rating scale," in *Recent developments in Parkinson's disease*, eds C. D. Marsden, S. Fahn, D. Calne, and M. Goldstein (Flora Park, NY: MacMillan Healthcare Information), 153–163.

Fineberg, N. A., Chamberlain, S. R., Goudriaan, A. E., Stein, D. J., Vanderschuren, L. J., Gillan, C. M., et al. (2014). New developments in human neurocognition: clinical, genetic and brain imaging correlates of impulsivity and compulsivity. *CNS Spectr.* 19, 69–89. doi: 10.1017/s1092852913000801

Fossati, A., Gratz, K. L., Borroni, S., Maffei, C., Somma, A., and Carlotta, D. (2015). The relationship between childhood history of ADHD symptoms and DSM-IV borderline personality disorder features among personality disordered outpatients: the moderating role of gender and the mediating roles of emotion dysregulation and impulsivity. *Compr. Psychiatry* 56, 121–127. doi: 10.1016/j.comppsych.2014.09.023

Gansler, D. A., Lee, A. K., Emerton, B. C., D'Amato, C., Bhadelia, R., Jerram, M., et al. (2011). Prefrontal regional correlates of self-control in male psychiatric patients: impulsivity facets and aggression. *Psychiatry Res.* 191, 16–23. doi: 10.1016/j.pscychresns.2010.09.003

Gvion, Y., Horresh, N., Levi-Belz, Y., Fischel, T., Treves, I., Weiser, M., et al. (2014). Aggression-impulsivity, mental pain and communication difficulties in medically serious and medically non-serious suicide attempters. *Compr. Psychiatry* 55, 40–50. doi: 10.1016/j.comppsych.2013.09.003

Hoehn, M. M., and Yahr, M. D. (1967). Parkinsonism: onset, progression and mortality. *Neurology* 17, 427–442. doi: 10.1212/wnl.17.5.427

Horn, N. R., Dolan, M., Elliott, R., Deakin, J. F. W., and Woodruff, P. W. R. (2003). Response inhibition and impulsivity: an fMRI study. *Neuropsychologia* 41, 1959–1966. doi: 10.1016/s0028-3932(03)00077-0

Hughes, A. J., Ben-Shlomo, Y., Daniel, S. E., and Lees, A. J. (1992). What features improve the accuracy of clinical diagnosis in Parkinson's disease: a clinicopathologic study. *Neurology* 42, 1142–1146. doi: 10.1212/wnl.42.6.1142

Jahanshahi, M. (2013). Effects of deep brain stimulation of the subthalamic nucleus on inhibitory and executive control over prepotent responses in Parkinson's disease. *Front. Syst. Neurosci.* 7:118. doi: 10.3389/fnsys.2013.00118

Kerr, K. L., Avery, J. A., Barcalow, J. C., Moseman, S. E., Bodurka, J., Bellgowan, P. S. F., et al. (2015). Trait impulsivity is related to ventral ACC and amygdala activity during primary reward anticipation. *Soc. Cogn. Affect. Neurosci.* 10, 36–42. doi: 10.1093/scan/nsu023

Kessler, J., Markowitsch, H. J., and Denzler, P. (2000). *Mini-Mental-Status-Test (MMST).* Göttingen: Beltz Test GMBH.

Kim, E. J., Sidhu, M., Gaus, S. E., Huang, E. J., Hof, P. R., Miller, B. L., et al. (2012). Selective frontoinsular von economo neuron and fork cell loss in early behavioral variant frontotemporal dementia. *Cereb. Cortex* 22, 251–259. doi: 10.1093/cercor/bhr004

Klupp, E., Forster, S., Grimmer, T., Tahmasian, M., Yakushev, I., Sorg, C., et al. (2014). In Alzheimer's disease, hypometabolism in low-amyloid brain regions may be a functional consequence of pathologies in connected brain regions. *Brain Connect.* 4, 371–383. doi: 10.1089/brain.2013.0212

Klupp, E., Grimmer, T., Tahmasian, M., Sorg, C., Yakushev, I., Yousefi, B. H., et al. (2015). Prefrontal hypometabolism in Alzheimer disease is related to longitudinal amyloid accumulation in remote brain regions. *J. Nucl. Med.* 56, 399–404. doi: 10.2967/jnumed.114.149302

Kringelbach, M. L. (2005). The human orbitofrontal cortex: linking reward to hedonic experience. *Nat. Rev. Neurosci.* 6, 691–702. doi: 10.1038/nrn1747

Kühner, C., Bürger, C., Keller, F., and Hautzinger, M. (2007). [Reliability and validity of the revised beck depression inventory (BDI-II). Results from german samples]. *Nervenarzt* 78, 651–656. doi: 10.1007/s00115-006-2098-7

Lee, T. Y., Kim, S. N., Jang, J. H., Shim, G., Jung, W. H., Shin, N. Y., et al. (2013). Neural correlate of impulsivity in subjects at ultra-high risk for psychosis. *Prog. Neuropsychopharmacol. Biol. Psychiatry* 45, 165–169. doi: 10.1016/j.pnpbp.2013.04.008

Lee, J. Y., Kim, J. M., Kim, J. W., Cho, J., Lee, W. Y., Kim, H. J., et al. (2010). Association between the dose of dopaminergic medication and the behavioral disturbances in Parkinson disease. *Parkinsonism Relat. Disord.* 16, 202–207. doi: 10.1016/j.parkreldis.2009.12.002

Leeman, R. F., and Potenza, M. N. (2012). Similarities and differences between pathological gambling and substance use disorders: a focus on impulsivity and compulsivity. *Psychopharmacology (Berl)* 219, 469–490. doi: 10.1007/s00213-011-2550-7

Lucignani, G., and Nobili, F. (2010). FDG-PET for early assessment of Alzheimer's disease: isn't the evidence base large enough? *Eur. J. Nucl. Med. Mol. Imaging* 37, 1604–1609. doi: 10.1007/s00259-010-1535-9

Matsuda, H., Mizumura, S., Nemoto, K., Yamashita, F., Imabayashi, E., Sato, N., et al. (2012). Automatic voxel-based morphometry of structural MRI by SPM8 plus diffeomorphic anatomic registration through exponentiated lie algebra improves the diagnosis of probable alzheimer disease. *AJNR Am. J. Neuroradiol.* 33, 1109–1114. doi: 10.3174/ajnr.a2935

Matsuo, K., Nicoletti, M., Nemoto, K., Hatch, J. P., Peluso, M. A., Nery, F. G., et al. (2009a). A voxel-based morphometry study of frontal gray matter correlates of impulsivity. *Hum. Brain Mapp.* 30, 1188–1195. doi: 10.1002/hbm.20588

Matsuo, K., Nicoletti, M. A., Peluso, M. A., Hatch, J. P., Nemoto, K., Watanabe, Y., et al. (2009b). Anterior cingulate volumes associated with trait impulsivity in individuals with bipolar disorder. *Bipolar Disord.* 11, 628–636. doi: 10.1111/j.1399-5618.2009.00732.x

Nandagopal, J. J., Fleck, D. E., Adler, C. M., Mills, N. P., Strakowski, S. M., and DelBello, M. P. (2011). Impulsivity in adolescents with bipolar disorder and/or attention-deficit/hyperactivity disorder and healthy controls as measured by the barratt impulsiveness scale. *J. Child Adolesc. Psychopharmacol.* 21, 465–468. doi: 10.1089/cap.2010.0096

Napier, T. C., Corvol, J. C., Grace, A. A., Roitman, J. D., Rowe, J., Voon, V., et al. (2015). Linking neuroscience with modern concepts of impulse control disorders in Parkinson's disease. *Mov. Disord.* 30, 141–149. doi: 10.1002/mds.26068

Owsley, C., McGwin, G., Jr., and McNeal, S. F. (2003). Impact of impulsiveness, venturesomeness and empathy on driving by older adults. *J. Safety Res.* 34, 353–359. doi: 10.1016/j.jsr.2003.09.013

Patton, J. H., Stanford, M. S., and Barratt, E. S. (1995). Factor structure of the barratt impulsiveness scale. *J. Clin. Psychol.* 51, 768–774. doi: 10.1002/1097-4679(199511)51:6<768::aid-jclp2270510607>3.0.co;2-1

Perry, J. L., Joseph, J. E., Jiang, Y., Zimmerman, R. S., Kelly, T. H., Darna, M., et al. (2011). Prefrontal cortex and drug abuse vulnerability: translation to prevention and treatment interventions. *Brain Res. Rev.* 65, 124–149. doi: 10.1016/j.brainresrev.2010.09.001

Probst, C. C., and Van Eimeren, T. (2013). The functional anatomy of impulse control disorders. *Curr. Neurol. Neurosci. Rep.* 13:386. doi: 10.1007/s11910-013-0386-8

Qiu, Y. W., Jiang, G. H., Su, H. H., Lv, X. F., Tian, J. Z., Li, L. M., et al. (2013). The impulsivity behavior is correlated with prefrontal cortex gray matter volume reduction in heroin-dependent individuals. *Neurosci. Lett.* 538, 43–48. doi: 10.1016/j.neulet.2013.01.019

Ray, N., and Strafella, A. P. (2010). Dopamine, reward and frontostriatal circuitry in impulse control disorders in Parkinson's disease: insights from functional imaging. *Clin. EEG Neurosci.* 41, 87–93. doi: 10.1177/155005941004100208

Rushworth, M. F., Behrens, T. E., Rudebeck, P. H., and Walton, M. E. (2007). Contrasting roles for cingulate and orbitofrontal cortex in decisions and social behavior. *Trends Cogn. Sci.* 11, 168–176. doi: 10.1016/j.tics.2007.01.004

Schoenbaum, G., Takahashi, Y., Liu, T. L., and McDannald, M. A. (2011). Does the orbitofrontal cortex signal value? *Ann. N Y Acad. Sci.* 1239, 87–99. doi: 10.1111/j.1749-6632.2011.06210.x

Schultz, W., Tremblay, L., and Hollerman, J. R. (2000). Reward processing in primate orbitofrontal cortex and basal ganglia. *Cereb. Cortex* 10, 272–283. doi: 10.1093/cercor/10.3.272

Sebastian, A., Jung, P., Krause-Utz, A., Lieb, K., Schmahl, C., and Tüscher, O. (2014). Frontal dysfunctions of impulse control - a systematic review in borderline personality disorder and attention-deficit/hyperactivity disorder. *Front. Hum. Neurosci.* 8:698. doi: 10.3389/fnhum.2014.00698

Seguin, J. R. (2004). Neurocognitive elements of antisocial behavior: relevance of an orbitofrontal cortex account. *Brain Cogn.* 55, 185–197. doi: 10.1016/s0278-2626(03)00273-2

Stanford, M. S., Mathias, C. W., Dougherty, D. M., Lake, S. L., Anderson, N. E., and Patton, J. H. (2009). Fifty years of the barratt impulsiveness scale: an update and review. *Pers. Individ. Dif.* 47, 385–395. doi: 10.1016/j.paid.2009.04.008

Tahmasian, M., Bettray, L. M., Van Eimeren, T., Drzezga, A., Timmermann, L., Eickhoff, C. R., et al. (2015a). A systematic review on the applications of resting-state fMRI in Parkinson's disease: does dopamine replacement therapy play a role? *Cortex* 73, 80–105. doi: 10.1016/j.cortex.2015.08.005

Tahmasian, M., Pasquini, L., Scherr, M., Meng, C., Förster, S., Mulej Bratec, S., et al. (2015b). The lower hippocampus global connectivity, the higher its local metabolism in alzheimer disease. *Neurology* 84, 1956–1963. doi: 10.1212/WNL.0000000000001575

Tahmasian, M., Knight, D. C., Manoliu, A., Schwerthöffer, D., Scherr, M., Meng, C., et al. (2013). Aberrant intrinsic connectivity of hippocampus and amygdala overlap in the fronto-insular and dorsomedial-prefrontal cortex in major depressive disorder. *Front. Hum. Neurosci.* 7:639. doi: 10.3389/fnhum.2013.00639

Trost, S., Diekhof, E. K., Zvonik, K., Lewandowski, M., Usher, J., Keil, M., et al. (2014). Disturbed anterior prefrontal control of the mesolimbic reward system and increased impulsivity in bipolar disorder. *Neuropsychopharmacology* 39, 1914–1923. doi: 10.1038/npp.2014.39

Tzourio-Mazoyer, N., Landeau, B., Papathanassiou, D., Crivello, F., Etard, O., Delcroix, N., et al. (2002). Automated anatomical labeling of activations in SPM using a macroscopic anatomical parcellation of the MNI MRI single-subject brain. *Neuroimage* 15, 273–289. doi: 10.1006/nimg.2001.0978

Van Eimeren, T., Ballanger, B., Pellecchia, G., Miyasaki, J. M., Lang, A. E., and Strafella, A. P. (2009). Dopamine agonists diminish value sensitivity of the orbitofrontal cortex: a trigger for pathological gambling in Parkinson's disease? *Neuropsychopharmacology* 34, 2758–2766. doi: 10.1038/sj.npp.npp2009124

Van Eimeren, T., Pellecchia, G., Cilia, R., Ballanger, B., Steeves, T. D., Houle, S., et al. (2010). Drug-induced deactivation of inhibitory networks predicts pathological gambling in PD. *Neurology* 75, 1711–1716. doi: 10.1212/WNL.0b013e3181fc27fa

Van Hilten, J. J., Van Der Zwan, A. D., Zwinderman, A. H., and Roos, R. A. (1994). Rating impairment and disability in Parkinson's disease: evaluation of the unified Parkinson's disease rating scale. *Mov. Disord.* 9, 84–88. doi: 10.1002/mds.870090113

Voon, V., Gao, J., Brezing, C., Symmonds, M., Ekanayake, V., Fernandez, H., et al. (2011a). Dopamine agonists and risk: impulse control disorders in Parkinson's disease. *Brain* 134, 1438–1446. doi: 10.1093/brain/awr080

Voon, V., Sohr, M., Lang, A. E., Potenza, M. N., Siderowf, A. D., Whetteckey, J., et al. (2011b). Impulse control disorders in Parkinson disease: a multicenter case--control study. *Ann. Neurol.* 69, 986–996. doi: 10.1002/ana.22356

Voon, V., Thomsen, T., Miyasaki, J. M., De Souza, M., Shafro, A., Fox, S. H., et al. (2007). Factors associated with dopaminergic drug-related pathological gambling in Parkinson disease. *Arch. Neurol.* 64, 212–216. doi: 10.1001/archneur.64.2.212

Wehrl, H. F., Hossain, M., Lankes, K., Liu, C. C., Bezrukov, I., Martirosian, P., et al. (2013). Simultaneous PET-MRI reveals brain function in activated and resting state on metabolic, hemodynamic and multiple temporal scales. *Nat. Med.* 19, 1184–1189. doi: 10.1038/nm.3290

Weintraub, D., Koester, J., Potenza, M. N., Siderowf, A. D., Stacy, M., Voon, V., et al. (2010). Impulse control disorders in Parkinson disease: a cross-sectional study of 3090 patients. *Arch. Neurol.* 67, 589–595. doi: 10.1001/archneurol.2010.65

Weiss, H. D., and Marsh, L. (2012). Impulse control disorders and compulsive behaviors associated with dopaminergic therapies in Parkinson disease. *Neurol. Clin. Pract.* 2, 267–274. doi: 10.1212/cpj.0b013e318278be9b

Wilbertz, T., Deserno, L., Horstmann, A., Neumann, J., Villringer, A., Heinze, H. J., et al. (2014). Response inhibition and its relation to multidimensional impulsivity. *Neuroimage* 103, 241–248. doi: 10.1016/j.neuroimage.2014.09.021

Winstanley, C. A., Theobald, D. E. H., Cardinal, R. N., and Robbins, T. W. (2004). Contrasting roles of basolateral amygdala and orbitofrontal cortex in impulsive choice. *J. Neurosci.* 24, 4718–4722. doi: 10.1523/jneurosci.5606-03.2004

Conflict of Interest Statement: The authors declare that the research was conducted in the absence of any commercial or financial relationships that could be construed as a potential conflict of interest.

Permissions

All chapters in this book were first published in ARNDAANAUS, by Frontiers Media SA; hereby published with permission under the Creative Commons Attribution License or equivalent. Every chapter published in this book has been scrutinized by our experts. Their significance has been extensively debated. The topics covered herein carry significant findings which will fuel the growth of the discipline. They may even be implemented as practical applications or may be referred to as a beginning point for another development.

The contributors of this book come from diverse backgrounds, making this book a truly international effort. This book will bring forth new frontiers with its revolutionizing research information and detailed analysis of the nascent developments around the world.

We would like to thank all the contributing authors for lending their expertise to make the book truly unique. They have played a crucial role in the development of this book. Without their invaluable contributions this book wouldn't have been possible. They have made vital efforts to compile up to date information on the varied aspects of this subject to make this book a valuable addition to the collection of many professionals and students.

This book was conceptualized with the vision of imparting up-to-date information and advanced data in this field. To ensure the same, a matchless editorial board was set up. Every individual on the board went through rigorous rounds of assessment to prove their worth. After which they invested a large part of their time researching and compiling the most relevant data for our readers.

The editorial board has been involved in producing this book since its inception. They have spent rigorous hours researching and exploring the diverse topics which have resulted in the successful publishing of this book. They have passed on their knowledge of decades through this book. To expedite this challenging task, the publisher supported the team at every step. A small team of assistant editors was also appointed to further simplify the editing procedure and attain best results for the readers.

Apart from the editorial board, the designing team has also invested a significant amount of their time in understanding the subject and creating the most relevant covers. They scrutinized every image to scout for the most suitable representation of the subject and create an appropriate cover for the book.

The publishing team has been an ardent support to the editorial, designing and production team. Their endless efforts to recruit the best for this project, has resulted in the accomplishment of this book. They are a veteran in the field of academics and their pool of knowledge is as vast as their experience in printing. Their expertise and guidance has proved useful at every step. Their uncompromising quality standards have made this book an exceptional effort. Their encouragement from time to time has been an inspiration for everyone.

The publisher and the editorial board hope that this book will prove to be a valuable piece of knowledge for researchers, students, practitioners and scholars across the globe.

List of Contributors

Kathinka Evers
Centre for Research Ethics and Bioethics (CRB), Uppsala University, Uppsala, Sweden

Karl Sallin
Centre for Research Ethics and Bioethics (CRB), Uppsala University, Uppsala, Sweden
Department of Women's and Children's Health, Division of Neonatology, Karolinska Institute, Solna, Sweden

Hugo Lagercrantz
Department of Women's and Children's Health, Division of Neonatology, Karolinska Institute, Solna, Sweden

Ingemar Engström
School of Health and Medical Sciences, Örebro University, Örebro, Sweden

Anders Hjern
Centre for Health and Equity Studies (CHESS), Karolinska Institute and Stockholm University, Stockholm, Sweden

Predrag Petrovic
Department of Clinical Neuroscience, Karolinska Institute, Solna, Sweden

F. Xavier Castellanos
Department of Child and Adolescent Psychiatry, the Child Study Center at NYU Langone Medical Center, New York, NY, USA
Nathan Kline Institute for Psychiatric Research, Orangeburg, NY, USA

Raymond C. K. Chan
Neuropsychology and Applied Cognitive Neuroscience Laboratory, Key Laboratory of Mental Health, Institute of Psychology, Chinese Academy of Sciences, Beijing, China

Morten L. Kringelbach
Department of Psychiatry, University of Oxford, Oxford, UK
Center for Music in the Brain (MIB), Aarhus University, Aarhus, Denmark
Nuffield Department of Surgical Sciences, John Radcliffe Hospital, Oxford, UK

Liangwei Xia
Medical Psychological Institute, Second Xiangya Hospital, Central South University, Changsha, Hunan, China

Shuqiao Yao
Medical Psychological Institute, Second Xiangya Hospital, Central South University, Changsha, Hunan, China
National Technology Institute of Psychiatry, Changsha, Hunan, China

Amy R. Bland, Heather Boland and Rebecca Elliott
Neuroscience and Psychiatry Unit, University of Manchester, Manchester, UK

Jonathan P. Roiser
Institute of Cognitive Neuroscience, University College London, London, UK

Mitul A. Mehta
Institute of Psychiatry, Psychology and Neuroscience, Kings College London, London, UK

Thea Schei
Department of Psychology, University of Cambridge, Cambridge, UK

Daniel K. Campbell-Meiklejohn
School of Psychology, University of Sussex, Brighton, UK

Richard A. Emsley
Institute of Population Health, University of Manchester, Manchester, UK

Marcus R. Munafo and Ian S. Penton-Voak
School of Experimental Psychology, University of Bristol, Bristol, UK

Essi Viding
Psychology and Language Sciences, University College London, London, UK

Ana Seara-Cardoso
Psychology and Language Sciences, University College London, London, UK
School of Psychology, University of Minho, Guimaraes, Portugal

Valerie Voon and Barbara J. Sahakian
Department of Psychiatry, University of Cambridge, Cambridge, UK

Behavioural and Clinical Neuroscience Institute, University of Cambridge, Cambridge, UK

Trevor W. Robbins
Department of Psychology, University of Cambridge, Cambridge, UK
Behavioural and Clinical Neuroscience Institute, University of Cambridge, Cambridge, UK

Alice M. S. Durieux, Declan Murphy and Grainne McAlonan
Department of Forensic and Neurodevelopmental Sciences, Institute of Psychiatry, Psychology and Neuroscience, King's College London, London, UK

Cathy Fernandes
Social, Genetic and Developmental Psychiatry Centre, Institute of Psychiatry, Psychology and Neuroscience, King's College London, London, UK

Marie Anais Labouesse
Physiology and Behaviour Laboratory, Swiss Federal Institute of Technology, Schwerzenbach, Switzerland

Sandra Giovanoli and Urs Meyer
Physiology and Behaviour Laboratory, Swiss Federal Institute of Technology, Schwerzenbach, Switzerland
Institute of Pharmacology and Toxicology, University of Zurich-Vetsuisse, Zurich, Switzerland

Qi Li
Department of Psychiatry, Li Ka Shing Faculty of Medicine, The University of Hong Kong, Hong Kong, China

Po-Wah So
Department of Neuroimaging, Institute of Psychiatry, Psychology and Neuroscience, King's College London, London, UK

Tim J. van Hartevelt
Department of Psychiatry, University of Oxford, Oxford, UK
Center of Functionally Integrative Neuroscience (CFIN), Aarhus University, Aarhus, Denmark

Arne Møller
Center of Functionally Integrative Neuroscience (CFIN), Aarhus University, Aarhus, Denmark

Joana Cabral
Department of Psychiatry, University of Oxford, Oxford, UK
Center of Brain and Cognition, Theoretical and Computational Neuroscience Group, Universitat Pompeu Fabra, Barcelona, Spain

Tipu Z. Aziz
Department of Psychiatry, University of Oxford, Oxford, UK
Nuffield Department of Surgical Sciences, John Radcliffe Hospital, Oxford, UK

Alexander L. Green and James J. FitzGerald
Nuffield Department of Surgical Sciences, John Radcliffe Hospital, Oxford, UK

Gustavo Deco
Center of Brain and Cognition, Theoretical and Computational Neuroscience Group, Universitat Pompeu Fabra, Barcelona, Spain
Institució Catalana de la Recerca i Estudis Avançats (ICREA), Universitat Pompeu Fabra, Barcelona, Spain

Xuebing Li, Jie Chen and Xinying Li
Key Laboratory of Mental Health, Institute of Psychology, Chinese Academy of Sciences, Beijing, China

Haiyang Geng
Key Laboratory of Mental Health, Institute of Psychology, Chinese Academy of Sciences, Beijing, China
State Key Laboratory of Cognitive Neuroscience and Learning, Beijing Normal University, Beijing, China

Ruolei Gu
Key Laboratory of Behavioral Science, Institute of Psychology, Chinese Academy of Sciences, Beijing, China

Barbara Gawda
Department of Psychology of Emotion and Cognition, University of Maria Curie Sklodowska, Lublin, Poland

Ewa Szepietowska
Department of Clinical Psychology and Neuropsychology of Maria Curie-Sklodowska, Lubin, Poland

Susanne Erk
Division of Mind and Brain Research, Department of Psychiatry and Psychotherapy, Charité Universitätsmedizin Berlin Berlin, Germany

Vera U. Ludwig, Corinde E. Wiers and Henrik Walter
Division of Mind and Brain Research, Department of Psychiatry and Psychotherapy, Charité Universitätsmedizin Berlin Berlin, Germany
Berlin School of Mind and Brain, Humboldt Universität zu Berlin, Berlin, Germany

Corinna Nüsser
Division of Medical Psychology, University of Bonn, Bonn, Germany
Department of Psychology, Technische Universität Dresden, Dresden, Germany

Thomas Goschke
Department of Psychology, Technische Universität Dresden, Dresden, Germany

Dina Wittfoth-Schardt
Institute of Neuroradiology, Hannover Medical School, Hannover, Germany
NICA—NeuroImaging and Clinical Applications, Hannover, Germany

Björn H. Schott
Division of Mind and Brain Research, Department of Psychiatry and Psychotherapy, Charité Universitätsmedizin Berlin Berlin, Germany
Leibniz-Institute for Neurobiology, Magdeburg, Germany

Ludger Tebartz van Elst, Max Fleck, Susanne Bartels, Andreas Riedel, Swantje Matthies, Bernd Feige, Evgeniy Perlov and Dominique Endres
Section for Experimental Neuropsychiatry, Department for Psychiatry and Psychotherapy, University Medical Center Freiburg, Freiburg, Germany

Dirk-Matthias Altenmüller
Department of Neurosurgery, Freiburg Epilepsy Center, University Medical Center Freiburg, Freiburg, Germany

Emanuel Bubl
Department for Psychiatry and Psychotherapy, Saarland University Medical Center, Homburg, Germany

Hongmei Wang, Tahir Mehmood Shakir, Cuiping Mao, Xuan Niu, Chen Niu, Liping Guo, Ming Zhang and Chenwang Jin
Department of Medical Imaging, the first Affiliated Hospital of Medical College, Xi'an Jiaotong University, Xi'an, China

Kai Yuan
School of Life Science and Technology, Xidian University, Xi'an, China

Engineering Research Center of Molecular and Neuro Imaging Ministry of Education, Xi'an, China

Naomi I. Eisenberger
Social and Affective Neuroscience Laboratory, University of California, Los Angeles, Los Angeles, CA, USA

Katarina Dedovic
Social and Affective Neuroscience Laboratory, University of California, Los Angeles, Los Angeles, CA, USA
Addiction Research Studies and Laboratory, Douglas Hospital Research Centre, McGill University, Montreal, QC, Canada

George M. Slavich and Michael R. Irwin
Cousins Center for Psychoneuroimmunology and Department of Psychiatry and Biobehavioral Sciences, University of California, Los Angeles, Los Angeles, CA, USA

Keely A. Muscatell
The Robert Wood Johnson Foundation Health and Society Scholars Program, University of California, San Francisco/University of California, Berkeley, San Francisco, CA, USA
Department of Psychology, University of California, Berkeley, Berkeley, CA, USA

Michihiko Koeda, Woochan Kim, Amane Tateno and Yoshiro Okubo
Department of Neuropsychiatry, Graduate School of Medicine, Nippon Medical School, Tokyo, Japan

Atsushi Watanabe and Banyar Than Naing
Division of Personalized Genetic Medicine, Nippon Medical School Hospital, Tokyo, Japan
Department of Biochemistry and Molecular Biology, Graduate School of Medicine, Nippon Medical School, Tokyo, Japan

Takashi Shimada
Department of Biochemistry and Molecular Biology, Graduate School of Medicine, Nippon Medical School, Tokyo, Japan

Kumiko Tsuda, Miwako Matsumoto and Masato Matsuura
Department of Biofunctional Informatics, Tokyo Medical and Dental University, Tokyo, Japan

Yumiko Ikeda and Hiroyuki Karibe
Department of Pediatric Dentistry, Nippon Dental University, Tokyo, Japan

Hidenori Suzuki
Department of Pharmacology, Graduate School of Medicine, Nippon Medical School, Tokyo, Japan

Yi Wang and Raymond C. K. Chan
Neuropsychology and Applied Cognitive Neuroscience Laboratory, Key Laboratory of Mental Health, Institute of Psychology, Chinese Academy of Sciences, Beijing, China

Wen-hua Liu
School of Health Management, Guangzhou Medical University, Guangzhou, China

Zhi Li
Neuropsychology and Applied Cognitive Neuroscience Laboratory, Key Laboratory of Mental Health, Institute of Psychology, Chinese Academy of Sciences, Beijing, China
University of Chinese Academy of Sciences, Beijing, China

Xin-hua Wei and Xin-qing Jiang
Department of Radiology, Guangzhou First People's Hospital, Guangzhou, China

David H. K. Shum and David L. Neumann
Menzies Health Institute Queensland and School of Applied Psychology, Griffith University, Gold Coast, QLD, Australia

Eric F. C. Cheung
Castle Peak Hospital, Hong Kong, China

Ji-Woo Seok and Jin-Hun Sohn
Department of Psychology, Brain Research Institute Chungnam National University, Daejeon, South Korea

Brian D. Vickers, Stephanie D. Preston, Richard Gonzalez and Andrea M. Angott
Department of Psychology, University of Michigan, Ann Arbor, MI, USA

Raymond C. K. Chan
Neuropsychology and Applied Cognitive Neuroscience Laboratory, Key Laboratory of Mental Health, Institute of Psychology, Chinese Academy of Sciences, Beijing, China

Chao Yan
Key Laboratory of Brain Functional Genomics (MOE and STCSM), School of Psychology and Cognitive Science, East China Normal University, Shanghai, China

Wei-Zhen Xie
Department of Psychology, University of California, Riverside, CA, USA

Ke Li, Ya-Wei Zeng and Zhen Jin
MRI Center, Hospital 306 of PLA, Beijing, China

Luisa Rochhausen, Franziska Maier, Kim L. Williamson, Lars Timmermann and Carsten Eggers
Department of Neurology, University Hospital of Cologne, Cologne, Germany

Thilo Van Eimeren
Department of Neurology, University Hospital of Cologne, Cologne, Germany
Department of Nuclear Medicine, University Hospital of Cologne, Cologne, Germany

Alexander Drzezga
Department of Nuclear Medicine, University Hospital of Cologne, Cologne, Germany

Masoud Tahmasian
Department of Neurology, University Hospital of Cologne, Cologne, Germany
Department of Nuclear Medicine, University Hospital of Cologne, Cologne, Germany
Sleep Disorders Research Center, Kermanshah University of Medical Sciences (KUMS), Kermanshah, Iran

Index

www.ingramcontent.com/pod-product-compliance
Lightning Source LLC
LaVergne TN
LVHW060553210926
848485LV00005B/1309